Ligamentous Injuries of the Foot and Ankle

Pieter D'Hooghe • Kenneth J. Hunt
Jeremy J. McCormick
Editors

Ligamentous Injuries of the Foot and Ankle

Diagnosis, Management and Rehabilitation

Springer

Editors
Pieter D'Hooghe
Department of Orthopedic Surgery
Aspetar Orthopaedic and Sports
Medicine Hospital
Doha, Qatar

Kenneth J. Hunt
Department of Orthopedic Surgery
University of Colorado School
of Medicine
Aurora, CO, USA

Jeremy J. McCormick
Department of Orthopaedic Surgery
Washington University School
of Medicine
St. Louis, MO, USA

ISBN 978-3-031-08681-6 ISBN 978-3-031-08682-3 (eBook)
https://doi.org/10.1007/978-3-031-08682-3

This Springer imprint is published by the registered company Springer Nature Switzerland AG
The registered company address is: Gewerbestrasse 11, 6330 Cham, Switzerland

Foreword: Land of Ligaments Text

Ligament injuries of the foot and ankle occur commonly in the athletic or active individual and no joint is spared a possible disruption. Mechanisms accounting for these "sprains" are diverse and often seemingly minor. While many of these ligament injuries present with gross dislocation or joint diastasis, there are just as many that are quite subtle, not apparent on routine exam or imaging. Instability, whether obvious or not, requires early detection and protection to minimize chondral injury and the long-term consequences of arthritis and malalignment.

It is exciting for me to see that what began as an Instructional Course Lecture series for the AAOS has now expanded into print. ***The Land of Ligaments***, the title given to this Academy lecture series, was extremely well received and provided valuable information to the general orthopedist, as well as the subspecialist managing ankle injuries in the active patient. Drs. Hunt, McCormick, and D'Hooghe, the editors of this text, have provided us a more in-depth platform with which to educate the readership to the specifics of a variety of ligament injuries in the foot and ankle. They have enlisted numerous renowned foot and ankle specialists with expertise in this arena, and I am honored to have served as a contributor. The editors had the foresight to create a much-needed text dealing with the complexities of these injuries and basically developing a comprehensive guide to the treatment opportunities. The chapters include a thorough description of not only techniques best utilized for a variety of scenarios but also a thorough description of indications and contraindications. Pertinent anatomy, evaluation pearls, decision-making tips, treatment algorithms, postoperative and rehabilitation protocols are provided for the athlete at all levels of participation. Whether managing the weekend warrior or elite athlete, an understanding of these concepts is necessary—the only real difference being decision-making on the impact of return to play and what risks may be present.

This textbook is extremely timely, given the large number of patients affected by these ligament injuries and those that have suffered the long-term consequences of a missed, underappreciated, or neglected diagnosis. Too often, many foot and ankle providers are challenged by the retired athlete presenting with end-stage arthritis and deformity as a result of an inadequately managed "sprain." I do believe that this text and multiple high-level contributions will heighten the awareness of the practicing orthopedist to the multiple presentations of ligament injuries in the foot and ankle with the end result being a decreased incidence of late disability.

I am proud to have been asked to write the Foreword for this valuable contribution, but most proud given that two of the editors (Drs. Hunt and McCormick) were former fellows of mine. It is a tribute to one's career when the mentor is surpassed by his students, or when the mentor becomes the student. I applaud the editors for guiding this project through and advancing the education and knowledge base of those that follow. Their motivation was to create a platform to enhance the level of understanding to the many potential ligament injuries in the foot and ankle. Overall, this will inspire the reader to be more enlightened, creative, and innovative when managing these particular entities.

Titletown Sports Medicine and Orthopedics
Green Bay, WI, USA

Green Bay Packers
Green Bay, WI, USA

Robert B. Anderson

Acknowledgments

This book on managing ligament injuries in the foot and ankle is a product of a tremendous teamwork and collaboration. Topic experts from around the globe have dedicated time, effort, and intellectual energy to share their knowledge and experience with the reader.

We thank all the authors that agreed with passion and enthusiasm to contribute to this project.

As in all such undertakings, the completion and publication of a scientific text requires multiple supporting energies.

We thank all of the chairs, speakers, and moderators who have participated in the AAOS Land of Ligaments Instructional Course Lecture (ICL). Many of these speakers have contributed to this text. This book is dedicated to them.

We acknowledge Dr. Steve Haddad who had the inspiration for the Land of Ligaments ICL and served as its first course chairman. When Steve recruited Dr. Bob Anderson, Dr. Tom Clanton, and Dr. Chris Coetzee as the first course faculty, we suspect that group never thought the ICL would evolve into the text it has become today.

In particular, we thank Dr. Bob Anderson who has been a thought leader and pioneer in the arena of ligamentous injuries to the foot and ankle, serving as a mentor to the editors of this text and countless others.

We must thank and commend Carolyn Jones for her extraordinary help and effort coordinating the completion of each chapter and collaborating with Springer staff.

We thank our families for supporting us in our practices and academic activities. We could not do this without their support and inspiration.

Finally, we thank the Springer team that has backed us in the production of this book dedicated to optimizing the management of ligament injuries in the foot and ankle.

Pieter D'Hooghe
Kenneth J. Hunt
Jeremy J. McCormick

Contents

1 **Introduction** 1
Kenneth J. Hunt

2 **Anatomy and Biomechanics of the Foot and Ankle** 5
Alberto Grassi and Massimiliano Mosca

3 **Imaging of Ligamentous Injuries in the Foot and Ankle** 17
Michael Durst

4 **Alignment and Instability: Managing Mechanical Contributors to Recurrent Ligament Injury and Instability** . . . 31
Caitlin M. Rugg, Richard Amendola, and Annunziato Amendola

5 **Rehabilitating the Elite Athlete with Ligamentous Injury of the Foot and Ankle** 47
Steven M. Short and Gretchen M. Short

6 **Lateral Ankle Sprains: Injury Epidemiology and Nonoperative Treatment** 61
Nasef Mohamed Nasef Abdelatif

7 **Lateral Ankle Sprains: Subtalar Instability** 75
Kateryna Barg, Jesse Steadman, Megan Mills, and Alexej Barg

8 **Lateral Ankle Instability: The Modified Brostrom** 91
Lorraine Boakye, Cortez Brown, Nia James, and MaCalus V. Hogan

9 **Lateral Ankle Instability: Arthroscopic Broström and Minimally Invasive Techniques** 97
Kenneth J. Hunt and Francisco Rodriguez-Fontan

10 **Lateral Ankle Instability: Tendon Transfers and Grafts** 105
Marissa D. Jamieson and Thomas O. Clanton

11 **Lateral Ankle Instability: The Role of Synthetic Ligament Augmentation** 115
Richard J. Lamour and Troy S. Watson

12 Lateral Ankle Instability: Rehab and Return to Sport 125
Christopher Neville, Erin Haggerty, Jeannie Park, Robert Carrier, and Eric Giza

13 Syndesmosis Injury: Classification, Evaluation, and Prevention 137
Umile Giuseppe Longo, Giovanna Stelitano, Bart Lubberts, Christopher W. Di Giovanni, Niek van Dijk, and Vincenzo Denaro

14 Syndesmosis Injuries: Surgical Indications, Techniques, and Outcomes 147
Kenneth J. Hunt and Stephen Blake Wallace

15 Syndesmotic Injuries in Athletes: Return to Play and Rehabilitation 159
Pieter D'Hooghe, Frederique Neys, Jonathan Bartolomei-Aguillar, and Kenneth J. Hunt

16 Deltoid Ligament Injury: When to Repair, Reconstruct, or Let It Heal 171
Matteo Guelfi and Jordi Vega

17 Spring Ligament Injuries and Instability: Repair/Reconstruction Indications and Techniques 181
Gordon Mackay and William Ribbans

18 Posterior Ankle Ligaments: The Role of Posterior Talofibular Ligament, Flexor Retinaculum, Posterior Talocalcaneal Ligament, and Fibulotalocalcaneal Ligament in Posterior Ankle Impingement 195
Gian Luigi Canata and Valentina Casale

19 Lisfranc Injuries of the Foot and Ankle: Diagnosis and Treatment Indications 201
Jeremy J. McCormick and Brian M. Fisher

20 Lisfranc Injuries in Athletes: Surgical Treatment Techniques 215
David A. Porter and Gregory J. Schmidt

21 Lisfranc Injury in Athletes: Return to Play and Rehabilitation 249
Ahmed K. Attia and Pieter D'Hooghe

22 Management of Turf Toe and Sesamoid Injuries 259
Benjamin J. Ebben and Robert B. Anderson

23 Lesser Toe Plantar Plate Injuries and Angular Deformities: Indications, Techniques, and Outcomes 273
James R. Jastifer, Christopher Traynor, and Homer Stryker

24 Returning to Sport: Tips and Techniques for Safe Transition to Sports Participation 285
Norman E. Waldrop III, Charles C. Pitts Jr, and Yvonne C. Conway

Index 301

Contributors

Nasef Mohamed Nasef Abdelatif Previously Orthopedics and Foot and Ankle Reconstructive Surgery, Bani Suef University, Bani Suef, Egypt

Orthopedic Foot and Ankle Reconstructive Surgery, DrNasef OrthoClinic Medical Center, Cairo, Egypt

Annunziato Amendola Orthopaedic Surgery, Division of Sports Medicine, Urbaniak Sports Sciences Institute, Athletic Department, Duke University, Durham, NC, USA

Richard Amendola Department of Orthopedic Surgery, SUNY Upstate Medical University, NY, USA

Robert B. Anderson Titletown Sports Medicine & Orthopedics, Green Bay, WI, USA

Ahmed K. Attia Department of Orthopaedic Surgery, Hamad General Hospital, Hamad Medical Corporation, Doha, Qatar

Alexej Barg Department of Orthopaedics, Trauma and Reconstructive Surgery, University Medical Center Hamburg-Eppendorf, Hamburg, Germany

Department of Orthopaedics, University of Utah, Salt Lake City, UT, USA

Kateryna Barg Department of Orthopaedics, Trauma and Reconstructive Surgery, University Medical Center Hamburg-Eppendorf, Hamburg, Germany

Jonathan Bartolomei-Aguillar Department of Physiotherapy, Move to Cure, Antwerpen, Belgium

Lorraine Boakye Department of Orthopaedic Surgery, University of Pittsburgh Medical Center, Pittsburgh, PA, USA

Cortez Brown Department of Orthopaedic Surgery, University of Pittsburgh Medical Center, Pittsburgh, PA, USA

Florida State University College of Medicine, Tallahassee, FL, USA

Gian Luigi Canata Centre of Sports Traumatology, Koelliker Hospital, Torino, TO, Italy

Robert Carrier Department of Physical Therapy Education, Upstate Medical University, Rochester, NY, USA

Valentina Casale Centre of Sports Traumatology, Koelliker Hospital, Torino, TO, Italy

Thomas O. Clanton Orthopedic Surgery Foot and Ankle, Steadman Clinic, Vail, CO, USA

Yvonne C. Conway Department of Orthopaedic Surgery, University of Alabama—Birmingham, Birmingham, AL, USA

Vincenzo Denaro Research Unit of Orthopaedic and Trauma Surgery, Fondazione Policlinico Universitario Campus Bio-Medico, Roma, Italy

Research Unit of Orthopaedic and Trauma Surgery, Department of Medicine and Surgery, Università Campus Bio-Medico di Roma, Roma, Italy

Pieter D'Hooghe Department of Orthopaedic Surgery, Aspetar Orthopaedic and Sports Medicine Hospital, Doha, Qatar

Niek van Dijk Department of Orthopedic Surgery, University of Amsterdam, Amsterdam, The Netherlands

FIFA Medical Centre of Excellence Ripoll-De Prado Sport Clinic, Madrid, Spain

FIFA Medical Centre of Excellence Clínica do Dragão, Porto, Portugal

Christopher W. Di Giovanni Massachusetts General Hospital, Harvard Medical School, Boston, MA, USA

Michael Durst Musculoskeletal Imaging and Intervention, Department of Radiology, University of Colorado, Aurora, CO, USA

Benjamin J. Ebben Department of Orthopedics and Rehabilitative Medicine, University of Wisconsin School of Medicine and Public Health, Madison, WI, USA

Department of Orthopedics, University of Colorado School of Medicine, Aurora, CO, USA

Brian M. Fisher Department of Orthopedic Surgery, Prisma Health-Upstate, University of South Carolina School of Medicine Greenville, Greenville, SC, USA

Eric Giza Department of Orthopedics, University of California, Davis, Sacramento, CA, USA

Alberto Grassi IIa Clinica Ortopedica e Traumatologica, IRCCS Istituto Ortopedico Rizzoli, Bologna, Italy

Matteo Guelfi Casa di Cura Villa Montallegro, Genoa, Italy

Department of Orthopaedic Surgery "Gruppo Policlinico di Monza", Clinica Salus, Alessandria, Italy

Human Anatomy and Embryology Unit, Department of Morphological Sciences, Universitat Autònoma de Barcelona, Barcelona, Spain

Erin Haggerty Department of Orthopedics, University of California, Davis, Sacramento, CA, USA

MaCalus V. Hogan Department of Orthopaedic Surgery, University of Pittsburgh Medical Center, Pittsburgh, PA, USA

Kenneth J. Hunt Department of Orthopedic Surgery, University of Colorado School of Medicine, Aurora, CO, USA

Nia James Department of Orthopaedic Surgery, University of Pittsburgh Medical Center, Pittsburgh, PA, USA

Marissa D. Jamieson Orthopedic Surgery Division of Foot and Ankle, University of Colorado, Denver, CO, USA

James R. Jastifer Ascension Borgess Orthopaedics, Kalamazoo, MI, USA

School of Medicine, Department of Orthopaedic Surgery, Western Michigan University, Kalamazoo, MI, USA

Richard J. Lamour Olympia Orthopaedic Associates, Olympia, WA, USA

Umile Giuseppe Longo Research Unit of Orthopaedic and Trauma Surgery, Fondazione Policlinico Universitario Campus Bio-Medico, Roma, Italy

Research Unit of Orthopaedic and Trauma Surgery, Department of Medicine and Surgery, Università Campus Bio-Medico di Roma, Roma, Italy

Bart Lubberts Foot & Ankle Research and Innovation Laboratory, Massachusetts General Hospital/Harvard Medical School, Boston, MA, USA

Gordon Mackay University of Stirling, Stirling, UK

Jeremy J. McCormick Department of Orthopaedic Surgery, Washington University School of Medicine, St. Louis, MO, USA

Megan Mills Department of Radiology and Imaging Sciences, University of Utah, Salt Lake City, UT, USA

Massimiliano Mosca IIa Clinica Ortopedica e Traumatologica, IRCCS Istituto Ortopedico Rizzoli, Bologna, Italy

Christopher Neville Department of Physical Therapy Education, Upstate Medical University, Rochester, NY, USA

Frederique Neys Department of Orthopaedic Surgery, UC Health Anschutz Medical Campus, Aurora, CO, USA

Jeannie Park Department of Orthopedics, University of California, Davis, Sacramento, CA, USA

Charles C. Pitts Jr Department of Orthopaedic Surgery, University of Alabama—Birmingham, Birmingham, AL, USA

David A. Porter Purdue University, Butler University, Wabash College, Indianapolis, IN, USA

Department of Orthopedics, Voluntary Clinical Faculty, Indiana University, Carmel, IN, USA

William Ribbans University of Northampton, Northampton, UK

Francisco Rodriguez-Fontan Department of Orthopedics, University of Colorado Anschutz Medical Campus, Aurora, CO, USA

Caitlin M. Rugg Division of Sports Medicine, Department of Orthopaedic Surgery, Duke University, Durham, NC, USA

Gregory J. Schmidt Department of Orthopedics, Indiana University, Indianapolis, IN, USA

Gretchen M. Short Select Physical Therapy, Physical Therapy, The Sisu Project, Golden, CO, USA

The Sisu Project, Arvada, CO, USA

Steven M. Short Physical Therapy & High Performance, Denver Nuggets Basketball Club, Physical Therapy, The Sisu Project, Denver, CO, USA

The Sisu Project, Arvada, CO, USA

Jesse Steadman Department of Orthopaedics, University of Utah, Salt Lake City, UT, USA

Giovanna Stelitano Research Unit of Orthopaedic and Trauma Surgery, Fondazione Policlinico Universitario Campus Bio-Medico, Roma, Italy

Research Unit of Orthopaedic and Trauma Surgery, Department of Medicine and Surgery, Università Campus Bio-Medico di Roma, Roma, Italy

Homer Stryker School of Medicine, Department of Orthopaedic Surgery, Western Michigan University, Kalamazoo, MI, USA

Christopher Traynor School of Medicine, Department of Orthopaedic Surgery, Western Michigan University, Kalamazoo, MI, USA

Jordi Vega Laboratory of Arthroscopic and Surgical anatomy, Department of Pathology and Experimental Therapeutics (Human Anatomy Unit), University of Barcelona, Barcelona, Spain

Foot and Ankle Unit, iMove Traumatology-Clinica Tres Torres, and Hospital Quirón Barcelona, Barcelona, Spain

MIFAS by GRECMIP, Merignac, France

Clinique Montchoisi, Lausanne, Switzerland

Norman E. Waldrop III Andrews Sports Medicine, American Sports Medicine Institute, Birmingham, AL, USA

Stephen Blake Wallace Department of Orthopaedic Surgery, University of Colorado School of Medicine, Aurora, CO, USA

Troy S. Watson Las Vegas Orthopaedic Foot and Ankle Fellowship, Desert Orthopaedic Center, Las Vegas, NV, USA

Orthopaedic Surgery Residency, Valley Hospital Medical Center/OPTI West, Las Vegas, NV, USA

Introduction

1

Kenneth J. Hunt

Biology of Ligament Healing

Acute ligament injuries are most often caused by extrinsic traumatic injuries that overload a ligament beyond its failure load (or that of the ligament's insertion). Rapid acceleration-deceleration movements are commonly associated with acute sports-related injuries. As a result, lower extremity ligament injuries at work or during sport-related activities are incredibly common and account for more than 20% of all emergency department visits annually [1]. Chronic degenerative changes in ligaments also can lead to susceptibility for ligament rupture or tear. Managing ligament injuries requires at least a general understanding of how ligaments heal. In the foot and ankle, there is significant variation in the ability of some ligaments to heal properly. For example, most high-grade lateral ankle sprains heal without surgical repair, whereas high-grade syndesmosis and Lisfranc injuries often require surgical stabilization in order to assure proper healing and prevent long-term degenerative changes due to a change in joint biomechanics. The location and severity of the injury will also impact treatment and outcomes, such as restoration of joint motion, management of stiffness, swelling, and adhesion formation, and prevention of chronic conditions [2].

Unlike fractures of bones, ligaments do not heal by tissue regeneration but rather through a wound healing process that follows a predictable healing pathway. This includes an early phase, reparative phase, and a remodeling phase that increases repaired tendon tensile properties. The early phase consists of hematoma formation, inflammation, and initiation of cell proliferation at the injury site. The reparative phase consists of proliferating cells from surrounding tissues that begin to heal the ruptured ligament by formation of fibrous tissue that contains a high proportion of type III collagen. This reparative phase can last for many weeks during which time the healing ligament remains mechanically weak and more readily subject to reinjury. During the remodeling phase, the fibrous repair tissue becomes less cellular, and the proportion of type I collagen increases [3]. Eventually, the collagen fibers align with the direction of stress to increase the repaired ligament tensile strength. In some cases, the remodeling phase can last several months. Factors that mediate inflammation, angiogenesis, cell proliferation, and extracellular matrix remodeling seem to be involved in the different phases of healing based on gene expression studies. However, the mechanisms that coordinate these gene expression events are not well understood.

It is also important to recognize that chronic instability may be very different from a ligament

K. J. Hunt (✉)
Department of Orthopedic Surgery, University of Colorado School of Medicine, Aurora, CO, USA
e-mail: Kenneth.j.hunt@cuanschutz.edu

P. D'Hooghe et al. (eds.), *Ligamentous Injuries of the Foot and Ankle*,
https://doi.org/10.1007/978-3-031-08682-3_1

healing perspective than acute injuries. An example related to the knee was discovered by Brophy et al. who analyzed gene expression between anterior cruciate ligaments that had been torn less than 3 months (acute), between 3 and 12 months (intermediate), or greater than 12 months (chronic) [4]. They harvested a small piece from the ends of the torn ligaments during surgical repair and found that genes involved in extracellular matrix reorganization were expressed in the acute samples, whereas the chronic specimens showed reductions in collagen gene expression a 30-fold decline in periostin expression. Thus, in cases of chronic ligamentous instability conditions, it cannot necessarily be expected that normal ligament healing will occur. Special considerations to supplement a repair with additional material (e.g., collagen-based grafts) or orthobiologics (e.g., concentrated progenitor cells) make sense in these cases, but clinical data is sparse.

Treatment Decision-Making

The vast majority of ligamentous injuries to the foot and ankle heal without surgical intervention, even in cases with complete ligamentous disruption. Immobilization and POLICE (protect, optimally load, ice, compress, elevate) [5] can be a helpful means of accelerating recovery and mitigating pain and gait irregularities during mobility as ligaments heal. However, for some ligamentous injuries in the foot and ankle, long-term consequences can ensue if they are not identified early with proper management initiated. In some cases, surgical intervention is required in order to restore normal (or close to normal) joint kinematics and function and to prevent long-term sequelae associated with some complete ligamentous injuries [6]. In most cases, skilled physical therapy can be an important adjunct to guiding recovery and facilitating return to sports participation [7]. It is critical for the treating clinician to understand surgical treatment considerations for injuries meeting that threshold, including indications, techniques, recovery times, and risks. This should be a shared decision-making process with the patient and their relevant support network. The ligamentous injuries in the foot and ankle that most commonly warrant surgical decision-making are the subject of this text and include lateral ankle sprains, syndesmosis injuries, Lisfranc injuries, turf toe, and plantar plate injuries.

The Role of the Orthopedic Surgeon

The orthopedic surgeon plays an important role in guiding the diagnostic algorithm for ligamentous injuries and determining which injuries warrant consideration for surgical intervention. Further, the orthopedic surgeon must remain up to date on the rapidly evolving milieu of surgical techniques and rehabilitation protocols. There are, and always will be, controversies and differences of opinion with regard to optimal treatment. In most cases, there are no singe right or wrong answers. As we see improvement in the quality of basic science and clinical outcomes data to support various treatments, more broadly accepted best practices emerge. Still, it may not be sufficient to know which treatment approach is appropriate in a given situation but also to have skill and proficiency in surgical and rehabilitation techniques. It is for this reason that foot and ankle subspecialists are increasingly involved in the acute and long-term management of foot and ankle injuries even in the sports arena. It is critical to remain up to date on the literature, skill set, and outcomes data for each injury type.

The Role of the Physical Therapist

While not all ligament injuries require formal physical therapy, most cases at minimum see a benefit from guided formal physical therapy. For many chronic instability conditions and higher-grade injuries, formal physical therapy can be necessary to restore normal joint and gait kinematics and to monitor progression to mitigate the risk of reactive tendinopathies. Thorough exploration of specific rehabilitation modalities is generally beyond the scope of this text. However, each section incorporates current practices in rehabilitation and return to sport considerations for each injury type.

References

1. De Boer AS, Schepers T, Panneman MJ, Van Beeck EF, Van Lieshout EM. Health care consumption and costs due to foot and ankle injuries in the Netherlands, 1986-2010. BMC Musculoskelet Disord. 2014;15:128.
2. Cottrell JA, Turner JC, Arinzeh TL, O'Connor JP. The biology of bone and ligament healing. Foot Ankle Clin. 2016;21(4):739–61.
3. Sakai H, Koibuchi N, Ohtake H, et al. Type I and type III procollagen gene expressions in the early phase of ligament healing in rabbits: an in situ hybridization study. J Orthop Res. 2001;19(1):132–5.
4. Brophy RH, Tycksen ED, Sandell LJ, Rai MF. Changes in transcriptome-wide gene expression of anterior cruciate ligament tears based on time from injury. Am J Sports Med. 2016;44(8):2064–75.
5. Schwitzguebel AJ, Muff G, Naets E, Karatzios C, Saubade M, Gremeaux V. The acute management of muscle injuries in 2018. Rev Med Suisse. 2018;14(613):1332–9.
6. Gribble PA, Bleakley CM, Caulfield BM, et al. Evidence review for the 2016 international ankle consortium consensus statement on the prevalence, impact and long-term consequences of lateral ankle sprains. Br J Sports Med. 2016;50(24):1496–505.
7. Pearce CJ, Tourne Y, Zellers J, et al. Rehabilitation after anatomical ankle ligament repair or reconstruction. Knee Surg Sports Traumatol Arthrosc. 2016;24(4):1130–9.

2 Anatomy and Biomechanics of the Foot and Ankle

Alberto Grassi and Massimiliano Mosca

Introduction

The foot and the ankle form a complex anatomical system that has evolved to allow bipedal walking with minimal energy expenditure and maximum performance during normal daily activities. The 26 bony segments of the foot (28 including distal tibia and fibula if we consider also the ankle), in fact, create a vaulted architecture, supported by three main arches, which discharges the weight on the ground through three support points. In turn, we can distinguish four main regions: the ankle (distal tibia and fibula and talus), the hindfoot (talus and calcaneus), the midfoot (navicular, cuboid, medial, intermediate, and lateral cuneiforms), and forefoot (metatarsals and phalanges of the five rays) (Fig. 2.1). The fifth metatarsal base represents an important structure from a traumatic and surgical perspective since is it the insertion of the peroneus brevis tendon and the location of common fractures (Fig. 2.2).

This complex anatomical structure allows the foot and ankle to dynamically vary its conformation during the gait cycle, thanks to the possibility of winding during the push-off phase to have a more rigid and propulsive conformation (supination), and unwinding during the mid-stance phase to enjoy a conformation that adapts to the soil and acts as a receptor organ (pronation).

To allow these physiological conformation changes while maintaining adequate stability, bone congruence and tenacious ligamentous and tendon structures are needed.

Distal Tibiofibular Syndesmosis

A fibrous joint in which two bone segments are held together by strong ligamentous structures represents the syndesmosis. This definition also applies to distal tibio-peroneal syndesmosis, consisting of a bone portion represented by the distal tibia and fibula and fundamental ligamentous components. In joint characterized by a relatively low mobility, its normal kinematics is important during the load and the extra-rotation [1]. In fact, when the syndesmosis is intact, regarding the distal fibula movements of only 2°–5° in extra-rotation, 0–2.5 mm in medial translation and 1–3.1 mm in posterior translation have been detected [2, 3].

The bone anatomy is characterized by the joint relationship between the convex surface of the distal fibula and the lateral tibial incisura (*incisura fibularis tibiae*). About 6–8 cm from the level of the tibiotarsal joint, the tibial interosseous crest forks in caudal direction in an anterior margin, more voluminous, ending in the Chaput's tubercle, and in a posterior margin, more elusive,

A. Grassi (✉) · M. Mosca
IIa Clinica Ortopedica e Traumatologica, IRCCS
Istituto Ortopedico Rizzoli, Bologna, Italy
e-mail: alberto.grassi@ior.it;
massimiliano.mosca@ior.it

P. D'Hooghe et al. (eds.), *Ligamentous Injuries of the Foot and Ankle*,
https://doi.org/10.1007/978-3-031-08682-3_2

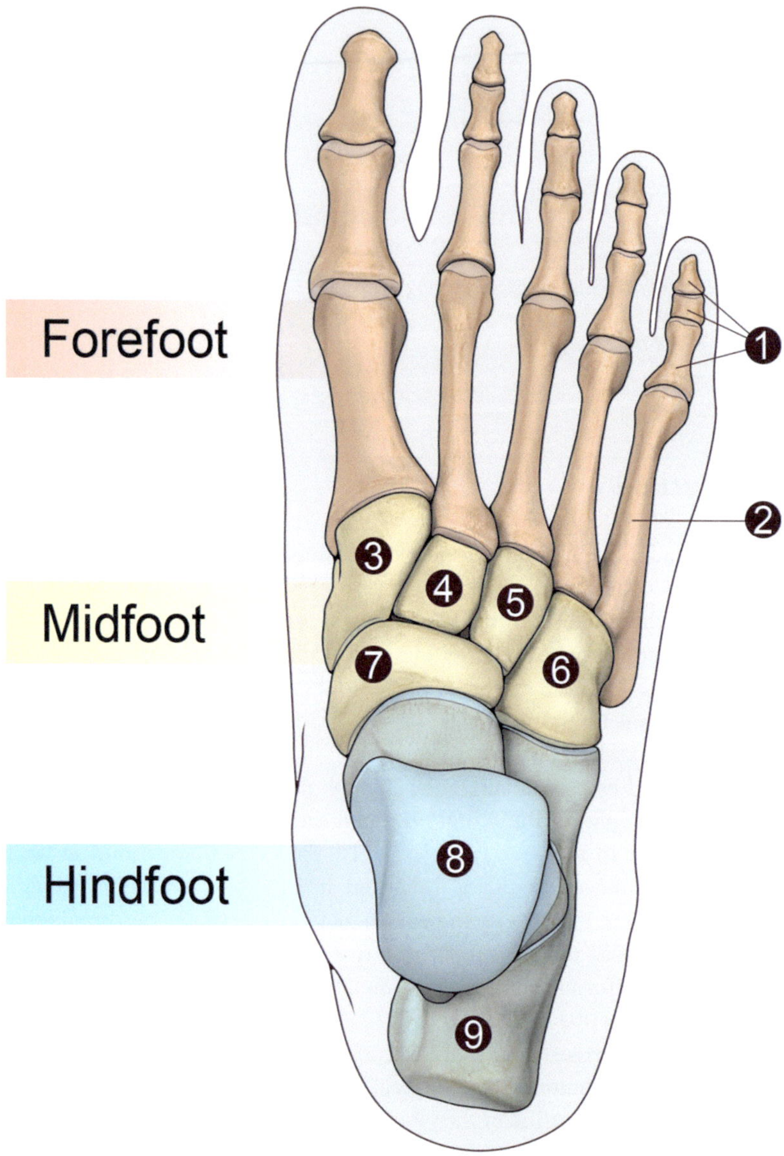

Fig. 2.1 The bony structures of the foot. (1) Phalanxes, (2) metatarsal bones, (3) medial cuneiform, (4) intermediate cuneiform, (5) lateral cuneiform, (6) cuboid, (7) navicular, (8) talus, and (9) calcaneus

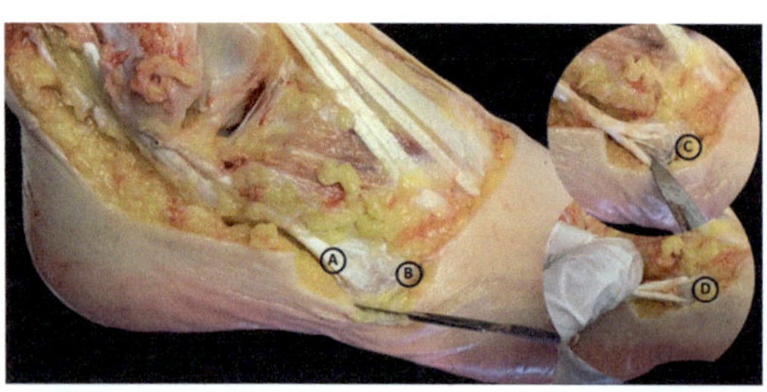

Fig. 2.2 Anatomic specimen of the fifth metatarsal base: (**a**) insertion of peroneus brevis tendon, (**b**) base of the fifth metatarsus, (**c**) bone surface after longitudinal split of the tendon insertion, and (**d**) preserved traction after debridement of fifth metatarsal apex

ending in the Volkmann's tubercle. The base of the triangular peroneal articular surface is formed by the anterior tubercle of Wagstaffe-Le Fort [4].

The stability of the distal tibiofibular syndesmosis is the result in part of the bone congruence of the tibia and fibula. The size and depth of the *incisura tibialis* can vary [5] and are clinically relevant. After a high-ankle sprain, a shallow *incisura tibialis* may predispose to a syndesmosis injury, with the less prominent posterior tubercle serving as the fulcrum for excessive rotation of the distal fibula around its longitudinal axis [6].

A small area of direct contact between fibula and distal tibia, at the base of the syndesmosis, has been described. This area is covered with a thin layer of hyaline cartilage of about 0.5–1 mm [4, 7]. In addition, a synovial recess almost always extends between the fibula and the distal tibia from the tibiocrural joint. Such "recessus tibiofibularis" can have different anatomical characteristics from subject to subject, with a depth that can vary from 4 to 25 mm [4]. The clinical relevance of this finding is represented by the risk of being crossed by K wires, fiches of external fixators or excessively long screws, becoming an entry door in the joint and increasing the risk of septic arthritis [8, 9].

The stabilizers of the distal tibiofibular syndesmosis are four: the anterior inferior tibiofibular ligament (AITFL), the posterior inferior tibiofibular ligament (PITFL), the interosseous ligament (IOL), and the inferior transverse ligament (ITL) (Fig. 2.3). These ligaments, associated with the bone congruence, contribute to axial, rotational, and translational stability.

The anterior inferior tibiofibular ligament (AITFL) runs obliquely from the proximal-medial to the distal-lateral, from the tibial Chaput's tubercle to the anterior tubercle of the distal fibula, crossing the superolateral angle of the tibiocrural joint. Macroscopically, the ligament is composed of three main fascicles (of which the intermediate one is the most resistant), which give it a trapezoidal shape, and has a length between 20 and 30 mm, an average width of about 18 mm and a thickness between 2 and 4 mm [4, 10]. The AITFL represents the weakest of the four syndesmotic ligaments and results often in injured high-ankle sprains (Fig. 2.4).

The Bassett's ligament, an accessory bundle, is present between 21% and 92% of anatomical specimens or MRI imaging, depending on authors [4]. This runs below the AITFL, and it is oblique and intra-articular and frequently crosses the superolateral angle of the tibiocrural joint (Fig. 2.5). The clinical relevance lies in the fact that during the dorsiflexion of the ankle, it comes into contact with the talar trochlea and can be the cause of pain and anterior impingement in the presence of an intact AITFL. Its arthroscopic release does not affect the stability of the syndesmosis and reduces the painful symptoms [11, 12].

The posterior inferior tibiofibular ligament (PITFL) is a particularly resistant ligament, both for its elasticity and for its amplitude. It extends from the posterior malleolus of the tibia to the posterior tubercle of the fibula, running from proximal-medial to distal-lateral. It has a fan shape, like its anterior counterpart, and converges on the posterior portion of the distal fibula [4, 10]. It is clinically important to remember that due to the strength of its fibers, during an ankle sprain, the excessive stress results more often in a fracture-avulsion of the posterior tibial malleolus than in a complete rupture of PITFL [13].

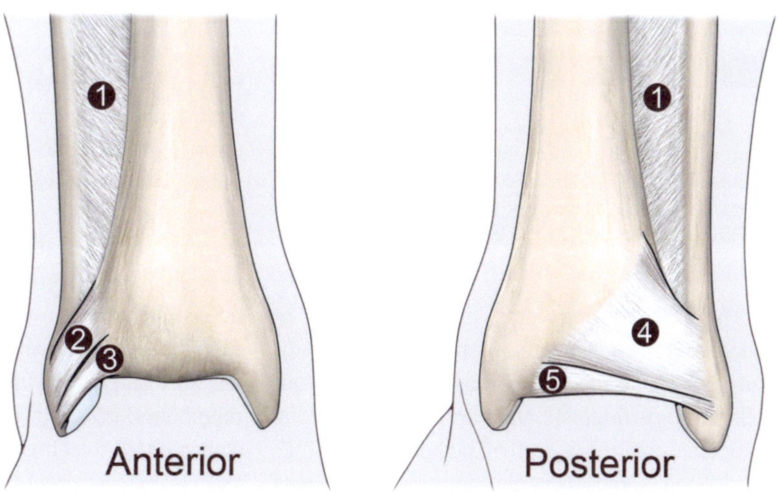

Fig. 2.3 Ligamentous complex of the distal tibiofibular syndesmosis. (1) Interosseous ligament (IOL), (2) anterior inferior tibiofibular ligament (AITFL), (3) Bassett's ligament, (4) posterior inferior tibiofibular ligament (PITFL), and (5) inferior transverse ligament (ITL)

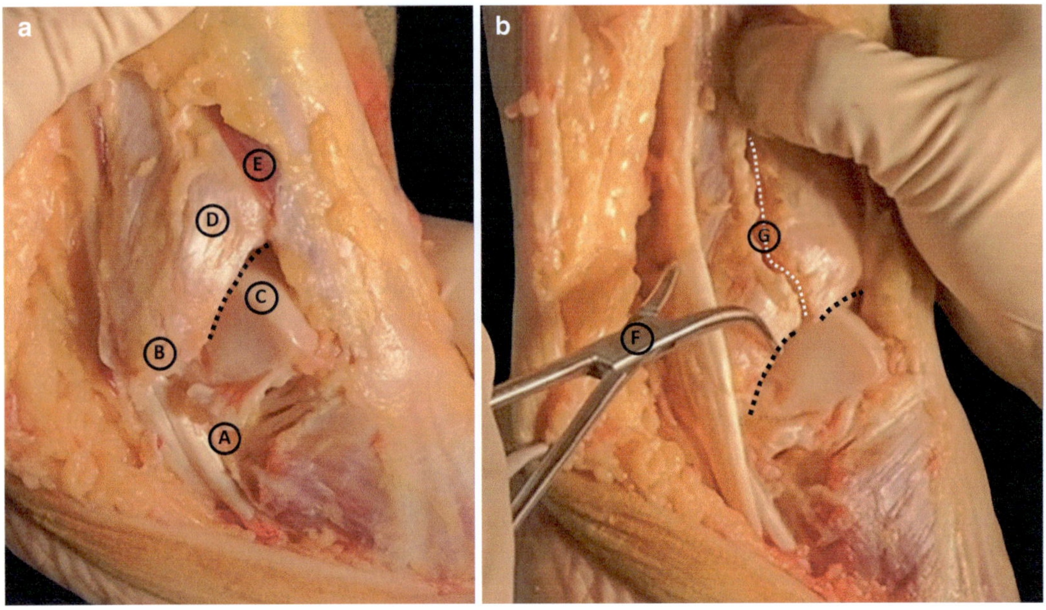

Fig. 2.4 Anatomic specimen of the distal tibiofibular syndesmosis. Figure "**a**" shows the intact syndesmosis (black dotted line), (**a**) cut and reflected anterior talofibular ligament (ATFL), (**b**) apex of lateral malleolus, (**c**) talus surface, (**d**) anterior inferior tibiofibular ligament (AITFL), and (**e**) peroneus tertius. Figure "**b**" shows the disrupted syndesmosis (black dotted line), with the traction of the forceps (**f**) that produces a separation between the tibia and fibula (white dotted line) and a visible gap (**g**)

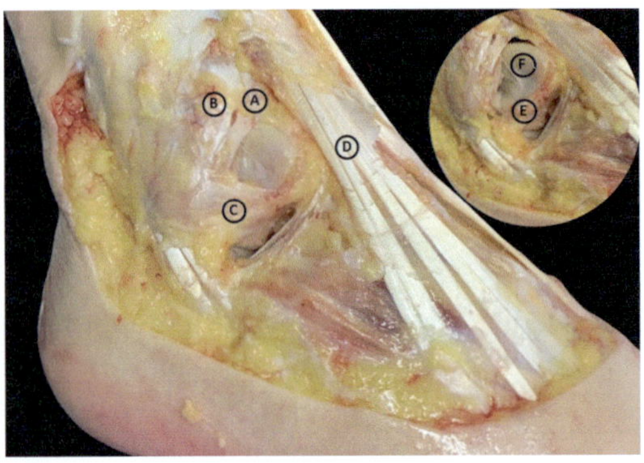

Fig. 2.5 Anatomic specimen of tibial, fibular, and talar ligaments: (**a**) Basset's ligament, (**b**) anterior inferior tibiofibular ligament (AITFL), (**c**) anterior talofibular ligament (ATFL), and (**d**) extensor tendons. After cutting the ATFL (**e**), the talar surface can be displaced (**f**)

The inferior transverse ligament (ITL), of roundish appearance, runs horizontally immediately below the PITFL, making them sometimes difficult to distinguish, and can reach the medial malleolus creating a sort of posterior "labrum." In addition, some fibers can merge with those of PITFL giving rise to what is called intermalleolar ligament (IML) [4, 10]. Controversies over the distinction of individual components are still present in the literature.

The interosseous ligament (IOL) is formed by a thickening of the most distal interosseous membrane portion. It extends deeply between the tibia and fibula and creates a pyramidal space filled with adipose tissue and fibrous fascicles. The most distal bundles originate from the anterior tubercle of the tibia and insert distally on the fibula immediately above the talocrural joint. Its presence is erratic, and in some subjects, it is absent while in others, it is really evident. When present, the space below the IOL is occupied by the syndesmotic recess [4, 10]. The IOL acts both as reinforcement, neutralizing the forces that are created during the heel-strike phase in gait cycle and stabilizing the tibiocrural joint during loading. In this regard, it has been shown how the IOL and the interosseous membrane are subjected to stress throughout the stance phase, placing a rational to the breaking of syndesmotic screws [4, 10, 14].

Lateral Collateral Ligaments of the Ankle

The tibiotalar joint is composed by the talar body, wedge-shaped, which articulates within the tibiofibular mortise. The normal movement of the ankle consists of dorsiflexion and plantarflexion through an oblique axis passing through the apex of the internal and external malleoli. Varus and valgus movements are allowed, within physiological limits, except in case of maximum dorsiflexion.

Joint stability is guaranteed, under normal conditions, both by intrinsic elements such as bone congruence and by extrinsic elements such as a complex ligament apparatus, divided into two main compartments: the lateral compartment and the medial compartment. The high bone congruence also allows to unload the important force vectors to which the joint is subjected on a wider loading area, reducing joint stress; some authors consider these biomechanical characteristics even better expressed than in the hip or knee [15, 16]. In addition, ligamentous structures also contribute to ankle stability through proprioceptive functions [17].

The ankle lateral ligament complex consists of three ligaments: the anterior talofibular ligament (ATFL), the calcaneofibular ligament (CFL), and the posterior talofibular ligament (PTFL) (Fig. 2.6).

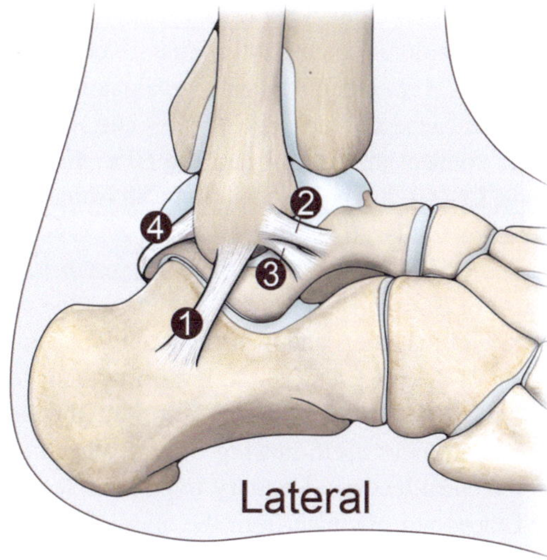

Fig. 2.6 The ankle lateral ligament complex. (1) Calcaneofibular ligament (CFL), (2) superior fascicle of the anterior talofibular ligament (ATFLsf), (3) inferior fascicle of the anterior talofibular ligament (ATFLif), and (4) posterior talofibular ligament (PTFL)

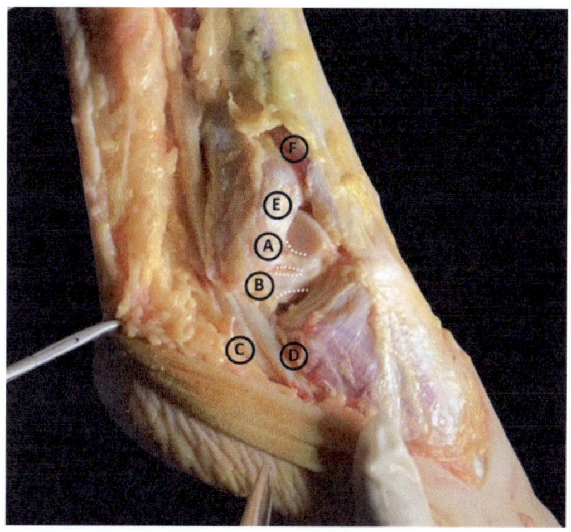

Fig. 2.7 Anatomic specimen of the ankle lateral ligament and tendon complex: (**a**) anterior talofibular ligament upper fascicle (ATFLsf), (**b**) anterior talofibular ligament lower fascicle (ATFLlf), (**c**) peroneus longus tendon, (**d**) peroneus brevis tendon, (**e**) anterior inferior tibiofibular ligament (AITFL), and (**f**) peroneus tertius

The ATFL, closely related to the anterolateral ankle capsule, typically consists of two bundles [18] separated by a "vascular window" (Fig. 2.7), though in literature, single-bundle or three-bundle variants have been described [19]. About 15–20 mm long, it originates from the anterior side of the distal fibula, at about 10 mm proximal to the apex of the lateral malleolus, and it inserts on the lateral side of the talus, immediately anterior to the lateral facet. This is more proximal than the lateral talar neck.

Its two fascicles are distinguished in the lower fascicle (ATFLif), extra-articular, and in the upper fascicle (ATFLsf), intra-articular. Overall, the ligament is virtually horizontal with the ankle in neutral position, facing upward with the dorsiflexed ankle and downward during plantarflexion. Only in the latter case, the ligament is tense and placed under stress, becoming vulnerable during sprains [19, 20] (Fig. 2.5). Recently in the literature, a close connection has been reported between the ATFLif and the CFL, which form what has been defined by Vega J. et al. [20] the lateral fibulotalocalcaneal ligament complex (TCLFL). This complex can be evaluated from the lateral aspect of the ankle where some arcuate fibers connect the ATFLif and the CFL. In this study, LFTCL has been shown to be an isometric structure, unlike ATFLsf [21].

The CFL, positioned anatomically just below the ATFLif, originates from the anterior edge of the lateral malleolus and is inserted on the lateral aspect of the calcaneus, at the level of a tubercle placed supero-posteriorly to the peroneal tubercle of the calcaneus itself, flowing into the sheath of the peroneal tendons. Contrary to popular belief, CFL does not originate from the apex of lateral malleolus [22]. From 2 to 3 cm long and about 4–8 mm wide, it runs in a medium-lateral and proximal-distal direction from its origin [23]. The angle between the CFL and the ATFL is about 104°, which can result to be useful in case of surgical reconstruction [23]. In case of chronic lateral ankle instability in which both ATFL and CFL are damaged, there is disagreement on the usefulness of repairing the CFL [24]. D'Hooghe P et al. [25], in a recent study on cadaver, compared biomechanics in case of isolated repair of ATFL to combined repair of ATFL/CFL. Immediately after an isolated or combined repair, the biomechanical characteristics of the ankle have not changed with respect to the previous "injured ankle." In addition, greater stiffness was highlighted in the case of combined repair, compared to isolated repair, and the CFL proved to be vulnerable immediately after repair, failing before the ATFL.

Anatomical variants have been described in literature. In 35% of cases, the CFL is reinforced by fibers from the lateral talocalcaneal ligament; only in 23%, the two ligaments are totally distinct; and in 42% of the cases, the lateral talocalcaneal ligament is absent and is replaced by anterior talocalcaneal ligament (in the latter case, it is evident that CFL acquires greater biomechanical importance) [19].

PTFL originates from the medial surface of the lateral malleolus and runs horizontally as far as the posterior side of the talus. Its length is about 3 cm and thickness from 5 to 8 mm [26]. Its insertion is wide and involves almost the entire posterior labrum of the talus. Due to its multifascicular structure, its insertion is not well defined, ending at the posterior surface of the talus, on the os trigonum, and merging with the posterior intermalleolar ligament, a consistent finding in dissections [26]. The posterior intermalleolar ligament is located between the ITL and the PTFL, running obliquely from lateral to medial and from downward to upward, finding its clinical relevance as a possible cause of posterior impingement of ankle [19, 27].

Dalmau-Pastor M. et al. [28] has recently pointed out that these ligamentous structures present variable interconnections seen on the medial side. In his study, constant connections between ATFLif and PTFL, ATFL and CFL, and CFL and PTFL were described in all specimens. Only in 42.5% were reported fibrous connections between ATFLsf and PTFL. Connections between ATFLif and CFL (LFTCL complex) have been highlighted in all dissections as arciform formations that cross the lateral aspect of the subtalar joint. These data raise doubts if the lateral ligamentous structures of the ankle are indeed a complex anatomical unit, rather than isolated structures, and the actual possibility of an isolated lesion of a single ligamentous component after an ankle sprain.

Medial Collateral Ligaments of the Ankle

The tears of the deltoid ligament are historically considered rare, according to some authors limited to 5% of ligamentous lesions of the ankle [29], but the incidence could be greater, and with the improvement of diagnostic tools, lesions of the deltoid ligament are being highlighted more often [30].

The deltoid ligament is a robust, multifascicled ligamentous complex that spreads distally from the medial malleolus with a large, fan-shaped insertional area. The ligamentous components are contiguous, difficult to distinguish in classic anatomical specimens, and closely connected to the capsular structures and to the adjacent tendons [19].

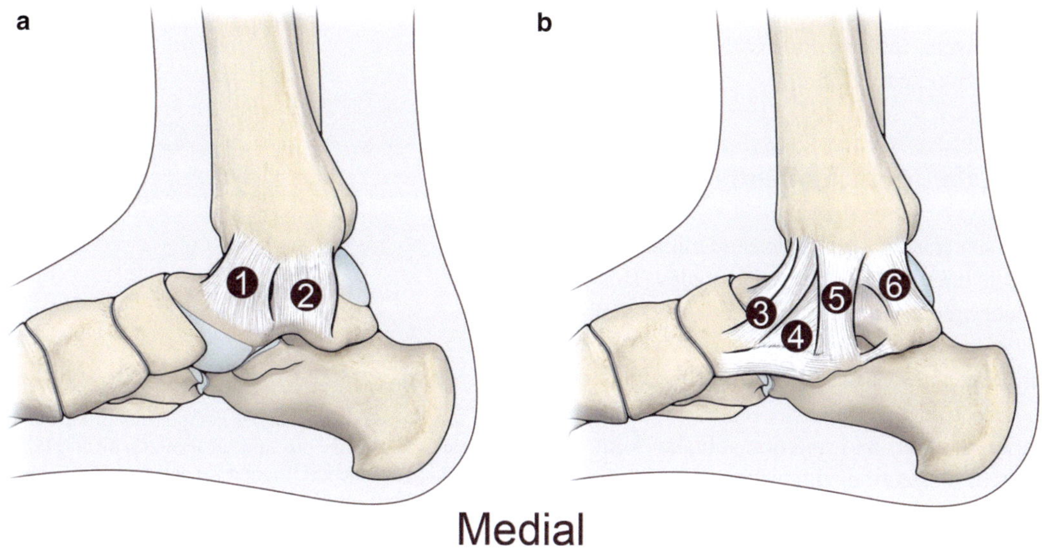

Fig. 2.8 (**a**) Deep layer of the deltoid ligament: (1) deep anterior tibiotalar ligament (DATTL) and (2) deep posterior tibiotalar ligament (DPTTL). (**b**) Superficial layer of the deltoid ligament: (3) tibionavicular ligament (TNL), (4) tibiospring ligament (TSL), (5) tibiocalcaneal ligament (TCL), and (6) superficial posterior tibiotalar ligament (SPTTL)

The literature, however, agrees in distinguishing two layers and six ligamentous components [31] (Fig. 2.8).

The superficial layer, which originates from the anterior colliculum of the tibial malleolus, is composed of four bundles with distinct insertions: the superficial posterior tibiotalar ligament (SPTTL), the tibiocalcaneal ligament (TCL), the tibiospring ligament (TSL), and the tibionavicular ligament (TNL). Only the last two are constant anatomical findings in anatomical specimens, while SPTTL and TCL may vary. In this regard, in a recent study, Amaha K et al. [32] anatomically examined the medial ankle joint, focusing on the deltoid ligament in perspective of the joint capsule. The authors highlighted how the medial capsule can be detached as a continuous layer and consists of three different types of tissues. The fibrous part of the capsule could correspond to the deltoid ligament and the cartilaginous part to the superior part of the spring ligament. This could explain why the number of bundles and the morphology of the deltoid ligament are variable in literature.

Other authors have pointed out that the TCL is to be considered anatomically constant, and where apparently absent, an anatomical variant of the TSL with a Y-shaped configuration serves as a connection between the tibial malleolus and the calcaneus, inserting both on the sustentaculum tali and at the level of the spring ligament [33].

Clinically, the superficial layer helps to maintain the correct alignment of the ankle and the hindfoot as well as to oppose excessive extra-rotation and abduction.

The deep layer consists of fibers that run between the medial malleolus and the medial aspect of the talus in two main bundles: the deep posterior tibiotalar ligament (DPTTL), constant, and the deep anterior tibiotalar ligament (DATTL), inconstant. These ligaments, shorter and thicker, flow into the medial capsule of the tibiotalar joint [30, 32].

The orientation of the deep-layer fibers prevents lateral displacement and external rotation of the talus, acting as the main stabilizing mechanism in plantarflexion [30].

Also, after the section of both superficial and deep layers, the anterior instability of the ankle does not increase [22].

Subtalar Joint Ligaments

The subtalar joint has awakened clinical and scientific interest only in recent decades. This joint, which represents an important and complex interface between the lower surface of the talus and the upper surface of the calcaneus, is composed of three articular facets that form the posterior, middle, and anterior subtalar joint. The current literature distinguishes the talocalcaneonavicular articulation (TCN) and the posterior talocalcaneal (TC) joint as two separate entities, separated by sinus tarsi, using the term subtalar only for the posterior TC articulation. Together, they form a functional unit that allows a triplanar movement [34] and is designed to pass from a flexible conformation, suitable to absorb shocks, to a more rigid one, suitable for propulsion.

Although the actual incidence is not known, it is thought that, generally, most subtalar capsuloligamentous lesions occur concurrently with lesions of the ligamentous complex of the ankle. It is estimated that 10% of patients with lateral ankle instability actually present a combined tibiotarsal and subtalar instability [35].

The subtalar ligaments can be divided into intrinsic (cervical ligament, CL; interosseous talocalcaneal ligament, ITCL; the roots of the inferior extensor retinaculum; the anterior talocalcaneal ligament, ATCL or ACaL) (Fig. 2.9) and extrinsic (calcaneofibular ligament, CFL; tibiocalcaneal fascicle of the deltoid ligament).

The extrinsic CFL and deltoid ligament have been previously discussed.

The intrinsic component probably plays a fundamental role in the stability of the subtalar joint, but the literature concerning the anatomy of these ligaments is still somewhat confusing [36].

The inferior extensor retinaculum (also known as "frondiform ligament" or "ligament of Retzius") is a reinforced portion of the ankle and foot fascia, with a typically Y-shaped stem consisting of a superficial and a deep lamina, inserted on the upper surface of the heel through three roots (medial, intermediate, and lateral) (Fig. 2.10). The medial root is a particularly complex and high-variability structure that originates from the deepest fibers of the inferior extensor retinaculum and inserts immediately behind the CL. In rare cases, the medial root may be absent [37]. The lateral root runs from the superficial lamina to the lateral aspect of the calcaneus, immediately posterior to the origin of the extensor digitorum brevis muscle. The intermediate root originates from the deep lamina and inserts on the floor of the sinus tarsi.

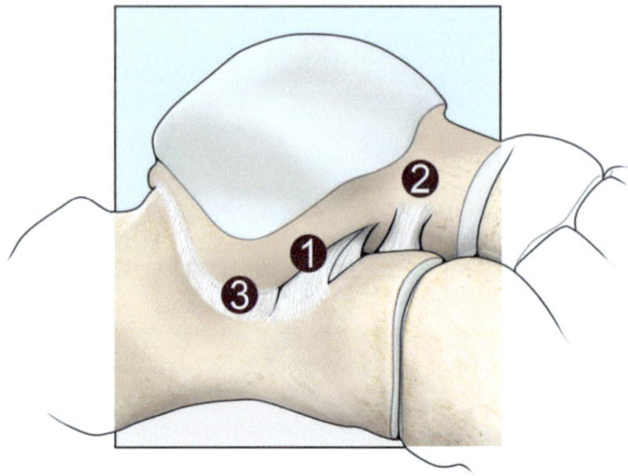

Fig. 2.9 Intrinsic ligamentous components of the subtalar joint. (1) Interosseous talocalcaneal ligament (ITCL), (2) cervical ligament (CL), and (3) anterior talocalcaneal ligament (ATCL or ACaL)

The CL, a robust quadrangular ligament of the anterolateral region of sinus tarsi, runs obliquely at 45°, from the talar neck to the calcaneus, inserting on its footprint at the level of the floor of sinus tarsi ("cervical tubercle") [38]. It usually consists of a single bundle though sometimes two [38] or multiple [36] bundles have been described.

The ITCL is a broad and flattened ligament consisting of two lamellae that run obliquely from the sulcus tali to the calcaneal sulcus, with an oblique axis of 35° on the coronal plane [38, 39]. In the central region of the sinus tarsi, the more lateral fibers cross the medial root of the lower extensor retinaculum. Three main morphologies can be distinguished: the band type (93%), the fan type (5%), and the multiple type (3%) [40]. It represents one of the main passive stabilizers of the subtalar joint and, together with

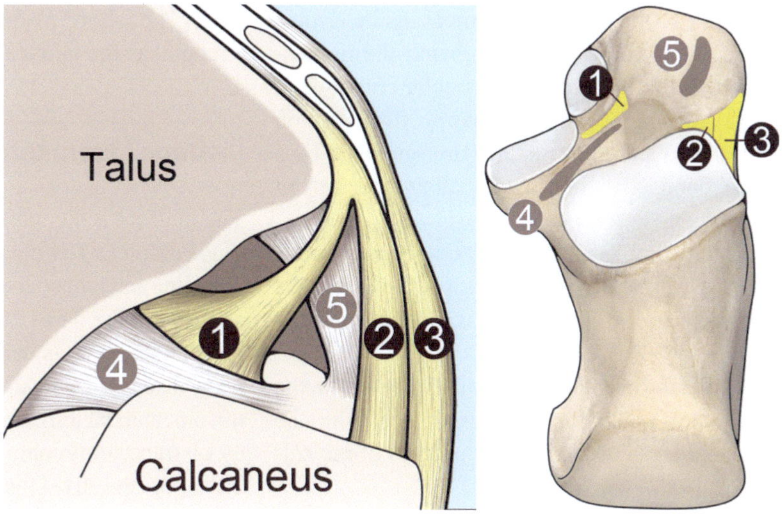

Fig. 2.10 Intrinsic ligamentous components of the subtalar joint, particularly of the inferior extensor retinaculum (coronal view of the sinus tarsi and posterior view of the calcaneus). (1) Medial root, (2) intermediate root, (3) lateral root, (4) interosseous talocalcaneal ligament (ITCL), and (5) cervical ligament (CL)

its proprioceptive characteristics, can be considered as the cruciate ligament of the knee.

The ATCL is represented by a flattened and rectangular bundle and corresponds to a thickening of the anterior capsule of the posterior subtalar joint. Some authors consider the ATCL to be part of the ITCL, and for others, it is a capsular reinforcement. It originates from the anterior edge of the posterior articular facet of the talus, and by running vertically, it is inserted to the front of the anterior edge of the posterior articular facet of the calcaneus [34]. The ATCL is put in tension during foot inversion and during the anterior drawer of the heel.

A recent study showed on cadaver that the intrinsic ligaments of the subtalar articulation present consistent location, presence, morphology, and dimensions, highlighting an important role of the CL and ATCL in joint stability [36].

Chopart Joint Ligamentous Complex

The midtarsal joint complex, or Chopart joint, represents the anatomical connection between the midfoot and the hindfoot, allowing the latter to adapt to the ground while the forefoot remains fixed during the inversion and eversion movements. It is formed by the talocalcaneonavicular joint and the calcaneocuboid joint.

The talocalcaneonavicular joint consists of the anterior articular surface of the talar head, the concave posterior surface of the navicular, and the anterior talar articular facet of the calcaneum. This particular joint morphology has been associated to the hip joint, gaining the name of "coxa pedis," [41] contained by a single capsule.

The calcaneocuboid joint is formed by the triangular surface of the anterior apophysis of the calcaneus and its articular surface of the cuboid.

There are various ligamentous structures that allow the stability of this complex biomechanical structure, often fused into capsular components. They can be subdivided for convenience in ligaments of talocalcaneonavicular pertinence (spring ligament complex, bifurcate ligament, and dorsal talonavicular ligament) and of calcaneocuboid pertinence (dorsal calcaneocuboid ligament and plantar calcaneocuboid ligament).

Among the main ligament structures of the foot, the one of greater anatomical and biomechanical complexity is represented by the spring ligament complex (SLC), also called plantar calcaneonavicular ligament. It is formed by the superomedial ligament, the medioplantar oblique ligament, and inferoplantar longitudinal ligament.

The superomedial bundle has a triangular shape, originating from the anterior margin of the sustentaculum tali, and inserts widely on the navicular tuberosity and on the tibiospring component of the deltoid ligament. Its innermost surface is fibrocartilaginous, giving the impression of being in front of an articular component. Its relationships with the posterior tibial tendon are known, and the structures are separated by a loose connective tissue that allows reciprocal sliding.

The medioplantar oblique bundle, more plantar, runs from the coronoid fossa of the calcaneus and projects medially to the navicular, immediately below the tuberosity.

The inferoplantar longitudinal bundle is the most thick and robust and originates from the coronoid fossa of the anterior process of the calcaneus [42].

SLC is often involved in ankle eversion injuries, producing distraction across the medial aspect of the Chopart joint. The medial distraction may cause traction injury from the superomedial bundle of the SLC, avulsion of the inferoplantar longitudinal bundle of the SLC, and fractures of the navicular bone [43].

The bifurcate ligament is composed of a medial calcaneonavicular bundle and a lateral calcaneocuboid bundle and creates support for the talonavicular and calcaneocuboid joints. The first runs between the intermediary tubercle and the dorsal surface of the cuboid, inserting at about 1.5 cm from the calcaneocuboid joint. The second one extends from the intermediary tubercle of the calcaneus to the posterosuperior slope of the navicular. The bifurcate ligament is placed before the cervical ligament and at the origin of the extensor digitorum brevis muscle.

The dorsal talonavicular ligament represents a capsular thickening stretched between the dorsal slope of the talar neck and the dorsal surface of the navicular bone [44].

The dorsal calcaneocuboid ligament is represented by a thin bundle that runs between the superolateral slope of the anterior calcaneal apophysis, medial to the lateral component of the bifurcate ligament, and the dorsal surface of the cuboid bone.

The plantar calcaneocuboid ligament consists of two components, the long and the short plantar ligaments, and stabilizes the calcaneocuboid joint. The long plantar ligament is more superficial and originates from the plantar surface of the heel. The short plantar ligament merges and strengthens the joint capsule [42].

Lisfranc Ligamentous Complex

The midfoot is composed of a bone and ligamentous complex. Ten bones form the bony component: the navicular, the cuboid, three cuneiform bones, and the bases of the five metatarsals. The proximal portion is called Chopart joint that has been discussed above. The distal portion is the tarsometatarsal joint complex (TMT), also known as Lisfranc joint complex, that encompasses the bases of the five metatarsal bones and their respective joint surfaces for the three cuneiform bones and cuboid [45].

From a biomechanical point of view, Lisfranc's joint represents the point of passage between the midfoot and the forefoot. Its asymmetrical Roman arch structure, with a keystone represented by the base of the second metatarsal, plays a fundamental role in walking, in particular on uneven terrain [46]. In this regard, the stability of the joint complex is essential for a normal gait cycle, and to this end, a complex ligamentous system stabilizes and strengthens the joint capsules.

This joint complex has been described in literature, such as by De Palma et al. [47], based on its position with respect to bone structures in dorsal, plantar, and interosseous.

The seven ligaments that form the dorsal ligamentous complex lie on the dorsal side, uniting cuneiforms and metatarsals.

The interosseous system involves lateral, central, and medial longitudinal ligaments. The medial compartment, also called "Lisfranc ligament," runs distally and laterally between the lateral surface of the medial cuneiform and the medial slope of the second metatarsal (Fig. 2.11). It represents the most voluminous ligament of the joint complex, with its 10 mm of length and 6 mm of thickness. Its importance has been demonstrated by the fact that an isolated lesion of this ligament can lead to instability of the Lisfranc complex [48, 49]. Other ligaments that are part of the interosseous complex are represented by intertarsal ligaments that run between the cunei-

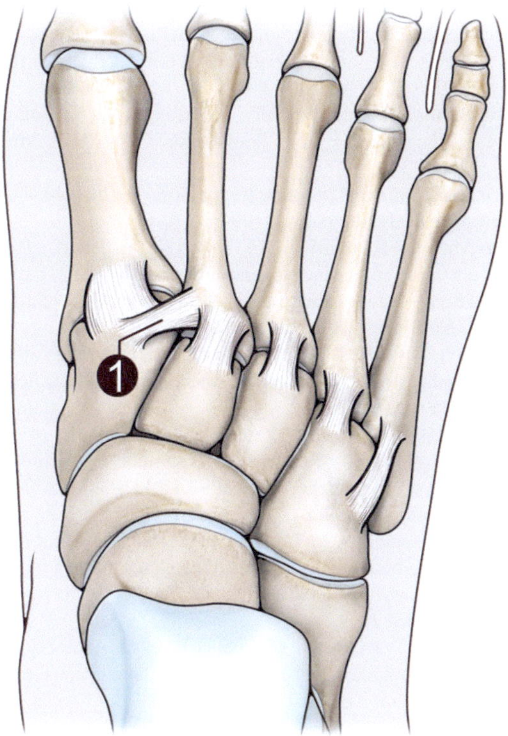

Fig. 2.11 The "Lisfranc ligament" (1), medial component of the tarsometatarsal joint interosseous system

forms and the cuboid and the three intermetatarsal interosseous ligaments that run between the bases of the metatarsals.

The plantar system is variable in number and layout but is arranged on the plantar side and, as interosseous, includes intertarsal and intermetatarsal ligaments.

Acknowledgments Authors would like to thank **Dr. Silvio Caravelli, MD** (II Clinic of Orthopedics and Traumatology, IRCCS Istituto Ortopedico Rizzoli, Bologna) and **Dr. Maria Pia Cumani** (Scuola di Disegno Anatomico, IRCCS Istituto Ortopedico Rizzoli, Bologna) for artwork and figures.

References

1. Beumer A, Valstar ER, Garling EH, et al. Kinematics of the distal tibiofibular syndesmosis: radiostereometry in 11 normal ankles. Acta Orthop Scand. 2003;74(3):337–43.
2. Yuen CP, Lui TH. Distal tibiofibular syndesmosis: anatomy, biomechanics, injury and management. Open Orthop J. 2017;11(4):670–7.
3. Peter RE, Harrington RM, Henley MB, et al. Biomechanical effects of internal fixation of the distal tibiofibular syndesmotic joint: comparison of two fixation techniques. J Orthop Trauma. 1994;8(3):215–9.
4. Hermans JJ, Beumer A, de Jong TAW, et al. Anatomy of the distal tibiofibular syndesmosis in adults: a pictorial essay with a multimodality approach. J Anat. 2010;217(6):633–45.
5. Elgafy H, Semaan HB, Blessinger B, et al. Computed tomography of normal distal tibiofibular syndesmosis. Skelet Radiol. 2010;39:559–64.
6. Ebraheim NA, Lu J, Yang H, et al. The fibular incisure of the tibia on CT scan: a cadaver study. Foot Ankle Int. 1998;19:318–21.
7. Ebraheim NA, Taser F, Shafiq Q, et al. Anatomical evaluation and clinical importance of the tibiofibular syndesmosis ligaments. Surg Radiol Anat. 2006;28:142–9.
8. Kim S, Huh YM, Song HT, et al. Chronic tibiofibular syndesmosis injury of ankle: evaluation with contrast-enhanced fat-suppressed 3D fast spoiled gradient-racalled acquisition in the steady state MR imaging. Radiology. 2007;242:225–35.
9. Lee PT, Clarke MT, Bearcroft PW, et al. The proximal extent of the ankle capsule and safety for the insertion of percutaneous fine wires. J Bone Joint Surg Br. 2005;87:668–71.
10. D'Hooghe P. Syndesmosis injuries. In: Canata GL, d'Hooghe P, Hunt KJ, et al., editors. Sport injuries of foot and ankle: a focus on advanced surgical techniques. New York: Springer, ISAKOS; 2019.
11. Akseki D, Pinar H, Bozkurt M, et al. The distal fascicle of the anterior inferior tibio-fibular ligament as a cause of anterolateral ankle impingement: results of arthroscopic resection. Acta Orthop Scand. 1999;70:478–82.
12. Subhas N, Vinson EN, Cothran RL, et al. MRI appearance of surgically proven abnormal accessory anterior-inferior tibiofibular ligament (Bassett's ligament). Skelet Radiol. 2008;37:27–33.
13. Van de Perre S, Vanhoenacker FM, De Vuyst D, et al. Imaging anatomy of the ankle. JBR-BTR. 2004;87:310–4.
14. Haraguchi N, Armiger RS, Myerson MS, et al. Prediction of three-dimensional contact stress and ligament tension in the ankle during stance determined from computational modelling. Foot Ankle Int. 2009;30:177–85.
15. Brockett CL, Chapman GJ. Biomechanics of the ankle. Orthop Traumatol. 2016;30(3):232–8.
16. Hunt KJ, Lawson P. Acute ankle ligament injuries. In: Canata GL, d'Hooghe P, Hunt KJ, et al., editors. Sport injuries of foot and ankle: a focus on advanced surgical techniques. New York: Springer, ISAKOS; 2019. p. 3–12.
17. Mosca M, Caravelli S, Massimi S, et al. Evaluation of proprioception and postural control at a minimum 1 year follow-up after ankle capsuloligamentous lateral plasty with Brostrom technique: a cohort study. Medicine (Baltimore). 2020;99(17):e19862.

18. Sarrafian SK. Anatomy of the foot and ankle. In: Descriptive, topographic, functional. 2nd ed. Philadelphia: Lippincott. p. 159–217.
19. Golanò P, Vega J, de Leeuw PAJ, et al. Anatomy of the ankle ligaments: a pictorial essay. Knee Surg Sports Traumatol Arthrosc. 2010;18:557–69.
20. Brostrom L. Sprained ankles V. Treatment and prognosis in recent ligament ruptures. Acta Chir Scand. 1966;132:537–50.
21. Vega J, Malagelada F, Manzanares Cèspedes MD, Dalmau-Pastor M. The lateral fibulotalocalcaneal ligament complex: an ankle stabilizing isometric structure. Knee Surg Sports Traumatol Arthrosc. 2020;28(1):8–17.
22. Clanton TO, Waldrop NE. Athletic injuries to the soft tissues of the foot and ankle. In: Coughlin MJ, Saltzman CL, Anderson RB, editors. Mann's surgery of the foot and ankle. 9th ed. Amsterdam: Elsevier; 2014.
23. Baxter DE. Traumatic injuries to the soft tissues of the foot and ankle. In: Mann RA, editor. Surgery of the foot. 5th ed. Maryland Heights, Missouri: Mosby; 1986.
24. Michels F, Pereira H, Calder J, et al. Searching for consensus in the approach to patients with chronic lateral ankle instability: ask the expert. Knee Surg Sports Traumatol Arthrosc. 2018;26(7):2095–102.
25. D'Hooghe P, Pereira H, Kelley J, et al. The CFL fails before the ATFL immediately after combined ligament repair in a biomechanical cadaveric model. Knee Surg Sports Traumatol Arthrosc. 2020;28:253–61.
26. Golanò P, Mariani PP, Rodriguez-Niedenfuhr M, et al. Arthroscopic anatomy of the posterior ankle ligaments. Arthroscopy. 2002;18:353–8.
27. Nikolopoulus CE, Tsirikos AI, Sourmelis S, et al. The accessory anteroinferior tibiofibular ligament as a cause of talar impingement. A cadaveric study. J Sports Med. 2004;32:389–95.
28. Dalmau-Pastor M, Malagelada F, Calder J, et al. The lateral ankle ligaments are interconnected: the medial connecting fibres between the anterior talofibular, calcaneofibular and posterior talofibular ligaments. Knee Surg Sports Traumatol Arthrosc. 2020;28:34–9.
29. Waterman BR, Belmont PJ Jr, Cameron KL, et al. Risk factors for syndesmotic and medial ankle sprain: role of sex, sport, and level of competition. Am J Sports Med. 2011;39(5):992–8.
30. Savage-Elliot I, Murawski CD, Smyth NA, et al. The deltoid ligament: an in-depth review of anatomy, function, and treatment strategies. Knee Surg Sports Traumatol Arthrosc. 2013;21:1316–27.
31. Boss AP, Hintermann B. Anatomical study of the medial ankle ligament complex. Foot Ankle Int. 2002;23(6):547–53.
32. Amaha K, Nimura A, Yamaguchi R, et al. Anatomic study of the medial side of the ankle base on the joint capsule: an alternative description of the deltoid and spring ligament. J Exp Orthop. 2019;6(1):2.
33. Guerra-Pinto F, Fabian A, Mota T, et al. The tibiocalcaneal bundle of the deltoid ligament - prevalence and variations. Foot Ankle Surg. 2020;S1268-7731(20):30052–7.
34. Bartonicek J, Rammelt S, Nanka O. Anatomy of the subtalar joint. Foot Ankle Clin North Am. 2018;23:315–40.
35. Renstrom AFH. Persistently painful sprained ankle. J Am Acad Orthop Surg. 1994;2:270–80.
36. Michels F, Matricali G, Vereecke E, et al. The intrinsic subtalar ligaments have a consistent presence, location and morphology. Foot Ankle Surg. 2020;S1268-7731(20):30040.
37. Schmidt HM. Gestalt und Befestigung der Bandsysteme in Sinus und Canalis tarsi des Menschen. Acta Anat. 1978;102:184–94.
38. Mabit C, Boncoeur-Martel MP, Chaudruc JB, et al. Anatomic and MRI study of the subtalar ligamentous support. Surg Radiol Anat. 1997;19:111–7.
39. Candela V, Longo UG, Salvatore G, et al. Subtalar joint instability. In: Canata GL, d'Hooghe P, Hunt KJ, et al., editors. Sport injuries of foot and ankle: a focus on advanced surgical techniques. New York: Springer, ISAKOS; 2019.
40. Jotoku T, Kinoshita M, Okuda R, et al. Anatomy of the ligamentous structures in the tarsal sinus and canal. Foot Ankle Int. 2006;27:533–8.
41. Pisani G. "Coxa pedis" today. Foot Ankle Surg. 2016;22(2):78–84.
42. Walter WR, Hirschmann A, Alaia EF, et al. Normal anatomy and traumatic injury of the midtarsal (Chopart) joint complex: an imaging primer. Radiographics. 2019;39:136–52.
43. Walter WR, Hirschmann A, Alaia EF, et al. MRI evaluation of midtarsal (Chopart) sprain in the setting of acute ankle injury. AJR Am J Roentgenol. 2018;210(2):386–95.
44. Walter WR, Hirschmann A, Tafur M, et al. Imaging of Chopart (midtarsal) joint complex: normal anatomy and posttraumatic findings. AJR. 2018;211:416–25.
45. Ewalefo SO, Jones SM, Boakye L, et al. Lisfranc Complex Injuries. In: Canata GL, d'Hooghe P, Hunt KJ, et al., editors. Sport injuries of foot and ankle: a focus on advanced surgical techniques. New York: Springer; 2019.
46. Lau S, Bozin M, Thillainadesan T. Lisfranc fracture dislocation: a review of a commonly missed injury of the midfoot. Emerg Med J. 2017;34(1):52–6.
47. De Palma L, Santucci A, Sabetta SP, et al. Anatomy of the Lisfranc joint complex. Foot Ankle Int. 1997;18(6):356–64.
48. Mulcahy H. Linfranc injury: current concepts. Radiol Clin N Am. 2018;56:859–76.
49. Panchbhavi VK, Andersen CR, Vallurupalli S, et al. A minimally disruptive model and three-dimensional evaluation of Lisfranc joint diastasis. J Bone Joint Surg Am. 2008;90(12):2707–13.

Imaging of Ligamentous Injuries in the Foot and Ankle

3

Michael Durst

Introduction

Ligamentous injury of the foot and ankle is a commonly encountered injury in the United States with approximately two million ankle sprains occurring per year, with an estimated incidence rate of approximately 2–7 per 1000 based on emergency room data [1]. The diagnosis commonly relies on a physical exam; however, the utilization of imaging to aid in the diagnosis and treatment is increasingly common [2]. Magnetic resonance imaging has become increasingly utilized for the diagnosis of ligamentous injuries and, in some cases, may help to determine conservative versus surgical management [3].

This chapter will introduce the imaging modalities of utility in the evaluation of ligamentous injuries to the foot and ankle, describe the appropriate utilization of imaging, and provide an overview of the imaging appearance of both the normal and abnormal anatomy associated with these injuries.

M. Durst (✉)
Musculoskeletal Imaging and Intervention, Department of Radiology, University of Colorado, Aurora, CO, USA
e-mail: michael.durst@cuanschutz.edu

Imaging Modalities

Many imaging modalities lie at the disposal of the orthopedic surgeon when evaluating and diagnosing suspected ligamentous injury to the foot and ankle. Often, the availability, invasiveness, cost-effectiveness, and image resolution dictate the use of each modality [4].

Conventional Radiography

Conventional radiography, or "x-ray," serves as the first-line modality in the evaluation of acute foot and ankle pain. X-ray serves as the quickest and most cost-effective way to evaluate for bony injury, readily demonstrating the presence of a fracture or dislocation. Conventional radiography is of limited clinical utility in the diagnosis of ligamentous injuries, however, often only demonstrating secondary signs of soft tissue injury such as swelling, joint effusions, or associated avulsion fractures [4] (Fig. 3.1). Additionally, stress radiographs can be clinically useful to evaluate for laxity and instability of the foot and ankle [2].

Computed Tomography (CT)

Computed tomography (CT) is often helpful in evaluating traumatic injury to the extremity and

P. D'Hooghe et al. (eds.), *Ligamentous Injuries of the Foot and Ankle*,
https://doi.org/10.1007/978-3-031-08682-3_3

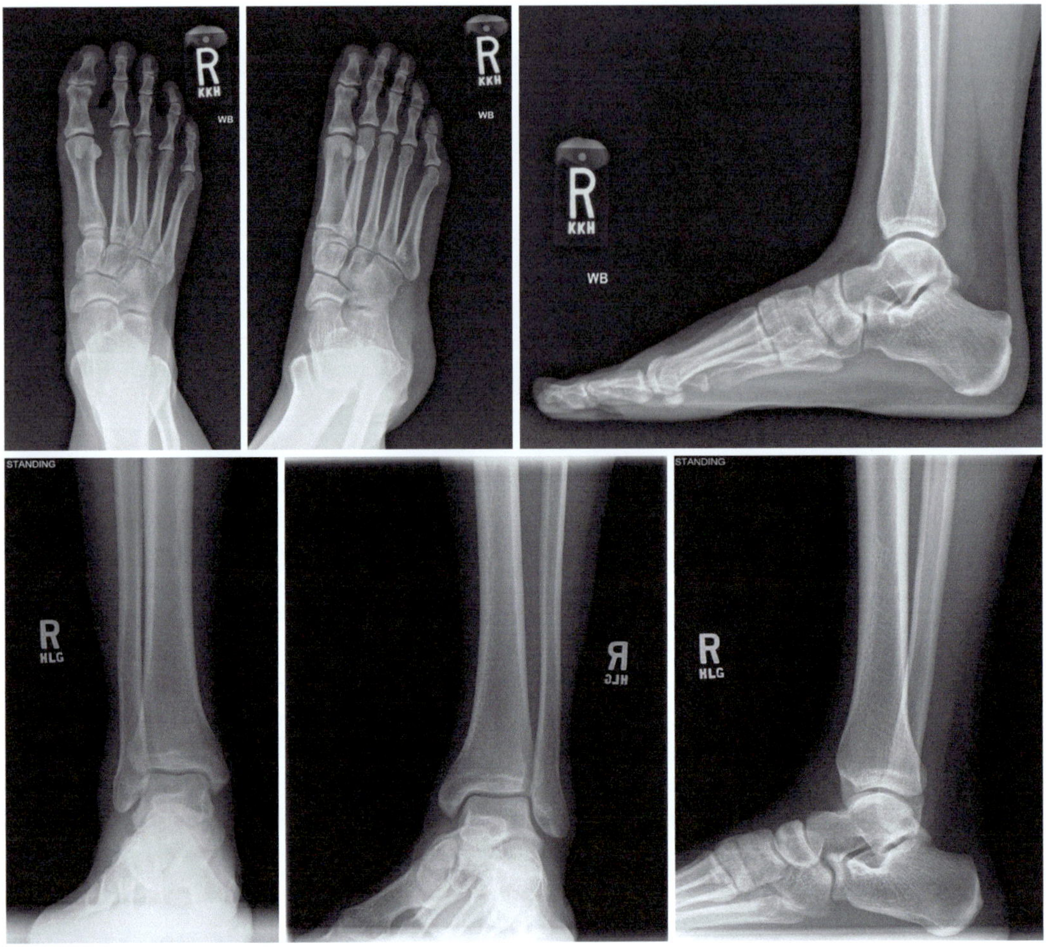

Fig. 3.1 Standard radiographic evaluation of the foot and ankle. Top row demonstrates weight-bearing images of the foot in the AP, oblique, and lateral projections. Bottom row demonstrates weight-bearing images of the ankle in AP, mortise, and lateral projections

allows for cross-sectional and three-dimensional evaluation of the site of injury (Fig. 3.2). CT provides much greater bony detail than conventional radiography and is useful in the evaluation of small joints as well as in the setting of clinical concern for non-displaced or occult fractures [4]. Soft tissue detail on CT is also improved over conventional radiography; however, subtle contrast differences between adjacent soft tissue structures limit the utility of CT in detecting ligamentous injuries of the ankle and foot. As with conventional radiography, much of the clinical utility rests in the identification of secondary signs of soft tissue injury.

Imaging soft tissue injuries with CT may be appropriate, however, in the setting of metallic orthopedic hardware that often severely degrades MR image quality or in individuals with contraindications to MRI, such as non-MR-compatible pacemakers [5].

Ultrasound

Ultrasound (US) utilizes the interaction of high-frequency sound waves within tissues to create imaging. This allows for good resolution and evaluation of soft tissue structures and allows

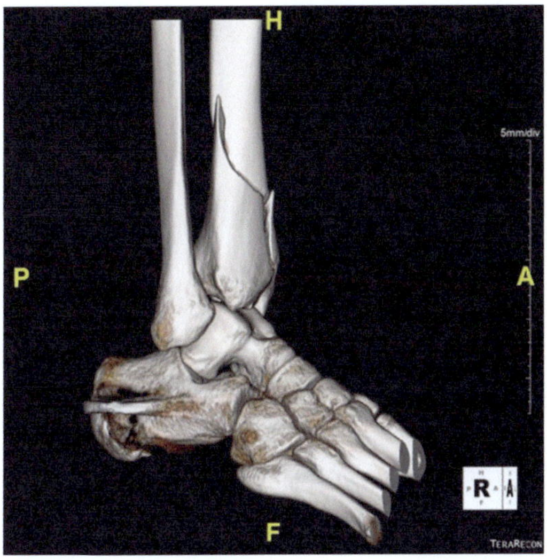

Fig. 3.2 Computed tomography allows 3D reconstructions that can be useful for preoperative planning, particularly in the setting of trauma

for the evaluation of these structures in real time with dynamic examinations [6]. In low-grade ligament sprains, ultrasound may detect subtle intra-substance hypoechogenicity or loss of normal ligament striations. In severe high-grade sprains, complete tear of the ligament may be identified centrally or at the peripheral attachments. Dynamic ultrasound shows an absence of normal tension across the ligament during stress maneuvers.

Magnetic Resonance Imaging (MRI)

The advent of magnetic resonance imaging (MRI) has revolutionized the imaging evaluation of the foot and ankle. MRI has allowed for the evaluation of complex and previously unidentified or missed structures within the foot and ankle. MRI utilizes strong magnetic fields that effect the protons (predominately water and lipid) within the body causing them to align along this field. The degree to which these protons align ultimately results in a signal that is detected by the MRI and produces the final image [3]. Because the signal that is produced is unique to the composition of each structure, this allows us to differentiate soft tissue in exquisite detail.

Although many different unique MR sequences exist, two main sequence categories will be discussed in this article, T1 and fluid-sensitive (T2, PD, STIR) sequences. A T1-weighted sequence is uniquely configured to fat signal. Fat-containing structures such as subcutaneous soft tissues and bone marrow will appear bright ("high signal") on T1-weighted imaging. Fluid by contrast on T1-weighted imaging appears dark ("low signal"). T1-weighted imaging offers excellent spatial resolution and bone detail. The identification of fracture lines, for example, is optimized with a T1-weighted sequence.

Fluid-sensitive sequences are uniquely configured to emphasize fluid and edema. Fluid such as synovial fluid will appear bright on all fluid-sensitive sequences. It is important to understand, however, that macroscopic fat also has a high water content and will appear bright on fluid-sensitive sequences unless a fat saturation (FS) is applied. Fat saturation is a technique that nulls fat signal making these structures (subcutaneous fat, marrow, etc.) appear dark. This additional step is important especially when evaluating for bone and subcutaneous edema that could easily be masked by a background of high-signal fat.

The increasing availability of MRI has resulted in the increased utility and applicability in the clinical setting. MRI has quickly become the gold standard and modality of choice for the evaluation of ligamentous injury to the foot and ankle.

MR Arthrogram (MRA) (Fig. 3.3)

MR arthrogram (MRA) is a variation of MRI which involves the direct injection of a solution of contrast material (gadolinium) mixed with local anesthetic, iodinated contrast, and saline into the joint in question. This results in expansion of the joint capsule allowing for improved visualization of ligamentous and capsular structures, which may be closely apposed. Additionally, injected contrast can also demonstrate abnormal communication between space or dehiscence of the capsule [7]. With the advent of improved magnets and larger field strengths, MRA is rarely required, and the risk of intervention must always be weighed against the diagnostic utility of the test.

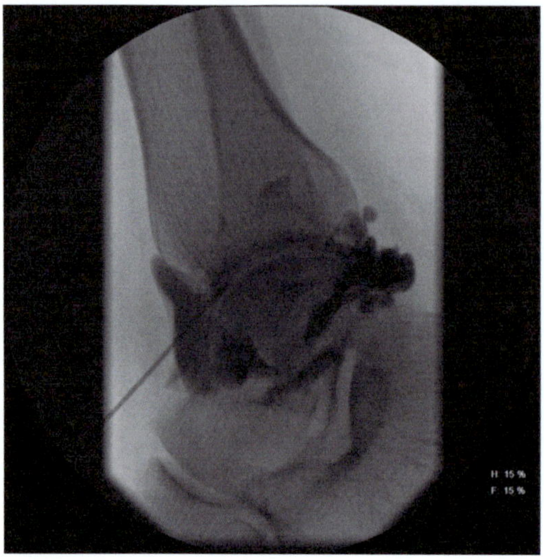

Fig. 3.3 Arthrography is an invasive technique utilizing image guidance to inject contrast material (either for CT or MR) directly into the joint. This single fluoroscopic image demonstrates an anterior approach to the tibiotalar joint for injection of contrast in preparation for MR arthrography

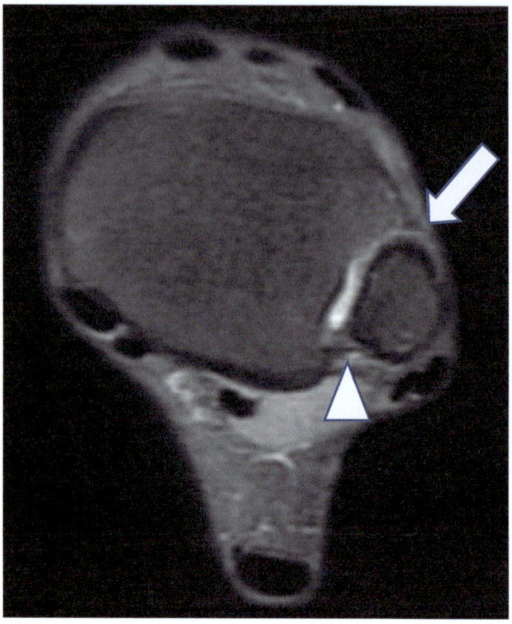

Fig. 3.4 Single axial proton density (PD) image through the ankle mortise demonstrating the normal appearance of the anterior tibiofibular (solid arrow) and the posterior tibiofibular (arrowhead) ligaments

Ankle

Imaging Anatomy of the Ankle Ligaments

Syndesmotic Ligaments

The proximal (superior) lateral ankle ligaments are comprised of the anterior inferior tibiofibular (AITFL) and posterior inferior tibiofibular ligaments (PITFL). When taken together with the interosseous ligament and transverse tibiofibular ligament, they form the syndesmotic ligament group [8]. These ligaments are best evaluated on T2-weighted axial images [9]. The AITFL and PITFL are identified on imaging at or slightly above the tibiotalar articulation. On axial imaging, these ligaments appear as short, taut, low-signal structures (Fig. 3.4).

The posterior inferior tibiofibular ligament is often surrounded by joint fluid on sagittal imaging, giving the appearance of an intra-articular body, and should not be confused as such [3].

The interosseous ligament represents a distal continuation of the interosseous membrane and acts as the main restraint to proximal migration of the talus.

Lateral Ankle Ligaments

The distal (inferior) lateral ankle ligaments are the anterior talofibular (ATFL), posterior talofibular (PTFL), and calcaneofibular ligaments (CFL). The ATFL and PTFL ligaments are again best evaluated on axial T2-weighted imaging below the tibiotalar joint, emanating from the concavity of the fibula called the malleolar fossa [3].

The ATFL appears as a low-signal thickening of the anterior joint capsule and is readily identified in the presence of a joint effusion. The ligament extends from the anteroinferior border of the fibula and extends to the neck of the talus [3] (Fig. 3.5).

The PTFL is a fan-shaped ligament with predominantly low-signal intensity interspersed with high-signal striations. This ligament extends from the posterior border of the fibula and inserts on the posterolateral tubercle of the talus, running perpendicular to the longitudinal axis of the tibia [9] (Fig. 3.5).

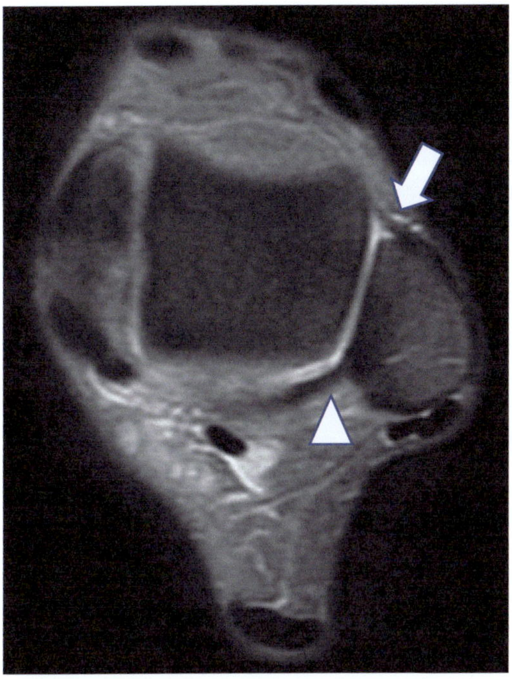

Fig. 3.5 Single axial PD MR image demonstrating the normal appearance of the anterior talofibular (solid arrow) and posterior talofibular ligaments (arrowhead)

The calcaneofibular ligament (CFL) is best identified on coronal T2-weight images. It is located just deep to the peroneal tendons and appears as a thin, low-signal intense structure extending obliquely between the anterior fibula proximal to the fibular tip to the lateral aspect of the calcaneus distal to the subtalar joint [9].

The posterior intermalleolar ligament is a normal anatomic variant of the posterior ankle. This variant is variable in size and can measure anywhere between 1–8 mm wide and 5–8 mm in diameter. While the posterior intermalleolar ligament is present in approximately 50% of the general population, it is only identified by MRI in about 20% of cases. The ligament itself is visualized on both coronal and axial sequences and appears as a distinct low-signal band traversing between the PITFL and the PTFL, originating from the posterior tibial margin, and the lateral fibers blend with the posterior tibiofibular ligament. The ligament courses downward and laterally and inserts on the fibula superior to the attachment of the posterior talofibular ligament [3].

Medial Ankle Ligaments

The deltoid ligament, or medial collateral ligamentous complex, is a broad band-like ligament that lies deep the flexor tendons. It is comprised of the tibiotalar, tibiocalcaneal, talonavicular, and plantar calcaneonavicular (spring) ligaments [3].

The tibiotalar component of the deltoid ligament complex is best identified on coronal T2-weighted imaging, appearing as low-signal structures extending between the medial malleolus and the talus. On axial imaging, it has a striated appearance [9].

The tibiocalcaneal component of the deltoid ligament appears as a low-signal band extending between the medial malleolus and calcaneus, most easily identified on coronal imaging as well. This ligament has a more vertical course, running deep to the flexor retinaculum but superficial to the tibiotalar component [9] (Fig. 3.6a).

The calcaneonavicular (spring) ligament is a thick triangular sheet that arises from the undersurface of the sustentaculum tali and attaches to the inferior and medial surfaces of the navicular. This structure is a vital stabilizer of the longitudinal arch of the foot, filling the gap between the anterior calcaneus and the navicular [10]. Because of the complex orientation of the spring ligament, it cannot be imaged in a single plane and should best be evaluated in two parts: The medial more vertical component, which is contiguous with the deltoid, is best visualized on axial imaging, and the horizontal component, which is contiguous with the bifurcate and short plantar ligaments, is best seen in the coronal plane. Care should be taken to distinguish the spring ligament from the adjacent expansion of the posterior tibialis tendon [9] (Fig. 3.6b).

Imaging Findings of Ligamentous Injury to the Ankle

Syndesmotic Injuries

Syndesmotic injuries comprise approximately 1–20% of all lateral ligament sprains [11]. The proposed mechanism resulting in syndesmotic injury is due to a forced external rotation of the foot with a combined internal rotation of the leg. Syndesmotic,

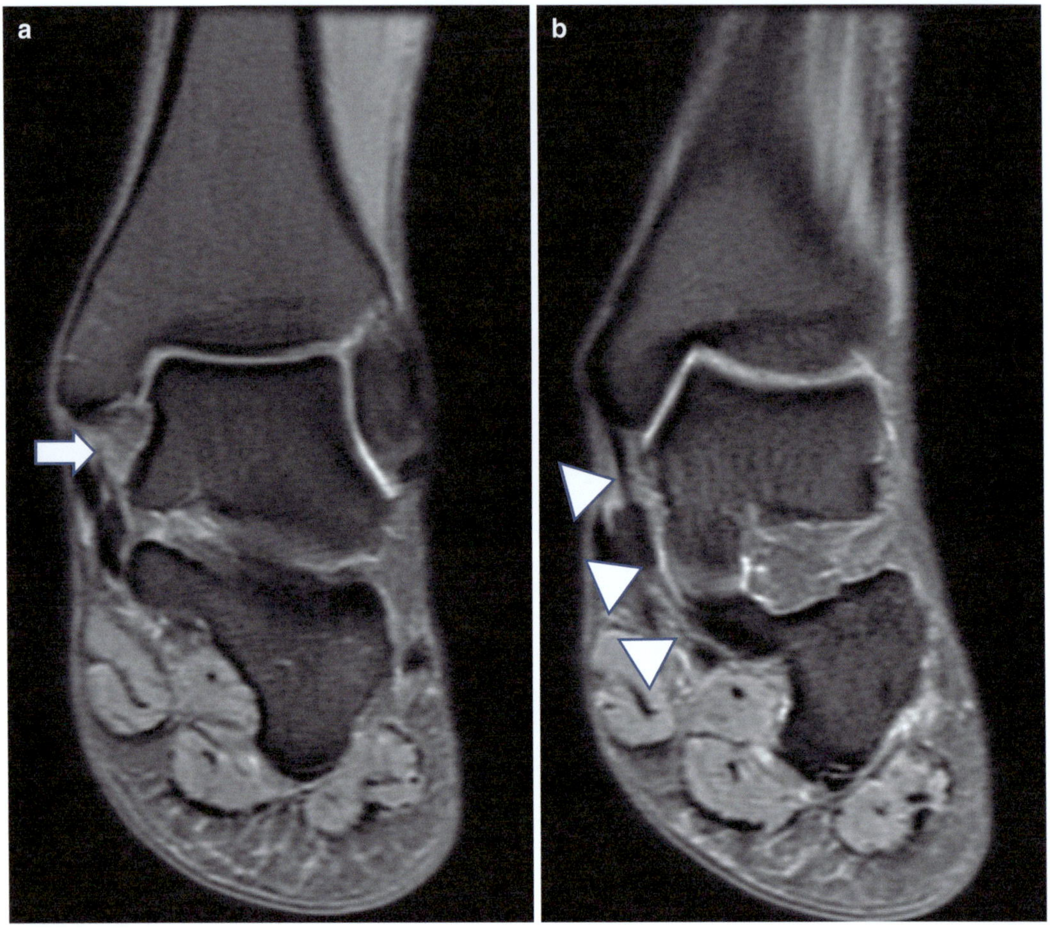

Fig. 3.6 Coronal PD MR images demonstrating the normal appearance of the medial ankle ligaments. Image (**a**) demonstrates the deltoid ligament (solid arrow). Image (**b**) highlights the calcaneonavicular (spring) ligament as it wraps around the head of the talus (arrowheads)

or high-ankle, injuries often have a longer recovery time and poor rehabilitation outcomes, resulting in chronic ankle dysfunction [11].

The initial imaging evaluation of suspected syndesmotic injury begins with three-view conventional radiography (anterior-posterior, lateral, and mortise views). Additional imaging of the proximal tibia/fibula is sometimes necessary to evaluate for proximal fibular injury. Stress radiographs may be useful in demonstrating mortise instability from ligamentous injury [4]. As discussed previously, conventional x-rays serve as a good first examination as they can identify or exclude osseous injury [4].

Injury to the syndesmotic ligaments is best characterized by MRI evaluation of the ankle. Injury appears as thickening, intersubstance T2 signal, and/or discontinuity of one or both syndesmotic ligaments [11] (Fig. 3.7).

Syndesmotic injuries are most commonly seen in concert with ligamentous injury of the lateral ankle ligaments, the anterior talofibular ligament being most common concomitant injury. Additional secondary injuries that are readily identified by MRI include bone contusions/fractures, osteochondral injuries, incongruity of the distal tibiofibular joint, and increased height of the tibiofibular recess [11] (Fig. 3.7).

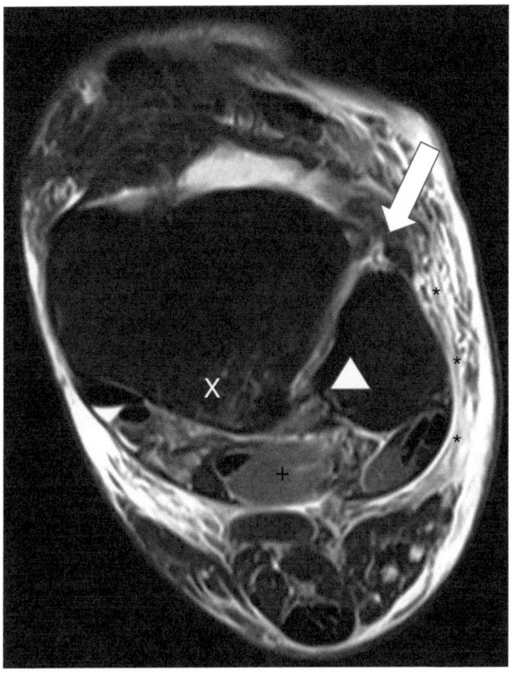

Fig. 3.7 Axial PD MR image through the level of the syndesmosis demonstrating discontinuity, thickening, and edema of both the anterior talofibular (solid arrow) and posterior talofibular (arrowhead) ligaments. Additional findings of extensive overlying soft tissue edema (asterisk), bone contusion (X), and muscle strain (plus symbol) are also present

Lateral Ankle Ligamentous Injuries

The most commonly injured ligament of the ankle is the anterior talofibular ligament [12]. The ATFL is frequently torn in isolation, but with more severe trauma, the other lateral ligaments will tear in a predictable order. The calcaneofibular ligament is often the next to tear, followed rarely by injury to the PTFL [9].

Evaluation of suspected lateral ankle ligament injury again begins with conventional radiography with standard projections (AP, lateral, and mortise views) to evaluate for osseous injury.

MRI is the gold standard in evaluating lateral ligamentous injury. The anterior talofibular ligament is easily identified as a thickening of the anterior joint capsule [3]. The ligament often appears attenuated and high in signal in the setting of acute injury. With complete rupture of the ligament, there is focal discontinuity of the ligament, often with joint fluid extending beyond the capsule into the overlying anterolateral soft tissues (Fig. 3.8a).

Injury of the calcaneofibular ligament is best demonstrated on coronal T2-weighted fat-saturated MR imaging [12]. The ligament appears high in signal with acute sprain and demonstrates focal discontinuity (often with redundancy) in the setting of complete rupture (Fig. 3.8b, c).

The posterior talofibular ligament is the strongest of the lateral ankle ligaments and is rarely involved in low ankle sprains. The normal appearance of the PTFL is fan-shaped with intersubstance, high T2-weighted striations that should not be confused with injury [9].

Medial Ankle Ligamentous Injuries

Injuries to the deltoid ligament, or medial collateral ligament complex, are becoming increasingly recognized as a result of the widespread use and availability of MRI [13]. Mechanism of injury most often involves pronation-eversion and extreme rotation. Injuries to the deltoid ligament complex often involve concomitant ankle fractures and lateral ligamentous injuries. Patient commonly present with a medial ankle hematoma and tenderness along the course of the deltoid.

Initial imaging evaluation of suspected deltoid ligament injuries begins with routine conventional radiography of the ankle, particularly given the association with lateral ankle fractures. Stress radiographs are particularly useful in demonstrating incompetence of the medial ankle ligaments, evidenced by widening of the medial clear space [4].

MRI is the imaging modality of choice for evaluating the medial ligaments of the ankle. This allows for more precise identification and characterization of the injury. Injuries should be characterized as involving the superficial portion, deep portion, or both. Additional characterization of the injury as proximal (Type I, most common), intermediate (Type II), or distal (Type III) can be clinically useful [13].

Low-grade deltoid injury on MRI appears as amorphous intersubstance signal and loss of normal ligament striation related to hemorrhage and focal fiber discontinuity. In higher-grade injuries, there is increased T2-weighted signal with fluid-filled intraligamentous gaps or frank discontinuity [13] (Fig. 3.9a).

The calcaneonavicular (spring ligament) plays a major role in the stability of the hindfoot [10] as

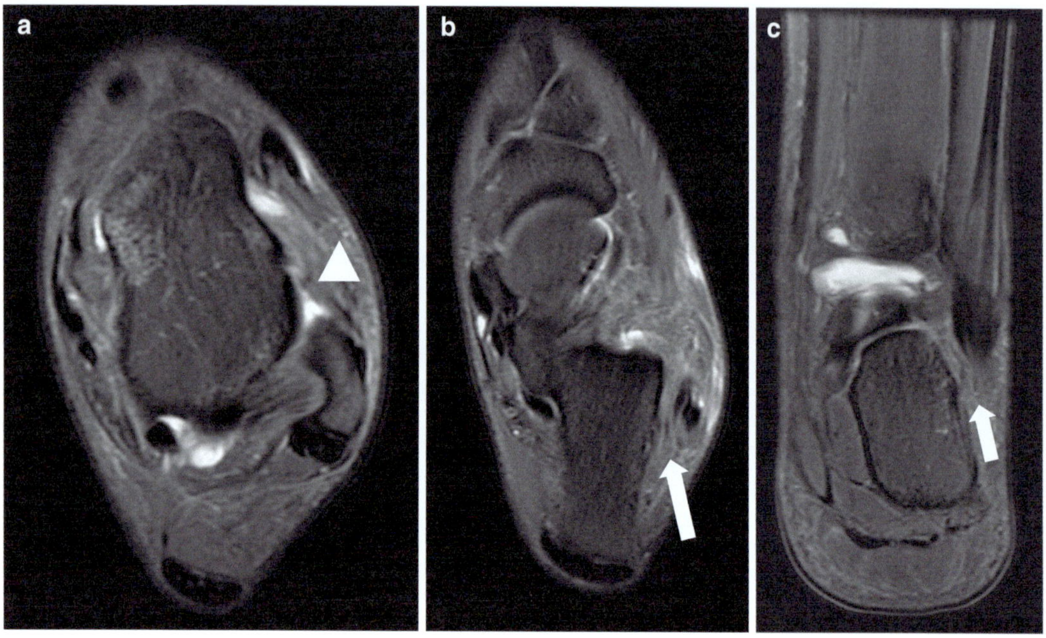

Fig. 3.8 Lateral ligamentous injuries. (**a**) Axial PD MRI of the ankle at the level of the plafond demonstrating discontinuity of the anterior talofibular ligament (arrowhead) with surrounding edema of the lateral soft tissues. (**b**) Axial PD MRI of the ankle showing discontinuity of the calcaneofibular ligament (solid arrow) with detachment from its distal calcaneal attachment and extensive surrounding edema. (**c**) Coronal PD MRI of the ankle also showing injury of the calcaneofibular ligament (solid arrow)

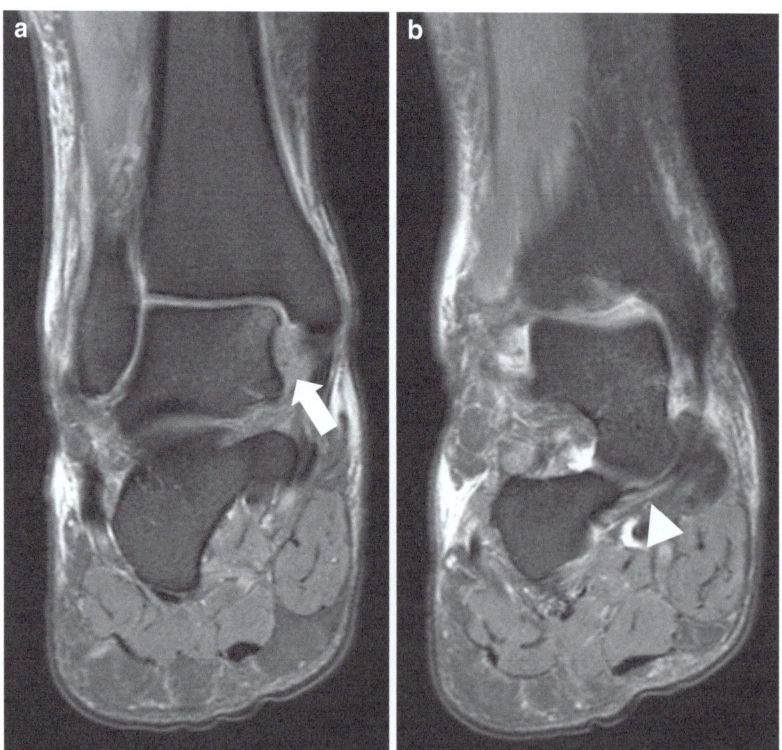

Fig. 3.9 Injury of the medial ankle ligaments. (**a**) Coronal PD MRI of the ankle demonstrating loss of normal striated appearance of the deltoid with extensive surrounding edema (solid arrow) consistent with a low-grade injury. (**b**) Coronal PD MRI of the ankle with thickening and periligamentous edema throughout the calcaneonavicular (spring) ligament (arrowheads)

well as the longitudinal arch of the midfoot. Injury to the spring ligament can result in the development of a flatfoot deformity, and ligamentous deficiency typically follows posterior tibial tendon dysfunction in a predictable pattern. Acute rupture of the spring ligament has been reported but remains a rare injury pattern [10].

Imaging evaluation of the spring ligament begins with conventional radiography and is often inferred from secondary radiographic findings such as midfoot sag and the development of pes planus. Conventional radiography is also useful in evaluating for bony injury resulting in hindfoot pain and flatfoot deformity.

MRI is again the modality of choice for evaluation of the spring ligament. Dysfunction of the spring ligament is usually a long-standing process, and the imaging characteristics reflect this [10]. Imaging demonstrates an increase in the normal caliber of the ligament, increased signal/heterogeneity, and often exhibits redundancy/waviness. Additional imaging findings include a full-thickness ligament gap in the setting of complete rupture. Adjacent posterior tibial tendinopathy has also been described [14] (Fig. 3.9b).

Foot

Imaging Anatomy of the Foot Ligaments

Lisfranc Joint Complex

The tarsometatarsal, or Lisfranc, joint complex is a complicated skeletal and capsuloligamentous structure that provides stability to the mid- and forefoot. The normal anatomy of the Lisfranc joint complex consists of nine bones—five metatarsals, three cuneiforms, and the cuboid. Three separate synovial articulations subdivide the forefoot into medial, middle, and lateral columns. The medial column is formed by the articulation of the first metatarsal on the medial cuneiform. The middle column is formed by the articulation of the second and third metatarsals on the middle and lateral cuneiform. The medial and the middle columns are rigid, which allows the foot to act as a lever and facilitates a normal gait. The lateral column is formed by the articulation of the fourth and fifth metatarsals on the cuboid. The lateral column is mobile, which is protective against significant injury and degeneration [15].

Additional stability to the Lisfranc joint complex is provided by a complex ligamentous arrangement, which is divided into dorsal, interosseous, and plantar components [16]. The Lisfranc ligament complex is composed of three distinct obliquely oriented structures: the Lisfranc ligament proper, which is the interosseous component connecting the medial cuneiform to the base of the second metatarsal (Fig. 3.10b); the dorsal component, connecting the medial cuneiform to the second metatarsal dorsally; and the plantar component, which typically has a single origin from the base of the medial cuneiform, with two attachments—one each on the bases of the second and third metatarsals. The interosseous and plantar components provide the primary ligamentous stability of the joint. Injury to the interosseous and plantar components is the primary cause of transverse instability and resultant tarsometatarsal widening with injury. The dorsal component is the weakest and accounts for the dorsal displacement that is often seen with Lisfranc injuries [15].

There are three cuneometatarsal ligaments that connect the cuneiforms to the first, second, and third metatarsals. The first cuneometatarsal ligament extends along the plantar surface between the medial cuneiform and the lateral aspect of the first metatarsal. The second cuneometatarsal ligament is triangularly shaped and extends between either the intermediate or lateral cuneiforms to attach to the second and third metatarsals. The third cuneometatarsal, or lateral longitudinal, ligament attaches the lateral aspect of the lateral cuneiform to the third metatarsal [15].

There are intermetatarsal ligaments that run along the plantar aspect of the second through fifth metatarsals (Fig. 3.10a). There is no dorsal intermetatarsal ligament connecting the first and second metatarsals, which likely accounts for the tendency of the second to fifth metatarsals to diverge as a group with injury [15].

Finally, thick intertarsal ligaments connect the cuneiforms and cuboid (Fig. 3.10b). The intertar-

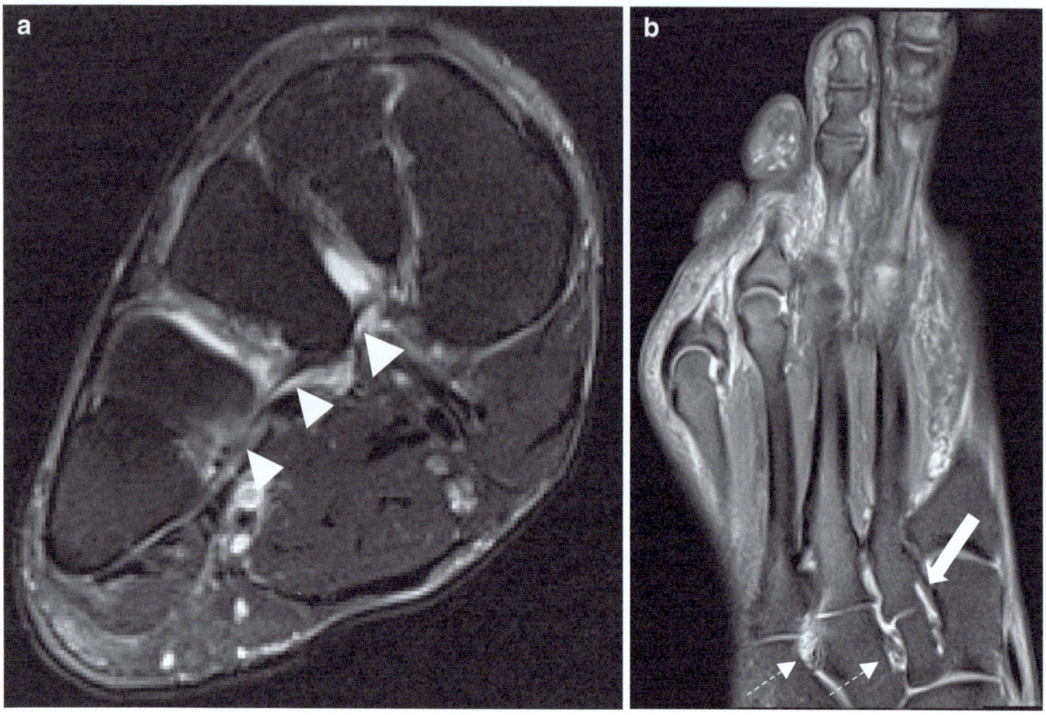

Fig. 3.10 Ligamentous anatomy of the Lisfranc. (**a**) Short-axis PD MRI through the bases of the metatarsals demonstrating the normal intermetatarsal ligament along the plantar surface of the second through fifth metatarsals. (**b**) Long-axis PD MRI demonstrating the proper Lisfranc ligament (solid arrow) and the intertarsal ligaments (dashed arrows)

sal ligament between the medial and intermediate cuneiform contributes to longitudinal instability and leads to intercuneiform widening when injured [15].

Plantar Plate

The plantar plate of the foot is a fibrocartilaginous structure formed by the plantar aponeurosis and the plantar capsule, which extends from the metatarsal neck and inserts on the plantar aspect of the base of the proximal phalanges [3]. The general structure of the plantar plate is similar between the great and lesser toes; however, important anatomic differences exist [17].

The first metatarsal head is wider than tall and has two separate articular surfaces. The superior articular surface forms broad articulation with the base of the first proximal phalanx. The plantar aspect of the first metatarsal head has a sagittal ridge called the crista which divides the articular surface into two grooves – one each for the sesamoids. Sagittal stability of the first MTP is provided by the glenosesamoid apparatus, which is comprised of the two sesamoids embedded in thick fibrous tissue combined with musculature of the hallux [17]. The plantar plate anchors to the base of the first proximal phalanx near the attachments of the intrinsic and extrinsic musculature of the hallux and envelopes the sesamoids. The plantar plate receives contributions from the deep fibers of the flexor hallucis brevis, the lateral deep metatarsal ligament, plantar fascia, and suspensory ligaments [17]. Dorsally, the MTP is supported by the extensor hallucis tendons and the extensor hood composed of oblique and transverse fibers extending around the capsule to blend with the plantar plate and deep transverse intermetatarsal ligament [17] (Fig. 3.11a, b).

The anatomy of the lesser MTP joints is simpler than the first. The fibrocartilaginous plantar plate extends from the metatarsal heads and firmly inserts on the bases of the proximal pha-

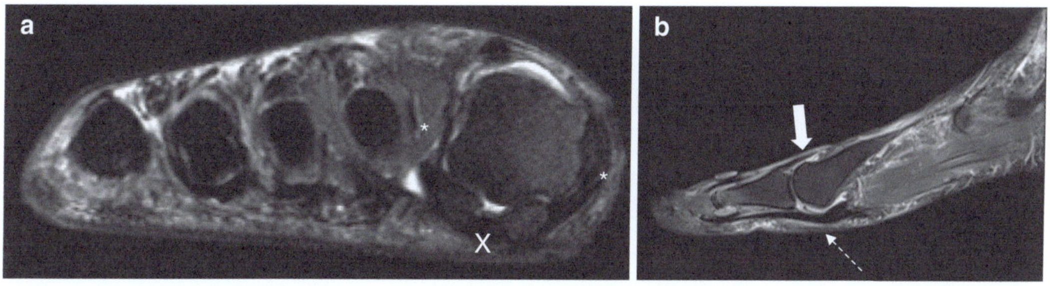

Fig. 3.11 Plantar plate. (**a**) Short-axis PD MRI of the first metatarsophalangeal joint demonstrating the normal appearance of the plantar plate structures including the medial and lateral metatarsosesamoid (asterisks) and intersesamoid (X) ligaments. (**b**) Sagittal PD MRI of the first metatarsophalangeal joint showing the fibrocartilaginous makeup of plantar plate (dotted arrow) with its insertion on the base of the first proximal phalanx. Additionally, the dorsal support apparatus with the extensor hallucis tendons and extensor hood are visualized (solid arrow)

langes. The plantar plate is composed of contributions from the plantar fascia, suspensory ligaments, and deep transverse intermetatarsal ligaments. The dorsal and plantar interossei muscle attachments at the proximal phalangeal bases provide additional support. The extensor digitorum brevis and longus tendons cross the joint under the extensor hood to provide dorsal support of the joint [17].

Imaging Findings of Ligamentous Injury of the Foot

Lisfranc Joint Complex

Injuries to the Lisfranc joint complex remain relatively rare, with a reported incidence in the United States of approximately 1 in 55,000. However, despite their uncommon nature, the morbidity of Lisfranc injuries is high, resulting in post-traumatic arthritis in approximately 50% of cases. An estimated 20% of Lisfranc injuries are initially underdiagnosed, often as a result of their subtle presentation or concurrent polytrauma. Because of this, imaging often plays an important role in the diagnosis of Lisfranc injuries [15].

The initial evaluation of suspected midfoot injury begins with conventional radiography. In the setting of trauma, AP, lateral, and internally rotated oblique images are obtained. Conventional x-rays are useful for evaluating for obvious fractures and dislocations. Findings of suspected Lisfranc injury can be subtle on non-weight-bearing images, with a small chip fracture (fleck sign) at the base of the second metatarsal or medial cuneiform considered to be virtually pathognomonic for high-impact injuries [15].

In the setting of clinically suspected Lisfranc injury, evaluation with weight-bearing radiographs is recommended. The most reliable imaging indicator of a Lisfranc injury is malalignment at the second tarsometatarsal articulation, with lateral displacement of the second metatarsal base relative to the intermediate cuneiform [15]. On AP radiographs, a diastasis of more than 2 mm between the first and second metatarsals is indicative of injury and instability [15] (Fig. 3.12a).

Computed tomography is an ideal modality for the evaluation of subtle fractures and has been advocated in the setting of high-velocity injury. CT is useful for the identification of radiographically occult fractures and subluxations, allowing for better visualization of osseous structures. CT also allows for 3D reconstruction, which is helpful with preoperative planning.

Magnetic resonance imaging is superior to all other modalities in the evaluation of soft tissue and ligamentous injury to the Lisfranc joint complex. The Lisfranc ligament is best seen on the horizontal long-axis and short-axis planes and appears homogenous or striated with predominately low to intermediate signal.

The most common MRI findings of Lisfranc injury include frank ligamentous disruption, ligament elongation, and periligamentous edema [15].

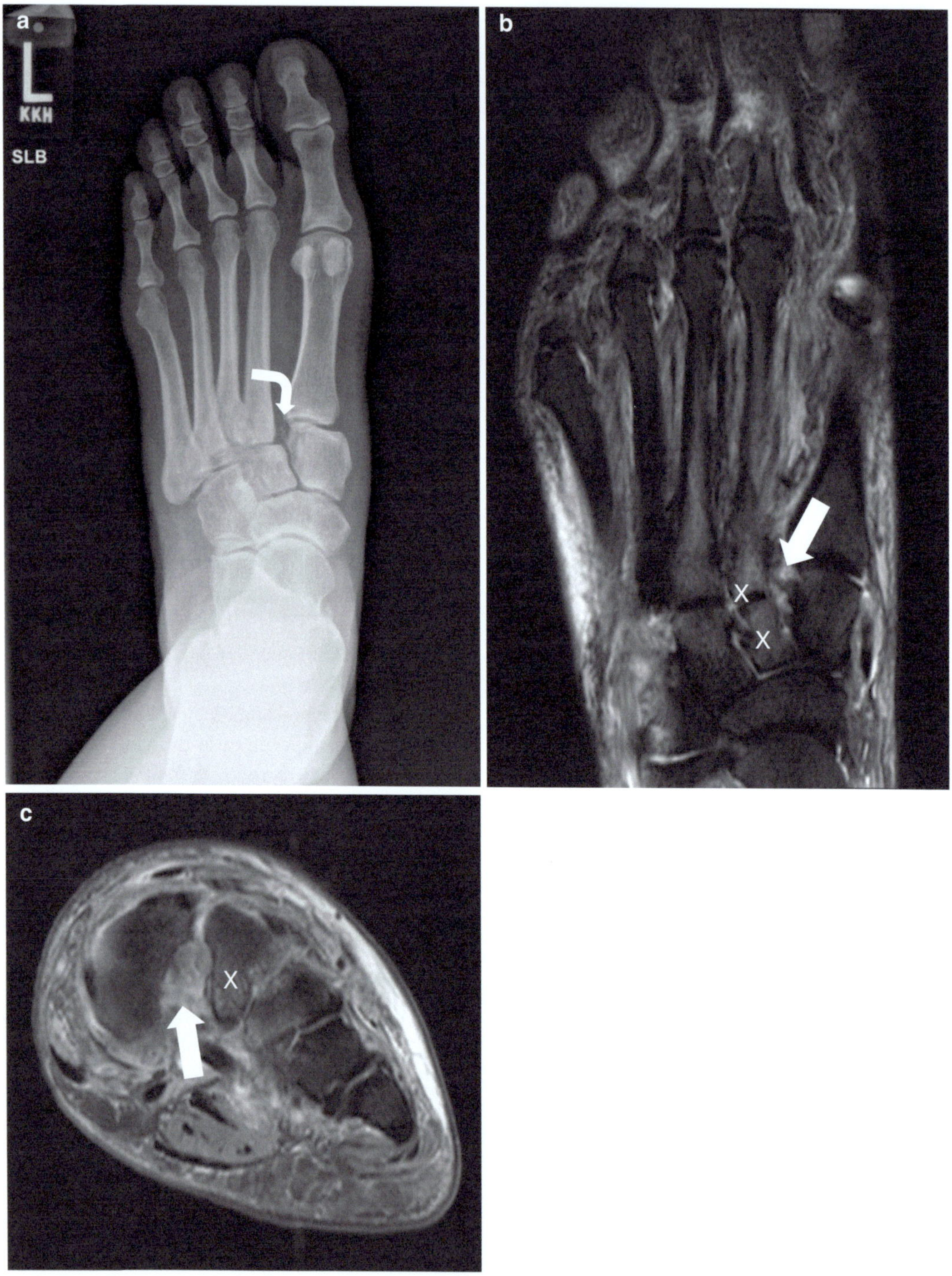

Fig. 3.12 Lisfranc injury. (**a**) Weight-bearing AP radiograph of the foot showing widening of the medial cuneiform-second metatarsal distance with lateral subluxation of the metatarsals. Small ossific fragments at the medial cuneiform compatible with associated fracture ("fleck sign") (curved arrow). (**b**) Long-axis PD MRI of the foot shows discontinuity of the proper Lisfranc ligament (straight arrow) with surrounding soft tissue and bone marrow edema (X). (**c**) Short-axis PD MRI of the foot shows discontinuity of the proper Lisfranc ligament (straight arrow) with surrounding soft tissue and bone marrow edema (X)

Additionally, bone marrow edema at the base of the second metatarsal or middle cuneiform may be present (Fig. 3.12b, c). MR imaging is also useful in the evaluation of other tarsal injuries to the cuboid, calcaneus, and talus, which are frequently reported to be coincident.

Plantar Plate

Injury to the capsuloligamentous structures of the first metatarsophalangeal joint, termed turf toe, is a relatively common entity among athletes reported to affect up to 40% of American football players [18]. This injury is classically described as a hyperextension injury in which axially applied force results in injury to the glenosesamoid apparatus and plantar ligaments [17]. Severity and grading of the injury are related to the degree of axial force applied and can range from a mild strain to a complete rupture [19].

Imaging diagnosis of first MTP plantar plate injury often begins with weight-bearing conventional radiography, which can demonstrate avulsion fractures of the proximal phalanx as well as secondary signs of ligamentous injury such as proximal migration of the sesamoids. Dedicated sesamoid views can be useful to evaluate for diastasis or fracture [19].

Magnetic resonance imaging is the imaging modality of choice for the diagnosis of plantar plate injury, readily demonstrating the soft tissue and cartilaginous abnormalities. Multiplanar imaging is necessary for complete evaluation, with the coronal short axis and sagittal sequences being the most useful [19]. The capsuloligamentous structures appear as low-signal structures on fluid-sensitive sequences. With injury, the imaging appearance correlates with severity. In grade I injuries, there is mild periligamentous edema, which appears as increased bright signal on fat-saturated fluid-sensitive sequences. Grade II injuries are partial tears, and imaging demonstrates partial disruption of the ligamentous fibers with increased surrounding fluid signal. Grade III injuries are complete tears, which appear as discontinuity of the ligaments and significant surrounding edema and swelling. Often, grade III injuries are associated with sesamoid fracture or diastasis [19] (Fig. 3.13a, b).

Pain and instability involving the lesser MTP joints is a common problem and is more often related to a chronic degenerative process rather than an acute injury [18]. MR imaging is useful in the evaluation of the capsuloligamentous structures of these joints, and imaging findings have been described. Pericapsular fibrosis ("pseudoneuroma" sign) appears on MRI as an intermediate signal intensity, ill-defined nodule, which is asymmetric within the interspace and abutting the plantar-lateral aspect of the MTP joint. An additional imaging finding associated with lesser plantar plate injuries includes widening of the plantar plate-proximal phalanx distance, with a cutoff value of 0.275 cm yielding the greatest specificity. Classic direct signs of injury such as partial or complete tear are also observed [19].

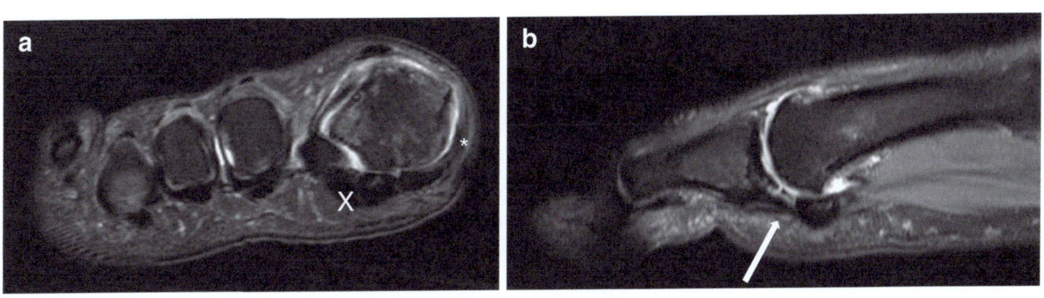

Fig. 3.13 Plantar plate injury – "turf toe." (**a**) Short-axis PD MR image showing edema and thickening of the medial metatarsosesamoid ligament (asterisk) resulting in subluxation of the tibial hallux sesamoid. Irregularity and redundancy of the intersesamoid ligament is also noted (X). (**b**) Sagittal PD MRI demonstrating focal discontinuity of the plantar plate from its insertion on the base of the first proximal phalanx (solid arrow)

Conclusion

Knowledge and understanding of the anatomy and imaging appearance of normal and abnormal ligamentous structures about the foot and ankle are critical to the appropriate management of these complex cases. Imaging should be used wisely and appropriately to help characterize these lesions in the most efficient and cost-effective manner.

References

1. Herzog M, et al. Epidemiology of Ankle sprains and chronic Ankle instability. J Athl Train. 2019;54(6):603–10.
2. Linklater J, et al. Acute Capsuloligamentous Sports Injuries in the Ankle and Foot. Radiology. 2017;283(3):644–62.
3. Spouge A, Pope T. Practical MRI of the foot and ankle. Boca Raton, Florida: CRC Press; 2001. p. 97–115.
4. Soto J, Lucey B. Emergency radiology. 1st ed. . Chapter 4. Maryland Heights, Missouri: Mosby Elsevier; 2009. p. 112–61.
5. Dean DG. The role of MRI in musculoskeletal practice: a clinical perspective. J Man Manip Ther. 2011;19(3):152–61. https://doi.org/10.1179/2042618611Y.0000000009.
6. Jacobson J. Fundamentals of musculoskeletal ultrasound. 3rd ed. Amsterdam: Elsevier; 2018.
7. Crim J, Morrison W. Specialty imaging: arthrography. 1st ed. Salt Lake City, Utah: Amirsys; 2009.
8. Manaster BJ, et al. Diagnostic and surgical imaging anatomy: knee, Ankle. 1st ed. Salt Lake City, Utah: Foot Amirsys; 2007.
9. Major N, et al. Musculoskeletal MRI. 3rd ed. Elsevier; 2020. Chapter 16
10. Toye L, et al. MRI of spring ligament tears. Am J Roentgenol. 2005;184:1475–80.
11. Brown K, et al. MRI findings associated with distal tibiofibular syndesmosis injury. Am J Roentgenol. 2004;182:131–6.
12. Rosenberg Z, et al. MR imaging of the Ankle and Foot. Radiographics. 2000;20:153–79.
13. Chhabra A, et al. MR imaging of deltoid ligament pathologic findings and associated impingement syndromes. Radiographics. 2010;30:751–61.
14. Balen P, Helms C. Association of Posterior Tibial Tendon Injury with spring ligament injury, sinus tarsi, and plantar fasciitis on MR imaging. Am J Roentgenol. 2001;176:1137–43.
15. Siddiqui N, et al. Evaluation of the tarsometatarsal joint using conventional radiography, CT and MR Imaging. Radiographics. 2004;34:514–31.
16. Palma L, et al. Anatomy of the Lisfranc joint complex. Foot Ankle Int. 1997;18(6):356–64.
17. Nery C, et al. MR imaging of the plantar plate: Normal anatomy, turf toe and other Injuries. Magn Reson Imaging Clin N Am. 2017;25:127–44.
18. Hallinan J, et al. High Resolution MRI of the first metatarsophalangeal joint: gross anatomy and injury characterization. Radiographics. 2020;40:1107–24.
19. Yamada A, et al. Second and third metatarsophalangeal plantar plate tears: diagnostic performance of direct and indirect MRI features using surgical findings as the reference standard. Am J Roentgenol. 2017;209:W100–8.

4 Alignment and Instability: Managing Mechanical Contributors to Recurrent Ligament Injury and Instability

Caitlin M. Rugg, Richard Amendola, and Annunziato Amendola

Introduction

Ankle sprains are a common clinical problem in the general population and in athletes. For patients presenting to the emergency room, there is an incidence rate of 2.15 per 1000 person-years in the United States [1]; however, this is likely an underestimation of the true incidence as many injuries are managed outside of the emergency room. Ankle sprains make up 7–15% of all injuries in collegiate athletes [2, 3]. These injuries have a wide severity, with 44% of collegiate athletes able to return to play in less than 24 h. However, recurrence is common, with rates reported from 5 to 47% [4]. One of the strongest risk factors for a future lateral ankle sprain is a history of prior ankle sprain, which has been demonstrated in the military cadet population [5] and in athletic populations [6, 7].

C. M. Rugg
Division of Sports Medicine, Department of Orthopaedic Surgery, Duke University, Durham, NC, USA
e-mail: Caitlin.rugg@duke.edu

R. Amendola
Department of Orthopedic Surgery, SUNY Upstate Medical University, NY, USA

A. Amendola (✉)
Orthopaedic Surgery, Division of Sports Medicine, Urbaniak Sports Sciences Institute, Athletic Department, Duke University, Durham, NC, USA
e-mail: Ned.amendola@duke.edu

Chronic lateral ankle instability may develop in 32–74% of patients experiencing lateral ankle instability [8]. Proposed mechanisms for recurrence include functional ligamentous laxity, decreased proprioception and neuromuscular control, and predisposing mechanical alignment [8–11]. In this chapter, we will focus on the association between foot and ankle alignment and chronic lateral ankle instability.

Hindfoot malalignment has been recognized as risk factor for recurrent lateral ankle instability for decades. This has been most heavily studied in the Charcot-Marie-Tooth (CMT) population, for whom soft tissue imbalances progress to fixed hindfoot cavus and forefoot equinus [12, 13]. While CMT is the most common cause for adult cavovarus deformity, more subtle, idiopathic cavovarus deformity has also been described in association with recurrent lateral ankle sprains [14–16]. The epidemiology of subtle cavovarus malalignment in the recurrent ankle instability population has been examined in multiple retrospective studies. In a study of 118 patients undergoing lateral ligament reconstruction, 17% were found to have hindfoot varus requiring calcaneal osteotomy, and 3% were found to have a hyperplantarflexed first ray requiring soft tissue release [17]. In a population of military patients undergoing modified Broström-Gould lateral ankle ligament reconstructions for chronic ankle instability, 8% of patients had varus hindfoot alignment [11]. Larsen et al. compared foot and ankle

P. D'Hooghe et al. (eds.), *Ligamentous Injuries of the Foot and Ankle*,
https://doi.org/10.1007/978-3-031-08682-3_4

radiographs in patients with ankle instability to healthy controls and found increased rates of hindfoot varus and pes cavus in the ankle instability population [18].

In this chapter, we will review the biomechanical evaluation of the foot and ankle, physical examination and imaging evaluation, treatment options for patients with ankle instability and hindfoot malalignment, and outcomes in this population.

Biomechanical Evaluation of the Foot and Ankle

The gait cycle is divided into the stance phase and the swing phase. The stance phase is composed of heel contact, midstance, terminal stance, and pre-swing. The shape and flexibility of the foot are critical in a normal gait cycle. At heel strike, there is a medial rotation of the forefoot and inversion of the heel. In the midstance phase of the gait cycle, the subtalar joint shifts into valgus (eversion), unlocking the midtarsal joints to allow for stress distribution. In terminal stance and in pre-swing phases, there is metatarsophalangeal dorsiflexion and locking of the midtarsal joints, which provides a rigid foot as a lever to push off. In normal gait mechanics, the foot rotates around the talus and the cuboid follows the calcaneus. The force vector of the posterior compartment and the Achilles normally applies a neutral plantarflexing force through the ankle joint [19].

Cavovarus deformity is defined as a varus hindfoot, high calcaneal pitch, high-pitched midfoot, and a plantarflexed and adducted forefoot. Since the calcaneus is internally rotated under the talus and there is a decrease in the anteroposterior talocalcaneal angle, the navicular is in a position superior to the cuboid and is forced into a locked position, and furthermore, the midtarsal joints are unable to function normally in midstance phase. The hindfoot is unable to go into eversion during stance and, with the foot in a varus alignment, creates predisposition to recurrent inversion ankle sprain episodes. This leads to the numerous consequences of cavovarus deformity, including chronic ankle instability and peroneal tendon overload [10, 19].

Cavovarus foot can be related to an underlying neuromuscular disorder but most commonly is idiopathic. It can be forefoot driven starting with a rigid plantarflexion of the first ray and subsequent hindfoot varus with weight-bearing, or it can be driven by the hindfoot with compensatory forefoot pronation. Figure 4.1 demonstrates this finding.

In a forefoot-driven hindfoot varus type of cavovarus feet, the plantarflexion of the first ray leads to relative dorsiflexion of the talus within the ankle mortise. Residual dorsiflexion is restricted causing increase contact forces in the anteromedial ankle. With subsequent varus malalignment of the hindfoot, the Achilles tendon insertion medializes relative to the ankle joint. This force vector worsens the alignment of the varus ankle and exacerbates the problem. The peroneus brevis is commonly weak in comparison to peroneus longus in neuromuscular cavovarus foot. With recurrent ankle sprains, it typically degenerates as well [10, 19].

Physical Examination

Patients should be examined with their bilateral lower extremities exposed and barefoot. Gait should be evaluated in clinic from in front and behind. Biomechanical evaluation is imperative. The normal hindfoot is aligned with 5–10 degrees of varus. Typically, it is difficult to discern subtle varus from the back, but the "peekaboo heel" sign is sensitive from the front. In a normal foot, the heel pad is not visible on the medial side of the foot from the front. The amount of heel pad visible correlates with the severity and can be compared from one side to the other easily. The "peekaboo heel" sign can give a false positive a large heel pad or if the patient is externally rotating their hips to compensate for severe metatarsus adductus [14].

The Coleman block test is used to differentiate between forefoot- and hindfoot-driven varus. It is performed starting with examination from behind noting the natural hindfoot varus with weight-

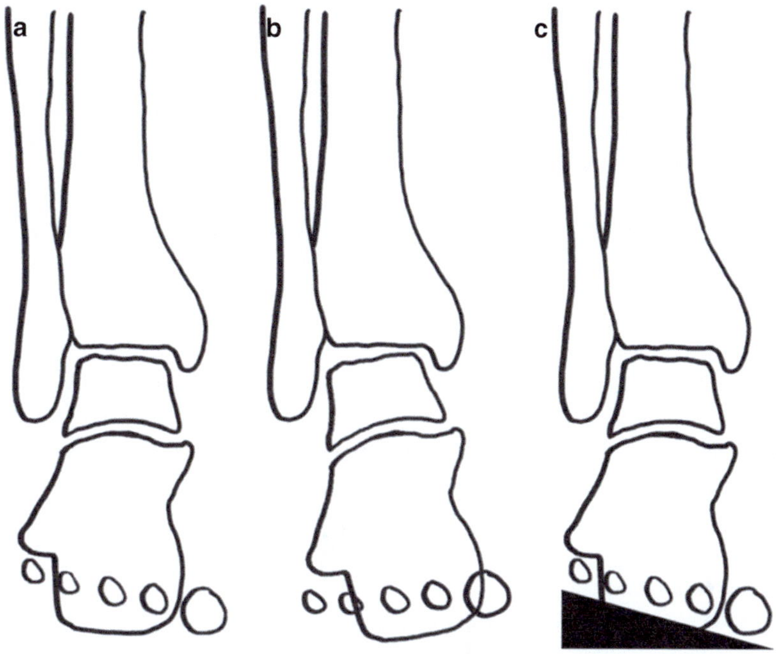

Fig. 4.1 Diagram of the effect of forefoot-driven hindfoot varus. (**a**) Non-weight-bearing with hindfoot in neutral with dropped first ray/ forefoot valgus. (**b**) Weight-bearing with forefoot-driven hindfoot varus. (**c**) Weight-bearing with lateral forefoot posting orthosis correcting hindfoot varus

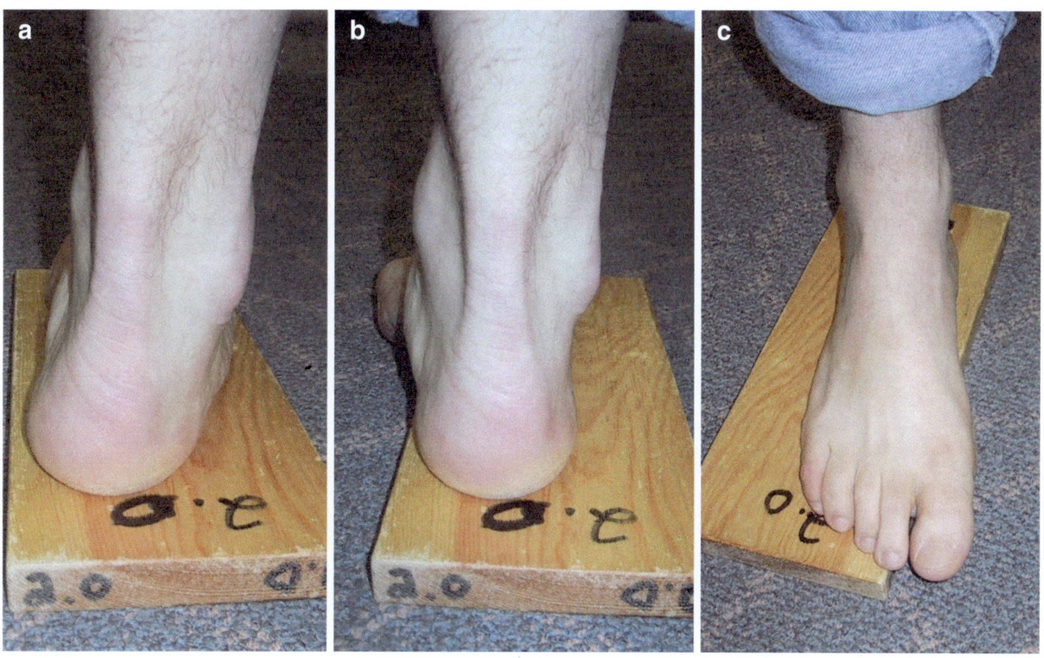

Fig. 4.2 This is an 18-year-old male collegiate athlete presenting with bilateral recurrent lateral ankle sprains. (**a**) Weighted posterior view of the right foot demonstrates varus hindfoot alignment. (**b**) Hindfoot varus corrects to neutral with Coleman block testing, indicating forefoot-driven varus. (**c**) Neutral alignment of the ankle viewed from the front with Coleman block testing

bearing. A 1-inch block is placed under the lateral aspect of the foot with the great toe and the first metatarsal hanging over the side. If the hindfoot varus is corrected, the examiner knows that the hindfoot deformity is flexible and it is driven by the plantarflexed first ray [20]. Figure 4.2a–c demonstrate Coleman block testing in a patient with a plantarflexed first ray.

Lateral ligamentous examination should be performed. The anterior drawer test is used to test the integrity of the anterior talofibular ligament. It is performed with the knee flexed and ankle plantarflexed comfortably to relax the musculature, grasping the calcaneus posteriorly with the index and long fingers and the anterior ankle with the thumb, and translating the hindfoot/talus anteriorly relative to the tibia. Increased laxity compared to the contralateral side is a positive result. The lateral talar tilt test is used to test the integrity of the calcaneal fibular ligament. It is performed with one hand on the talus and calcaneus and the other hand on the tibia. Using a supination force on the hindfoot, a positive result is increased laxity compared to the normal side.

Other supplemental exam features include assessment of arch height, which is typically evaluated from the side of the patient looking at their contralateral foot. Silfverskiöld test is performed to examine the presence and severity of equinus [21]. Location of calluses on the feet can help discern the loading pattern during weight-bearing. A full neurologic assessment should be performed to discriminate between neuromuscular and idiopathic cavovarus deformity.

Imaging Studies

Standard imaging studies in the setting of chronic ankle instability include weight-bearing anteroposterior, mortise, and lateral ankle radiographs. Supplemental studies in the setting of suspected hindfoot and/or forefoot deformity include bilateral weight-bearing hindfoot alignment views and anteroposterior, lateral, and oblique views of the foot. Saltzman hindfoot alignment views are shown in Fig. 4.3. Dynamic fluoroscopic examination of the ankle can also be used in the workup

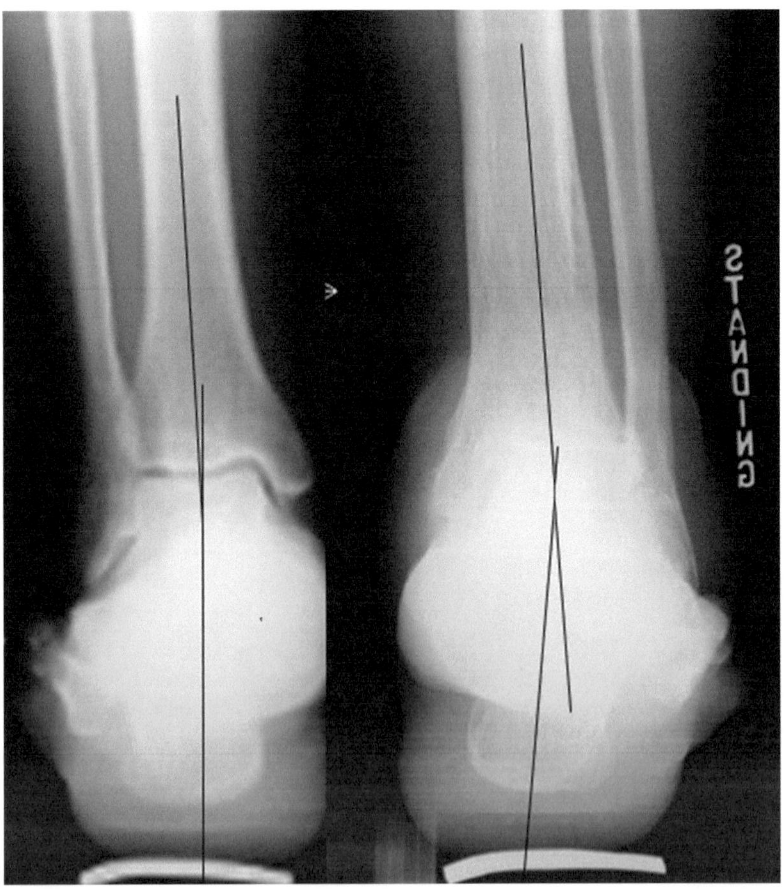

Fig. 4.3 Saltzman hindfoot alignment view demonstrating significant hindfoot varus compared to the contralateral limb

of ankle instability [22]. Dynamic tests include talar tilt, anterior drawer, and dorsiflexion/external rotation testing to detect instability.

Angular measurements can be made on two-dimensional lateral radiograph to describe a cavovarus deformity. Calcaneal pitch indicates the angle between the horizontal and a line along the undersurface of the calcaneus from the inferior tubercle to the inferior anterior process. Cavovarus deformity is defined as an increase over 30 degrees. The angle of Meary is the angle between the long axis of the talus and the axis of the first metatarsal. Normally, this angle is 0 degrees ±4 degrees; in cavovarus deformity, the angle is greater than 4 degrees plantarflexion of the first metatarsal. Navicular height may be measured from the plantar surface of the foot to the inferior, distal navicular. Hibbs angle is the angle formed between the axis of the calcaneus and the axis of the first metatarsal, and values greater than 45 degrees indicate a cavus deformity. Finally, lateral radiographs of cavovarus feet can exhibit a more posterior position of the fibula relative to the tibia, a flat-topped or double-domed talus, and a sinus tarsi see-through sign, which are artifactual due to the external rotation of the ankle in cavovarus feet [19].

The concept of the Tripod Index allows for quantitative assessment of complex foot deformities [23]. It provides a single measurement that describes the additive or compensatory effects of deformities at different levels of the foot. The measurement is made on an AP radiograph using the relationship between the center of the talar head and the foundation of the tripod composed of the center of the heel and medial/lateral borders of the forefoot. It is shown to have high accuracy as a quantitative assessment in the diagnosis of a symptomatic flatfoot and cavovarus foot.

Advanced imaging is considered for patients with recurrent ankle instability who do not have resolution of their symptoms with at least 6 weeks of standard ankle rehabilitation or those with suspected pathology not detected on radiographs. Magnetic resonance imaging (MRI) is routinely obtained if surgical management is being considered to evaluate for intra-articular pathology such as osteochondral lesions, bone edema, loose bodies, ligament injury, scar tissue, synovitis, and peroneal tendon pathology [24, 25]. Weight-bearing computed tomography (CT) of the ankle is a novel imaging method that can detect subtle alignment abnormalities and has been used to retrospectively show subtle varus hindfoot alignment as a risk factor for chronic lateral ankle instability when compared to healthy controls [26].

Nonoperative Management

Nonoperative management is the mainstay of treatment for both acute and recurrent ankle sprains. Typical rest, ice, compression, and elevation are successful in the vast majority of cases. This includes but is not limited to activity modification, physical therapy with balance, stretching and strengthening programs, orthoses, and bracing. It is of the author's opinion that a dedicated physical therapy program with focus on peroneal tendon strengthening and proprioceptive exercises combined with proper orthoses and bracing should be attempted for 3–6 months before considering surgical intervention. A recent network meta-analysis showed that the highest level of data found moderate strength evidence supporting a 4-week supervised multimodal rehabilitation program. In the setting of forefoot-driven varus with a flexible hindfoot, custom corrective orthotics with lateral forefoot posting will control the hindfoot varus and help patients feel more stable (Fig. 4.1). However, persistent symptoms of pain, swelling, or recurrent instability should prompt further inquiry in the form of repeat examination and advanced imaging as described above. Based on imaging findings, further nonoperative rehabilitation can be pursued, or surgical management may be indicated.

Indications for Surgical Management

Initial management of instability in the setting of chronic instability with malalignment should consist of nonoperative treatment as mentioned above. Many cases are slowly progressive, with a well-compensated foot prior to an acute injury. In cases in which patients have exhausted the aforementioned nonoperative treatment options and optimal rehabilitation, surgical intervention may be indicated. A variety of procedures are available to address malalignment, instability, or both depending on the patient and findings.

In primary surgical treatment of recurrent ankle instability in athletes with mild hindfoot varus, most surgeons would opt to just treat the instability without bony realignment. It is a much easier decision to correct the varus alignment in cases of failed lateral ligament surgery. In cases with significant malignment, soft tissue surgery alone will not hold up in the long run and will eventually give way to recurrent instability.

Cavovarus foot deformity may be hindfoot driven, forefoot driven, or a combination of the two as described previously. The goals of surgical management in the setting of cavovarus deformity should be to restore lateral ligamentous stability while creating a biomechanical construct, which results in inherent stability of the foot tripod. Indications for lateral ligamentous repair or reconstruction will be covered elsewhere, and in this chapter, we will focus on indications for adjuvant realignment procedures to address the mechanical contributors to the deformity [27].

The first step in surgical planning is assessment of the flexibility of the cavovarus deformity. When the hindfoot is fixed in varus, the varus does not correct with Coleman block testing. In this case, calcaneal osteotomy is indicated to address the fixed hindfoot varus. Deformities that correct with Coleman block testing indicate that the hindfoot is flexible, and the deformity is forefoot driven. Indicated procedures address the forefoot and plantarflexed first ray.

Operative Technique

The patient is placed supine on a radiolucent table and moved to the end of the bed. A bump is placed under the ipsilateral hip to aid in internal rotation of the leg and easy access to the lateral aspect of the foot and ankle. Examination under anesthesia is performed to confirm the Silfverskiöld findings, the anterior drawer examination, the talar tilt examination, and hindfoot and forefoot flexibility.

Prior to addressing the malalignment, gastrocnemius and Achilles contractures are first addressed. This allows for more accurate assessment of flexibility of the remainder of the foot. Our preferred technique for gastrocnemius recession is endoscopic. If necessary, our preferred technique for Achilles tendon contracture release is a Hoke percutaneous triple hemisection. The ankle is then manipulated to break up residual attachments, and dorsiflexion as well as varus deformity is reassessed.

In fixed hindfoot cavovarus deformity, the next step is addressing the hindfoot varus. Calcaneal osteotomy is the preferred technique to address this, with lateralization and closing wedge as options to realign the hindfoot. Radiographs from a representative case are shown in Fig. 4.4a–c, and MRI findings are shown in Fig. 4.5a–c. There are a number of different techniques described for calcaneal osteotomy.

Our preferred technique is the modified Dwyer calcaneal osteotomy, a closing wedge, lateralizing osteotomy. A 4-cm lateral oblique incision is made in line with the superior anterior aspect of the calcaneal tuberosity to the plantar anterior aspect of the tuberosity. Dissection is taken down to the bone. The periosteum is incised sharply and elevated with a periosteal elevator anteriorly and posteriorly. Small Hohmann retractors are placed superiorly and inferiorly between the calcaneal bone and surrounding soft tissues. A 30-mm oscillating saw blade is then used to score the cortex in two parallel lines with the desired width of the closing wedge. The saw is then used to complete the two cuts, which converge at the medial cortex. The wedge of bone is removed using osteotomes. In the classic Dwyer osteotomy, closing of the wedge is then performed and affixed [28]. In the modified version, the osteotomy is lateralized in addition to closed. If not already complete, the osteotomy is completed medially with osteotomes. A periosteal elevator is then used to elevate the periosteum off the medial cortex of the proximal and distal calcaneus to improve mobility of the fragments. The fragments are then manually reduced with simultaneous closure of the lateral wedge osteotomy and lateralization of the posterior tuberosity fragment to the desired distance. Two parallel guidewires are placed in the tuberosity aimed toward the posterior facet of the calcaneus. The reduction is checked under fluoroscopy using lateral and Harris heel views. The wires are overdrilled, and two headless compression screws are used to compress across the osteotomy, with the heads buried just under the posterior cortex. Figure 4.6a–e demonstrate our technique. Figure 4.7a–e demonstrate adjuvant procedures performed in the same patient, including peroneus brevis repair and modified Broström-Gould lateral ligament repair.

Alterative calcaneal osteotomy techniques include the oblique lateralizing calcaneal osteotomy without closing wedge, in which a single cut is made using a similar approach. Another alternative is the Malerba step-cut osteotomy, in

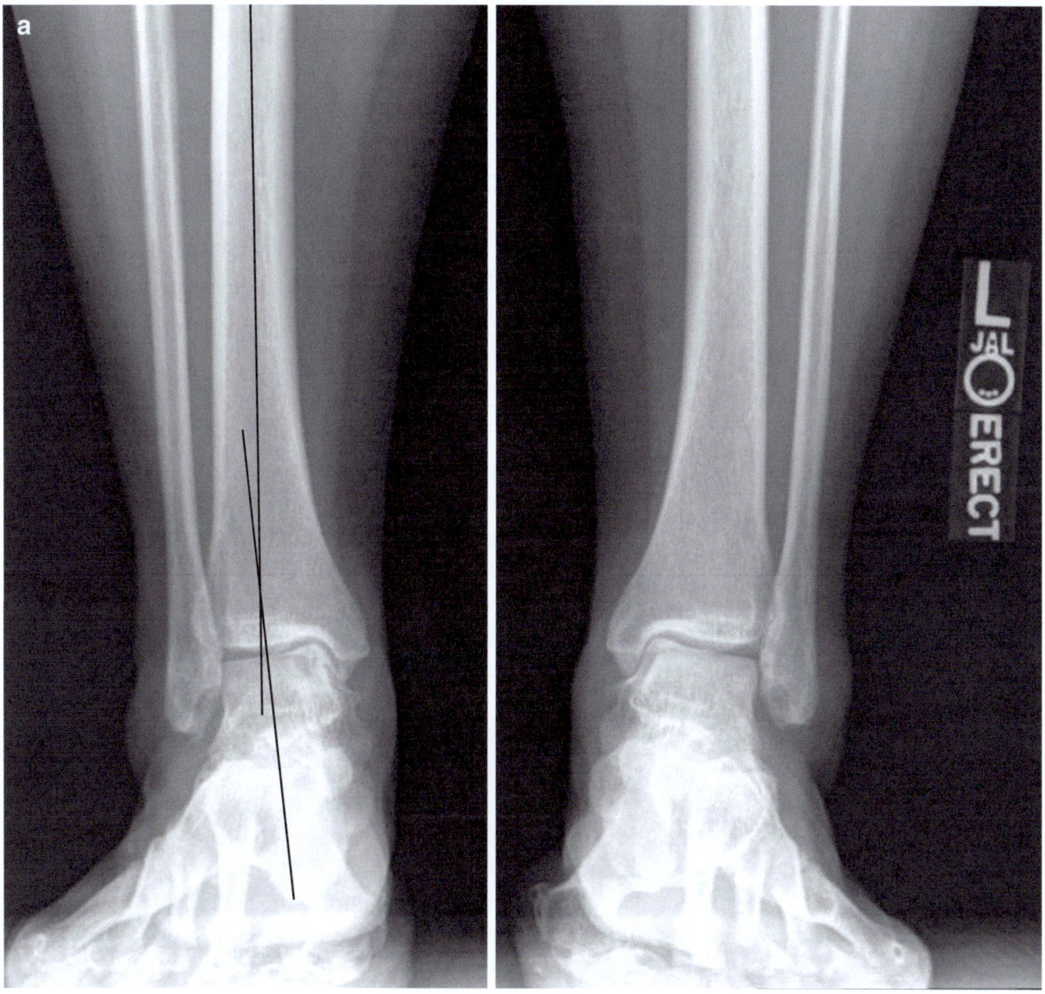

Fig. 4.4 Fixed, hindfoot-driven varus in a 57-year-old woman with recurrent right lateral ankle instability. (**a**) Weight-bearing AP radiographs measure 9 degrees of hindfoot varus, medial joint space narrowing, and osteophyte formation. (**b**) Weight-bearing mortise view of the right ankle demonstrating varus talar alignment, medial joint space narrowing, and osteophytes. (**c**) Lateral radiograph demonstrates anterior and posterior distal tibial osteophytes and dorsal talar osteophyte. The patient does not demonstrate forefoot cavus

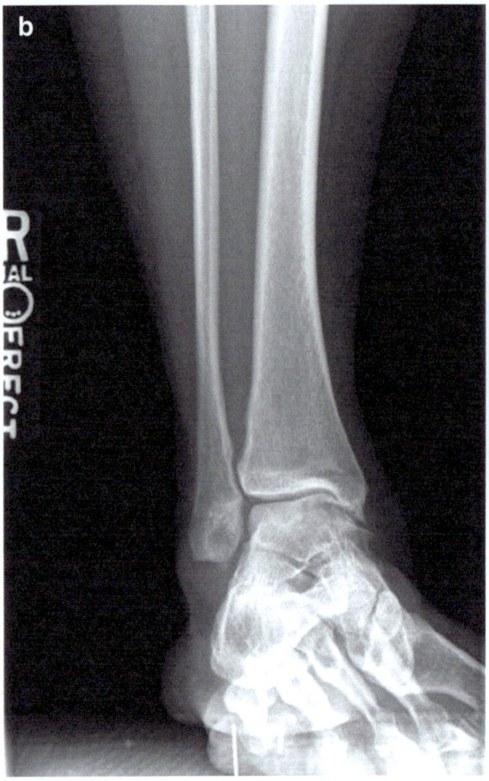

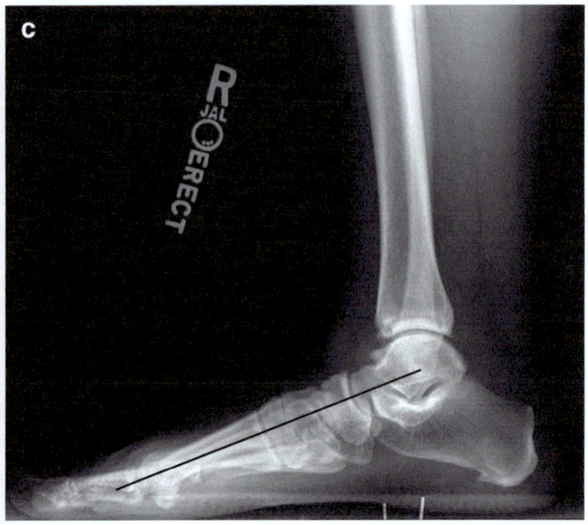

Fig. 4.4 (continued)

which a horizontal step cut is made with a z-configuration, and closing of a 2- to 6-mm wedge plus lateralization is performed [29]. In a comparative three-dimensional digital model analysis, Cody et al. found that the modified Dwyer osteotomy resulted in the most improvement in hindfoot alignment and translation [30].

In hindfoot-driven varus, following calcaneal osteotomy, the forefoot is examined for a plantarflexed first ray and associated forefoot valgus. In forefoot-driven varus, these procedures may be done in isolation without calcaneal osteotomy. Forefoot equinus may be flexible or fixed. Initially, peroneal overdrive may dynamically cause the plantarflexed first ray, but over time, this deformity becomes fixed [14, 31]. In the setting of flexible first ray deformity, peroneus longus to brevis transfer may be employed to remove the deforming force.

More commonly, forefoot equinus is fixed and is primarily managed with bony realignment with first ray dorsiflexion osteotomy. Figures 4.2a–c and 4.8a–c demonstrate the Coleman block testing findings and preoperative radiographic findings for a patient with forefoot-driven hindfoot varus. First ray dorsiflexion osteotomy may be accomplished with either a dorsally closing wedge osteotomy of the medial cuneiform or first metatarsal or with arthrodesis through the first tarsometatarsal or tarsocuneiform joints.

Our preferred technique in the absence of midfoot arthritis is closing wedge osteotomy of the base of the first metatarsal. Advantages of this technique include ease of surgical dissection, reliable healing, and joint-sparing nature. A dorsal incision is made overlying the first metatarsal from the distal medial cuneiform to the midshaft of the first metatarsal. The extensor hallucis is retracted medially or laterally and protected. The tarsometatarsal joint is identified, and the planned osteotomy is localized 1.5 cm distal to the joint. The periosteum is incised and elevated of the metatarsal base medially and laterally, and Hohmann retractors are used to protect the sur-

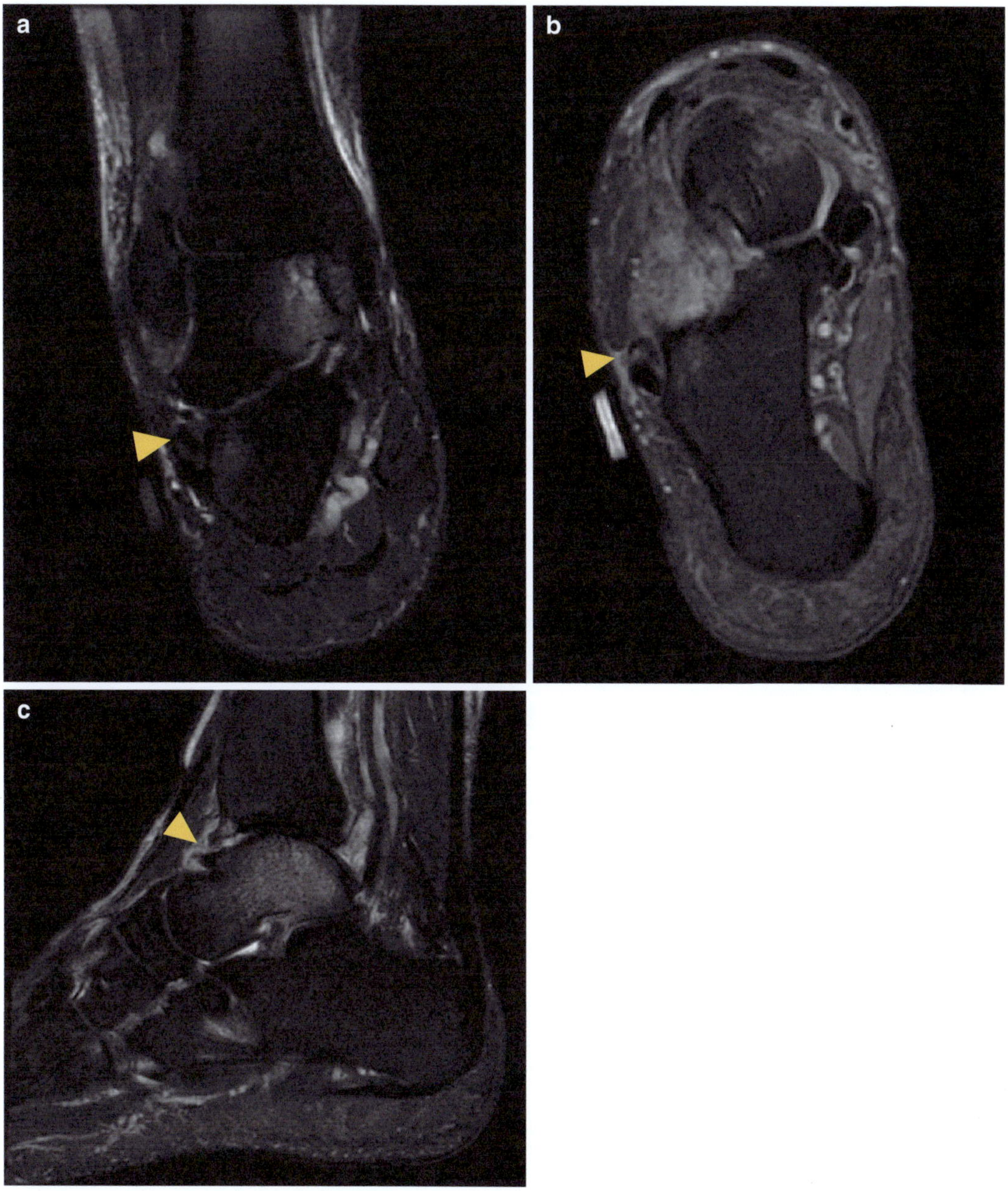

Fig. 4.5 Magnetic resonance imaging (MRI) of the right ankle. (**a**). Coronal T2-weighted MR image demonstrates medial talar edema and cyst formation, narrowing of the medial joint space, and osteophytes along the medial malleolus. Arrow indicates peroneus brevis tendon. (**b**) Axial T2-weighted MR image demonstrating split tear of the peroneus brevis tendon, marked with the arrow. (**c**) Sagittal T2-weighted MR image at the level of the medial talar body, demonstrating edema in the talar body and prominent anterior distal tibial and dorsal talar neck spurs with associated synovitis, marked with an arrow

rounding structures. A dorsal closing wedge osteotomy is planned with the proximal portion of the osteotomy parallel to the joint surface and the amount of bone removed from the dorsal surface depending on the degree of correction desired. A saw is used to score the cortex and create the osteotomies, and osteotome is used to further open the osteotomy. The osteotomy can then be

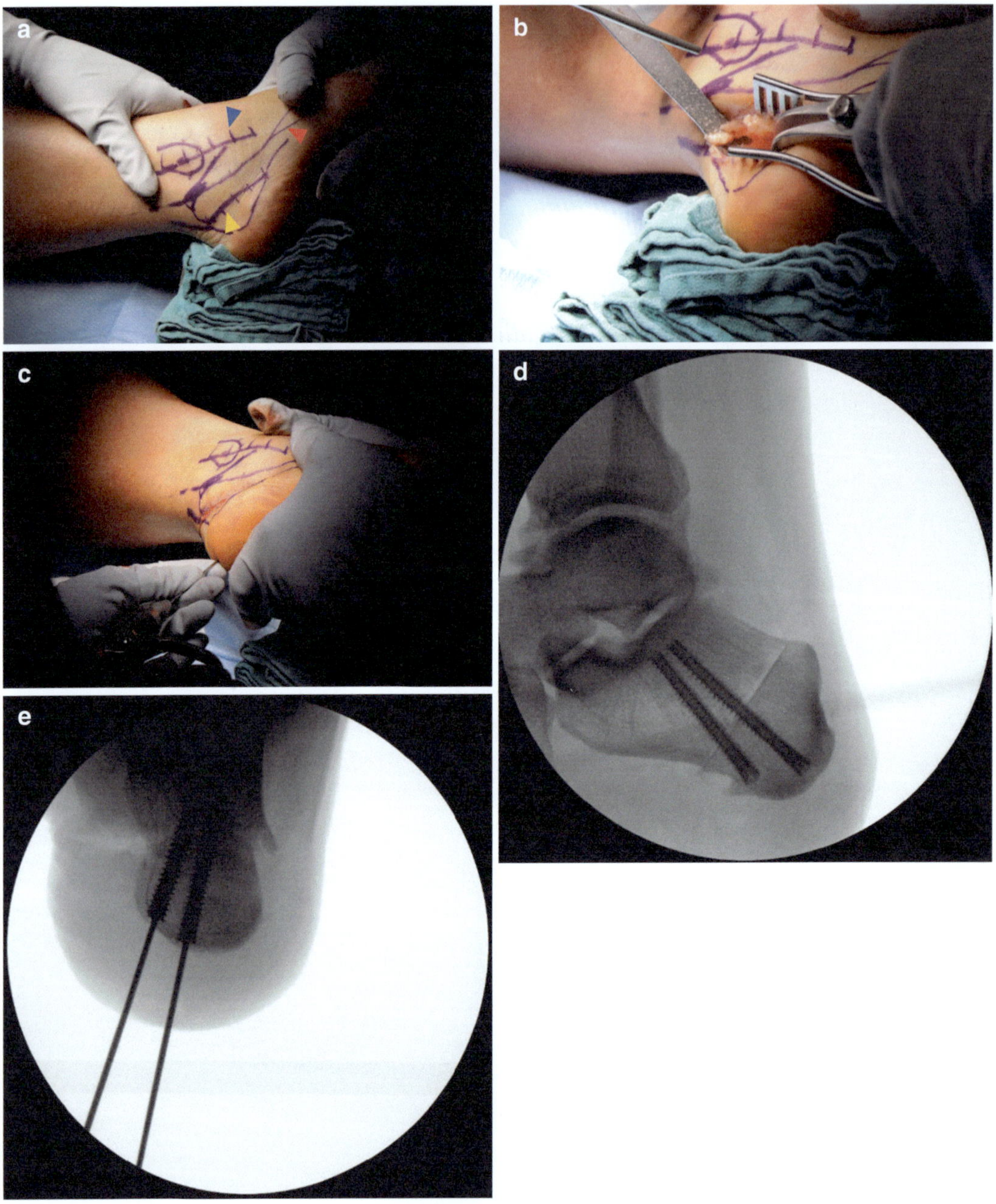

Fig. 4.6 Intraoperative photographs from lateralizing calcaneal osteotomy. (**a**) Planned incisions for calcaneal osteotomy (yellow arrow), peroneal repair, and modified Broström-Gould procedure (blue arrow). Sural nerve outlined and indicated with red arrow. (**b**) Exposing calcaneal osteotomy. Following elevation of the periosteum along the osteotomy, baby Hohmann and Weitlaner retractors are placed. The osteotomy is completed with saw and osteotomes. A laminar spreader is then inserted into the osteotomy to facilitate elevation of the medial periosteum, allowing for mobilization of the tubercle. (**c**). The modified Dwyer osteotomy is then manually closed laterally (closing wedge) and lateralized. Guidewires are placed distal to the Achilles insertion on the calcaneus crossing the osteotomy. (**d**) Intraoperative fluoroscopy demonstrates 5.5-mm headless compression screws placed across the osteotomy with closure of the wedge. The heads are buried under the posterior cortex. (**e**) Intraoperative Harris heel view demonstrates lateralization of the calcaneus by approximately 6 mm and closure of the wedge. The heads of the screws are just beneath the cortex

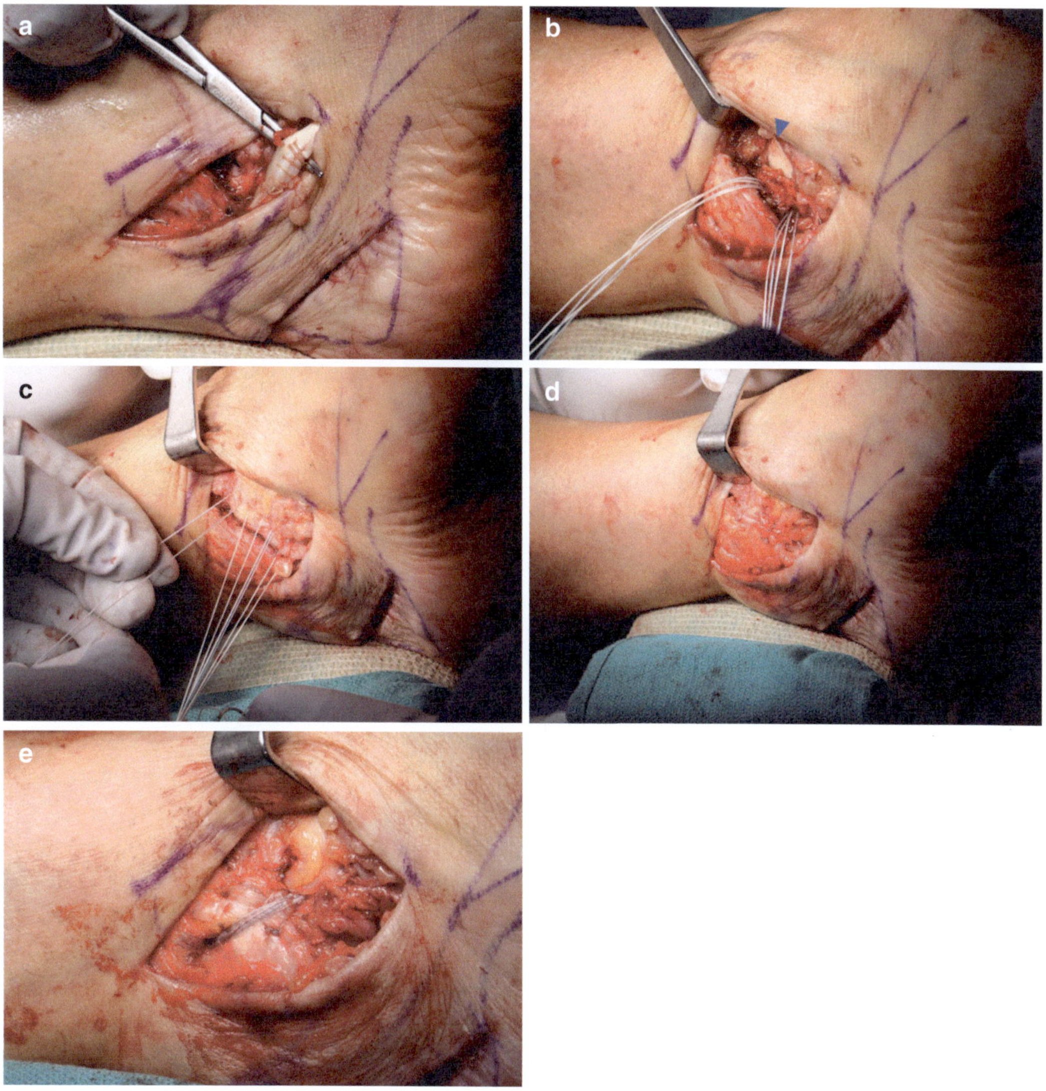

Fig. 4.7 Intraoperative images of adjuvant procedures to lateralizing calcaneal osteotomy. (**a**) Peroneus brevis tendon split tear repair with absorbable suture. (**b**) Modified Broström-Gould lateral ligament reconstruction. Two double-loaded suture anchors are placed in the distal fibula. The talar cartilage is visible medially (blue arrow). (**c**) Following passage of the eight suture limbs through the distal sleeve of ATFL and extensor retinaculum in horizontal mattress fashion. (**d**) One limb from each pair of the tied horizontal mattress suture is then passed proximally through the remnant ligamentous tissue on the fibula in simple fashion. (**e**) A nonabsorbable braided suture tape (Arthrex Internal Brace) is then placed overlying the repair with anchors in the fibula between the two suture anchors and the talus

manually closed, or Kirschner wires can be used with compressor to close the osteotomy. The osteotomy is then affixed with a low-profile, dorsal 2.7-mm locking T-plate, which is joint sparing and stable. Figure 4.9a–c demonstrate postoperative radiographs in a patient following first metatarsal base dorsiflexion osteotomy with this technique. Cortical screw fixation crossing the osteotomy is also an option.

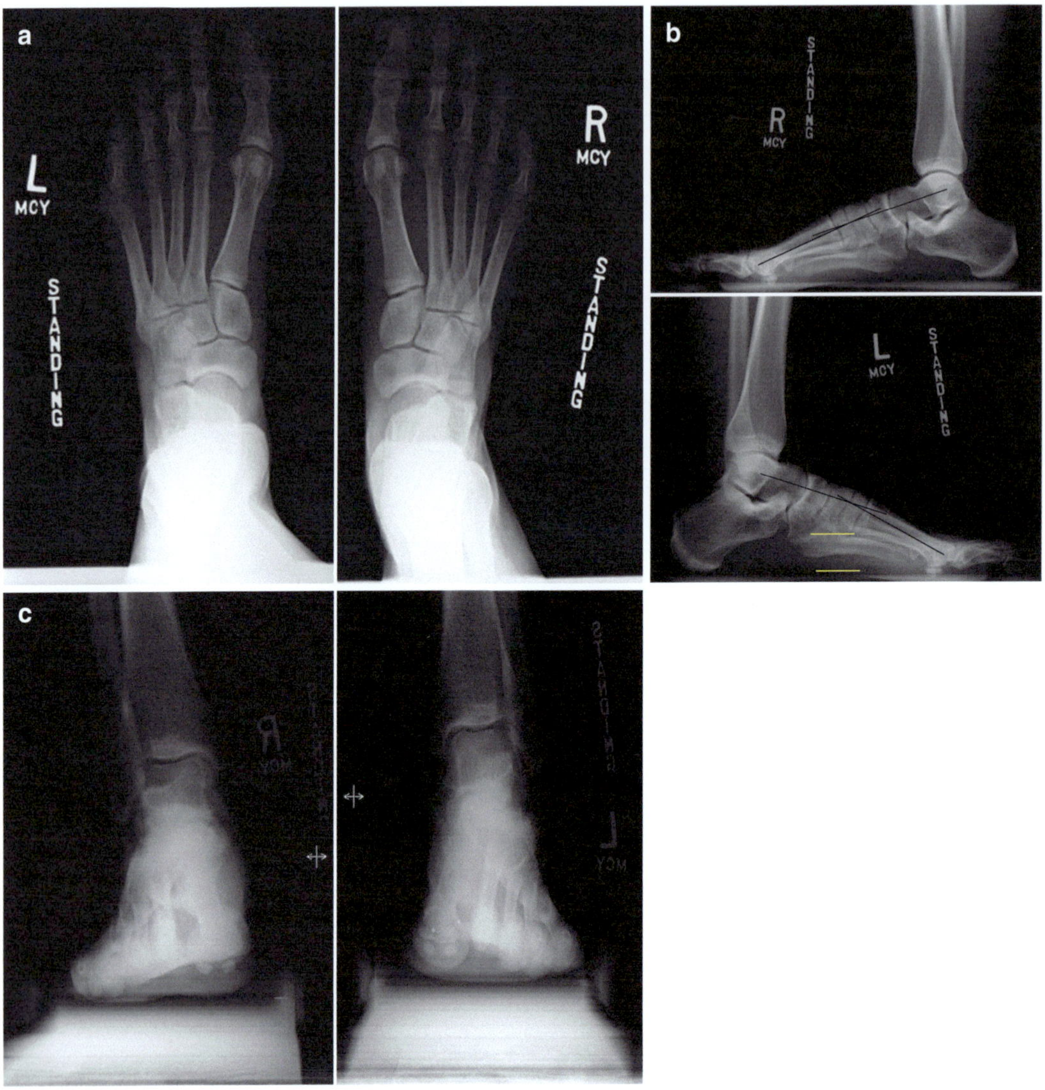

Fig. 4.8 Radiographs of an 18-year-old collegiate athlete with bilateral forefoot-driven varus ankle alignment and recurrent instability. (**a**) Standing AP views of the bilateral feet. (**b**) Standing lateral views of the bilateral feet demonstrating forefoot cavus with positive Meary's angle and signs of ankle varus on the left including see-through sign and double dome sign. Navicular height is also elevated on the left (yellow lines). (**c**) Standing AP radiographs of the ankle and hindfoot demonstrating bilateral hindfoot varus with a plantarflexed first ray

Outcomes

Patients with chronic lateral ankle instability are at risk for failure if an underlying cavovarus deformity is not addressed. Multiple authors have reported clinical failure following lateral ligament repair or reconstruction in patients with a cavovarus deformity [32, 33]. In a study of Broström-Gould procedures performed in a military population, one-quarter of revisions were performed in patients with untreated concomitant varus malalignment [11]. These studies emphasize the need for comprehensive preoperative evaluation in the patient with chronic ankle instability.

There are few studies examining outcomes among patients with chronic lateral ankle instability and malalignment. In a case series of 15 patients with subtle cavovarus deformity who underwent modified Broström procedures, Shim et al. reported that isolated lateral closing wedge osteotomy was required in four patients, isolated first metatarsal dorsiflexion osteotomy was performed in eight patients, and both procedures were performed in three patients, two of whom also underwent gastrocnemius recession. At average 58-month follow-up, there were no episodes of recurrent instability, and patient reported outcomes were significantly improved [16]. Vienne et al. reported on eight patients with cavovarus deformity treated for recurrent chronic lateral ankle instability who had failed prior operative intervention. Lateralizing calcaneal osteotomy and peroneus longus to peroneus brevis transfer were performed in all patients, and a Broström ligament reconstruction was performed in four patients. At average 37-month follow-up, all patients were satisfied and final radiographs demonstrated restoration of a valgus hindfoot alignment. In a case series of 23 patients (29 feet) with

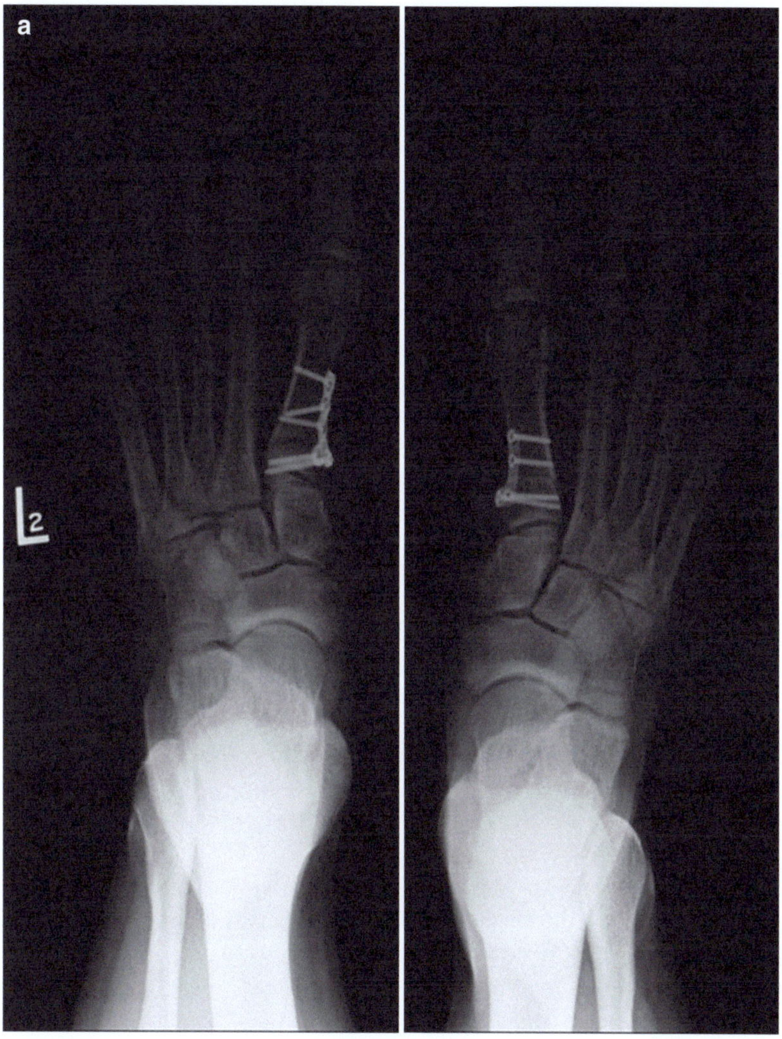

Fig. 4.9 Postoperative imaging following bilateral first ray dorsiflexion osteotomies with a plate. (**a**) AP of the bilateral feet demonstrates plate fixation of bilateral first metatarsal osteotomies. (**b**) Lateral views of the bilateral feet demonstrate closed dorsal wedge osteotomy of the first metatarsal and neutral Meary's angle. (**c**) Standing AP views of the ankle and hindfoot demonstrate neutral ankle alignment

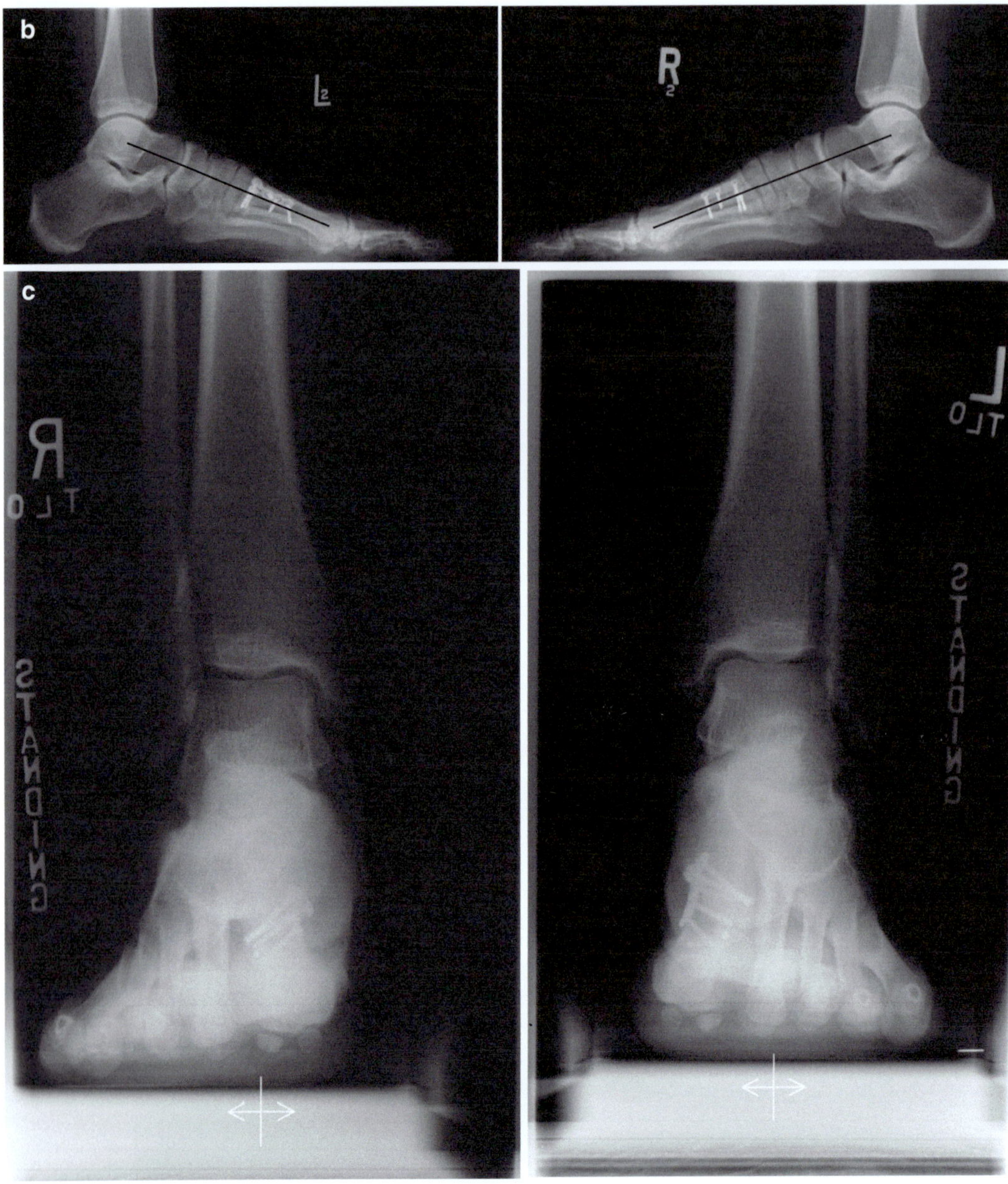

Fig. 4.9 (continued)

lateral ankle instability and subtle cavovarus foot deformities, Maskill et al. performed lateralizing calcaneal osteotomies in 100% of patients, peroneal transfer and dorsiflexion first metatarsal osteotomy in 86% of patients, tendo-Achilles lengthening in 28% of patients, and gastrocnemius recession in 17% of patients [15]. Additionally, 17% of patients received ankle ligament reconstruction. At average 4.4 years of follow-up, there were no patients with recurrent instability or nonunion; 34% of patients had undergone removal of hardware.

Conclusion

Chronic lateral ankle instability is clinically common, but recognition of underlying anatomic factors contributing to instability is paramount to proper management. The physical exam and radiographs provide important information regarding the source and degree of deformity. Conservative management remains the mainstay of treatment, but patients with anatomic predisposition may be more likely to go on to chronic instability after an ankle sprain. In hindfoot-driven varus, calcaneal osteotomy is the primary intervention to address the deformity. In forefoot-driven varus, both bony and soft tissue procedures may be performed to elevate the first ray. Proper recognition and surgical management of cavovarus deformity in chronic lateral ankle instability result in high patient satisfaction and low recurrence of instability.

References

1. Waterman BR, Owens BD, Davey S, Zacchilli MA, Belmont PJ Jr. The epidemiology of ankle sprains in the United States. J Bone Joint Surg Am. 2010;92(13):2279–84.
2. Hootman JM, Dick R, Agel J. Epidemiology of collegiate injuries for 15 sports: summary and recommendations for injury prevention initiatives. J Athl Train. 2007;42(2):311–9.
3. Roos KG, Kerr ZY, Mauntel TC, Djoko A, Dompier TP, Wikstrom EA. The epidemiology of lateral ligament complex ankle sprains in National Collegiate Athletic Association Sports. Am J Sports Med. 2017;45(1):201–9.
4. Herzog MM, Kerr ZY, Marshall SW, Wikstrom EA. Epidemiology of ankle sprains and chronic ankle instability. J Athl Train. 2019;54(6):603–10.
5. Kucera KL, Marshall SW, Wolf SH, Padua DA, Cameron KL, Beutler AI. Association of Injury History and Incident Injury in cadet basic military training. Med Sci Sports Exerc. 2016;48(6):1053–61.
6. Clifton DR, Koldenhoven RM, Hertel J, Onate JA, Dompier TP, Kerr ZY. Epidemiological patterns of ankle sprains in youth, high school, and college football. Am J Sports Med. 2017;45(2):417–25.
7. McKay GD, Goldie PA, Payne WR, Oakes BW. Ankle injuries in basketball: injury rate and risk factors. Br J Sports Med. 2001;35(2):103–8.
8. Gribble PA, Bleakley CM, Caulfield BM, et al. Evidence review for the 2016 international ankle consortium consensus statement on the prevalence, impact and long-term consequences of lateral ankle sprains. Br J Sports Med. 2016;50(24):1496–505.
9. Hiller CE, Nightingale EJ, Lin CW, Coughlan GF, Caulfield B, Delahunt E. Characteristics of people with recurrent ankle sprains: a systematic review with meta-analysis. Br J Sports Med. 2011;45(8):660–72.
10. Krause F, Seidel A. Malalignment and lateral ankle instability: causes of failure from the varus tibia to the Cavovarus foot. Foot Ankle Clin. 2018;23(4):593–603.
11. Strauss JE, Forsberg JA, Lippert FG 3rd. Chronic lateral ankle instability and associated conditions: a rationale for treatment. Foot Ankle Int. 2007;28(10):1041–4.
12. Bernasconi A, Cooper L, Lyle S, et al. Pes cavovarus in Charcot-Marie-tooth compared to the idiopathic cavovarus foot: a preliminary weightbearing CT analysis. Foot Ankle Surg. 2021;27(2):186–95.
13. Rose KJ, Hiller CE, Mandarakas M, Raymond J, Refshauge K, Burns J. Correlates of functional ankle instability in children and adolescents with Charcot-Marie-tooth disease. J Foot Ankle Res. 2015;8:61.
14. Manoli A 2nd, Graham B. The subtle cavus foot, "the underpronator". Foot Ankle Int. 2005;26(3):256–63.
15. Maskill MP, Maskill JD, Pomeroy GC. Surgical management and treatment algorithm for the subtle cavovarus foot. Foot Ankle Int. 2010;31(12):1057–63.
16. Shim DW, Suh JW, Park KH, Lee JW, Byun J, Han SH. Diagnosis and operation results for chronic lateral ankle instability with subtle Cavovarus deformity and a peek-A-boo heel sign. Yonsei Med J. 2020;61(7):635–9.
17. Araoye I, De Cesar NC, Cone B, Hudson P, Sahranavard B, Shah A. Results of lateral ankle ligament repair surgery in one hundred and nineteen patients: do surgical method and arthroscopy timing matter? Int Orthop. 2017;41(11):2289–95.
18. Larsen E, Angermann P. Association of ankle instability and foot deformity. Acta Orthop Scand. 1990;61(2):136–9.
19. Aminian A, Sangeorzan BJ. The anatomy of cavus foot deformity. Foot Ankle Clin. 2008;13(2):191–8.
20. Coleman SS, Chesnut WJ. A simple test for hindfoot flexibility in the cavovarus foot. Clin Orthop Relat Res. 1977;123:60–2.
21. Singh D. Nils Silfverskiöld (1888-1957) and gastrocnemius contracture. Foot Ankle Surg. 2013;19(2):135–8.
22. Lee KM, Chung CY, Kwon SS, et al. Relationship between stress ankle radiographs and injured ligaments on MRI. Skelet Radiol. 2013;42(11):1537–42.
23. Arunakul M, Amendola A, Gao Y, Goetz JE, Femino JE, Phisitkul P. Tripod index: a new radiographic parameter assessing foot alignment. Foot Ankle Int. 2013;34(10):1411–20.
24. Magee TH, Hinson GW. Usefulness of MR imaging in the detection of talar dome injuries. AJR Am J Roentgenol. 1998;170(5):1227–30.
25. Michels F, Pereira H, Calder J, et al. Searching for consensus in the approach to patients with chronic lat-

eral ankle instability: ask the expert. Knee Surg Sports Traumatol Arthrosc. 2018;26(7):2095–102.
26. Lintz F, Bernasconi A, Baschet L, Fernando C, Mehdi N, de Cesar NC. Relationship between chronic lateral ankle instability and hindfoot varus using weight-bearing Cone beam computed tomography. Foot Ankle Int. 2019;40(10):1175–81.
27. Vienne P, Schöniger R, Helmy N, Espinosa N. Hindfoot instability in cavovarus deformity: static and dynamic balancing. Foot Ankle Int. 2007;28(1):96–102.
28. Dwyer FC. Osteotomy of the calcaneum for pes cavus. J Bone Joint Surg Br. 1959;41(1):80–6.
29. Malerba F, De Marchi F. Calcaneal osteotomies. Foot Ankle Clin. 2005;10(3):523–40.
30. Cody EA, Kraszewski AP, Conti MS, Ellis SJ. Lateralizing calcaneal osteotomies and their effect on calcaneal alignment: a three-dimensional digital model analysis. Foot Ankle Int. 2018;39(8):970–7.
31. Mosca VS. The cavus foot. J Pediatr Orthop. 2001;21(4):423–4.
32. Broström L, Sprained ankles. V. Treatment and prognosis in recent ligament ruptures. Acta Chir Scand. 1966;132(5):537–50.
33. Brunner R, Gaechter A. Repair of fibular ligaments: comparison of reconstructive techniques using plantaris and peroneal tendons. Foot Ankle. 1991;11(6):359–67.

Rehabilitating the Elite Athlete with Ligamentous Injury of the Foot and Ankle

5

Steven M. Short and Gretchen M. Short

The entry point to patient-centered rehabilitative management of ankle and foot injuries is the subjective and subsequent correlative objective examination. Detailed gathering of information, including communication with adjunct medical providers, allows for the comprehensive evaluation and accumulation of clinical impairments that will drive clinical reasoning [1, 2]. Consistently reevaluating the clinical findings and the patient's response to respective interventions via reasoning feedback loops will allow the clinician to assist in the progression throughout their course of care [1].

An important metric that the clinician must first consider is appropriate tissue healing timelines and the natural history of the injury. Both the extent (severity, irritability) and the nature (tissue type, stage) of the injury will impact the individual recovery and resultant progression of therapeutic activity [3, 4]. Distinct tissues have been identified to have unique healing pathways. Ligamentous injury has varying timelines with collagen fiber response demonstrating remodeling to grossly "normal" after 7 weeks. However, the collagen composition in the remodeled ligament has been documented to be irregular from uninjured ligaments, with related disadvantageous biomechanical properties that remain abnormal on long-term follow-up [4]. Beyond structure, associated functional impairments (laxity, loss of balance, etc.) and reinjury risk last often beyond 1 year [5]. Concomitant pathology and postoperative conditions may exist and warrant further consideration for management and prognosis.

Treatment of ligamentous injury is often accompanied by a varying period of relative immobilization, which is necessary to protect, stabilize, and augment the immediate inflammatory and healing cascade. This may be promoted with assistive devices such as tape, braces, boots, crutches, and walkers to keep the patient locally protected. To maximize the acute rehabilitation period, a focus should be on what can be trained on the individual as opposed to what they must be restricted from. A phased rehabilitation protocol (periodized strength and reconditioning) is recommended to progress through the stages and allow return to play [6–8].

Periodized rehabilitation can typically be broken down into three- or five-phase programs. A three-phase program is typically defined by acute, subacute, and functional reconditioning phases that conclude in a return to function [9–11]. A five-phase program provides increased detail to treat functional impairments, with a goal of pro-

S. M. Short (✉)
Physical Therapy & High Performance, Denver Nuggets Basketball Club, Physical Therapy, The Sisu Project, Denver, CO, USA

The Sisu Project, Arvada, CO, USA
e-mail: Steven.short@nuggets.com

G. M. Short
Select Physical Therapy, Physical Therapy, The Sisu Project, Golden, CO, USA

The Sisu Project, Arvada, CO, USA

P. D'Hooghe et al. (eds.), *Ligamentous Injuries of the Foot and Ankle*,
https://doi.org/10.1007/978-3-031-08682-3_5

gramming a more adequate training stimulus to bridge the gap from returning to play to true athletic performance. The initial phases can still typically be defined as acute, subacute, and/or proliferation. More functionally, these early phases place an emphasis on improving global human capacity and local tissue healing. Describing the final three phases is a matter of the desired physical adaptations required to recover from injury and restore sport-specific qualities. Common terminology of the final three phases can include, but are not limited to, accumulation, transmutation or reconditioning, and realization, respectively [7, 12]. These terms are applied from classic strength and conditioning periodization models and can be modified to suit the demands of the injured athlete and their respective sporting goals. As opposed to a strict linear progression of achieving one construct goal before progressing, an undulating program design will allow separate construct criteria to be trained simultaneously, often promoting progression efficiency and potentially augmenting outcomes [6]. For example, loading the triceps surae via an eccentric-biased heel raise program can facilitate both improvements in pain [13], muscle fascicle length [13, 14], strength [13], function [13], and ankle range of motion over a blocked time course [15].

Early active interventions, as opposed to delayed, are shown to result in superior outcomes [16, 17]. It is recommended that the early management of these injuries follow the POLICE acronym (protect, optimally load, ice, compress, and elevate) [18]. While protecting the injury is essential in initial management, shifting the focus to load management methods and safe exercise prescription will promote local and systemic healing [5].

Additional early-stage goals often consist of controlling pain and inflammation, improving local and regional mobility, and restoring the function of activities of daily living (i.e., ambulation, stair negotiation, self-care, etc.). While there is limited evidence supporting passive treatment strategies on long term outcomes, the use of modalities such as cryotherapy, compression, and manual therapy may serve a purpose in the acute and sub-acute phases of injury management. Manual therapy interventions offer low-risk pain reduction while assisting in early motion and associated return to function goals while facilitating the tissue-sensitive healing process through mechanotransduction [19]. Common manual therapy techniques often focus on joint and soft tissue-based strategies and have been shown to improve range of motion and clinical outcomes [5, 20]. As with exercise, the appropriate dosage of manual therapy and early motion is important to achieve results. It is recommended to dose manual therapies pragmatically [21] to an improvement in concordant signs as no specific dosage of manipulative therapy has consistently shown superior outcomes [22–24] (Figs. 5.1 and 5.2).

While modalities such as electrotherapy, ultrasound, and laser therapies cannot currently be recommended to improve outcomes [25], the use

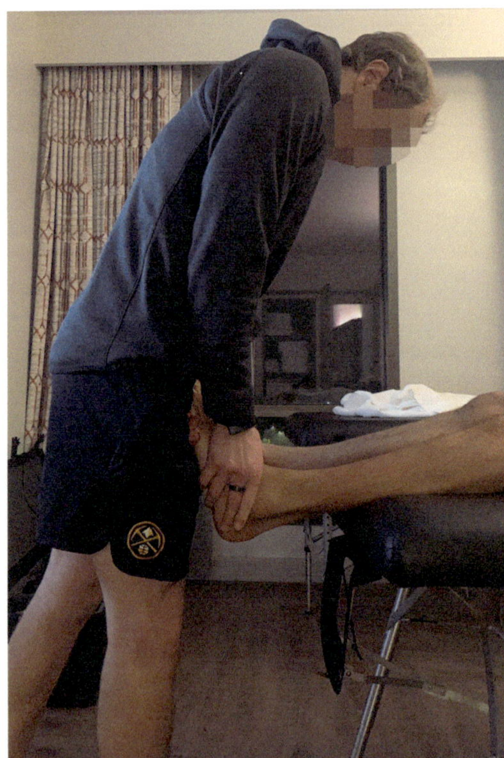

Fig. 5.1 Anterior to posterior mobilization of the talocrural joint. With the clinician's hands broadly placed across the talus, apply a graded and oscillating force in an anterior to posterior direction for decreases in pain and improved ankle mobility

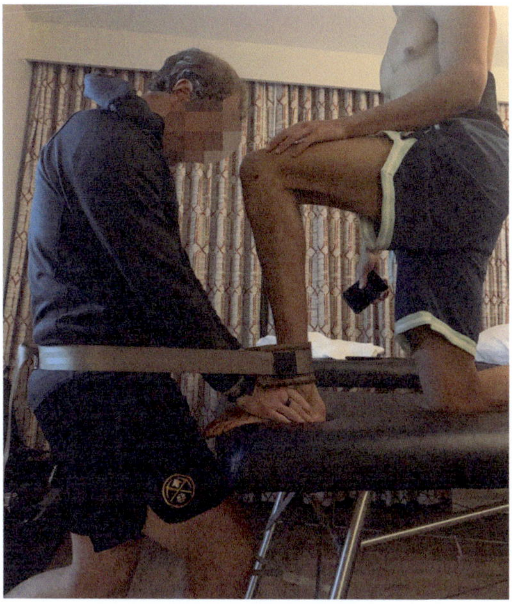

Fig. 5.2 Dorsiflexion mobilization with movement of the talocrural joint. With the clinician's hands broadly placed across the talus and a belt assisting the advancement of the shank, the clinician mobilizes the talus anterior to posterior while the patient in half kneeling advances the ankle through dorsiflexion

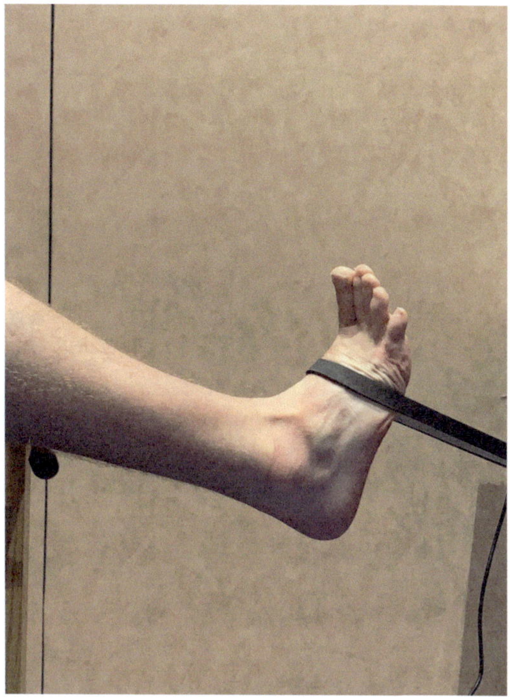

Fig. 5.3 Ankle four-way exercise variation with an emphasis on cueing eccentrically controlled inversion against combined ankle eversion-dorsiflexion resistance

of cryotherapy can be utilized as an adjunct low-cost, low-risk modality to manage pain [5, 26, 27]. Cryotherapy is often combined with varying forms of compression such as garment or pneumatic device [28]. Compression garments have been shown to expedite recovery of ankle sprains in select subgroups [29]. The effects of compression can be augmented by reducing the impact of gravity dependence positioning via elevation [30]. Cryo and compression-based treatment modalities, combined with manual therapy, have more efficacy in improving short-term outcomes while facilitating compound improvements between sessions to impact long-term outcomes [31]. Long-term management will move beyond assistive modalities and rely on patient education, self-efficacy, exercise, and self-management interventions [32–34].

Basic exercise principles are imposed in the acute stage of rehabilitation and throughout return to performance [12]. Early mobilization is encouraged and has been shown to result in improved outcomes that consider return to work, time loss from sport, and patient satisfaction in various conditions about the foot, ankle, and lower extremity as a whole [5, 35–37]. Imposing exercise principles must consider the tissue stress and often initially revolve around submaximal efforts, isometrics, active and/or passive range of motion with varying degrees of resistance, regionally related muscle groups, and compound movement interventions. The volume of these exercises generally must be quite high as the load that the tissue is able to safely tolerate is often below a standard recommended to cause physiological and structural change [38]. Movement-related pain improvements and cellular responses from neuromuscular excitation can still be achieved as part of low-level graded exposure to movement both locally and globally [39, 40] (Fig. 5.3).

According to the nature of injury, the affected limb may require significant period of unloading and protection, often prescribed as a non-weight-bearing and immobilized joint. Passive and active motion may be allowed depending on the nature of the injury and the course of surgical vs. conservative management. Consistent with early protection, local resistance training of the foot and ankle is often limited to open chain activity and required to be performed at subthreshold resistances. Adverse reactions to associated disuse include atrophy, impaired neuromuscular performance, and prolonged strength and power deficits locally and throughout the affected limb [41–43]. The atrophy signaling pathways of immobilization take effect within the first few days of disuse and begin to attenuate around 2 weeks [41]. While the clinical decision-making is dependent on the respective injury, lateral ankle sprains have been shown to have improved outcomes in those who initially progress weight-bearing as tolerated vs. non-weight-bearing immobilization as an example of early motion in pratice [5].

Strength impairments, both locally at the ankle [44] (inversion/eversion/plantarflexion) and regionally in the lower extremity [45] (hip), can be safely exercised in early-stage rehabilitation. Eccentric training of the ankle evertors improves strength and reaction time of the musculature, potentially providing a means to resist mechanisms of inversion injury and improve proprioceptive joint stability [46, 47]. Further eccentric training of the plantarflexor musculature through rehabilitation has been proposed to improve muscle coordination through neuromuscular mechanisms, making the ankle and foot unit more stiff and energy efficient for functional tasks [48]. Muscular foot intrinsic impairments have been identified in those both with lower extremity injury and foot and ankle injury [49]. It has been proposed that addressing these impairments may improve function in the acute and subacute phases (Fig. 5.4). Combing foot intrinsic drills and lower-level balance activities while barefoot or in minimalist conditions may promote an increase in mechanical and sensory stimuli [50, 51]. Implementing this proprioceptive effect [52] to improve flexor capacity may better force distribution about the ankle-foot unit and the kinetic chain [49, 53].

When a limb or joint requires significant unloading, utilization of concepts such as the of crossover effect, in which the unaffected limb is resistance trained, has been shown to provide positive adaptations to the contralateral extremity in an attempt to reduce the adverse reactions of disuse [54, 55]. Adjunct exercise-based modalities such as blood flow-restricted exercise (BFR) have been shown promote an anabolic cascade that simulates heavy resistance training and improve outcomes while still protecting the healing injury from excessive load [56, 57]. Additional benefits of BFR may include an increase bony metabolism during an unloading period [58]and intrasession pain improvements [59]. By either loading the unaffected limb at a stress level consistent with exercise recommendations that impose physiologic change [38] or

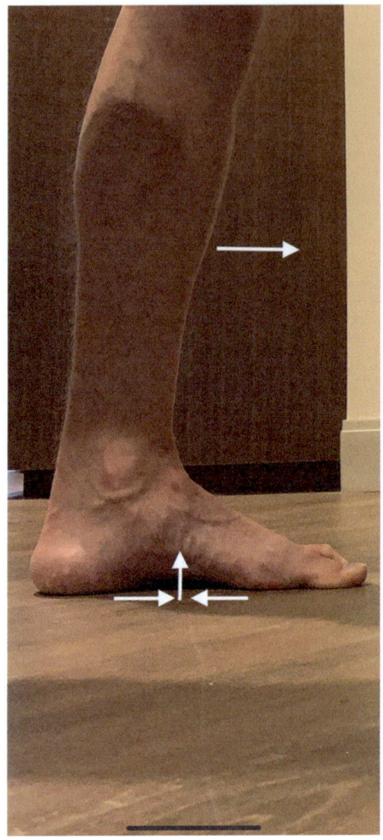

Fig. 5.4 Short foot intrinsic exercise. The patient is cued to draw the calcaneus and the base of the first metatarsophalangeal joint toward each other drawing up the arch of the foot. Challenges to foot posture can be advanced by displacing the center of mass forward or through maintaining posture through various single leg tasks such as balance perturbations or squatting

utilizing BFR at low loads (i.e., 20–30% 1RM), the patient may be able to achieve a desired exercise-related response.

As the individual progresses beyond the early phases, an increased emphasis is placed on graded, progressive loading. Scheduling these progressions typically takes place in linear or undulated programs [6, 12]. Loads and repetition schemes should attempt to hit a target stimulus to produce mechanotransduction-induced adaptions that include hypertrophy, strength, and power development [12, 19, 60] (Table 5.1). Each block of the training process may place a greater focus on different qualities as it respects the tissue and training status and history of the athlete. Within this exercise program, priority should be given to the exercises that will provide the most efficient benefit within the individual's session or home exercise program as exercise adherence has been shown to be a limiting factor in rehabilitation [61]. Moving from the subacute phase and beyond, focus often shifts from single joint isolation exercises (Fig. 5.5) to multi-joint compound exercises. Double limb and single leg exercise can be beneficial to both restoring limb capacity and developing physical qualities [62]. Partially supported exercises such as the rear-foot elevated split squat and unilaterally supported bilateral squat may assist in progressions while maintaining consideration of the injured limb [63–65]. Transitioning to single leg exercise can effectively elicit similar strength and neuromuscular improvement gains while simultaneously addressing balance and asymmetry deficits [66–68] (Figs. 5.6, 5.7, and 5.8).

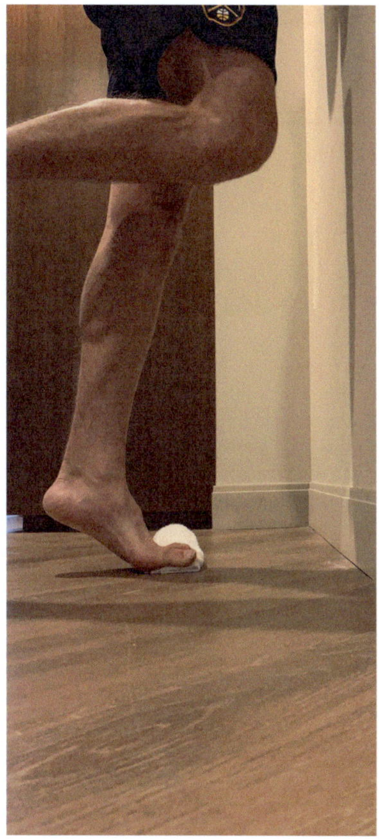

Fig. 5.5 Single leg heel raise. A towel is placed under the great toe, potentially increasing the demands on the plantar fascia and foot intrinsic musculature [99]

Table 5.1 Therapeutic exercise dosing principles. Primary and secondary resistance and plyometric exercise drills as demonstrated within the chapter and beyond should be dosed to the corresponding goals and requirements for physiologic adaptation

Exercise Repetitions	Percent 1 Repetition Max	Sets	Rehabilitation Target Stimulus
1	100	3–5	Strength/Power/NM
2	95	3–5	Strength/Power/NM
3	93	3–5	Strength/Power/NM
4	90	3–5	Strength/Power
5	87	3–5	Strength
6	85	3–4	Strength
7	83	3–4	Strewth
8	80	3–4	NM/Hypertrophy/Strength
9	77	1–3	NM/Hypertrophy
10	75	1–3	NM/Hypertrophy
15>	65<	1–3	Neuromuscular(NM)/Endurance

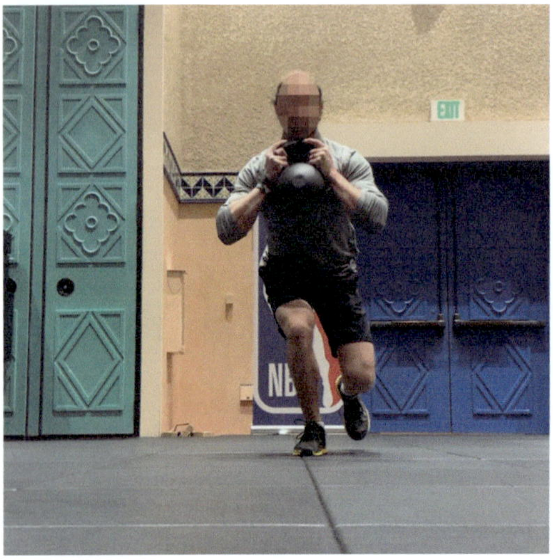

Fig. 5.6 Single leg exercise demonstrated as a single leg squat. Resistance is to be guided by the stage of rehabilitation and principles discussed in Table 5.1. Drills can be judiciously performed with less load, varying velocity, and on an unstable surface if the target stimulus is for proprioception and motor control as opposed to strength and power development

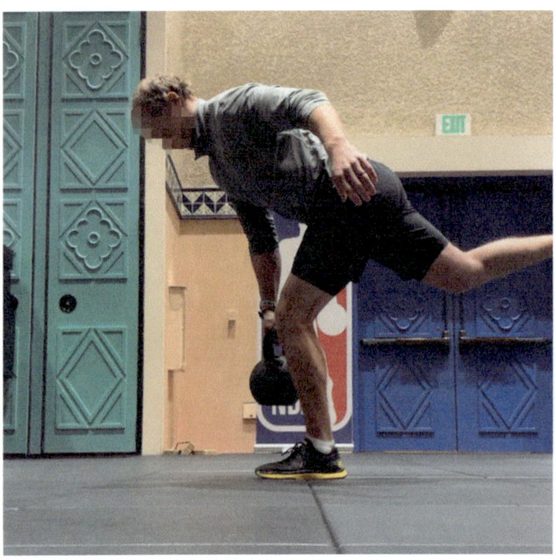

Fig. 5.7 Single leg exercise demonstrated as a single leg dead lift. Resistance is to be guided by the stage of rehabilitation and principles discussed in Table 5.1. Drills can be judiciously performed with less load, varying velocity, and on an unstable surface if the target stimulus is for proprioception and motor control as opposed to strength and power development

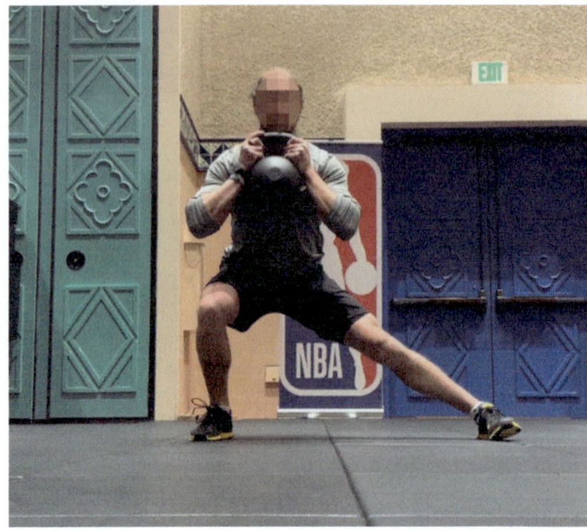

Fig. 5.8 Single leg dominant, triplanar exercise demonstrated as a lateral lunge. Resistance is to be guided by the stage of rehabilitation and principles discussed in Table 5.1 Drills can be judiciously performed with less load, varying velocity, and on an unstable surface if the target stimulus is for proprioception and motor control as opposed to strength and power development

Proprioception, motor control, balance, and neuromuscular training are all broad exercise terms that are recommended to improve clinical outcomes via exercise modes. Despite their widespread use [69] and broadly similar definitions, their pragmatic application is based heavily on clinical experience as opposed to rigorously supported data. With a lack of descriptive evidence to support therapeutic dosage [70], clinicians can rely on fundamental exercise principles such as mode, volume, intensity, and specificity to achieve the goals of limb stability and kinetic chain movement coordination and efficiency. Generally accepted constructs across terminology include varying degrees of single leg tasks that include reasonable dynamic function and movement positioning of the trunk and lower extremity that can be accomplished through a broad spectrum of exercise drills [71, 72].

A multifaceted program consists of addressing key constructs of mobility, strength, power, motor control [73, 74], balance [75], and goal-specific reconditioning [76] to not only restore function but to achieve tertiary reinjury prevention [77]. Objective testing within these parameters allows for a criteria-based progression through the rehabilitation. It has been proposed that appropriate objective measures, along with tradition healing and time-based measures and patient input, are key to improved outcomes [78]. Clinical measures such as rate of perceived exertion, repetitions in reserve, the soreness rules, basic dynamometry, repetitions to fatigue, repetition maximums (i.e., 10 repetition max) and limb symmetry indexes can be used to assess and progress therapeutic exercise dosage on an intra- and intersession basis [8, 12, 38, 79]. Single leg and proprioceptive balance training improvements can be tracked through simple clinical tools such as single limb squat test variations, Star Excursion Balance Test, or the Y Balance test, which has shown value in assessing current ability and future risk via composite and anterior reach metrics [80] (Fig. 5.9). While no single variable is completely demonstrative of outcomes, batteries of tests, including hop tests [74], may better evaluate the patient's progress. Functional test batteries may be externally valid and sensitive for assessing poor function, and their specificity may not be adequate to identify long-standing impairments beyond the tested task and resultant objective metric [81, 82] (Fig. 5.10) [74]. Tools such as force plates and movement analysis technology may provide detailed kinematic and kinetic data in dynamic tasks (countermovement jumps, drop jumps) and address potential limitations of practical field-based tests [81]. These tools are not commonly available in standard physiotherapy practice due to cost and application barriers (time, advanced training). There is a paucity of evidence regarding adequate criteria for patient return to function for specific ankle and foot pathologies; thus, a reliance on risk constructs and other regional recommendations are required to combine with patient goals to create evidence-informed criteria for progression [78, 79, 83].

Aerobic training is an important consideration for all stages of rehabilitation. The cardiovascular system is quickly and negatively impacted by periods of immobilization. Deconditioning has been identified by increases in resting heart rate

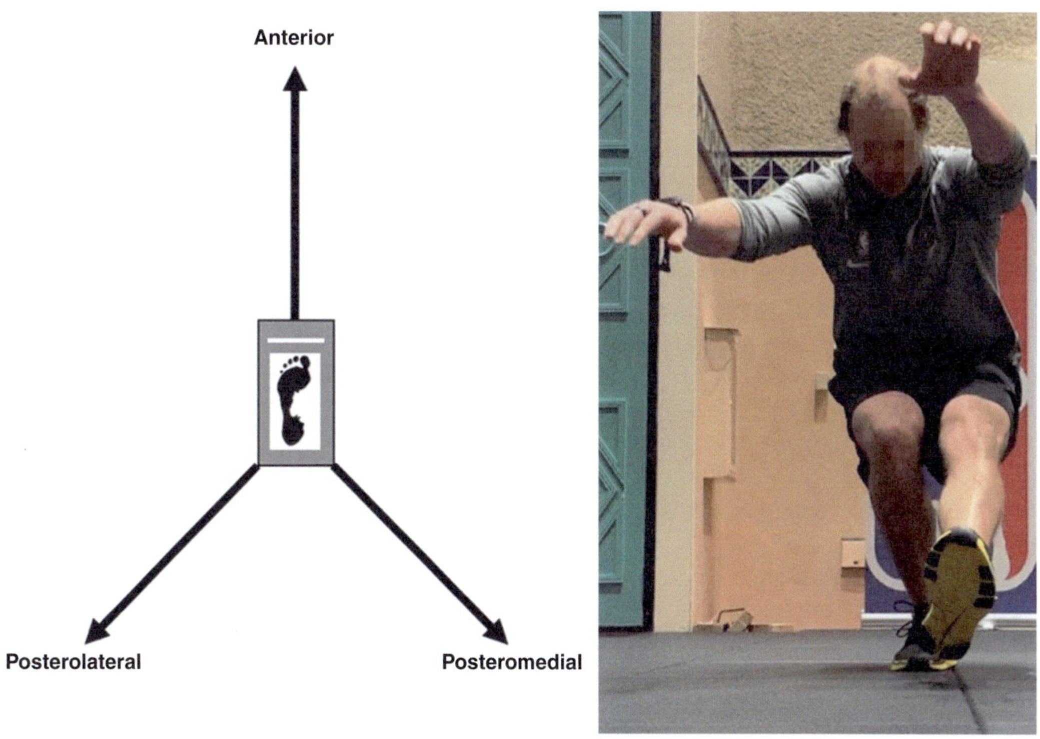

Fig. 5.9 Y Balance Test with anterior reach demonstration

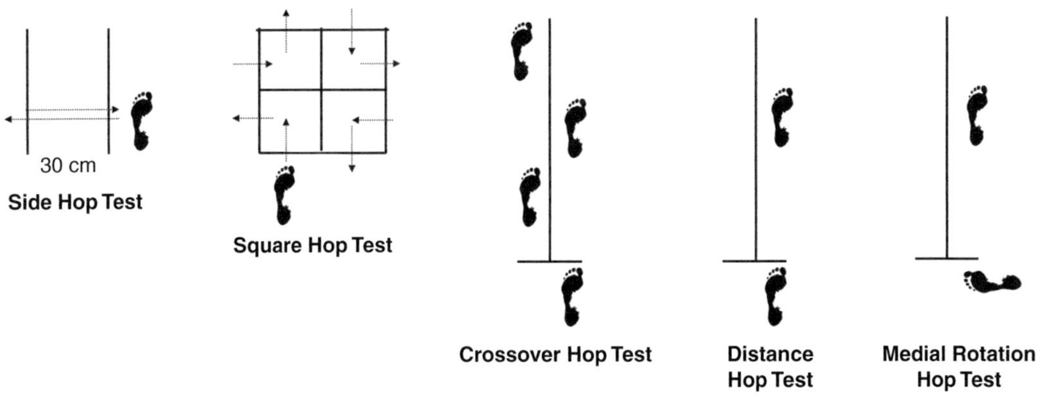

Fig. 5.10 Hop test battery including side hop, square hop, crossover, linear hop for distance, and medial rotation hop for distance tests

by 1–2 beats per minute per day in the initial stages of disuse [84, 85]. In the acute and global capacity phase, an emphasis on long, slow aerobic conditioning may help offset deconditioning as well as satellite cell availability and promote healing [8, 86]. Long-term development of the aerobic system is also a common method to protect against injury risk [76, 87]. Additional systemic effects such as pain reduction and increased blood perfusion may improve the individuals tolerance to other training stimulus provided in their rehabilitation program [88]. Baseline fitness can be achieved through basic tests such as the 6-min walk test or the timed sit-to-stand and step-up tests and cycling power assessments (i.e., Wingate Test).

Transitioning to overground training may be assisted by underwater or antigravity treadmill running and jumping and may have a positive improvement on the recovery of foot and ankle pathoanatomy [89]. As weight-bearing is allowed and progressed, integration into functional activity is recommended. Simple plyometric training can be performed as line hops or box jumps or even patient goal specific such as a basketball jump shot or football dribbling [90] (Fig. 5.11). Lesser volumes and intensities are recommended to progress in a rehabilitation setting [91] as opposed to traditional textbook definitions of plyometric volumes [90] as those may elicit too much load for rehabilitation progressions initially. Basic clinical strength (limb symmetry index) and dynamic tolerance criteria (hop testing battery) is recommended to be achieved before progressive running programs [79]. As the volume of an activity such as running is progressed, long-duration cardiovascular activity transitions to tempo, interval, repeat sprint, and agility training variants [8]. If the goal is to return to sport, simulating tasks such as defensive shuffling or basic sporting drills with appropriate work to rest ratios and durations are recommended to match training loads as the individual approaches return to sport [79]. Specific agility drills have not been identified as predicative of lower extremity outcomes or agility drills, and their multicomponent sport-specific and reactive nature make it challenging to assess true change of direction function in those returning to play [80, 92]. However, matching the overall stressors of activity and assisting the individual to train to prior levels activity or the desired return to functional activity reduce the risk of future injury [8] (Fig. 5.12).

Gradual introduction of multidirectional activity requires a similar objective criteria and can utilize sporting drills to reintroduce specific tasks. Progressive sporting agility and return to performance can be programmed on a "control-chaos" continuum, in that early extensive reconditioning drills are highly confined and protective at low percentage of competitive workload (low-impact individual sport-skill sessions) and gradually built up to unpredictable intensive drills with

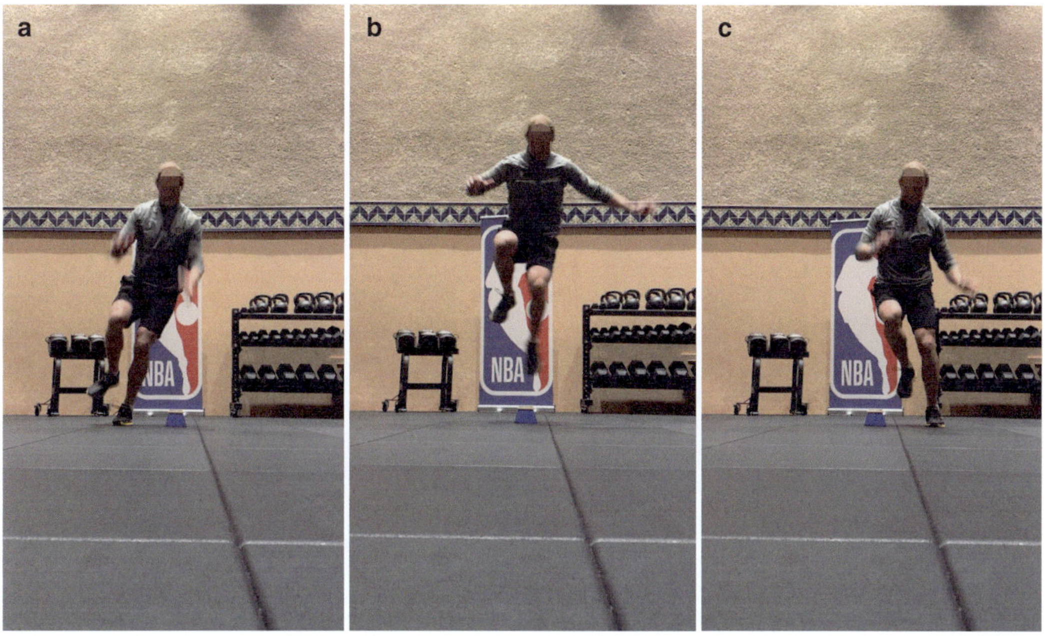

Fig. 5.11 (**a–c**) Lateral hurdle hop plyometric training drill. With the patient hopping over a hurdle, the clinician can cue for compliant and controlled landings or for speed and stiffness depending on the stage of the rehabilitation and the goal of the drill within the periodized rehabilitation block

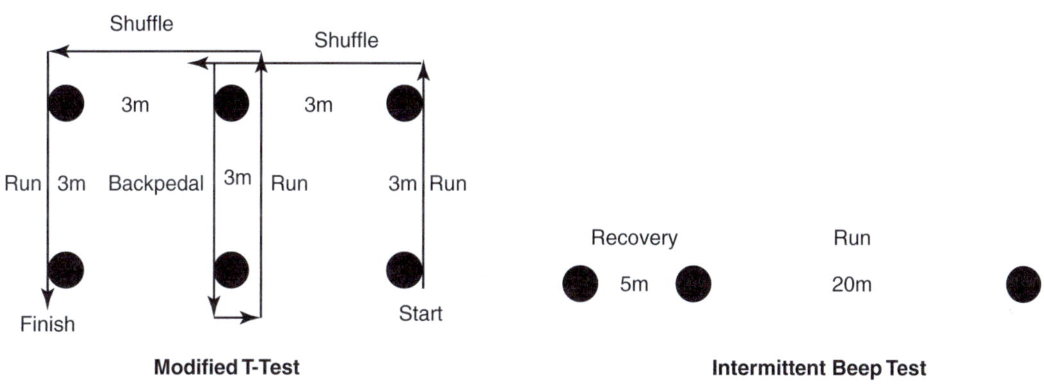

Fig. 5.12 Field-based agility and conditioning tests to be matched to energy system demands of sport

minimal confines with increasing percentage of sport-specific workloads (small-sided games) [93]. Internal (physiologic) and external (mechanical) workloads can be tracked to ensure that a satisfactory level of reconditioning has occurred prior to a return to work and sport. Common internal metrics include rating of perceived exertion, heart rate monitoring, and subjective recovery, while external metrics include volume measures such as distance, sprints, accelerations, decelerations, etc. [94–96]. If the patient's desired goal is less intense, the clinician should educate and promote methods for lifelong physical activity (exercise) and wellness (nutrition, sleep, mental health) habits that not only treat the current condition but contribute to the overall health and well-being of the individual in the future [34, 97, 98].

References

1. Jones M. Clinical reasoning and pain. Man Ther. 1995;1(1):17–24. https://doi.org/10.1054/math.1995.0245.
2. Gluyas H. Patient-centred care: improving healthcare outcomes. Nurs Stand. 2015;30(4):50–7; quiz 59. https://doi.org/10.7748/ns.30.4.50.e10186.
3. Jarvinen TA, Jarvinen TL, Kaariainen M, et al. Muscle injuries: biology and treatment. Am J Sports Med. 2005;33(5):745–64. https://doi.org/10.1177/0363546505274714.
4. Liu SH, Yang R-S, Al-Shaikh R, et al. Collagen in tendon, ligament, and bone healing: a current review. Clin Orthop Relat Res. 1995;318:265–78.
5. Martin RL, Davenport TE, Paulseth S, et al. Ankle stability and movement coordination impairments: ankle ligament sprains. J Orthop Sports Phys Ther. 2013;43(9):A1–40. https://doi.org/10.2519/jospt.2013.0305.
6. Blanchard S, Glasgow P. A theoretical model for exercise progressions as part of a complex rehabilitation programme design. Br J Sports Med. 2019;53(3):139–40. https://doi.org/10.1136/bjsports-2017-097486.
7. Lorenz DS, Reiman MP, Walker JC. Periodization: current review and suggested implementation for athletic rehabilitation. Sports Health. 2010;2(6):509–18. https://doi.org/10.1177/1941738110375910.
8. Morrison S, Ward P, duManoir GR. Energy system development and load management through the rehabilitation and return to play process. Int J Sports Phys Ther. 2017;12(4):697–710.
9. Wilk KE, Reinold MM, Dugas JR, et al. Current concepts in the recognition and treatment of superior labral (SLAP) lesions. J Orthop Sports Phys Ther. 2005;35(5):273–91. https://doi.org/10.2519/jospt.2005.35.5.273.
10. Anloague PA, Strack DS. Considerations in the diagnosis and accelerated return to sport of a professional basketball player with a triceps Surae injury: a case report. J Orthop Sports Phys Ther. 2018;48(5):388–97. https://doi.org/10.2519/jospt.2018.7192.
11. Short SM, Anloague PA, Strack DS. Rehabilitation and return to sport following surgical repair of the rectus abdominis and adductor longus in a professional basketball player: a case report. J Orthop Sports Phys Ther. 2016;46(8):697–706. https://doi.org/10.2519/jospt.2016.6352.
12. Lorenz D, Morrison S. Current concepts in periodization of strength and conditioning for the sports physical therapist. Int J Sports Phys Ther. 2015;10(6):734–47.
13. Murphy M, Rio E, Debenham J, et al. Evaluating the progress of mid-portion ACHILLES tendinopathy during rehabilitation: a review of outcome measures for muscle structure and function, tendon structure, and neural and pain associated mechanisms. Int J Sports Phys Ther. 2018;13(3):537–51.
14. Duclay J, Martin A, Duclay A, et al. Behavior of fascicles and the myotendinous junction of human medial gastrocnemius following eccentric strength training. Muscle Nerve. 2009;39(6):819–27. https://doi.org/10.1002/mus.21297.
15. Howe LP, Bampouras TM, North JS, et al. Improved ankle mobility after a 4-week training program affects landing mechanics: a randomized controlled trial. J Strength Cond Res. 2020; Publish Ahead of Print; https://doi.org/10.1519/jsc.0000000000003717.
16. McCormack R, Bovard J. Early functional rehabilitation or cast immobilisation for the postoperative management of acute Achilles tendon rupture? A systematic review and meta-analysis of randomised controlled trials. Br J Sports Med. 2015;49(20):1329–35. https://doi.org/10.1136/bjsports-2015-094935.
17. Deal JB, Patzkowski JC, Groth AT, et al. Early vs delayed weightbearing after microfracture of osteochondral lesions of the talus: a prospective randomized trial. Foot Ankle Orthop. 2019;4(2):2473011419838832. https://doi.org/10.1177/2473011419838832.
18. Bayer ML, Magnusson SP, Kjaer M. Early versus delayed rehabilitation after acute muscle injury. N Engl J Med. 2017;377(13):1300–1. https://doi.org/10.1056/NEJMc1708134.
19. Khan KM, Scott A. Mechanotherapy: how physical therapists' prescription of exercise promotes tissue repair. Br J Sports Med. 2009;43(4):247–52. https://doi.org/10.1136/bjsm.2008.054239.
20. Plaza-Manzano G, Vergara-Vila M, Val-Otero S, et al. Manual therapy in joint and nerve structures combined with exercises in the treatment of recurrent ankle sprains: a randomized, controlled trial. Man Ther. 2016;26:141–9. https://doi.org/10.1016/j.math.2016.08.006.
21. Roenz D, Broccolo J, Brust S, et al. The impact of pragmatic vs. prescriptive study designs on the outcomes of low back and neck pain when using mobilization or manipulation techniques: a systematic review and meta-analysis. J Man Manip Ther. 2018;26(3):123–35. https://doi.org/10.1080/10669817.2017.1398923.
22. Weerasekara I, Deam H, Bamborough N, et al. Effect of mobilisation with movement (MWM) on clinical outcomes in lateral ankle sprains: a systematic review and meta-analysis. Foot. 2020;43:101657. https://doi.org/10.1016/j.foot.2019.101657.
23. Pasquier M, Daneau C, Marchand A-A, et al. Spinal manipulation frequency and dosage effects on clinical and physiological outcomes: a scoping review. Chiropr Man Therap. 2019;27:23. https://doi.org/10.1186/s12998-019-0244-0.
24. Cleland JA, Mintken PE, McDevitt A, et al. Manual physical therapy and exercise versus supervised home exercise in the management of patients with inversion ankle sprain: a multicenter randomized clinical trial. J Orthop Sports Phys Ther. 2013;43(7):443–55. https://doi.org/10.2519/jospt.2013.4792.
25. Cleland JA, Abbott JH, Kidd MO, et al. Manual physical therapy and exercise versus electrophysical agents and exercise in the management of plantar heel

pain: a multicenter randomized clinical trial. J Orthop Sports Phys Ther. 2009;39(8):573–85. https://doi.org/10.2519/jospt.2009.3036.
26. Bleakley C, McDonough S, MacAuley D. The use of ice in the treatment of acute soft-tissue injury: a systematic review of randomized controlled trials. Am J Sports Med. 2004;32(1):251–61. https://doi.org/10.1177/0363546503260757.
27. Bleakley CM, Hopkins JT. Is it possible to achieve optimal levels of tissue cooling in cryotherapy? Phys Ther Rev. 2010;15(4):344–50. https://doi.org/10.1179/174328810X12786297204873.
28. Hansrani V, Khanbhai M, Bhandari S, et al. The role of compression in the management of soft tissue ankle injuries: a systematic review. Eur J Orthop Surg Traumatol. 2015;25(6):987–95. https://doi.org/10.1007/s00590-015-1607-4.
29. Bendahou M, Khiami F, Saïdi K, et al. Compression stockings in ankle sprain: a multicenter randomized study. Am J Emerg Med. 2014;32(9):1005–10. https://doi.org/10.1016/j.ajem.2014.05.054.
30. Tsang KKW, Hertel J, Denegar CR. Volume decreases after elevation and intermittent compression of Postacute ankle sprains are negated by gravity-dependent positioning. J Athl Train. 2003;38(4):320–4.
31. Cook CE, Showalter C, Kabbaz V, et al. Can a within/between-session change in pain during reassessment predict outcome using a manual therapy intervention in patients with mechanical low back pain? Man Ther. 2012;17(4):325–9. https://doi.org/10.1016/j.math.2012.02.020.
32. Lewis JS, Cook CE, Hoffmann TC, et al. The elephant in the room: too much medicine in musculoskeletal practice. J Orthop Sports Phys Ther. 2020;50(1):1–4. https://doi.org/10.2519/jospt.2020.0601.
33. Caneiro JP, Alaiti RK, Fukusawa L, et al. There is more to pain than tissue damage: eight principles to guide care of acute non-traumatic pain in sport. Br J Sports Med. 2020:bjsports-2019-101705. https://doi.org/10.1136/bjsports-2019-101705.
34. Skou ST, Pedersen BK, Abbott JH, et al. Physical activity and exercise therapy benefit more than just symptoms and impairments in people with hip and knee osteoarthritis. J Orthop Sports Phys Ther. 2018;48(6):439–47. https://doi.org/10.2519/jospt.2018.7877.
35. Karlsson J, Eriksson BI, Swärd L. Early functional treatment for acute ligament injuries of the ankle joint. Scand J Med Sci Sports. 1996;6(6):341–5. https://doi.org/10.1111/j.1600-0838.1996.tb00104.x.
36. Dettori JR, Pearson BD, Basmania CJ, et al. Early ankle mobilization, part I: the immediate effect on acute, lateral ankle sprains (a randomized clinical trial). Mil Med. 1994;159(1):15–20. https://doi.org/10.1093/milmed/159.1.15.
37. Lantto I, Heikkinen J, Flinkkila T, et al. Early functional treatment versus cast immobilization in tension after achilles rupture repair: results of a prospective randomized trial with 10 or more years of follow-up. Am J Sports Med. 2015;43(9):2302–9. https://doi.org/10.1177/0363546515591267.
38. Reiman MP, Lorenz DS. Integration of strength and conditioning principles into a rehabilitation program. Int J Sports Phys Ther. 2011;6(3):241–53.
39. Macaluso F, Myburgh KH. Current evidence that exercise can increase the number of adult stem cells. J Muscle Res Cell Motil. 2012;33(3–4):187–98. https://doi.org/10.1007/s10974-012-9302-0.
40. Cooper MA, Kluding PM, Wright DE. Emerging relationships between exercise, sensory nerves, and neuropathic pain. Front Neurosci. 2016;10:372. https://doi.org/10.3389/fnins.2016.00372.
41. Appell HJ. Muscular atrophy following immobilisation. A review. Sports Med. 1990;10(1):42–58. https://doi.org/10.2165/00007256-199010010-00005.
42. Campbell M, Varley-Campbell J, Fulfold J. Effect of immobilization on neuromuscular function: a systematic review. Sports Med. 2019;49(6):931–50. https://doi.org/10.1007/s40279-019-01088-8.
43. Brooks NE, Myburgh KH. Skeletal muscle wasting with disuse atrophy is multi-dimensional: the response and interaction of myonuclei, satellite cells and signaling pathways. Front Physiol. 2014;5:99. https://doi.org/10.3389/fphys.2014.00099.
44. Willems T, Witvrouw E, Verstuyft J, et al. Proprioception and muscle strength in subjects with a history of ankle sprains and chronic instability. J Athl Train. 2002;37(4):487–93.
45. Friel K, McLean N, Myers C, et al. Ipsilateral hip abductor weakness after inversion ankle sprain. J Athl Train. 2006;41(1):74–8.
46. Hanci E, Sekir U, Gur H, et al. Eccentric training improves ankle evertor and dorsiflexor strength and proprioception in functionally unstable ankles. Am J Phys Med Rehabil. 2016;95(6):448–58. https://doi.org/10.1097/phm.0000000000000421.
47. Keles SB, Sekir U, Gur H, et al. Eccentric/concentric training of ankle evertor and dorsiflexors in recreational athletes: muscle latency and strength. Scand J Med Sci Sports. 2014;24(1):e29–38. https://doi.org/10.1111/sms.12105.
48. O'Neill S, Watson PJ, Barry S. Why are eccentric exercises effective for achilles tendinopathy? Int J Sports Phys Ther. 2015;10(4):552–62.
49. McKeon PO, Hertel J, Bramble D, et al. The foot core system: a new paradigm for understanding intrinsic foot muscle function. Br J Sports Med. 2015;49(5):290. https://doi.org/10.1136/bjsports-2013-092690.
50. Goldmann J-P, Potthast W, Brüggemann G-P. Athletic training with minimal footwear strengthens toe flexor muscles. Footwear Sci. 2013;5(1):19–25. https://doi.org/10.1080/19424280.2012.744361.
51. Maurer C, Mergner T, Bolha B, et al. Human balance control during cutaneous stimulation of the plantar soles. Neurosci Lett. 2001;302(1):45–8. https://doi.org/10.1016/s0304-3940(01)01655-x.
52. Kavounoudias A, Roll R, Roll JP. Foot sole and ankle muscle inputs contribute jointly to human erect

posture regulation. J Physiol. 2001;532(Pt 3):869–78. https://doi.org/10.1111/j.1469-7793.2001.0869e.x.
53. Kelly LA, Cresswell AG, Racinais S, et al. Intrinsic foot muscles have the capacity to control deformation of the longitudinal arch. J R Soc Interface. 2014;11(93):20131188. https://doi.org/10.1098/rsif.2013.1188.
54. Cirer-Sastre R, Beltrán-Garrido JV, Corbi F. Contralateral effects after unilateral strength training: a meta-analysis comparing training loads. J Sports Sci Med. 2017;16(2):180–6.
55. Lee M, Carroll TJ. Cross education: possible mechanisms for the contralateral effects of unilateral resistance training. Sports Med. 2007;37(1):1–14. https://doi.org/10.2165/00007256-200737010-00001.
56. Hughes L, Paton B, Rosenblatt B, et al. Blood flow restriction training in clinical musculoskeletal rehabilitation: a systematic review and meta-analysis. Br J Sports Med. 2017;51(13):1003–11. https://doi.org/10.1136/bjsports-2016-097071.
57. Yow BG, Tennent DJ, Dowd TC, et al. Blood flow restriction training after Achilles tendon rupture. J Foot Ankle Surg. 2018;57(3):635–8. https://doi.org/10.1053/j.jfas.2017.11.008.
58. Bittar ST, Pfeiffer PS, Santos HH, et al. Effects of blood flow restriction exercises on bone metabolism: a systematic review. Clin Physiol Funct Imaging. 2018; https://doi.org/10.1111/cpf.12512.
59. Korakakis V, Whiteley R. 3 Low-load resistance exercise, blood flow restriction, or sham blood flow restriction for anterior knee pain. A three-arm pilot RCT. Br J Sports Med. 2019;53(Suppl 1):A1. https://doi.org/10.1136/bjsports-2019-scandinavianabs.3.
60. Dunn SL, Olmedo ML. Mechanotransduction: relevance to physical Therapist practice-understanding our ability to affect genetic expression through mechanical forces. Phys Ther. 2016;96(5):712–21. https://doi.org/10.2522/ptj.20150073.
61. McCall A, Dupont G, Ekstrand J. Injury prevention strategies, coach compliance and player adherence of 33 of the UEFA elite Club injury study teams: a survey of teams' head medical officers. Br J Sports Med. 2016;50(12):725–30. https://doi.org/10.1136/bjsports-2015-095259.
62. Appleby BB, Cormack SJ, Newton RU. Unilateral and bilateral lower-body resistance training does not transfer equally to Sprint and change of direction performance. J Strength Cond Res. 2020;34(1):54–64.
63. Helme M, Bishop C, Emmonds S, et al. Validity and reliability of the rear foot elevated Split squat 5 repetition maximum to determine unilateral leg strength symmetry. J Strength Cond Res. 2019;33(12):3269–75.
64. Helme M, Emmonds S, Low C. Is the Rear Foot Elevated Split Squat Unilateral? An Investigation Into the Kinetic and Kinematic Demands. J Strength Cond Res. 2020;Publish Ahead of Print
65. Jean LMY, Chiu LZF. Elevating the noninvolved limb reduces knee extensor asymmetry during squat exercise in persons with reconstructed anterior cruciate ligament. J Strength Cond Res. 2020;34(8)
66. Bogdanis GC, Tsoukos A, Kaloheri O, et al. Comparison between unilateral and bilateral plyometric training on single- and double-leg jumping performance and strength. J Strength Cond Res. 2019;33(3):633–40. https://doi.org/10.1519/jsc.0000000000001962.
67. Nijem RM, Galpin AJ. Unilateral versus bilateral exercise and the role of the bilateral force deficit. Strength Cond J. 2014;36(5):113–8.
68. Eliassen W, Saeterbakken AH, van den Tillaar R. Comparison of bilateral and unilateral squat exercises on barbell kinematics and muscle activation. Int J Sports Phys Ther. 2018;13(5):871–81. https://doi.org/10.26603/ijspt20180871.
69. Kaminski TW, Hertel J, Amendola N, et al. National Athletic Trainers' association position statement: conservative management and prevention of ankle sprains in athletes. J Athl Train. 2013;48(4):528–45. https://doi.org/10.4085/1062-6050-48.4.02.
70. Page P, Hoogenboom B, Voight M. Improving the reporting of therapeutic exercise interventions in rehabilitation research. Int J Sports Phys Ther. 2017;12(2):297–304.
71. Arundale AJH, Bizzini M, Giordano A, et al. Exercise-based knee and anterior cruciate ligament injury prevention. J Orthop Sports Phys Ther. 2018;48(9):A1–a42. https://doi.org/10.2519/jospt.2018.0303.
72. Thorborg K, Krommes KK, Esteve E, et al. Effect of specific exercise-based football injury prevention programmes on the overall injury rate in football: a systematic review and meta-analysis of the FIFA 11 and 11+ programmes. Br J Sports Med. 2017;51(7):562–71. https://doi.org/10.1136/bjsports-2016-097066.
73. Hegedus EJ, McDonough S, Bleakley C, et al. Physical performance tests predict injury in National Collegiate Athletic Association athletes: a three-season prospective cohort study. Br J Sports Med. 2016;50(21):1333–7. https://doi.org/10.1136/bjsports-2015-094885.
74. Caffrey E, Docherty CL, Schrader J, et al. The ability of 4 single-limb hopping tests to detect functional performance deficits in individuals with functional ankle instability. J Orthop Sports Phys Ther. 2009;39(11):799–806. https://doi.org/10.2519/jospt.2009.3042.
75. Hartley EM, Hoch MC, Boling MC. Y-balance test performance and BMI are associated with ankle sprain injury in collegiate male athletes. J Sci Med Sport. 2018;21(7):676–80. https://doi.org/10.1016/j.jsams.2017.10.014.
76. Murphy DF, Connolly DAJ, Beynnon BD. Risk factors for lower extremity injury: a review of the literature. Br J Sports Med. 2003;37(1):13–29. https://doi.org/10.1136/bjsm.37.1.13.
77. Wollin M, Thorborg K, Drew M, et al. A novel hamstring strain injury prevention system: post-match strength testing for secondary prevention in football.

Br J Sports Med. 2019:bjsports-2019-100707. https://doi.org/10.1136/bjsports-2019-100707.
78. Tassignon B, Verschueren J, Delahunt E, et al. Criteria-based return to sport decision-making following lateral ankle sprain injury: a systematic review and narrative synthesis. Sports Med. 2019;49(4):601–19. https://doi.org/10.1007/s40279-019-01071-3.
79. Lorenz D, Domzalski S. Criteria-based return to sprinting progression following lower extremity injury. Int J Sports Phys Ther. 2020;15(2):326–32.
80. Clanton TO, Matheny LM, Jarvis HC, et al. Return to play in athletes following ankle injuries. Sports Health. 2012;4(6):471–4. https://doi.org/10.1177/1941738112463347.
81. Kotsifaki A, Korakakis V, Whiteley R, et al. Measuring only hop distance during single leg hop testing is insufficient to detect deficits in knee function after ACL reconstruction: a systematic review and meta-analysis. Br J Sports Med. 2019; https://doi.org/10.1136/bjsports-2018-099918.
82. Batty LM, Feller JA, Hartwig T, et al. Single-leg squat performance and its relationship to extensor mechanism strength after anterior cruciate ligament reconstruction. Am J Sports Med. 2019;47(14):3423–8. https://doi.org/10.1177/0363546519878432.
83. Shrier I. Strategic assessment of risk and risk tolerance (StARRT) framework for return-to-play decision-making. Br J Sports Med. 2015;49(20):1311–5. https://doi.org/10.1136/bjsports-2014-094569.
84. Taylor HL, Henschel A, et al. Effects of bed rest on cardiovascular function and work performance. J Appl Physiol. 1949;2(5):223–39. https://doi.org/10.1152/jappl.1949.2.5.223.
85. Dittmer DK, Teasell R. Complications of immobilization and bed rest. Part 1: musculoskeletal and cardiovascular complications. Can Fam Physician. 1993;39:1428–37.
86. Joanisse S, Snijders T, Nederveen JP, et al. The impact of aerobic exercise on the muscle stem cell response. Exerc Sport Sci Rev. 2018;46(3):180–7. https://doi.org/10.1249/jes.0000000000000153.
87. Lisman PJ, de la Motte SJ, Gribbin TC, et al. A systematic review of the association between physical fitness and musculoskeletal injury risk: part 1-cardiorespiratory endurance. J Strength Cond Res. 2017;31(6):1744–57. https://doi.org/10.1519/jsc.0000000000001855.
88. Ote Karaca S, Demirsoy N, Gunendi Z. Effects of aerobic exercise on pain sensitivity, heart rate recovery, and health-related quality of life in patients with chronic musculoskeletal pain. Int J Rehabil Res. 2017;40(2):164–70. https://doi.org/10.1097/mrr.0000000000000212.
89. Kunz RI, Coradini JG, Silva LI, et al. Effects of immobilization and remobilization on the ankle joint in Wistar rats. Braz J Med Biol Res. 2014;47(10):842–9. https://doi.org/10.1590/1414-431x20143795.
90. Davies G, Riemann BL, Manske R. Current concepts of plyometric exercise. Int J Sports Phys Ther. 2015;10(6):760–86.
91. Verstegen M, Falsone S, Orr R, et al. Suggestions from the field for return to sports participation following anterior cruciate ligament reconstruction: American football. J Orthop Sports Phys Ther. 2012;42(4):337–44. https://doi.org/10.2519/jospt.2012.4031.
92. Myer GD, Schmitt LC, Brent JL, et al. Utilization of modified NFL combine testing to identify functional deficits in athletes following ACL reconstruction. J Orthop Sports Phys Ther. 2011;41(6):377–87. https://doi.org/10.2519/jospt.2011.3547.
93. Taberner M, Allen T, Cohen DD. Progressing rehabilitation after injury: consider the 'control-chaos continuum'. Br J Sports Med. 2019;53(18):1132. https://doi.org/10.1136/bjsports-2018-100157.
94. Gabbett TJ. Debunking the myths about training load, injury and performance: empirical evidence, hot topics and recommendations for practitioners. Br J Sports Med. 2018:bjsports-2018-099784. https://doi.org/10.1136/bjsports-2018-099784.
95. Impellizzeri FM, Marcora SM, Coutts AJ. Internal and external training load: 15 years on. Int J Sports Physiol Perform. 2019;14(2):270–3. https://doi.org/10.1123/ijspp.2018-0935.
96. Scanlan AT, Wen N, Tucker PS, et al. The relationships between internal and external training load models during basketball training. J Strength Cond Res. 2014;28(9):2397–405. https://doi.org/10.1519/jsc.0000000000000458.
97. O'Donoghue G, Cunningham C, Murphy F, et al. Assessment and management of risk factors for the prevention of lifestyle-related disease: a cross-sectional survey of current activities, barriers and perceived training needs of primary care physiotherapists in the Republic of Ireland. Physiotherapy. 2014;100(2):116–22. https://doi.org/10.1016/j.physio.2013.10.004.
98. Russell HC, Tracey J, Wiese-Bjornstal DM, et al. Physical activity in former competitive athletes: the physical and psychological impact of musculoskeletal injury. Quest. 2018;70(3):304–20. https://doi.org/10.1080/00336297.2017.1386114.
99. Rathleff MS, Mølgaard CM, Fredberg U, et al. High-load strength training improves outcome in patients with plantar fasciitis: a randomized controlled trial with 12-month follow-up. Scand J Med Sci Sports. 2015;25(3):e292–300. https://doi.org/10.1111/sms.12313.

6 Lateral Ankle Sprains: Injury Epidemiology and Nonoperative Treatment

Nasef Mohamed Nasef Abdelatif

Introduction

Acute ankle sprains are generally looked upon as one of the most commonly occurring orthopedic injuries. They occur more frequently in athletic populations but can also occur commonly in the general population. In addition, acute ankle sprains are notorious for their high rate of recurrence and can result in chronic ankle instability (CAI) with resultant ankle osteoarthrosis, degeneration, and debility. The combined liability of both acute ankle sprains and the possible long-term disabilities constitutes both financial and psychological burdens on the society as a whole. An understanding of the incidence and epidemiology of this very common injury and its sequalae might help in the improvement of patients' musculoskeletal well-being and reduce the burdens that this injury might generate.

N. M. N. Abdelatif (✉)
Orthopedic Foot and Ankle Reconstructive Surgery, DrNasef OrthoClinic Medical Center, Cairo, Egypt

Previously Orthopedics and Foot and Ankle Reconstructive Surgery, Bani Suef University, Bani Suef, Egypt
e-mail: wecare@drnasef.com

Overview and Incidence of Acute Ankle Sprains in the General Population

Acute ankle sprains are considered to be one of the most commonly occurring musculoskeletal injuries, and this incidence seems to be particularly high in physically active individuals [1–6]. It is estimated that in the United States of America (USA) alone, almost two million acute ankle sprains occur annually [1]. Sprains of the lateral ligament complex are the most commonly occurring sprains in the ankle [2, 3, 6–9]. Of these lateral ankle ligament complex sprains, it has been estimated that almost 73% are involving the anterior talofibular ligament [3, 7]. These are followed by calcaneofibular and, to lesser extent, the posterior talofibular ligaments [9, 10]. The remainder of the percentage is formed by the combined ratios of the deltoid ligament sprains or syndesmotic ligament injuries [11]. Emergency center data suggest that the incidence is approximately two to seven sprains per 1000 individuals [1, 3, 12]. However, that statistic in itself might be even considered an underestimate since not all individuals sustaining an acute ankle sprain might present to an emergency department or even seek medical care. This presentation to the emergency department has been found to be slightly different in different parts of the world. In Denmark, for example, it was reported to be ranging from 2.1 to 26.6 per 1000 persons [13],

P. D'Hooghe et al. (eds.), *Ligamentous Injuries of the Foot and Ankle*,
https://doi.org/10.1007/978-3-031-08682-3_6

while in the United Kingdom, another study reported this ratio to be 5.27 per 1000 individuals [14]. An interesting study performed in the Netherlands suggested that the true incidence of acute ankle sprains in the general population was 5.5 times higher than the data presented by the emergency departments [15]. Another study conducted in the USA suggested that over half of the patients presenting with acute ankle sprains were not actively participating in any sporting activity at the time of the injury, pointing to the fact that perhaps this injury might occur in a larger subset of individuals rather than just those with higher levels of activity or those individuals participating in active sports [1].

In a systematic review and meta-analysis of a more than 180 epidemiological studies of ankle sprains, it was reported that the incidence of acute ankle sprains is generally slightly higher in females (13.6–6.9 per 1000 people) [16]. Also, it seems that this incidence decreases with age as children demonstrated an incidence of 2.85 per 1000 exposures, adolescents 1.94 per 100 exposures, and adults 0.72 per 1000 exposures [16]. However, another article showed that the peak incidence might differ from females to males with the peak incidence reported as 10–14 years in females and 15–19 years in males [1].

It is apparent though that our true understanding of the incidence and epidemiology of ankle sprains in the general population is certainly lacking. This might be in part due to the limited data available and the extraction of this data from emergency departments or hospitals that might tend to receive the more higher grades of sprains, whereas the vast majority of individuals might not have sought any medical care for their injuries in the first place. Certainly, this is an area of research that could benefit from expanding the databases available and perhaps utilizing other records such as administrative data, primary care data, and general population surveys to name a few [17].

Incidence of Acute Ankle Sprains in the Athletic Population

Acute ankle sprains are common at all activity levels, ranging from recreational athletes to collegiate sports to elite competitions. Ankle sprain incidence in sports has been reported as between 0.324 and 9 per 1000 h of activity [16–19]. This variability is most likely due to different definitions of injury and of the examined population cohort. An incidence rate of 0.93 per 1000 athletic exposure (AE) has been reported in a meta-analysis, where the athletic exposure (AE) was defined as one athlete competing in one competition or in one practice [16]. In the USA in collegiate athletes, ankle sprains compromised approximately 15% of all injuries in this cohort [7, 20]. This was similar to the 15–17% reported for high school sports also in the USA [21]. When reviewing 15 different sports in the National Collegiate Athletic Association over a 15-year period, the incidence of acute ankle sprains ranged from 0.75 to 0.89 per 1000 athletic exposures. In comparison, anterior cruciate ligament injuries ranged from 0.11 to 0.17 per 1000 AEs, and concussions recorded a range of 0.15–0.41 per 1000 AEs [20]. Regarding high school sports, an interesting observation in one report was that the incidence of acute ankle sprains decreased from 4.6 per 10,000 AEs recorded in 2005–2006 to 3.1 per 10,000 AEs recorded in 2010–2011 [21].

A similar high incidence trend of acute ankle sprains was also observed in high-level competitive sporting activities. Acute ankle sprains were the most commonly reported injuries in the 2004 Olympic Games [22]. Similarly, ankle injuries were the most commonly reported injuries in international top-level football tournaments for the reported period between 1998 and 2012, with ankle sprains constituting 17% of all reported injuries [23].

High incidence rates of acute ankle sprains were also reported within the National Basketball Association (NBA) players, with an incidence of 3.2–3.5 per 1000 player games [24–26]. Comparatively, the next common injury was lumbar strain/spasm with an incidence of 1.1 per 1000 player games [25]. In another study performed on NBA players over a three-season period, ankle sprains were found to affect approximately 26% of players *each* season and accounted for a large proportion of missed games per season [27].

Equally, the incidence of acute ankle sprains in National Football League players was also high. Although an interesting point to note was that it seemed the incidence proportion for high ankle sprains or syndesmotic injuries was much higher than in other cohorts [28]. Syndesmotic sprains represented almost 40% of all ankle sprains in this specific population compared to 6% in other populations [11, 28]. A recent article looking at the incidence of lower extremity injuries in the NFL also reiterated the findings that acute ankle sprains were the second most common injuries sustained in this subset of athletes second to hamstring strains [29]. This study combined the NFL electronic health record database (EHR) with official NFL game statistics [29].

In Major League Baseball (MLB) players, it was similarly demonstrated that acute ankle sprains were the most commonly sustained injury and the one responsible for the most total missed days [30]. Recently, an epidemiological study carried out to assess leg and ankle injuries utilizing the recently implemented MLB Health and Injury Tracking system (HIT) also confirmed ankle sprains to be the second most common injury occurring in these subset of individuals (second only to "leg contusions") [31]. The collected data also pointed to the fact that anterior talofibular ligament injuries were the most common and resulted in the greatest number of total days missed, while injuries to the anterior tibiofibular ligament resulted in the greatest mean days missed [31].

Though reported to lesser degrees, but other less popular sports have also recorded similar high incidences of acute ankle sprains. For example, in high-level competing gymnastics during the Olympic Games, the most common diagnosis was also an ankle sprain compromising 14% of all injuries and 23% of time-loss injuries [32]. In English professional squash players, the majority of injuries were described as occurring around the ankle and heel (20.8%) [33].

These acute ankle sprain trends have also been similarly reported in other areas across the globe other than just the USA. A study of an English Premier League (EPL) club conducted over a 4-year period revealed that 20% of injuries were injuries of the foot and ankle with a resultant mean return to sport time of 54 days [34]. In a study examining Finnish basketball players, the ankle was the most commonly injured site with a percentage of 48%. Additionally, the number of recurrent injuries was high (28% of all injuries), and most of them were ankle sprains (35 of 44, 79%) [35]. Likewise, in a South Korean study conducted on the injuries sustained by youth soccer players, the ankle (26.6%) and knee joints (14.1%) were the most common sites of injury [36].

In addition to these specific individuals participating in particular sporting activities, other subsets of individuals exist that are also subjected to increased physical activities, such as the military personnel. In the USA, within active-duty military personnel, the incidence of acute ankle sprains was 58.3 injuries per 1000 person-years, which was much higher than the incidence reported in the general population [1, 11].

It might thus seem readily apparent upon comparing these rates in high-demand populations with the rates of ankle sprains in the general population that the incidence of these sprains is markedly higher in the high-demand population. However, similar to the drawbacks for general population data collection and analysis, the data among this cohort is also still largely lacking. Data collection from all levels of participation and across all types of sporting activity is urgently needed. In particular, the two ends of the spectrum within the athletic participation, namely the youth and the highly professional athletes, are significantly insufficient. The significance of these two particular groups is that the youth represent a majority and a larger percentage of the athletic population, while the professional high-level athletes represent more constant training and competitive conditions, and consequently, more reliable data could be extracted from this particular cohort and generalized upon other groups of athletes [17]. Another point worth noting is that most of the data already collected has focused on the more popular sporting activities and the more popular sporting teams, such as soccer, football, and basketball. More research is warranted for other athletic sporting activities.

Epidemiology of Ankle Sprain Reinjury Risk

When discussing the epidemiology of acute lateral ankle sprains, some authors agree that the high incidences reported are largely due to the frequency of reinjury following an initial acute sprain [7, 37]. Attenborough et al. in their systematic review stated that a large proportion of acute ankle sprains were actually recurrent. The incidences reported were 19% for soccer, 28% in basketball, 43% for American football, and 46% for volleyball [37]. Other investigators have reported ratios of 12%–47% [14, 34, 35, 38]. A single incident of a previous ankle sprain has been implicated to be one of the most important risk factors for developing another or recurrent lateral ankle sprains [5, 39, 40]. In a prospective study of almost 10,000 military cadets, individuals with a previous ankle sprain had an approximately 3.5 times increased risk of sustaining another ankle sprain than those with no previous history of sprains [41].

Similarly, it seems that the number of previous ankle sprains sustained by the athlete also plays a significant role. In recreational and elite basketball players in Australia, 73% had an ankle injury history, and their mean number of prior injuries was 3.5 with a standard deviation of 2.7 [5]. An epidemiological study carried out in China on athletes of different levels showed that 22% of all patients had sustained five or more prior sprains [42].

From the previous studies, it appears that acute, first time, and recurrent ankle sprains all play a role in the incidence rates of these populations, and consequently, these factors should be taken into consideration when planning injury prevention intervention protocols.

In spite of the fact that previous research has targeted the incidence of recurrence of ankle sprain injuries, research is still lacking when it comes to assessment of the time relation of that ankle sprain incident with the prediction of reinjury rates. Additionally, studies are also lacking regarding the correlation between severity of ankle sprain initial injuries and the development of long-term adverse effects as osteoarthrosis and chronic ankle instability (CAI) [17].

Epidemiology Related to Chronic Ankle Sprains

A major problem accompanying ankle injury is the high rate of recurrence associated with chronic ankle instability [9, 43]. Although the scope of this chapter is not chronic ankle sprains, however, due to the fact that chronic sprains can develop after a single ankle sprain, from repetitive injuries to the same anatomical structure or from other injury mechanisms [8, 37, 44], it would be therefore worthwhile to highlight briefly a few pertinent points regarding the epidemiology of chronic ankle sprains.

Recently, a review study showed that up to 70% of individuals sustaining an acute ankle sprain might be at risk for development of chronic ankle sprains within a short time following that injury [4]. Other investigators found a 40% prevalence of occurrence of a chronic ankle instability within 1 year following the initial acute ankle sprain although some critics might consider those percentages a continuum of symptoms and of disability duration [45]. A finding that has been reported with chronic ankle instability that is not so evident with acute ankle sprains is the higher prevalence in gymnastics and dancers than in other sports [4, 37]. When assessing CAI prevalence in high school and collegiate athletes, a higher incidence was discovered among females (32%) than males (17%) [46]. This same study found that the incidence was 31% among high school athletes compared to 19% within collegiate athletes. Another interesting fact was that almost two-thirds of the athletes suffering from chronic ankle instability (CAI) in that study did not report a prior ankle sprain [46].

The sheer proportions of individuals who later report chronic ankle instability or other disabilities following ankle sprains is a testament for further research to be conducted on this aspect. Studies such as the work of Doherty and coworkers should be expanded upon [45], and adequate screening tools to assess chronicity risk, and consequently prevention, should be further developed [17].

Injury Prevention

Injury prevention protocols focusing on improving biomechanics, increasing muscle strengthening, proprioception, and balancing have been shown to be beneficial for preventing musculoskeletal injuries and improving pain and dysfunction in patients following ankle sprains [47–54]. A randomized controlled study on multistation proprioceptive exercises caused a reduced rate of an ankle sprain injury by almost 65% compared to a control group [55]. Likewise, a 6-year prospective analysis of a proprioceptive exercise program showed a decrease of ankle sprains by 81% [56]. Similarly, other studies have also shown the effectiveness of proprioception and balance training programs in reducing risk of ankle sprains [49, 51, 54, 57, 58]. It is worthwhile to note that any of the studies proposed for injury prevention should not only investigate just the interventions proposed for reducing the injury incidence and severity. A cyclic four-step sequential approach to injury prevention has been proposed by van Mechelen et al. [59]. It describes the following steps: (1) identify the incidence and severity, (2) identify the causes of the injury, (3) introduce preventive measures, and (4) evaluate the effect of the proposed preventive measures [59]. Since acute ankle sprains occur across a wide distribution of the general population, future work should preferably measure injury prevention programs for modification and application among this general population.

Rehabilitation and adequate treatment after an initial ankle sprain might also act as an additional injury prevention program to prevent the recurrence of this injury. However, relatively limited data are available on the actual prevention of these recurrent injuries [60]. Additionally, prevention proposals to reduce the likelihood of progression to posttraumatic osteoarthritis are also urgently needed to reduce the long-term consequences of these injuries, and the possibly initial step toward progress in this area is the continuous scrutiny of the pathway from initial ankle sprain till posttraumatic osteoarthritis.

Nonoperative Management of Acute Ankle Sprains

The annual cost of ankle sprain management has been estimated to be just over 30 million US dollars per 1 million people [61]. The cost of treating an ankle sprain varies from 360 Euros [62] to 1100 Euros [63] per individual. In addition to this short-term burden, the possibility of developing long-term chronic conditions and complications also exists leading to further added costs.

Furthermore, as stated previously, this injury is one of the most commonly occurring musculoskeletal injuries seen in the emergency department. The socioeconomic burdens of the injury itself and its management are tremendous both financially and in terms of sick leaves and days away from work [4, 8]. It might therefore come as a slight surprise that in spite of these facts, in actuality, the initial management of acute ankle sprains is still not yet scientifically validated or proven [64]. It is apparent therefore that optimized management strategies and prevention will provide both economic benefits to the society as a whole, in addition to favorable clinical effects for the patients themselves.

Perhaps the most commonly used therapy applied in the initial treatment of acute ankle sprains is referred to as *RICE management*, namely rest, ice, compression, and elevation. A systematic review article performed by van den Bekerom and coworkers in 2012 actually showed that there was insufficient evidence from the collected randomized control studies to determine the effectiveness of each of these criteria in the initial treatment of acute ankle sprains [64]. Also, several studies have tried to determine the best methods of management of acute ankle sprains including several Cochrane reviews [65–68]. A recently conducted study also confirmed most of the statements described by van den Bekerom and colleagues [69]. Specifically, the following recommendations were stated.

Regarding RICE only, cryotherapy, or compression therapy alone, no evidence has been proven that these factors have a positive impact on pain, swelling, or function of patients following an acute ankle sprain [69].

Regarding *nonsteroidal anti-inflammatory drugs*, although they are commonly prescribed, however, likewise, there is no strong evidence to support its usage. Actually, level 2 evidence might suggest that care should be taken with the prescription of such drugs due to the complications associated with the intake, and additionally, they might actually delay the healing process [69].

Another important method of management is *immobilization*, or the lack of immobilization and, actually, mobility and exercise. It has been found that a period of 4 weeks or more of immobilization would result in less favorable outcomes than functional support and exercise [68, 70]. Consequently, the recommendations are if immobilization is to be applied, it should be only for short periods of time, and generally not exceeding 10 days, and after which functional therapy should be commenced immediately [69, 71, 72].

Functional supports in the form of ankle braces or ankle tape have been frequently used following ankle sprains. These have been found to be much more effective than rigid immobilization or other less adequate items as compression bandages [71, 73]. Superiority of one form of bracing over another has been extensively debated in literature [74–76]. A meta-analysis showed that a lace-up brace is superior to elastic bandage [68] and showed better results when compared with other types of functional support [69].

Similarly, *exercise programs* have been an important part of acute ankle sprain initial managements. These include neuromuscular and proprioceptive exercise protocols. It has been found that if initiated early, these exercise programs can reduce the recurrence of these injuries and even decrease the occurrence of functional ankle instability [77–80]. However, there is still contradictory evidence regarding whether or not these exercise programs should be supervised or not [69, 81].

Another useful management method is *manual mobilization* specially to allow for short-term increase in ankle dorsiflexion range of motion [78, 82]. Additionally, when combined with exercise programs, manual therapy has been shown to generate better results than exercise alone [83].

Various *other treatment modalities* have been suggested for the management of acute ankle sprains. However, generally, no effect on pain, edema, function, or return to activities has been documented for ultrasound [66, 67], laser therapy [84], electrotherapy [85], or shock wave therapy [86] in the management of acute ankle sprains. More recently, other modalities have been described. Acupuncture has conflicting reports, and thus, the evidence is inconclusive [87, 88]. Vibration therapy was reported to be beneficial in increasing dorsiflexion and eversion and reducing ankle stiffness [89]. Bioptron light therapy was also combined with cryotherapy in another study and was reported to be beneficial also [90]. However, these are still all lacking in strong evidence and thus still not recommended for acute ankle sprain treatment [69].

In light of all the previous data, it seems that peer-reviewed scientific data in the management of acute ankle sprains supports the utilization of progressive weight-bearing with or without very short periods of immobilization, if and when needed, as the treatment of choice [91, 92]. This is also the author's current preferred management protocol, namely RICE management under analgesic coverage for first few days to reduce pain and to enhance motion and progressive weight-bearing supplemented with a regimen of exercise-based rehabilitation (Figs. 6.1, 6.2, 6.3, 6.4, 6.5 and 6.6) whether supervised or home based. As has been previously stated, there are still no clear-cut guidelines on whether these exercise protocols should be supervised or not [69, 81]. Recently, a high-quality randomized controlled study showed that supervised rehabilitation had no value over standard care [93] even though that contradicts other level 1 studies

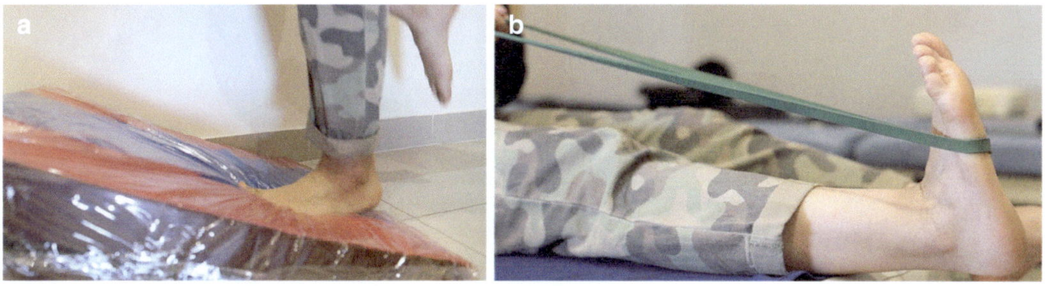

Fig. 6.1 Achilles stretching exercises, active (**a**) and passive (**b**)

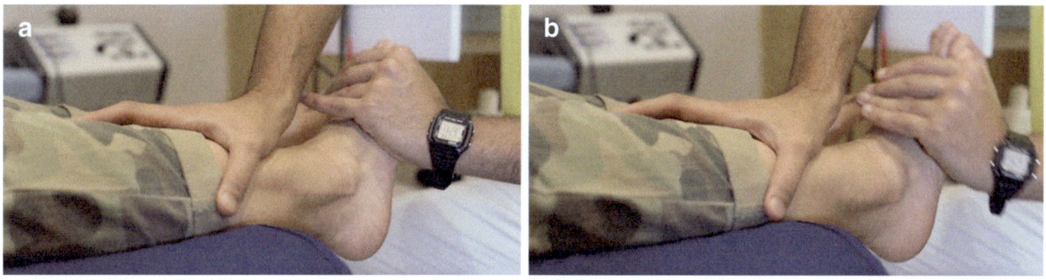

Fig. 6.2 Manually applied perturbation resisting inversion (**a**) and plantarflexion (**b**) by moving ankle into eversion and dorsiflexion

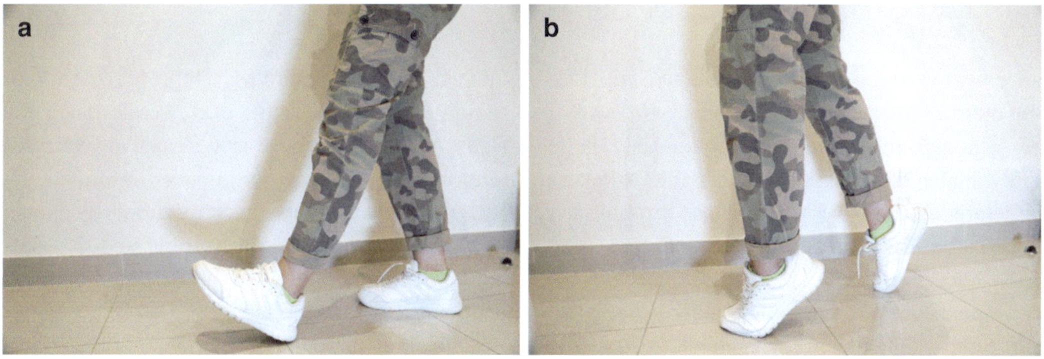

Fig. 6.3 Walking on heels (**a**) and toes (**b**) to assess ability to bear weight and maintain balance

on the same issue [94]. In fact, it seems that to date, there is still no consensus on the optimal exercise programs or content of these exercise rehabilitation protocols for the management of acute ankle sprains [95], and that is certainly another area that warrants extensive and meticulous research.

Generally, the goals of physiotherapy exercise treatment protocols should be to control the inflammatory process, regain full range of motion (ROM), and improve muscle strength and power while maintaining and improving proprioceptive abilities. The acronym POLICE (protection, optimal loading, ice compression, and elevation) has been used within the first 24–72 h after sustaining an ankle sprain [96]. Early functional rehabilitation should include ROM and isometric and isotonic strength training exercises [97]. Strengthening of the muscles would ensure a more rapid recovery as well as reduce further reinjury incidences [98]. Additionally, other authors have concluded that proprioceptive bal-

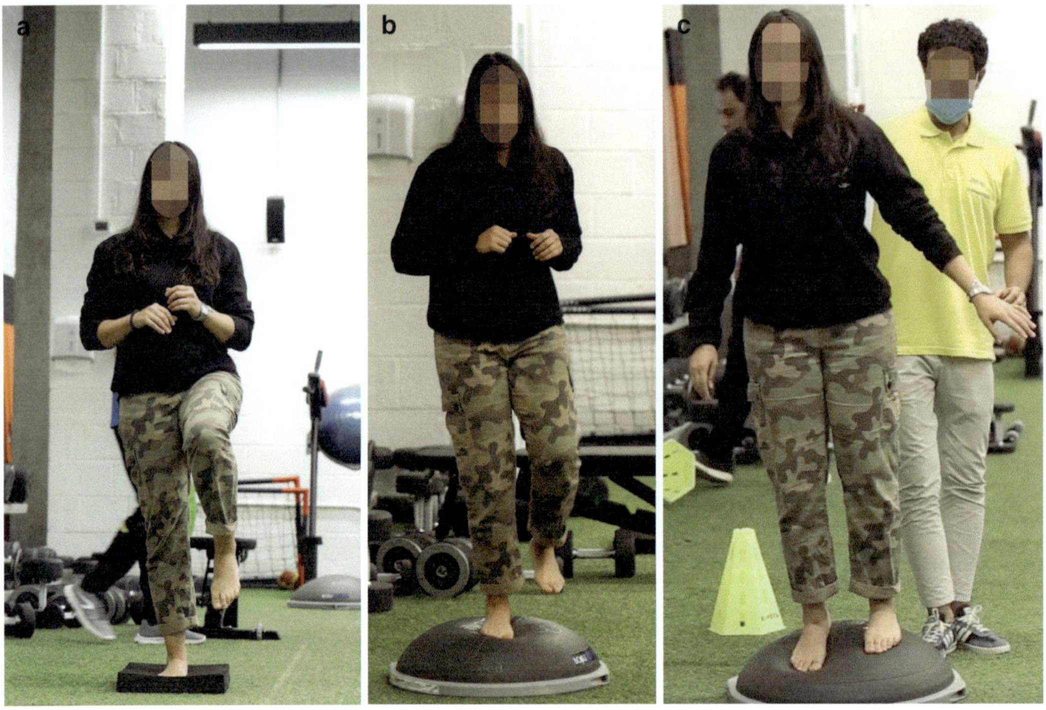

Fig. 6.4 Balance exercises done with different surfaces and with eyes open or closed (**a** and **b**) and gradually progressed to resisting externally generated stimuli (**c**)

ance board exercises are also effective in reducing these reinjury incidences [99].

Although rehabilitation programs are better individualized, yet it is also valuable to have a structured and progressive exercise program as a general baseline guide for treatment of acute ankle sprains.

Generally, once pain and swelling have subsided and ROM has been regained, one is ready to proceed to the *strengthening phase of rehabilitation*. It has been advised to concentrate on the peroneal muscle group during this stage of muscle strengthening as the relative weakness of this group has been associated with a higher incidence of recurrence and CAI [98]. However, all muscle groups and *both* sides should be targeted equally. Achilles tendon stretching exercises are also an important component of this phase (Fig. 6.1). Strengthening exercises begin with isometric against immobile objects in all directions of ankle motion and progress to dynamic resistive exercises using weights or rubber bands [97]. These same authors prefer clinician-assisted manual resistive exercises (Fig. 6.2). Another option for these resistive exercises is using the Daily Adjustable Progressive Resistive Exercises (DAPRE) that were originally described by Knight [100] and then later modified by Perrin and Gieck [101]. It has been suggested that during these exercises, the emphasis should be more on the eccentric component [102].

Once the patient is able to ambulate pain-free, and perhaps on both toes and heels (Fig. 6.3), one can then commence to the *proprioceptive and balance control phase of rehabilitation exercises*. The simplest and perhaps most commonly used for this is the wobble board device [103]. Balancing exercises can be progressed from non-weight-bearing to weight-bearing, from bilateral stance to unilateral stance, from eyes open to eyes closed, from firm to softer surfaces, and from stable even surfaces to uneven mobile surfaces (Fig. 6.4). These exercises would then be progressed to dynamic activities while maintaining balance and stability (Fig. 6.5).

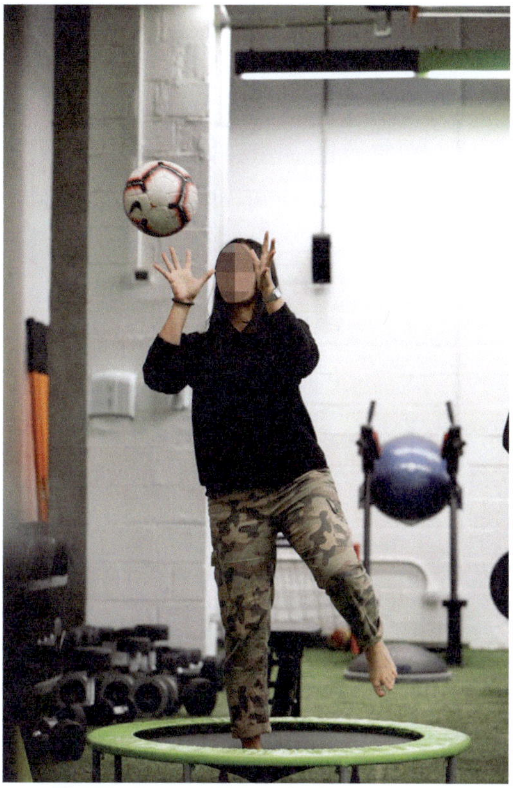

Fig. 6.5 Advanced balancing and functional exercises with performance of dynamic activities

During this stage, the presiding physiotherapist could alter the surrounding medium and the degree of resistance while performing these activities such as the utilization of water medium as pools or hydrotherapy (Fig. 6.6). This water resistance could also be increased by using turbine-driven water resistance forces. The variation of media and resistance forces can be quite varied.

The final rehabilitation stage would then be progression to *activity-specific rehabilitative exercises* [97]. This would probably commence when the subject could be able to walk for distances and is not limited by any pain. Hence, running and jogging could then be initiated. Additionally, backward running, pattern running, circles and figure-of-eight jogging, and jumping could be then employed. Naturally, the final phase of rehabilitation would be the ability to perform sport-specific exercises without pain and at intensity levels comparable to the patient's pre-injury state.

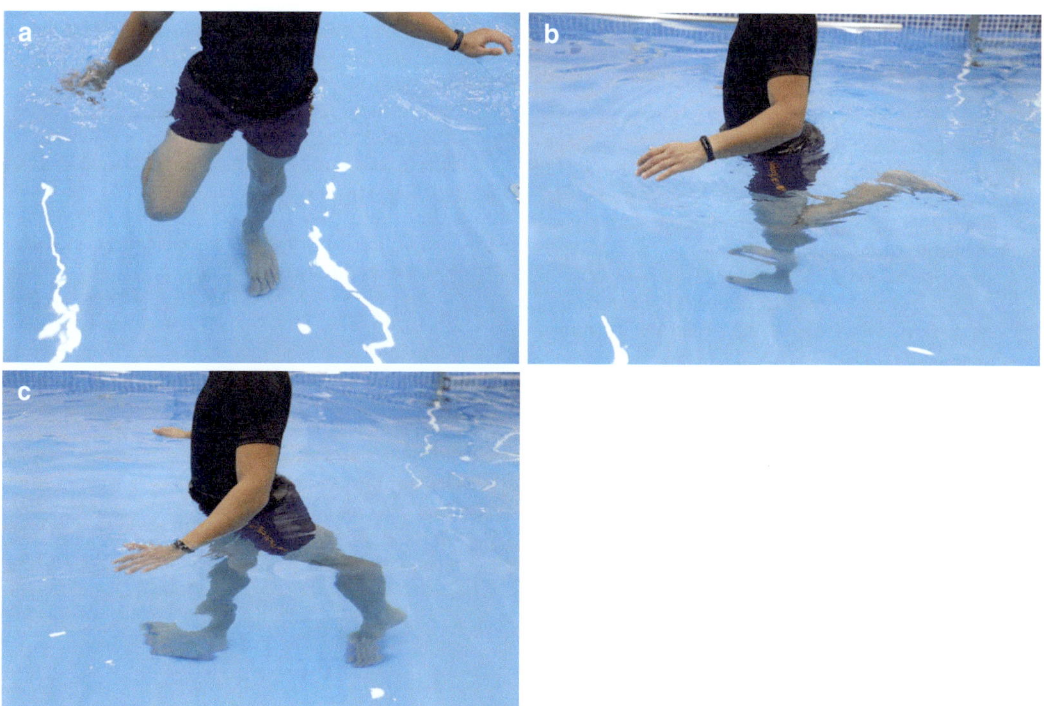

Fig. 6.6 Water exercises without resistance (**a**), with resistance (**b**), and functional exercises (**c**)

Conclusion

Acute ankle sprains are one of the most commonly occurring musculoskeletal injuries. The incidence of these injuries might vary slightly from the general population to the athletic population and indeed might even vary more in sport-specific activities. These injuries and more so the complications or long-term sequelae associated with them might pose a significant socioeconomic burden on the society. One should be aware of the proper management protocols for treating such common injuries and should closely follow up those patients at risk of development of these complications. In the immediate management of acute ankle sprains, generally the protocol consists of rest, protected mobilization, ice, and elevation and then progresses gradually through structured physiotherapy and exercise programs to sport-specific exercises and rehabilitation. It should be noted, however, that the exact specific exercises, duration, repetitions, and sequence of these protocols are yet to be scientifically validated.

References

1. Waterman BR, Owens BD, Davey S, Zacchilli MA, Belmont PJ Jr. The epidemiology of ankle sprains in the United States. J Bone Joint Surg Am. 2010;92(13):2279–84.
2. Cumps E, Verhagen E, Meeusen R. Prospective epidemiological study of basketball injuries during one competitive season: ankle sprains and overuse knee injuries. J Sports Sci Med. 2007;6(2):204–11.
3. Fong DT, Hong Y, Chan LK, Yung PS, Chan KM. A systematic review on ankle injury and ankle sprain in sports. Sports Med. 2007;37(1):73–94.
4. Gribble PA, Bleakley CM, Caulfield BM, Docherty CL, Fourchet F, Fong DT, Hertel J, Hiller CE, Kaminski TW, McKeon PO, Refshauge KM, Verhagen EA, Vicenzino BT, Wikstrom EA, Delahunt E. Evidence review for the 2016 international ankle consortium consensus statement on the prevalence, impact and long-term consequences of lateral ankle sprains. Br J Sports Med. 2016;50(24):1496–505.
5. McKay GD, Goldie PA, Payne WR, Oakes BW. Ankle injuries in basketball: injury rate and risk factors. Br J Sports Med. 2001;35(2):103–8.
6. Nelson AJ, Collins CL, Yard EE, Fields SK, Comstock RD. Ankle injuries among United States high school sports athletes, 2005–2006. J Athl Train. 2007;42(3):381–7.
7. Roos KG, Kerr ZY, Mauntel TC, Djoko A, Dompier TP, Wikstrom EA. The epidemiology of lateral ligament complex ankle sprains in National Collegiate Athletic Association sports. Am J Sports Med. 2017;45(1):201–9.
8. Gribble PA, Bleakley CM, Caulfield BM, Docherty CL, Fourchet F, Fong DT, Hertel J, Hiller CE, Kaminski TW, McKeon PO, Refshauge KM, Verhagen EA, Vicenzino BT, Wikstrom EA, Delahunt E. 2016 consensus statement of the International Ankle Consortium: prevalence, impact and long-term consequences of lateral ankle sprains. Br J Sports Med. 2016;50(24):1493–5.
9. Waterman BR, Belmont PJ Jr, Cameron KL, Deberardino TM, Owens BD. Epidemiology of ankle sprain at the United States Military Academy. Am J Sports Med. 2010;38(4):797–803.
10. Hertel J. Functional anatomy pathomechanics and pathophysiology of lateral instability. J Athl Train. 2002;37:364–75.
11. Waterman BR, Belmont PJ Jr, Cameron KL, Svoboda SJ, Alitz CJ, Owens BD. Risk factors for syndesmotic and medial ankle sprain: role of sex, sport, and level of competition. Am J Sports Med. 2011;39(5):992–8.
12. Shah S, Thomas AC, Noone JM, Blanchette CM, Wikstrom EA. Incidence and cost of ankle sprains in United States Emergency Departments. Sports Health. 2016;8(6):547–52.
13. Holmer P, Sondergaard L, Kondradsen L, Nielsen PT, Jørgensen LN. Epidemiology of sprains in the lateral ankle and foot. Foot Ankle Int. 1994;15(2):72–4.
14. Bridgman SA, Clement D, Downing A, Walley G, Phair I, Maffulli N. Population based epidemiology of ankle sprains attending accident and emergency units in the West Midlands of England, and a survey of UK practice for severe ankle sprains. Emerg Med J. 2003;20(6):508–10.
15. Kemler E, van de Port I, Valkenberg H, Hoes AW, Backx FJ. Ankle injuries in the Netherlands: trends over 10–25 years. Scand J Med Sci Sports. 2015;25(3):331–7.
16. Doherty C, Delahunt E, Caulfield B, Hertel J, Ryan J, Bleakley C. The incidence and prevalence of ankle sprain injury: a systematic review and meta-analysis of prospective epidemiological studies. Sports Med. 2014;44(1):123–40.
17. Herzog MM, Kerr ZY, Marshall SW, Wikstrom EA. Epidemiology of ankle sprains and chronic ankle instability. J Athl Train. 2019;54(6):603–10. https://doi.org/10.4085/1062-6050-447-17.
18. Cloke DJ, Ansell P, Avery P, Deehan D. Ankle injuries in football academies: a three-centre prospective study. Br J Sports Med. 2011;45(9):702–8.

19. Giza E, Fuller C, Junge A, Dvorak J. Mechanisms of foot and ankle injuries in soccer. Am J Sports Med. 2003;31(4):550–4.
20. Hootman JM, Dick R, Agel J. Epidemiology of collegiate injuries for 15 sports: summary and recommendations for injury prevention initiatives. J Athl Train. 2007;42(2):311–9.
21. Swenson DM, Collins CL, Fields SK, Comstock RD. Epidemiology of U.S. high school sports-related ligamentous ankle injuries, 2005/06–2010/11. Clin J Sport Med. 2013;23(3):190–6.
22. Junge A, Langevoort G, Pipe A, Peytavin A, Wong F, Mountjoy M, Beltrami G, Terrell R, Holzgraefe M, Charles R, Dvorak J. Injuries in team sport tournaments during the 2004 Olympic Games. Am J Sports Med. 2006;34(4):565–76.
23. Junge A, Dvorak J. Injury surveillance in the World Football Tournaments 1998-2012. Br J Sports Med. 2013;47(12):782–8. https://doi.org/10.1136/bjsports-2013-092205.
24. Deitch JR, Starkey C, Walters SL, Moseley JB. Injury risk in professional basketball players: a comparison of Women's National Basketball Association and National Basketball Association athletes. Am J Sports Med. 2006;34(7):1077–83.
25. Drakos MC, Domb B, Starkey C, Callahan L, Allen AA. Injury in the National Basketball Association: a 17-year overview. Sports Health. 2010;2(4):284–90.
26. Starkey C. Injuries and illnesses in the National Basketball Association: a 10-year perspective. J Athl Train. 2000;35(2):161–7.
27. Herzog MM, Mack CD, Dreyer NA, Wikstrom EA, Padua DA, Kocher MS, DiFiori JP, Marshall SW. Ankle sprains in the National Basketball Association, 2013-2014 through 2016-2017. Am J Sports Med. 2019;47(11):2651–8. https://doi.org/10.1177/0363546519864678.
28. Osbahr DC, Drakos MC, O'Loughlin PF, et al. Syndesmosis and lateral ankle sprains in the National Football League. Orthopedics. 2013;36(11):1378–84.
29. Mack CD, Kent RW, Coughlin MJ, Shiue KY, Weiss LJ, Jastifer JR, Wojtys EM, Anderson RB. Incidence of lower extremity injury in the National Football League: 2015 to 2018. Am J Sports Med. 2020;48(9):2287–94. https://doi.org/10.1177/0363546520922547.
30. Camp CL, Dines JS, van der List JP, Conte S, Conway J, Altchek DW, Coleman SH, Pearle AD. Summative report on time out of play for major and minor league baseball: an analysis of 49,955 injuries from 2011 through 2016. Am J Sports Med. 2018;46(7):1727–32.
31. Lucasti CJ, Dworkin M, Warrender WJ, Winters B, Cohen S, Ciccotti M, Pedowitz D. Ankle and lower leg injuries in professional baseball players. Am J Sports Med. 2020;48(4):908–15. https://doi.org/10.1177/0363546520902135.
32. Edouard P, Steffen K, Junge A, Leglise M, Soligard T, Engebretsen L. Gymnastics injury incidence during the 2008, 2012 and 2016 Olympic Games: analysis of prospectively collected surveillance data from 963 registered gymnasts during Olympic Games. Br J Sports Med. 2018;52(7):475–81.
33. Horsley Dr IG, O'Donnell V, Leeder J. The epidemiology of injuries in English professional squash; a retrospective analysis between 2004 and 2015. Phys Ther Sport. 2020;46:1–6. https://doi.org/10.1016/j.ptsp.2020.07.009.
34. Jain N, Murray D, Kemp S, Calder J. Frequency and trends in foot and ankle injuries within an English Premier League Football Club using a new impact factor of injury to identify a focus for injury prevention. Foot Ankle Surg. 2014;20:237–40.
35. Pasanen K, Ekola T, Vasankari T, Kannus P, Heinonen A, Kujala UM, Parkkari J. High ankle injury rate in adolescent basketball: a 3-year prospective follow-up study. Scand J Med Sci Sports. 2017;27(6):643–9.
36. Lee I, Jeong HS, Lee SY. Injury profiles in Korean youth soccer. Int J Environ Res Public Health. 2020;17(14):5125. https://doi.org/10.3390/ijerph17145125.
37. Attenborough AS, Hiller CE, Smith RM, Stuelcken M, Greene A, Sinclair PJ. Chronic ankle instability in sporting populations. Sports Med. 2014;44(11):1545–56.
38. Kemler E, Thijs KM, Badenbroek I, van de Port IG, Hoes AW, Backx FJ. Long-term prognosis of acute lateral ankle ligamentous sprains: high incidence of recurrences and residual symptoms. Fam Pract. 2016;33(6):596–600.
39. Beynnon BD, Murphy DF, Alosa DM. Predictive factors for lateral ankle sprains: a literature review. J Athl Train. 2002;37(4):376–80.
40. Clifton DR, Koldenhoven RM, Hertel J, Onate JA, Dompier TP, Kerr ZY. Epidemiological patterns of ankle sprains in youth, high school, and college football. Am J Sports Med. 2017;45(2):417–25.
41. Kucera KL, Marshall SW, Wolf SH, Padua DA, Cameron KL, Beutler AI. Association of injury history and incident injury in cadet basic military training. Med Sci Sports Exerc. 2016;48(6):1053–61.
42. Yeung MS, Chan KM, So CH, Yuan WY. An epidemiological survey on ankle sprain. Br J Sports Med. 1994;28(2):112–6.
43. Woods C, Hawkins R, Hulse M, Hodson A. The Football Association Medical Research Programme: an audit of injuries in professional football: an analysis of ankle sprains. Br J Sports Med. 2003;37(3):233–2388.
44. Thompson C, Schabrun S, Romero R, Bialocerkowski A, van Dieen J, Marshall P. Factors contributing to chronic ankle instability: a systematic review and meta-analysis of systematic reviews. Sports Med. 2018;48(1):189–205.
45. Doherty C, Bleakley C, Hertel J, Caulfield B, Ryan J, Delahunt E. Recovery from a first-time lateral ankle sprain and the predictors of chronic ankle instability:

a prospective cohort analysis. Am J Sports Med. 2016;44(4):995–1003.
46. Tanen L, Docherty CL, Van Der Pol B, Simon J, Schrader J. Prevalence of chronic ankle instability in high school and division I athletes. Foot Ankle Spec. 2014;7(1):37–44.
47. Baydogan SN, Tarakci E, Kasapcopur O. Effect of strengthening versus balance-proprioceptive exercises on lower extremity function in patients with juvenile idiopathic arthritis: a randomized, single blind clinical trial. Am J Phys Med Rehabil. 2015;94(6):417–24.
48. Collins NJ, Bisset LM, Crossley KM, Vicenzino B. Efficacy of nonsurgical interventions for anterior knee pain: systematic review and meta-analysis of randomized trials. Sports Med. 2012;42(1):31–49.
49. Emery CA, Rose MS, McAllister JR, Meeuwisse WH. A prevention strategy to reduce the incidence of injury in high school basketball: a cluster randomized controlled trial. Clin J Sport Med. 2007;17(1):17–24.
50. Hewett TE, Lindenfeld TN, Riccobene JV, Noyes FR. The effect of neuromuscular training on the incidence of knee injury in female athletes. A prospective study. Am J Sports Med. 1999;27(6):699–706.
51. LaBella CR, Huxford MR, Grissom J, Kim KY, Peng J, Christoffel KK. Effect of neuromuscular warm-up on injuries in female soccer and basketball athletes in urban public high schools: cluster randomized controlled trial. Arch Pediatr Adolesc Med. 2011;165(11):1033–40.
52. Longo UG, Loppini M, Berton A, Marinozzi A, Maffulli N, Denaro V. The FIFA 11 program is effective in preventing injuries in elite male basketball players: a cluster randomized controlled trial. Am J Sports Med. 2012;40(5):996–1005.
53. Rathleff MS, Roos EM, Olesen JL, Rasmussen S. Exercise during school hours when added to patient education improves outcome for 2 years in adolescent patellofemoral pain: a cluster randomized trial. Br J Sports Med. 2015;49(6):406–12.
54. Taylor JB, Ford KR, Nguyen AD, Terry LN, Hegedus EJ. Prevention of lower extremity injuries in basketball: a systematic review and meta-analysis. Sports Health. 2015;7(5):392–8.
55. Eils E, Schroter R, Schr¨oder M, Gerss J, Rosenbaum D. Multistation proprioceptive exercise program prevents ankle injuries in basketball. Med Sci Sports Exerc. 2010;42(11):2098–105.
56. Riva D, Bianchi R, Rocca F, Mamo C. Proprioceptive training and injury prevention in a professional men's basketball team: a six-year prospective study. J Strength Cond Res. 2016;30(2):461–75.
57. Hupperets MD, Verhagen EA, Heymans MW, Bosmans JE, van Tulder MW, van Mechelen W. Potential savings of a program to prevent ankle sprain recurrence: economic evaluation of a randomized controlled trial. Am J Sports Med. 2010;38(11):2194–200.
58. McGuine TA, Keene JS. The effect of a balance training program on the risk of ankle sprains in high school athletes. Am J Sports Med. 2006;34(7):1103–11.
59. van Mechelen W, Hlobil H, Kemper HC. Incidence, severity, aetiology and prevention of sports injuries. A review of concepts. Sports Med. 1992;14(2):82–99.
60. McKeon PO, Hertel J. Systematic review of postural control and lateral ankle instability, part I: can deficits be detected with instrumented testing? J Athl Train. 2008;43(3):293–304.
61. Zeegers AVCM. Supination injury of the ankle joint [dissertation]. Utrecht, The Netherlands: University of Utrecht; 1995.
62. Verhagen EA, van Tulder M, van der Beek AJ, Bouter LM, van Mechelen W. An economic evaluation of a proprioceptive balance board training programme for the prevention of ankle sprains in volleyball. Br J Sports Med. 2005;39(2):111–5.
63. Cooke MW, Marsh JL, Clark M, Nakash R, Jarvis RM, Hutton JL, Szczepura A, Wilson S, Lamb SE, CAST trial group. Treatment of severe ankle sprain: a pragmatic randomised controlled trial comparing the clinical effectiveness and cost-effectiveness of three types of mechanical ankle support with tubular bandage. The CAST trial. Health Technol Assess. 2009;13(13):iii, ix-x, 1-121
64. van den Bekerom MP, Struijs PA, Blankevoort L, Welling L, van Dijk CN, Kerkhoffs GM. What is the evidence for rest, ice, compression, and elevation therapy in the treatment of ankle sprains in adults? J Athl Train. 2012;47(4):435–43.
65. Kim TH, Lee MS, Kim KH, Kang JW, Choi TY, Ernst E. Acupuncture for treating acute ankle sprains in adults. Cochrane Database Syst Rev. 2014;6:1.
66. Van der Windt D, Van der Heijden G, Van den Berg S, Ter Riet G, De Winter AF, Bouter LM. Ultrasound therapy for acute ankle sprains. Cochrane Database Syst Rev. 2002;1:1.
67. van den Bekerom MP, van der Windt DA, ter Riet G, van der Heijden GJ, Bouter LM. Therapeutic ultrasound for acute ankle sprains. Cochrane Database Syst Rev. 2011;6:325.
68. Kerkhoffs G, Rowe BH, Assendelft W, Kelly K, Struijs P, Van Dijk C. Immobilisation and functional treatment for acute lateral ankle ligament injuries in adults. Cochrane Database Syst Rev. 2002;3:3.
69. Vuurberg G, Hoorntje A, Wink LM, van der Doelen BFW, van den Bekerom MP, Dekker R, van Dijk CN, Krips R, Loogman MCM, Ridderikhof ML, Smithuis FF, Stufkens SAS, Verhagen EALM, de Bie RA, Kerkhoffs GMMJ. Diagnosis, treatment and prevention of ankle sprains: update of an evidence-based clinical guideline. Br J Sports Med. 2018;52(15):956.
70. Naeem M, Rahimnajjad MK, Rahimnajjad NA, et al. Assessment of functional treatment versus plaster of Paris in the treatment of grade 1 and 2 lateral ankle sprains. J Orthop Traumatol. 2015;16:41–6.
71. Prado MP, Mendes AA, Amodio DT, Camanho GL, Smyth NA, Fernandes TD. A comparative,

prospective, and randomized study of two conservative treatment protocols for first-episode lateral ankle ligament injuries. Foot Ankle Int. 2014;35(3):201–6.
72. Bilgic S, Durusu M, Aliyev B, Akpancar S, Ersen O, Yasar SM, Ardic S. Comparison of two main treatment modalities for acute ankle sprain. Pak J Med Sci. 2015;31(6):1496–9.
73. Pijnenburg AC, Van Dijk CN, Bossuyt PM, Marti RK. Treatment of ruptures of the lateral ankle ligaments: a meta-analysis. J Bone Joint Surg Am. 2000;82(6):761–73.
74. Kerkhoffs GM, Struijs PA, Marti RK, Assendelft WJ, Blankevoort L, van Dijk CN. Different functional treatment strategies for acute lateral ankle ligament injuries in adults. Cochrane Database Syst Rev. 2002;(3):CD002938; Update in: Cochrane Database Syst Rev. 2013;3:CD002938
75. van den Bekerom MP, van Kimmenade R, Sierevelt IN, Eggink K, Kerkhoffs GM, van Dijk CN, Raven EE. Randomized comparison of tape versus semi-rigid and versus lace-up ankle support in the treatment of acute lateral ankle ligament injury. Knee Surg Sports Traumatol Arthrosc. 2016;24(4):978–84.
76. Kemler E, van de Port I, Schmikli S, Huisstede B, Hoes A, Backx F. Effects of soft bracing or taping on a lateral ankle sprain: a non-randomised controlled trial evaluating recurrence rates and residual symptoms at one year. J Foot Ankle Res. 2015;8:13.
77. Zech A, Hübscher M, Vogt L, Banzer W, Hänsel F, Pfeifer K. Neuromuscular training for rehabilitation of sports injuries: a systematic review. Med Sci Sports Exerc. 2009;41(10):1831–41.
78. van der Wees PJ, Lenssen AF, Hendriks EJ, Stomp DJ, Dekker J, de Bie RA. Effectiveness of exercise therapy and manual mobilisation in ankle sprain and functional instability: a systematic review. Aust J Physiother. 2006;52(1):27–37.
79. Bleakley CM, McDonough SM, MacAuley DC. Some conservative strategies are effective when added to controlled mobilisation with external support after acute ankle sprain: a systematic review. Aust J Physiother. 2008;54(1):7–20.
80. Postle K, Pak D, Smith TO. Effectiveness of proprioceptive exercises for ankle ligament injury in adults: a systematic literature and meta-analysis. Man Ther. 2012;17(4):285–91.
81. Feger MA, Herb CC, Fraser JJ, Glaviano N, Hertel J. Supervised rehabilitation versus home exercise in the treatment of acute ankle sprains: a systematic review. Clin Sports Med. 2015;34(2):329–46.
82. Loudon JK, Reiman MP, Sylvain J. The efficacy of manual joint mobilization/manipulation in treatment of lateral ankle sprains: a systematic review. Br J Sports Med. 2014;48:365–70.
83. Cleland JA, Mintken PE, McDevitt A, Bieniek ML, Carpenter KJ, Kulp K, Whitman JM. Manual physical therapy and exercise versus supervised home exercise in the management of patients with inversion ankle sprain: a multicenter randomized clinical trial. J Orthop Sports Phys Ther. 2013;43(7):443–55.
84. de Bie RA, de Vet HC, Lenssen TF, van den Wildenberg FA, Kootstra G, Knipschild PG. Low-level laser therapy in ankle sprains: a randomized clinical trial. Arch Phys Med Rehabil. 1998;79(11):1415–20.
85. Feger MA, Goetschius J, Love H, Saliba SA, Hertel J. Electrical stimulation as a treatment intervention to improve function, edema or pain following acute lateral ankle sprains: a systematic review. Phys Ther Sport. 2015;16(4):361–9.
86. Barker AT, Barlow PS, Porter J. A double-blind clinical trial of lower power pulsed shortwave therapy in the treatment of a soft tissue injury. Phys Ther. 1985;71:500–4.
87. Park J, Hahn S, Park JY, Park HJ, Lee H. Acupuncture for ankle sprain: systematic review and meta-analysis. BMC Complement Altern Med. 2013;13:55.
88. Kim TH, Lee MS, Kim KH, Kang JW, Choi TY, Ernst E. Acupuncture for treating acute ankle sprains in adults. Cochrane Database Syst Rev. 2014;(6):CD009065. https://doi.org/10.1002/14651858.CD009065.pub2.
89. Peer KS, Barkley JE, Knapp DM. The acute effects of local vibration therapy on ankle sprain and hamstring strain injuries. Phys Sportsmed. 2009;37(4):31–8.
90. Stasinopoulos D, Papadopoulos C, Lamnisos D, Stasinopoulos I. The use of Bioptron light (polarized, polychromatic, non-coherent) therapy for the treatment of acute ankle sprains. Disabil Rehabil. 2017;39(5):450–7.
91. van den Bekerom MP, Kerkhoffs GM, McCollum GA, Calder JD, van Dijk CN. Management of acute lateral ankle ligament injury in the athlete. Knee Surg Sports Traumatol Arthrosc. 2013;21:1390–5.
92. Kerkhoffs GM, van den Bekerom M, Elders LA, van Beek PA, Hullegie WA, Bloemers GM, de Heus EM, Loogman MC, Rosenbrand KC, Kuipers T, Hoogstraten JW, Dekker R, Ten Duis HJ, van Dijk CN, van Tulder MW, van der Wees PJ, de Bie RA. Diagnosis, treatment and prevention of ankle sprains: an evidence-based clinical guideline. Br J Sports Med. 2012;46(12):854–60. https://doi.org/10.1136/bjsports-2011-090490.
93. Brison RJ, Day AG, Pelland L, Pickett W, Johnson AP, Aiken A, Pichora DR, Brouwer B. Effect of early supervised physiotherapy on recovery from acute ankle sprain: randomised controlled trial. BMJ. 2016;355:i5650. https://doi.org/10.1136/bmj.i5650.
94. Doherty C, Bleakley C, Delahunt E, Holden S. Treatment and prevention of acute and recurrent ankle sprain: an overview of systematic reviews with meta-analysis. Br J Sports Med. 2017;51(2):113–25. https://doi.org/10.1136/bjsports-2016-096178.
95. Bleakley CM, Taylor JB, Dischiavi SL, Doherty C, Delahunt E. Rehabilitation exercises reduce reinjury post ankle sprain, but the content and parameters of an optimal exercise program have yet to be

established: a systematic review and meta-analysis. Arch Phys Med Rehabil. 2019;100(7):1367–75. https://doi.org/10.1016/j.apmr.2018.10.005.

96. Salim MNS, Umar MA, Shaharudin S. Effects of the standard physiotherapy programme on pain and isokinetic ankle strength in individuals with grade I ankle sprain. J Taibah Univ Med Sci. 2018;13(6):576–81.
97. Mattacola CG, Dwyer MK. Rehabilitation of the ankle after acute sprain or chronic instability. J Athl Train. 2002;37(4):413–29.
98. Thacker SB, Stroup DF, Branche CM, Gilchrist J, Goodman RA, Weitman EA. The prevention of ankle sprains in sports. A systematic review of the literature. Am J Sports Med. 1999;27:753–60.
99. Verhagen EA, van der Beek A, Twisk J, Bouter L, Bahr R, van Mechelen W. The effect of a proprioceptive balance board training program for the prevention of ankle sprains: a prospective controlled trial. Am J Sports Med. 2004;32(6):1385–93.
100. Knight KL. Knee rehabilitation by the daily adjustable progressive resistive exercise technique. Am J Sports Med. 1979;7:336–7.
101. Perrin DH, Gieck JH. Principles of therapeutic exercise. In: Perrin DH, editor. The injured athlete. 3rd ed. Philadelphia, PA: Lippincott-Raven; 1999. p. 123–39.
102. Hartsell HD, Spaulding SJ. Eccentric/concentric ratios at selected velocities for the invertor and evertor muscles of the chronically unstable ankle. Br J Sports Med. 1999;33:255–8.
103. Hintermann B. Biomechanics of the unstable ankle joint and clinical implications. Med Sci Sports Exerc. 1999;31(7 suppl):459–69.

Lateral Ankle Sprains: Subtalar Instability

7

Kateryna Barg, Jesse Steadman, Megan Mills, and Alexej Barg

Introduction

Subtalar joint instability (SJI) exists among lateral, medial, and rotational subtypes as the major instabilities of the hindfoot. However, the exact diagnosis and appropriate treatment of SJI remain challenging as this instability is commonly overlooked or misdiagnosed as "simple" lateral ankle instability [1–5]. The number of patients with this misdiagnosis who actually complain about SJI is estimated to be as high as 25% [1, 6]; however, the exact rate of false-positive cases remains unclear [2]. The challenge of correctly diagnosing SJI can be partially explained by its nonspecific and overlapping symptoms with chronic lateral ankle instability [3, 7].The management of SJI should begin with nonoperative treatment. However, in patients who have exhausted these conservative options, operative intervention including anatomic reconstruction of the ligamentous stabilizers of the subtalar joint is indicated. Concomitant problems (e.g., deformities) can also be corrected synchronously if necessary.

K. Barg
Department of Orthopaedics, Trauma and Reconstructive Surgery, University Medical Center Hamburg-Eppendorf, Hamburg, Germany

J. Steadman
Department of Orthopaedics, University of Utah, Salt Lake City, UT, USA
e-mail: jesse.steadman@hsc.utah.edu

M. Mills
Department of Radiology and Imaging Sciences, University of Utah, Salt Lake City, UT, USA
e-mail: megan.mills@hsc.utah.edu

A. Barg (✉)
Department of Orthopaedics, Trauma and Reconstructive Surgery, University Medical Center Hamburg-Eppendorf, Hamburg, Germany

Department of Orthopaedics, University of Utah, Salt Lake City, UT, USA
e-mail: al.barg@uke.de

Etiology of Subtalar Joint Instability

There is a paucity of evidence in literature reporting on the epidemiology of SJI. Conversely, general instability of the ankle joint has been highlighted in several clinical and epidemiological studies. Although low in quantity, the existing studies on SJI are in consensus that isolated cases are rare and most patients present with a combination of both subtalar and ankle instability [3]. Therefore, etiological data related to ankle instability can also be utilized to describe SJI in part. It has been demonstrated that 25–40% of all patients suffering an acute ankle sprain may develop painful chronic ankle instability [8–10]. Additionally, several risk factors have been identified that substantially contribute to the development of chronic ankle instability such as high body mass index [11], female sex [11], severity of injury [12], deltoid ligament involvement [13], and avulsion fracture of the distal fibula [14,

P. D'Hooghe et al. (eds.), *Ligamentous Injuries of the Foot and Ankle*,
https://doi.org/10.1007/978-3-031-08682-3_7

15]. Interestingly, patients with a post-traumatic lesion of the calcaneofibular ligament (CLF) are at a particularly higher risk of developing isolated symptomatic SJI [5, 16]. However, an acute ankle sprain rarely results in isolated trauma to the CFL with a reported incidence of less than 1% [17–19]. Therefore, these epidemiological findings may partially explain the low incidence of isolated SJI.

Acute Subtalar Dislocation

Acute ankle sprain is the most common cause of symptomatic chronic ankle instability especially in athletes [20, 21]. Therefore, the postulation that acute subtalar dislocation may be another risk factor for SJI is quite reasonable. Acute subtalar dislocation is a rare hindfoot injury with a reported incidence of 1–2% of all joint dislocations and up to 15% of all acute talar injuries (Fig. 7.1) [22–24]. Often both joints—subtalar and talonavicular—are simultaneously dislocated [25]. Interestingly, patients with an acute subtalar dislocation often develop the opposite of SJI—painful subtalar stiffness and arthrofibrosis [2, 24, 26]. Further clinically significant complications following an acute subtalar dislocation include avascular necrosis with an incidence as high as 10% and 50% in closed and open dislocations, respectively [24, 26, 27]. Additionally, post-traumatic subtalar osteoarthritis is commonly implicated in these cases with an incidence of 40–80% [28, 29].

Clinical Assessment of Subtalar Instability

Patients with SJI often have a positive history of one or more substantial hindfoot inversion injuries. Patients may report limitations in daily and sporting activities, persistent hindfoot swelling, painful and limited range of motion of the subtalar joint, diffuse hindfoot pain which is aggravated by sporting activities or walking on uneven ground, and impaired proprioception [3, 30–32]. However, these symptoms are unspecific and can also be reported by patients with lateral ankle instability. A more specific symptom that may aid in a diagnostic workup is lateral hindfoot pain along the posterior facet of the subtalar joint with substantial radiation into the sinus tarsi, especially in patients with any radiographic signs of subtalar joint degeneration [33].

Clinical assessment starts with detailed visualization of both lower extremities while the patient is standing, sitting, and walking. Special attention is given in the evaluation of overall hindfoot alignment—valgus, varus, or neutral (Fig. 7.2) [34, 35]. However, clinical assessment of the hindfoot is not always reliable and may appear neutral due to compensatory alignment in the subtalar joint [35]. Any abnormal clinical findings should be confirmed using conventional weight-bearing radiographs or weight-bearing computed tomography (WBCT) [36–38].

Overall hindfoot stability is assessed manually using the anterior drawer and talar tilt test with the patient in a seated position (Fig. 7.3) [39]. Based on the authors' experience, we recommend adding external rotation to the anterior drawer test. With this addition, supplementary pressure is applied to the CFL by the rotated talar body. This pressure can elicit additional symptoms which may help distinguish the extent of CFL involvement. Rammelt and Zwipp also described a specific clinical test for the assessment of SJI. They recommend stabilizing the tibiotalar joint in a dorsiflexed position resulting in natural "blocking" of the talus within the ankle mortise to impede tibiotalar motion while instability testing is being performed (Fig. 7.4) [32, 33]. Ultrasound- or fluoroscopy-guided injection of the subtalar joint may also help distinguish between sinus tarsi and SJI symptoms [40].

Radiographic Assessment of Subtalar Joint Instability

Basic radiographic assessment of this pathology includes a series of four weight-bearing radiographs: anteroposterior and lateral views

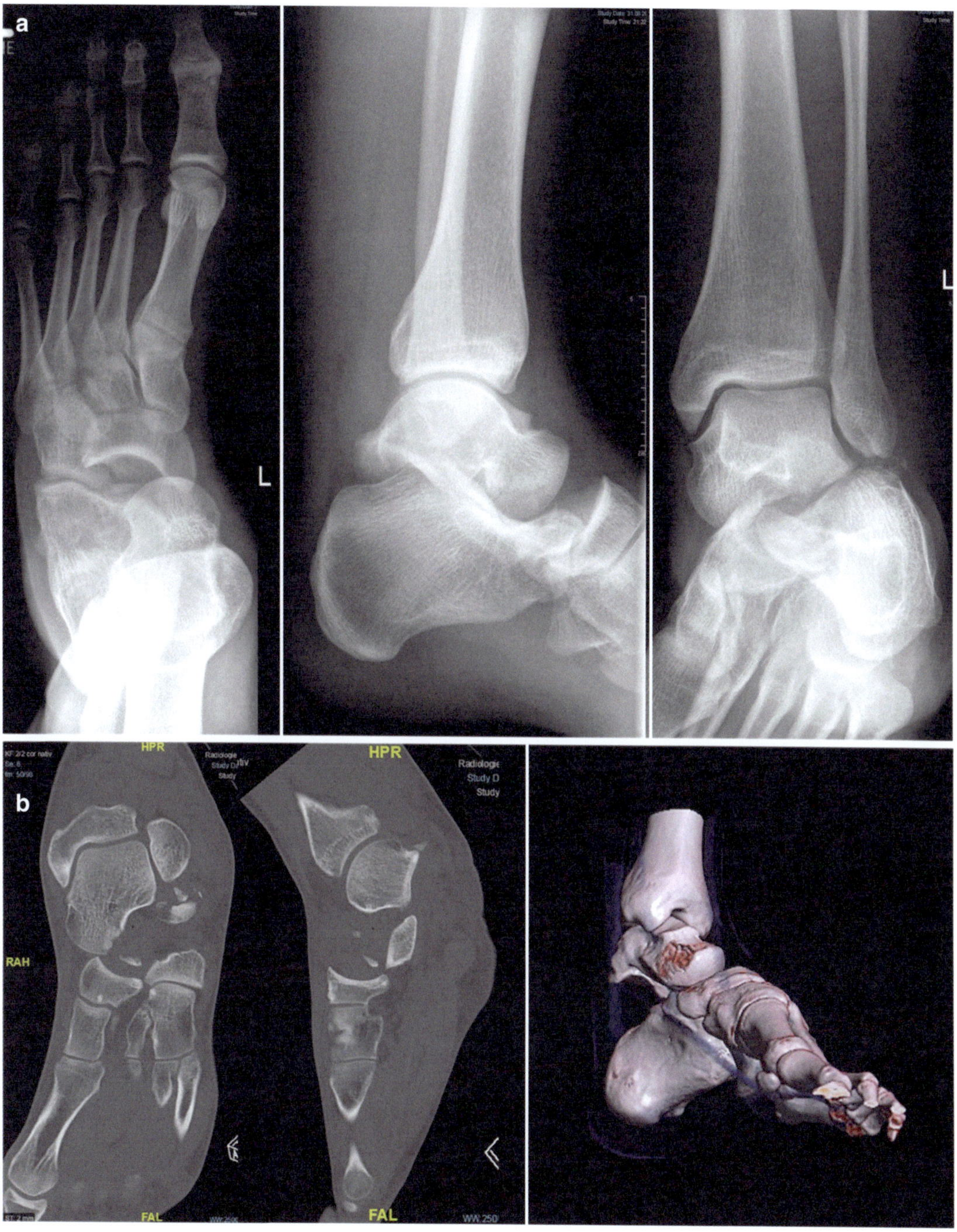

Fig. 7.1 Acute subtalar dislocation in a 17-year-old male who was involved in a biking accident. (**a**) Conventional radiographs demonstrate complete dislocation at the subtalar and talonavicular joints. (**b**) Computed tomography confirms the dislocation and demonstrates a lateral talus fracture

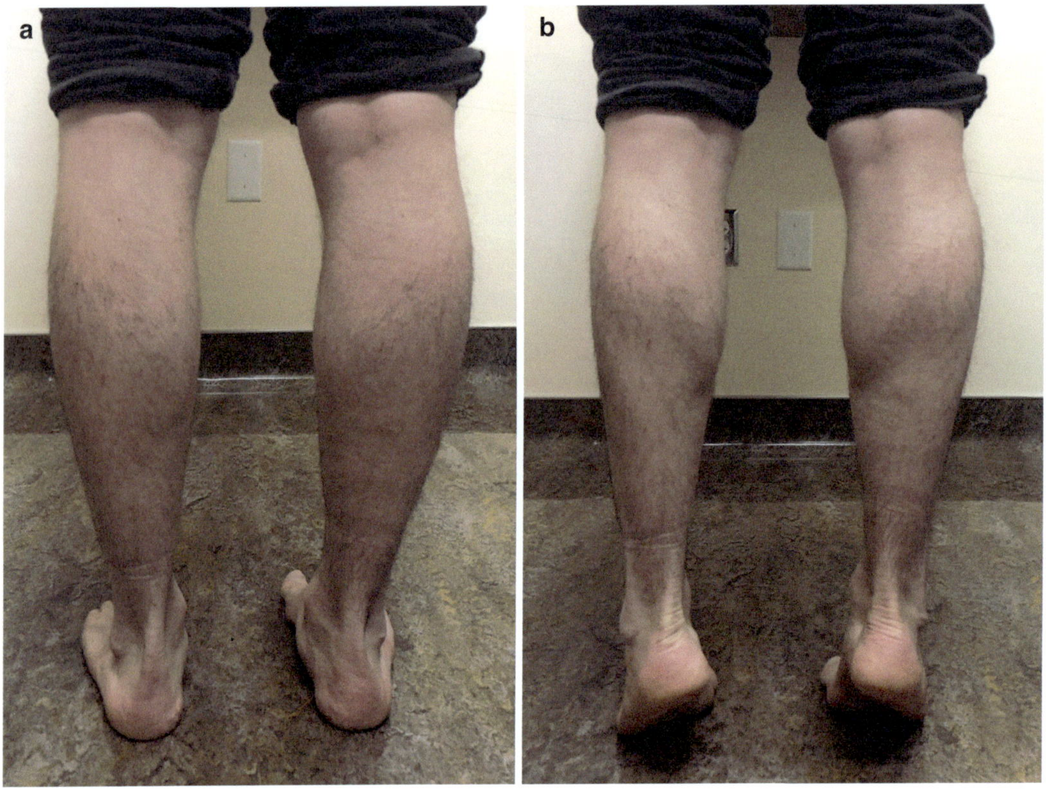

Fig. 7.2 Clinical assessment of hindfoot alignment. (**a**) A healthy male patient without any symptoms and mild valgus positioning of the heels. (**b**) Appropriate varization of the heels at tiptoeing, indicating appropriate function of the posterior tibial muscle

of the foot, a mortise view of the ankle, and a hindfoot alignment view (Fig. 7.5) [36, 41]. The Brodén view is a special image that can also be used in subtalar joint assessment [42]. This view is obtained with the ankle in a non-weight-bearing, neutral dorsiflexion position with the leg internally rotated 30° and the radiograph beam centered over the lateral malleolus with cephalad tube tilt varying between 10° and 40° for optimal assessment of the curved geometry present in the posterior facet of the subtalar joint (Fig. 7.6). Using these radiographic views, numerous quantitative parameters have been developed and published to assess for SJI (Fig. 7.7) [43].

Stress radiography is another imaging option available to investigate SJI [33, 44, 45]. Heilman et al. performed an anatomical study with ten specimens who underwent sectioning of the CFL, subtalar joint capsule, and ITFL [46]. Subtalar stability was assessed using 10°, 20°, 30°, and 40° Brodén stress views. Separation of the posterior facet greater than 7 mm was identified as an important indicator of SJI [46]. Lee et al. performed a clinical study with 66 patients to evaluate the diagnostic validity of manual supination-anterior drawer test radiographs in detecting SJI with concomitant ankle instability [47]. High interobserver and intraobserver reliability was found for measurements of talar rotation, anterior talar translation, and talar tilt angle. Diagnostic "cut-off" values, sensitivity, and specificity metrics were calculated for patients with combined lesions of the ATFL and CFL and were summarized as follows (cut-off value (sensitivity/specificity)): anterior talar translation, 0.755 (66.7%/28.6%); talar tilt angle, 0.670° (84.8%/42.0%); and talar rotation, 0.78% (66.7%/0.0%) [47]. Although these findings have

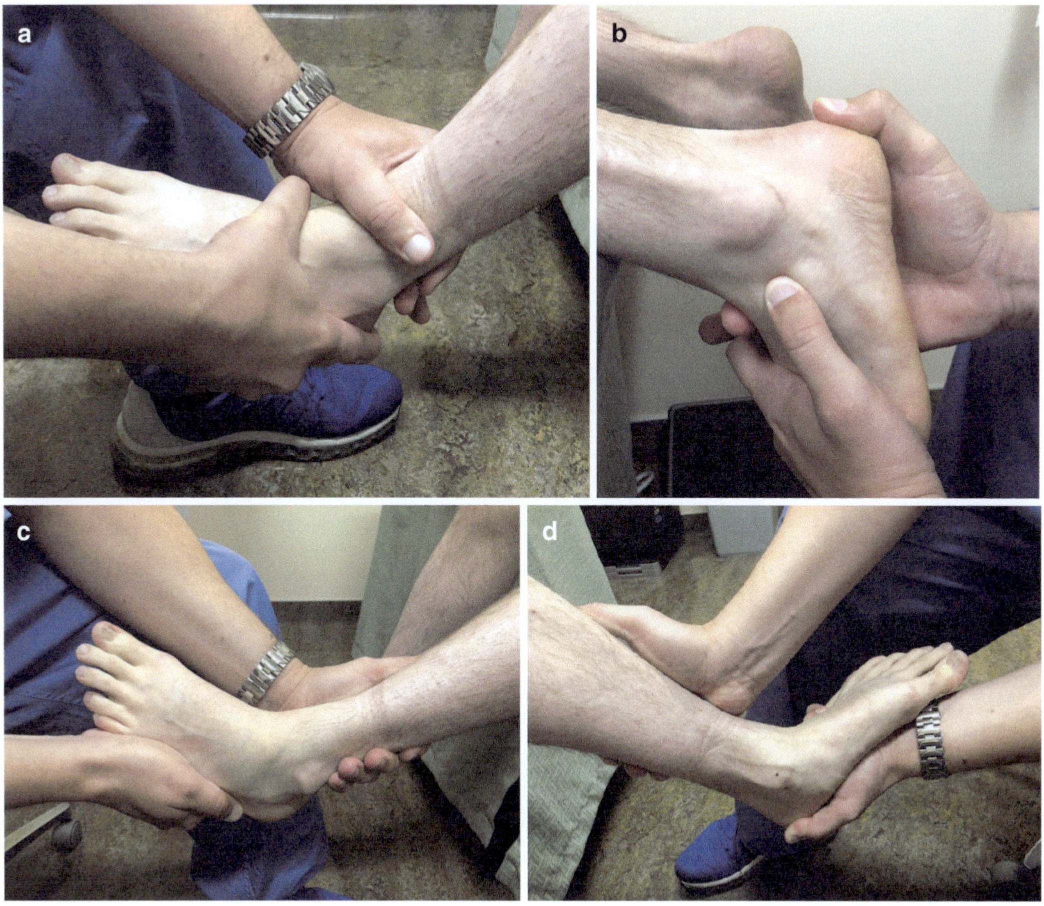

Fig. 7.3 Clinical assessment of hindfoot stability. Anterior drawer test in a sitting (**a**) and prone (**b**) position. Talar tilt test for clinical assessment of lateral (**c**) and medial (**d**) hindfoot stability

proved helpful in the diagnosis of SJI, stress radiography as a modality remains controversial for daily use as it can be painful to patients and provides a potential mechanism of iatrogenic cartilage damage of the subtalar joint.

Frequently, advanced imaging is necessary for appropriate diagnosis of SJI. Magnetic resonance imaging (MRI) is the advanced imaging modality of choice in patients with hindfoot instability (Figs. 7.8 and 7.9). Tochigi et al. evaluated MRIs of 24 patients who sustained an acute inversion ankle injury [48]. Among these patients, the following structures were lesioned: anterior talofibular ligament (ATFL) in 23/24 cases, CFL in 15/24, posterior talofibular ligament in 11/24, interosseous talocalcaneal ligament (ITCL) in 13/24, cervical ligament in 12/24, and the deltoid ligament in 8/24. Furthermore, authors found a statistically significant relationship between ITCL lesions and clinical symptoms including instability, pain, and a reduced ankle range of motion [48]. Park et al. evaluated the diagnostic accuracy of utilizing an oblique coronal MRI in a retrospective study of 91 patients with a confirmed CFL injury [49]. Sensitivity and accuracy of CFL injury detection were significantly higher in oblique than orthogonal images [49]. Kim et al. used a 3D isotropic ankle MRI in 23 patients with SJI [50]. Thickness and width of the anterior capsular ligament (ACL), ITCL, as well as thickness of the CFL and ATFL were measured and compared to results obtained in 23 age- and sex-matched control subjects without instability symptoms. The measurements of

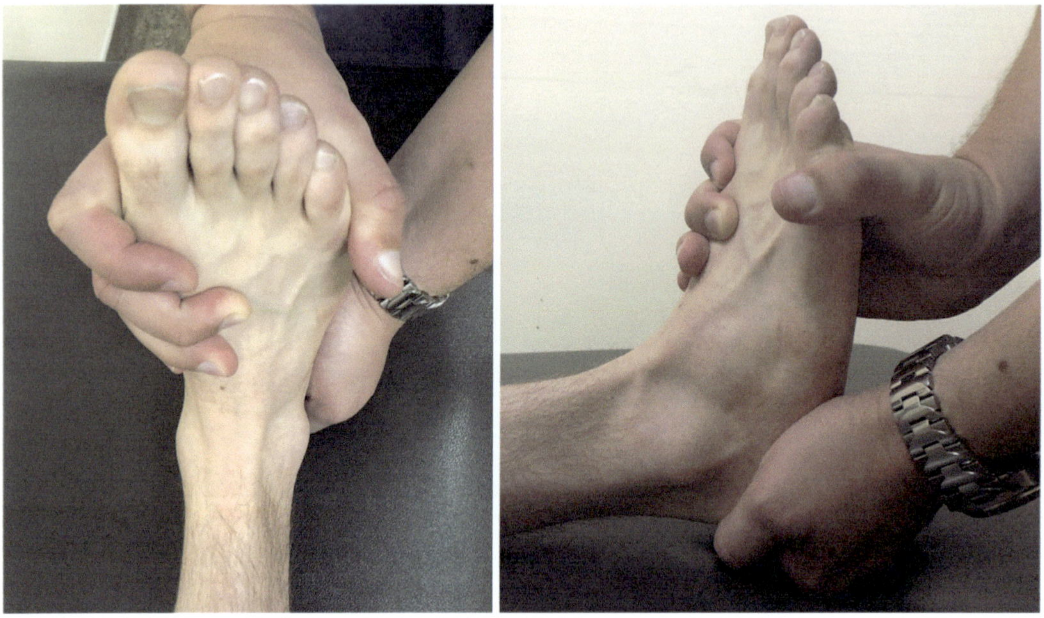

Fig. 7.4 Rammelt's test for manual assessment of anterolateral rotational stability of the subtalar joint with the ankle stabilized in a dorsiflexed position

ITCL, CFL, and ATFL were comparable in both groups; however, complete tear of CFL and ATFL was more common in the instability group. ACL thickness and width in the instability group was significantly smaller than the control group with values of 1.73 vs. 2.22 mm and 7.21 vs. 8.80 mm, respectively. Ringleb et al. performed a cadaver study with eight specimens that were tested intact, after dissecting the ATFL, after dissecting the ATFL and CFL, and finally after performing one of two reconstructive techniques to repair these lesions [51]. Three-dimensional stress MRI was used to assess the hindfoot stability while inversion and anterior drawer force was applied. Dissection of the ATFL and CFL resulted in a significant increase in hindfoot rotation while in inversion. The observed changes were reversed after Broström or Chrisman-Snook procedures were performed [51].

Computed tomography (CT) is another advanced imaging technique that can be used in the diagnosis of SJI. Sijbrandij et al. evaluated CTs in a cohort of 10 patients with SJI and compared the observed results with those obtained using the Brodén stress view [52]. Subtalar tilt was measured in the midportion and posteromedial areas of the talus. In the midpart, the tilt was 0° and 10.8° using CT and Brodén stress view, respectively. In the posteromedial aspect the subtalar tilt was 10.2° and 10.8° using CT and Brodén stress view, respectively [52].

WBCT is a novel imaging modality with several obvious advantages including assessment of a natural standing position, high-contrast and spatial resolution, fast image acquisition time, reasonable radiation dosage, a relatively small scanner size, and less capitalization cost than a conventional CT scan [53, 54]. In the last decade, literature addressing the use of WBCT in foot and ankle disorders has grown immensely [55]. Pertinently, Krähenbühl et al. performed a cadaver study to assess the question of whether WBCT imaging can be utilized to diagnose SJI [56].

Ultrasonography is another imaging tool which has been used to detect SJI. Waldecker et al. described a novel method for the assessment of SJI by using the well-described fibula-trochlear angle [57]. The measurements were performed in four cadaveric specimens with intact vs. sectioned lateral stabilizing structures in a neutrally positioned ankle as well as under inversion stress. An angle ratio of more than 1.6 was strongly cor-

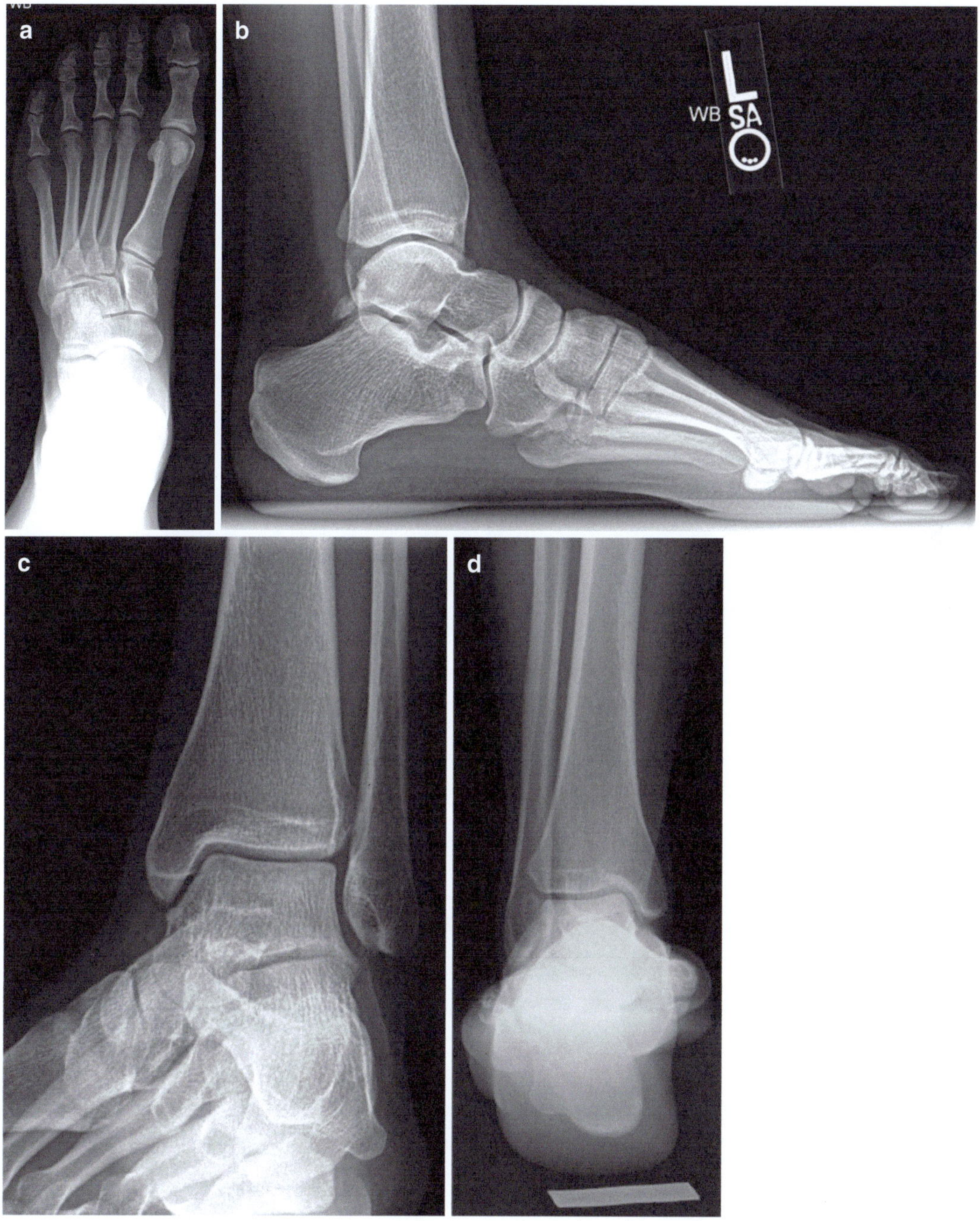

Fig. 7.5 Radiographic assessment in a 25-year-old female patient with post-traumatic subtalar instability including weight-bearing conventional radiographs: anteroposterior (**a**) and lateral (**b**) iews of the foot, a mortise view of the ankle (**c**), and a hindfoot alignment view (**d**)

related with a radiographically unstable subtalar joint [57]. Several radiographic parameters were measured utilizing digitally reconstructed radiographs obtained using WBCT at different sectioning levels including CFL, ITCL, and the deltoid ligament. Application of internal torque was demonstrated to be helpful in improving the accuracy of measurements [56]. WBCT can also be used

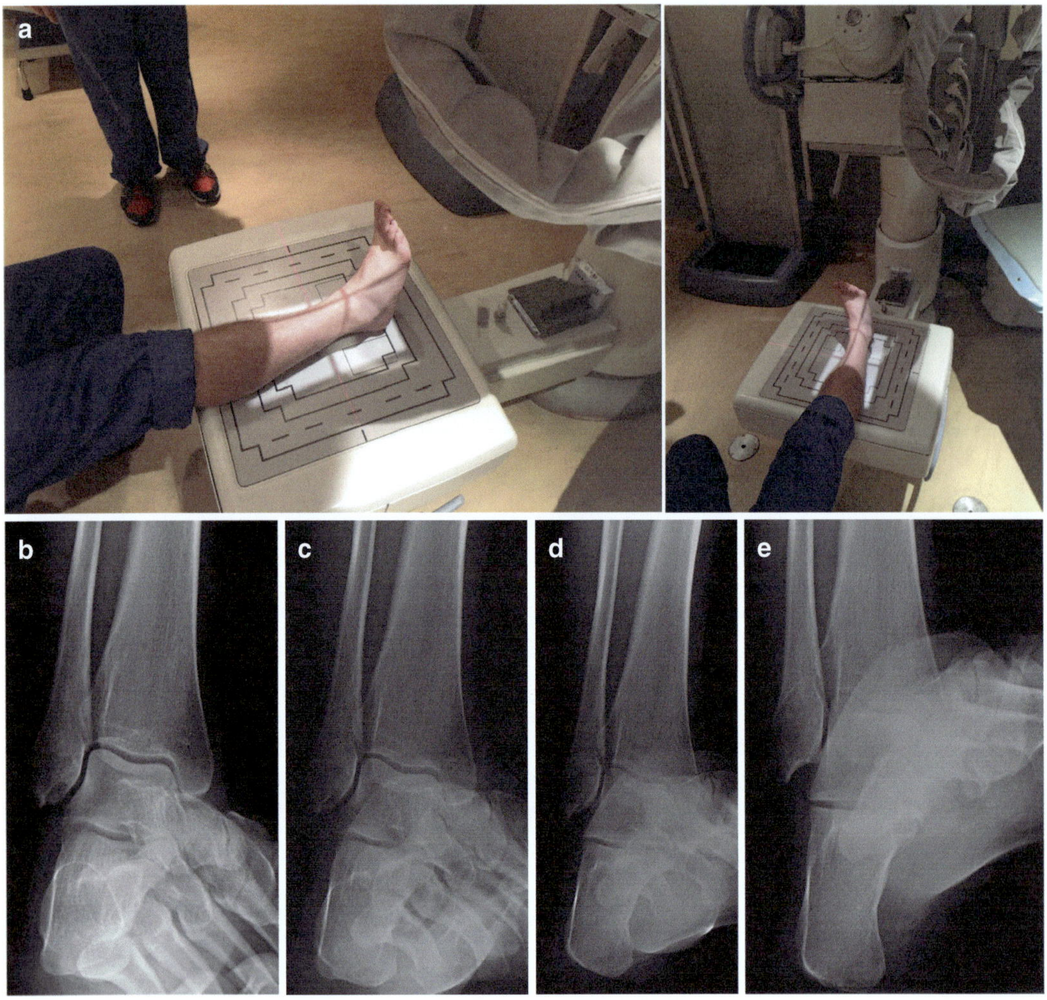

Fig. 7.6 The Brodén view for radiographic assessment of the posterior facet of the subtalar joint. (**a**) Radiographic technique (for details, please see the text). Different variants of the Brodén view with cephalad tube tilt of 10° (**b**), 20° (**c**), 30° (**d**), and 40° (**e**)

to assess the specific morphology of the subtalar joint which may also play a role in the etiology of SJI [58]. Krähenbühl et al. used WBCT to assess the orientation of the subtalar joint in 40 patients with ankle osteoarthritis vs. 20 healthy controls [59]. Assessment of the subtalar vertical angle was found to be at a very high level of reliability. In the analyzed cohort, varus osteoarthritis of the tibiotalar joint was associated with varus orientation of the subtalar joint whereas patients with valgus ankle osteoarthritis demonstrated valgus orientation of the subtalar joint [59]. Recently, Krähenbühl et al. performed a WBCT study of 27 asymptomatic healthy individuals to assess subtalar joint morphology using statistical shape modeling [60]. Parameters such as three-dimensional shape variation, coverage, space, and congruency of the subtalar joint were investigated. Considerable shape variation was observed within the analyzed cohort; however, the posterior and anteromedial articular facets demonstrated a highly consistent congruency [60].

Subtalar arthrography also possesses diagnostic value in patients with SJI. In 1988, Meyer

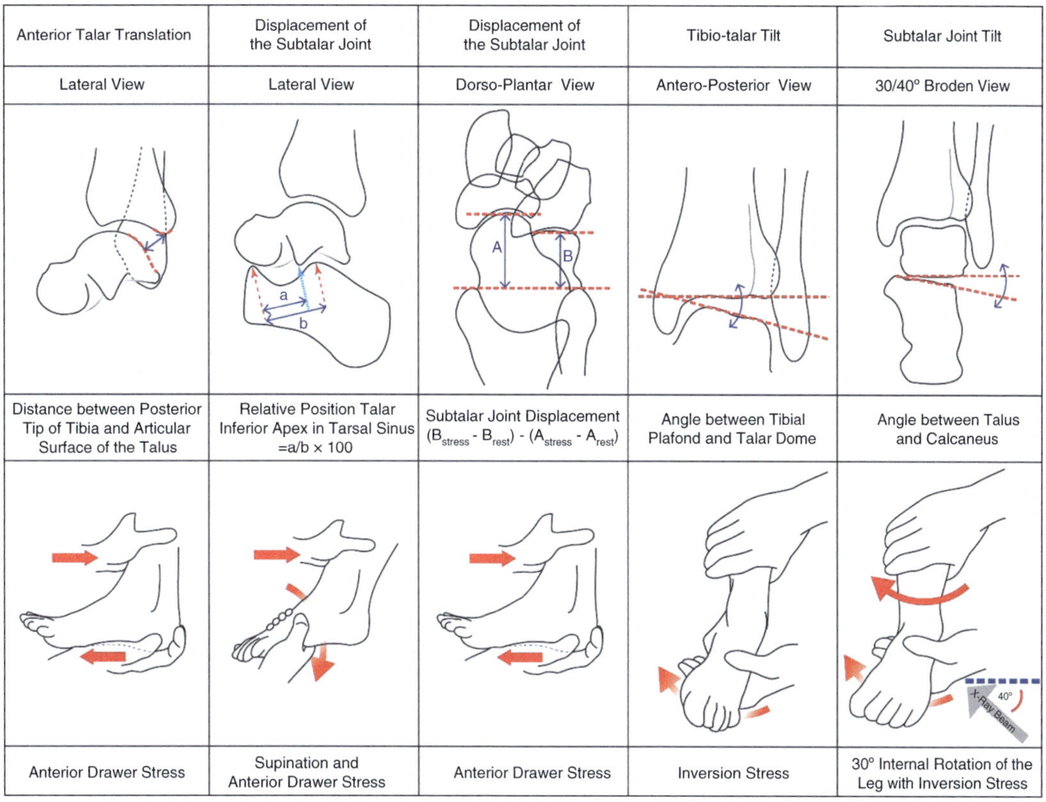

Fig. 7.7 Specific measurement methods using conventional radiographs as well as clinical methods for assessment of subtalar joint instability

et al. analyzed subtalar arthrograms and ankle stress films in 40 patients with subtalar and ankle sprains [61]. In 33 of 40 patients, contrast leak on the lateral aspect of the hindfoot was observed. Six patients with positive arthrograms demonstrated negative stress films confirming the usefulness of this invasive diagnostic method [61]. Sugimoto et al. used this imaging modality in 37 patients with chronic recurrent lateral hindfoot instability [62] as well as in 27 patients with acute injury of the CFL [18]. In the first study, the mean time interval between the initial injury and arthrography was slightly over 4 years with a range of 6 months to 22 years. In all patients, the condition of the CFL was assessed during surgery and was observed as ruptured in 13 of 37 feet. The incidence of leakage to the ankle and peroneal tendon sheath was different in both chronic and acute subgroups with 11 of 13 vs. 6 of 24 and 9 of 13 vs. 1 of 24 positive findings, respectively. The difference of leakage to the sinus tarsi did not reach statistical significance with 8 of 13 vs. 9 of 24 positive findings, respectively [62]. In the second study, the difference in contrast leakage was compared between 27 patients with a confirmed acute CFL injury and 43 patients without CFL damage [18]. The findings from the previous study [62] regarding leakage rate into the ankle, sinus tarsi, and peroneal tendon sheath were confirmed in this study [18].

Conservative Treatment of SJI

With new patients presenting to clinic and receiving a diagnosis of SJI, nonoperative treatment options are initiated and considered first line. These conservative treatments include physical

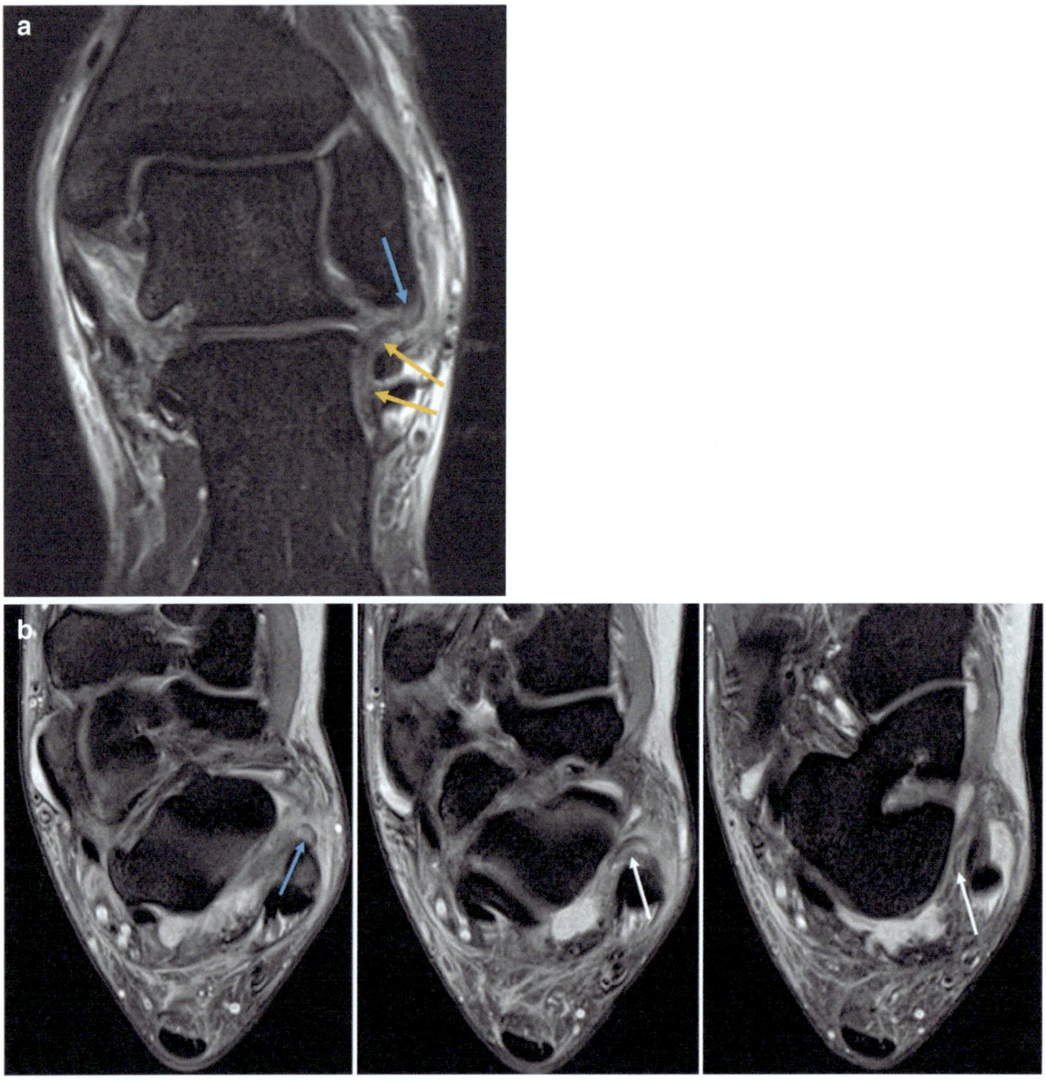

Fig. 7.8 Calcaneofibular ligament (CFL) injury in a 17-year-old male resulting in subtalar joint instability following an acute ankle sprain. (**a**) Coronal T2FS image shows increased signal and laxity of the CFL (orange arrows) with disruption of the ligament from the fibular attachment (blue arrow). (**b**) Sequential axial PDFS images from proximal (left) to distal (right). Images show disruption of the CFL from the fibular attachment (white arrow) with increased signal and abnormal morphology along the mid and distal aspects of the ligament (blue arrows)

therapy and shoe modifications or insoles for patients with concomitant hindfoot deformities. Physical therapy should have the following aims: active improvement of proprioception, active and passive improvement of hindfoot, and specifically subtalar, range of motion, strengthening of periarticular structures such as the peroneal muscles, and gait analysis and improvement if needed. Local physiotherapeutic measures may include the application of ultrasound and/or iontophoresis as well as lymph drainage to reduce hindfoot swelling. Bracing the hindfoot including kinesiotaping [63] may improve stability and proprioception, especially for sporting activities. Taping and kinesiotaping demonstrated promising results in patients with chronic ankle insta-

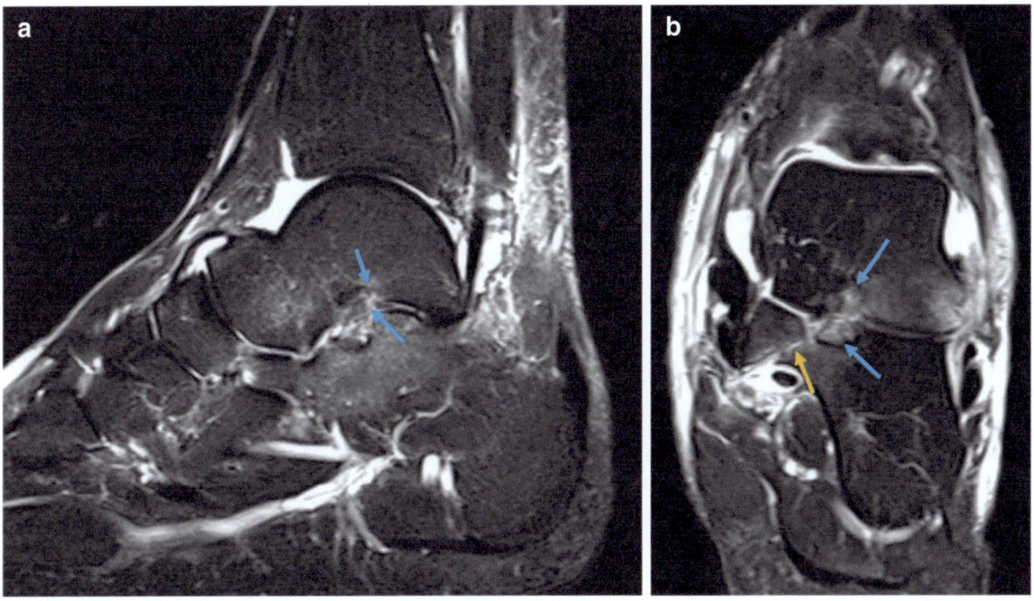

Fig. 7.9 A 40-year-old male with painful subtalar joint instability following an acute ankle sprain. (**a**) Sagittal and (**b**) coronal T2FS images through the sinus tarsi show disruption of the interosseous talocalcaneal ligament (blue arrows). A delayed sustentaculum tali fracture union is also present (orange arrow)

bility [63, 64]; however, the available literature is quite inconsistent [65, 66]. It should also be mentioned that the current, available evidence of physical therapy is based on studies including patients with chronic ankle instability and not specifically SJI [67–70].

Operative Treatment of Subtalar Joint Instability

In patients undergoing conservative treatment for 3–6 months seeing no improvement in signs and symptoms, operative intervention is indicated unless general or specific surgical contraindications are present. Surgical treatment of the SJI includes the following:

- Anterior ankle arthroscopy with arthroscopic assessment of instability and intra-articular debridement if needed.
- Anatomic reconstruction of lateral ligaments including CFL and ATFL.
- Surgical realigning procedures to address concomitant deformities if needed.

Anterior ankle arthroscopy is usually performed utilizing two established portals: anteromedial and anterolateral [71]. In patients with preoperatively diagnosed osteochondral lesion(s), the exact localization of the lesion needs to be analyzed prior to portal placement. In patients with a posteriorly localized osteochondral lesion, a posterior ankle arthroscopy should be performed to allow for intra-articular debridement [72–74]. An ankle arthroscopy procedure has diagnostic, as well as therapeutic, value. From a diagnostic standpoint, it can be used to assess intra-articular degeneration as well as any underlying dynamic deformity. From a therapeutic perspective, removal of loose bodies, intra-articular debridement, and/or debridement of an osteochondral lesion with or without microfracturing of subchondral bone can be performed if indicated.

As a second step, reconstruction of the lateral ATFL and CFL ligaments should be performed [75]. In current literature, numerous surgical techniques have been described to restore ligamentous stability of the ankle and hindfoot utilizing open [76, 77] and arthroscopic [78–80] procedures. In

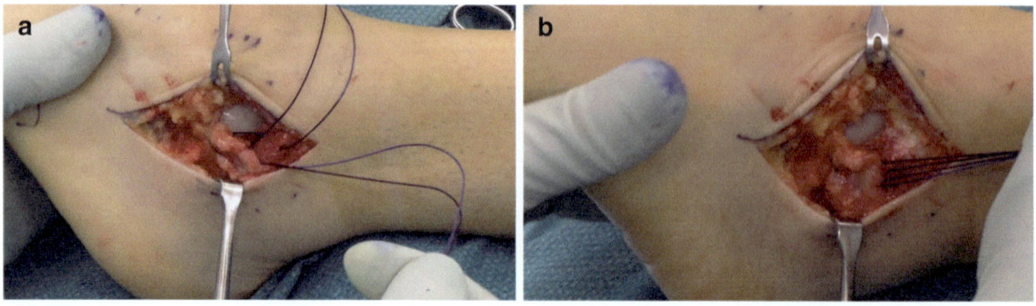

Fig. 7.10 Anatomic reconstruction of the lateral ligaments using the Broström-Gould procedure. (**a**) Transosseous sutures are used for fixation of ATFL and CFL. (**b**) Both sutures are tensioned to check the lateral ankle stability

our experience, the open Broström-Gould procedure has proved to be a reliable surgery to correct lateral ankle and hindfoot instability (Fig. 7.10) [76, 81–83]. In patients with concomitant medial ankle instability, anatomic reconstruction of the deltoid ligament should also be performed to address potential rotational instability [13, 75].

As numerous operative techniques for ankle ligament reconstruction have been described, no consensus has yet been established on a technique that yields the most reliable and superior outcomes. It has been shown that anatomic reconstruction has a great capacity to restore the kinematics and biomechanics of the ankle joint [84–87]. Choisne et al. compared anatomic ligament reconstruction with tenodesis in a cadaveric SJI model [88]. The Broström-Gould procedure demonstrated superior outcomes with regard to the restoration of subtalar and ankle joint kinematics. The tenodesis procedure resulted in a substantial restriction of internal rotation at the subtalar joint compared to intact conditions [88]. Behrens et al. analyzed both the traditional Broström and modified Broström-Gould procedures in a time-zero cadaveric instability model [84]. Both procedures demonstrated comparable restoration of biomechanical parameters of ankle stability [84]. In general, the favorable results observed in previously mentioned cadaveric studies have been confirmed by numerous clinical studies demonstrating very good mid- to long-term clinical outcomes [89–91]. Additionally, in the last 5 years, there has been an increasing number of publications describing arthroscopic reconstructive techniques to correct ankle instability [80, 90, 92–100].

Finally, in patients with substantial concomitant deformities, realignment procedures should be performed including supramalleolar [101, 102] and/or calcaneal [103] osteotomies, depending on which level the deformity is observed.

Conclusions

SJI remains a diagnostic challenge for orthopedic surgeons as it is the least studied type of hindfoot instability [2, 4, 5]. The subtalar joint belongs to the most complex structures in the hindfoot with remarkable interindividual variability regarding its shape [58, 60, 104, 105]. In current literature, there is still vibrant debate about which ankle ligament is the most important stabilizer of the subtalar joint resulting in two major partitions. One group believes the CFL has been identified as the primary ligament stabilizer of the subtalar joint [16, 106–111], while the other group names the ITCL as the most important subtalar stabilizing structure [31, 46, 48, 79, 88, 112–116]. This opinion is supported by various surgical techniques developed to restore the ITCL resulting in improvement of subtalar joint stability [40, 117–120]. However, the validity of this evidence is limited by small patient cohorts, short follow-up duration, and/or isolated surgical technique descriptions.

In conclusion, the diagnosis and treatment of SJI remain challenging. However, in the last decade, there have been substantial efforts to address this issue by innovative approaches, e.g., using weight-bearing computed tomography for better understanding of the subtalar joint [56, 60]. Clinical assessment of SJI includes careful and detailed examination of the entire lower extremity. Radiographic assessment should include weight-bearing radiographs often followed by advanced imaging including MRI and/or weight-bearing computed tomography. Concerning treatment, conservative management options should be exhausted initially. If this treatment fails, operative intervention is indicated and includes anatomic reconstruction of the lateral ligaments and synchronous correction of any concomitant problems or deformities.

References

1. Aynardi M, Pedowitz DI, Raikin SM. Subtalar instability. Foot Ankle Clin. 2015;20(2):243–52.
2. Barg A, Tochigi Y, Amendola A, Phisitkul P, Hintermann B, Saltzman CL. Subtalar instability: diagnosis and treatment. Foot Ankle Int. 2012;33(2):151–60.
3. Barg A, Weinberg MW, Burssens A, Saltzman CL, Krahenbuhl N. Subtalar instability: diagnosis and treatment options. Fuss Sprungg. 2018;16(2):253–63.
4. Mittlmeier T, Rammelt S. Update on subtalar joint instability. Foot Ankle Clin. 2018;23(3):397–413.
5. Mittlmeier T, Wichelhaus A. Subtalar joint instability. Eur J Trauma Emerg Surg. 2015;41(6):623–9.
6. Brantigan JW, Pedegana LR, Lippert FG. Instability of the subtalar joint. Diagnosis by stress tomography in three cases. J Bone Joint Surg Am. 1977;59(3):321–4.
7. Michels F, Pereira H, Calder J, Matricali G, Glazebrook M, Guillo S, et al. Searching for consensus in the approach to patients with chronic lateral ankle instability: ask the expert. Knee Surg Sports Traumatol Arthrosc. 2018;26(7):2095–102.
8. Chan KW, Ding BC, Mroczek KJ. Acute and chronic lateral ankle instability in the athlete. Bull NYU Hosp Jt Dis. 2011;69(1):17–26.
9. de Vries JS, Krips R, Sierevelt IN, Blankevoort L, van Dijk CN. Interventions for treating chronic ankle instability. Cochrane Database Syst Rev. 2011;(8):Cd004124.
10. van Rijn RM, van Os AG, Bernsen RM, Luijsterburg PA, Koes BW, Bierma-Zeinstra SM. What is the clinical course of acute ankle sprains? A systematic literature review. Am J Med. 2008;121(4):324–331.e6.
11. Hershkovich O, Tenenbaum S, Gordon B, Bruck N, Thein R, Derazne E, et al. A large-scale study on epidemiology and risk factors for chronic ankle instability in young adults. J Foot Ankle Surg. 2015;54(2):183–7.
12. Pourkazemi F, Hiller CE, Raymond J, Nightingale EJ, Refshauge KM. Predictors of chronic ankle instability after an index lateral ankle sprain: a systematic review. J Sci Med Sport. 2014;17(6):568–73.
13. Hintermann B, Valderrabano V, Boss A, Trouillier HH, Dick W. Medial ankle instability: an exploratory, prospective study of fifty-two cases. Am J Sports Med. 2004;32(1):183–90.
14. Ahn HW, Lee KB. Comparison of the modified Broström procedure for chronic lateral ankle instability with and without subfibular ossicle. Am J Sports Med. 2016;44(12):3158–64.
15. Choi WJ, Yoon HK, Yoon HS, Kim BS, Lee JW. Comparison of the proximal chevron and Ludloff osteotomies for the correction of hallux valgus. Foot Ankle Int. 2009;30(12):1154–60.
16. Weindel S, Schmidt R, Rammelt S, Claes L, v Campe A, Rein S. Subtalar instability: a biomechanical cadaver study. Arch Orthop Trauma Surg. 2010;130(3):313–9.
17. Rigby R, Cottom JM, Rozin R. Isolated calcaneofibular ligament injury: a report of two cases. J Foot Ankle Surg. 2015;54(3):487–9.
18. Sugimoto K, Samoto N, Takaoka T, Takakura Y, Tamai S. Subtalar arthrography in acute injuries of the calcaneofibular ligament. J Bone Joint Surg. 1998;80(5):785–90.
19. Usuelli FG, Mason L, Grassi M, Maccario C, Ballal M, Molloy A. Lateral ankle and hindfoot instability: a new clinical based classification. Foot Ankle Surg. 2014;20(4):231–6.
20. Chang SH, Morris BL, Saengsin J, Tourné Y, Guillo S, Guss D, et al. Diagnosis and treatment of chronic lateral ankle instability: review of our biomechanical evidence. J Am Acad Orthop Surg. 2021;29(1):3–16.
21. Lau BC, Barg A, Haytmanek CT, McCullough K, Amendola A. Evolution in surgical management of ankle instability in athletes. J Am Acad Orthop Surg. 2021;29(1):e5–e13.
22. Pennal GF. Fractures of the talus. Clin Orthop Relat Res. 1963;30:53–63.
23. Rammelt S, Bartoníček J, Park KH. Traumatic injury to the subtalar joint. Foot Ankle Clin. 2018;23(3):353–74.
24. Rammelt S, Goronzy J. Subtalar dislocations. Foot Ankle Clin. 2015;20(2):253–64.
25. Wagner R, Blattert TR, Weckbach A. Talar dislocations. Injury. 2004;35 Suppl 2:Sb36–45.
26. Zimmer TJ, Johnson KA. Subtalar dislocations. Clin Orthop Relat Res. 1989;238:190–4.
27. Goldner JL, Poletti SC, Gates HS 3rd, Richardson WJ. Severe open subtalar dislocations. Long-term results. J Bone Joint Surg Am. 1995;77(7):1075–9.
28. Bibbo C, Anderson RB, Davis WH. Injury characteristics and the clinical outcome of subtalar dislo-

cations: a clinical and radiographic analysis of 25 cases. Foot Ankle Int. 2003;24(2):158–63.
29. Heppenstall RB, Farahvar H, Balderston R, Lotke P. Evaluation and management of subtalar dislocations. J Trauma. 1980;20(6):494–7.
30. Karlsson J, Eriksson BI, Renstrom PA. Subtalar ankle instability. A review. Sports Med. 1997;24(5):337–46.
31. Keefe DT, Haddad SL, Subtalar instability. Etiology, diagnosis, and management. Foot Ankle Clin. 2002;7(3):577–609.
32. Zwipp H, Rammelt S, Grass R. Ligamentous injuries about the ankle and subtalar joints. Clin Podiatr Med Surg. 2002;19(2):195–229.
33. Zwipp H, Rammelt S. Ligamente: Rupturen und Luxationen. In: Zwipp H, Rammelt S, editors. Tscherne Unfallchirurgie Fuß. Heidelberg: Springer; 2014. p. 215–70.
34. Pagenstert GI, Hintermann B, Barg A, Leumann A, Valderrabano V. Realignment surgery as alternative treatment of varus and valgus ankle osteoarthritis. Clin Orthop Relat Res. 2007;462(1): 156–68.
35. Wang B, Saltzman CL, Chalayon O, Barg A. Does the subtalar joint compensate for ankle malalignment in end-stage ankle arthritis? Clin Orthop Relat Res. 2015;473(1):318–25.
36. Barg A. Conventional imaging of the hindfoot and Saltzman view. Fuss Sprungg. 2015; 13(2):58–77.
37. Burssens A, Peeters J, Buedts K, Victor J, Vandeputte G. Measuring hindfoot alignment in weight bearing CT: a novel clinical relevant measurement method. Foot Ankle Surg. 2016;22(4):233–8.
38. Richter M, Seidl B, Zech S, Hahn S. PedCAT for 3D-imaging in standing position allows for more accurate bone position (angle) measurement than radiographs or CT. Foot Ankle Surg. 2014;20(3):201–7.
39. Phisitkul P, Chaichankul C, Sripongsai R, Prasitdamrong I, Tengtrakulcharoen P, Suarchawaratana S. Accuracy of anterolateral drawer test in lateral ankle instability: a cadaveric study. Foot Ankle Int. 2009;30(7):690–5.
40. Pisani G, Pisani PC, Parino E. Sinus tarsi syndrome and subtalar joint instability. Clin Podiatr Med Surg. 2005;22(1):63–77.
41. Saltzman CL, el-Khoury GY. The hindfoot alignment view. Foot Ankle Int. 1995;16(9):572–6.
42. Broden B. Roentgen examination of the subtaloid joint in fractures of the calcaneus. Acta Radiol. 1949;31(1):85–91.
43. Krähenbühl N, Weinberg MW, Davidson NP, Mills MK, Hintermann B, Saltzman CL, et al. Currently used imaging options cannot accurately predict subtalar joint instability. Knee Surg Sports Traumatol Arthrosc. 2019;27(9):2818–30.
44. Zwipp H. Rekonstruktionsmaßnahmen nach veralteten Frakturen und Luxationen des Fußes. Der Orthopade. 2014;43(11):1025–40.
45. Zwipp H, Tscherne H. Die radiologische Diagnostik der Rotationsinstabilität im hinteren unteren Sprunggelenk. Unfallheilkunde. 1982;85:494–8.
46. Heilman AE, Braly WG, Bishop JO, Noble PC, Tullos HS. An anatomic study of subtalar instability. Foot Ankle. 1990;10(4):224–8.
47. Lee BH, Choi KH, Seo DY, Choi SM, Kim GL. Diagnostic validity of alternative manual stress radiographic technique detecting subtalar instability with concomitant ankle instability. Knee Surg Sports Traumatol Arthrosc. 2016;24(4):1029–39.
48. Tochigi Y, Yoshinaga K, Wada Y, Moriya H. Acute inversion injury of the ankle: magnetic resonance imaging and clinical outcomes. Foot Ankle Int. 1998;19(11):730–4.
49. Park HJ, Lee SY, Park NH, Kim E, Chung EC, Kook SH, et al. Usefulness of the oblique coronal plane in ankle MRI of the calcaneofibular ligament. Clin Radiol. 2015;70(4):416–23.
50. Kim TH, Moon SG, Jung HG, Kim NR. Subtalar instability: imaging features of subtalar ligaments on 3D isotropic ankle MRI. BMC Musculoskelet Disord. 2017;18(1):475.
51. Ringleb SI, Udupa JK, Siegler S, Imhauser CW, Hirsch BE, Liu J, et al. The effect of ankle ligament damage and surgical reconstructions on the mechanics of the ankle and subtalar joints revealed by three-dimensional stress MRI. J Orthop Res. 2005;23(4):743–9.
52. Sijbrandij ES, van Gils AP, van Hellemondt FJ, Louwerens JW, de Lange EE. Assessing the subtalar joint: the Broden view revisited. Foot Ankle Int. 2001;22(4):329–34.
53. Barg A, Bailey T, Richter M, de Cesar NC, Lintz F, Burssens A, et al. Weightbearing computed tomography of the foot and ankle: emerging technology topical review. Foot Ankle Int. 2018;39(3):376–86.
54. Lintz F, de Cesar NC, Barg A, Burssens A, Richter M. Weight-bearing cone beam CT scans in the foot and ankle. EFORT Open Rev. 2018; 3(5):278–86.
55. Richter M, Lintz F, de Cesar Netto C, Barg A, Burssens A, Ellis S. Weight bearing cone beam computed tomography (WBCT) in the foot and ankle: a scientific, technical and clinical guide. Cham: Springer; 2020.
56. Krähenbühl N, Burssens A, Davidson NP, Allen CM, Henninger HB, Saltzman CL, et al. Can weightbearing computed tomography scans be used to diagnose subtalar joint instability? A cadaver study. J Orthop Res. 2019;37(11):2457–65.
57. Waldecker U, Blatter G. Sonographic measurement of instability of the subtalar joint. Foot Ankle Int. 2001;22(1):42–6.
58. Krahenbuhl N, Horn-Lang T, Hintermann B, Knupp M. The subtalar joint: a complex mechanism. EFORT Open Rev. 2017;2(7):309–16.
59. Krahenbuhl N, Tschuck M, Bolliger L, Hintermann B, Knupp M. Orientation of the subtalar joint: mea-

surement and reliability using weightbearing CT scans. Foot Ankle Int. 2016;37(1):109–14.
60. Krähenbühl N, Lenz AL, Lisonbee RJ, Peterson AC, Atkins PR, Hintermann B, et al. Morphologic analysis of the subtalar joint using statistical shape modeling. J Orthop Res. 2020;38(12):2625–33.
61. Meyer JM, Garcia J, Hoffmeyer P, Fritschy D. The subtalar sprain. A roentgenographic study. Clin Orthop Relat Res. 1988;226:169–73.
62. Sugimoto K, Takakura Y, Samoto N, Nakayama S, Tanaka Y. Subtalar arthrography in recurrent instability of the ankle. Clin Orthop Relat Res. 2002;394:169–76.
63. Hadadi M, Haghighat F, Mohammadpour N, Sobhani S. Effects of kinesiotape vs soft and semirigid ankle orthoses on balance in patients with chronic ankle instability: a randomized controlled trial. Foot Ankle Int. 2020;41(7):793–802.
64. Sarvestan J, Ataabadi PA, Svoboda Z, Kovačikova Z, Needle AR. The effect of ankle Kinesio™ taping on ankle joint biomechanics during unilateral balance status among collegiate athletes with chronic ankle sprain. Phys Ther Sport. 2020;45:161–7.
65. Shin JC, Kim JH, Nam D, Park GC, Lee JS. Add-on effect of kinesiotape in patients with acute lateral ankle sprain: a randomized controlled trial. Trials. 2020;21(1):176.
66. Slevin ZM, Arnold GP, Wang W, Abboud RJ. Immediate effect of kinesiology tape on ankle stability. BMJ Open Sport Exerc Med. 2020;6(1):e000604.
67. Cain MS, Ban RJ, Chen YP, Geil MD, Goerger BM, Linens SW. Four-week ankle-rehabilitation programs in adolescent athletes with chronic ankle instability. J Athl Train. 2020;55(8):801–10.
68. Dejong AF, Koldenhoven RM, Hertel J. Proximal adaptations in chronic ankle instability: systematic review and meta-analysis. Med Sci Sports Exerc. 2020;52(7):1563–75.
69. Kwon YU, Harrison K, Kweon SJ, Williams DSB 3rd. Ankle coordination in chronic ankle instability, coper, and control groups in running. Med Sci Sports Exerc. 2020;52(3):663–72.
70. Molina-Rueda F, Cuesta-Gómez A, Carratalá-Tejada M, Koutsou A, Fernández-González P, Alguacil-Diego IM. Ankle muscle activation during the limits of stability test in subjects with chronic ankle instability. Phys Ther Sport. 2021;47:134–9.
71. Golano P, Vega J, Perez-Carro L, Gotzens V. Ankle anatomy for the arthroscopist. Part I: the portals. Foot Ankle Clin. 2006;11(2):253–73.
72. Barg A, Saltzman CL, Beals TC, Bachus KN, Blankenhorn BD, Nickisch F. Arthroscopic talar dome access using a standard versus wire-based traction method for ankle joint distraction. Arthroscopy. 2016;32(7):1367–74.
73. Nickisch F, Barg A, Saltzman CL, Beals TC, Bonasia DE, Phisitkul P, et al. Posterior ankle and hindfoot arthroscopy. JBJS Essent Surgn Tech. 2012;2(3):e15.
74. Nickisch F, Barg A, Saltzman CL, Beals TC, Bonasia DE, Phisitkul P, et al. Postoperative complications of posterior ankle and hindfoot arthroscopy. J Bone Joint Surg Am. 2012;94(5):439–46.
75. Hintermann B, Ruiz R. Foot and ankle instability: a clinical guide to diagnosis and surgical management. Cham: Springer; 2021.
76. Aicale R, Maffulli N. Chronic lateral ankle instability: topical review. Foot Ankle Int. 2020;41(12):1571–81.
77. Yasui Y, Shimozono Y, Kennedy JG. Surgical procedures for chronic lateral ankle instability. J Am Acad Orthop Surg. 2018;26(7):223–30.
78. Acevedo JI, Palmer RC, Mangone PG. Arthroscopic treatment of ankle instability: Brostrom. Foot Ankle Clin. 2018;23(4):555–70.
79. Matsui K, Burgesson B, Takao M, Stone J, Guillo S, Glazebrook M. Minimally invasive surgical treatment for chronic ankle instability: a systematic review. Knee Surg Sports Traumatol Arthrosc. 2016;24(4):1040–8.
80. Vega J, Dalmau-Pastor M. Editorial commentary: arthroscopic treatment of ankle instability is the emerging gold standard. Arthroscopy. 2021;37(1):280–1.
81. Brostrom L, Sprained ankles. V. Treatment and prognosis in recent ligament ruptures. Acta Chir Scand. 1966;132(5):537–50.
82. Gould N, Seligson D, Gassman J. Early and late repair of lateral ligament of the ankle. Foot Ankle. 1980;1(2):84–9.
83. Hunt KJ, Griffith R. Open Brostrom for lateral ligament stabilization. Curr Rev Musculoskelet Med. 2020;13(6):788–96.
84. Behrens SB, Drakos M, Lee BJ, Paller D, Hoffman E, Koruprolu S, et al. Biomechanical analysis of Brostrom versus Brostrom-Gould lateral ankle instability repairs. Foot Ankle Int. 2013;34(4):587–92.
85. Boey H, Verfaillie S, Natsakis T, Vander Sloten J, Jonkers I. Augmented ligament reconstruction partially restores Hindfoot and midfoot kinematics after lateral ligament ruptures. Am J Sports Med. 2019;47(8):1921–30.
86. Brown CA, Hurwit D, Behn A, Hunt KJ. Biomechanical comparison of an all-soft suture anchor with a modified Broström-Gould suture repair for lateral ligament reconstruction. Am J Sports Med. 2014;42(2):417–22.
87. Wainright WB, Spritzer CE, Lee JY, Easley ME, DeOrio JK, Nunley JA, et al. The effect of modified Brostrom-Gould repair for lateral ankle instability on in vivo tibiotalar kinematics. Am J Sports Med. 2012;40(9):2099–104.
88. Choisne J, Hoch MC, Alexander I, Ringleb SI. Effect of direct ligament repair and tenodesis reconstruction on simulated subtalar joint instability. Foot Ankle Int. 2017;38(3):324–30.
89. Brodsky AR, O'Malley MJ, Bohne WH, Deland JA, Kennedy JG. An analysis of outcome measures following the Brostrom-Gould procedure for

chronic lateral ankle instability. Foot Ankle Int. 2005;26(10):816–9.
90. Guelfi M, Zamperetti M, Pantalone A, Usuelli FG, Salini V, Oliva XM. Open and arthroscopic lateral ligament repair for treatment of chronic ankle instability: a systematic review. Foot Ankle Surg. 2018;24(1):11–8.
91. Matheny LM, Johnson NS, Liechti DJ, Clanton TO. Activity level and function after lateral ankle ligament repair versus reconstruction. Am J Sports Med. 2016;44(5):1301–8.
92. Feng SM, Maffulli N, Ma C, Oliva F. All-inside arthroscopic modified Broström-Gould procedure for chronic lateral ankle instability with and without anterior talofibular ligament remnant repair produced similar functional results. Knee Surg Sports Traumatol Arthrosc. 2021;29(8):2453–61.
93. Feng SM, Wang AG, Sun QQ, Zhang ZY. Functional results of all-inside arthroscopic Broström-Gould surgery with 2 anchors versus single anchor. Foot Ankle Int. 2020;41(6):721–7.
94. Guillo S, Odagiri H. All-inside endoscopic Broström-Gould technique. Arthrosc Tech. 2020;9(1):e79–84.
95. Martinelli N, Manfroni F, Bianchi A. Ankle lateral ligament augmentation versus the modified Broström-Gould procedure: letter to the editor. Am J Sports Med. 2019;47(10):Np51.
96. Nery C, Fonseca L, Raduan F, Moreno M, Baumfeld D. Prospective study of the "inside-out" arthroscopic ankle ligament technique: preliminary result. Foot Ankle Surg. 2018;24(4):320–5.
97. Vilá-Rico J, Cabestany-Castellà JM, Cabestany-Perich B, Núñez-Samper C, Ojeda-Thies C. All-inside arthroscopic allograft reconstruction of the anterior talo-fibular ligament using an accessory transfibular portal. Foot Ankle Surg. 2019;25(1):24–30.
98. Woo BJ, Lai MC, Koo K. Arthroscopic versus open Broström-Gould repair for chronic ankle instability. Foot Ankle Int. 2020;41(6):647–53.
99. Zeng G, Hu X, Liu W, Qiu X, Yang T, Li C, et al. Open Broström-Gould repair vs arthroscopic anatomical repair of the anterior Talofibular ligament for chronic lateral ankle instability. Foot Ankle Int. 2020;41(1):44–9.
100. Zhou YF, Zhang ZZ, Zhang HZ, Li WP, Shen HY, Song B. All-inside arthroscopic modified Broström technique to repair anterior Talofibular ligament provides a similar outcome compared with open Broström-Gould procedure. Arthroscopy. 2021;37(1):268–79.
101. Barg A, Saltzman CL. Single-stage supramalleolar osteotomy for coronal plane deformity. Curr Rev Musculoskelet Med. 2014;7(4):277–91.
102. Hintermann B, Knupp M, Barg A. Supramalleolar osteotomies for the treatment of ankle arthritis. J Am Acad Orthop Surg. 2016;24(7):424–32.
103. Tennant JN, Carmont M, Phisitkul P. Calcaneus osteotomy. Curr Rev Musculoskelet Med. 2014;7(4):271–6.
104. Krähenbühl N, Lenz AL, Lisonbee R, Deforth M, Zwicky L, Hintermann B, et al. Imaging of the subtalar joint: a novel approach to an old problem. J Orthop Res. 2019;37(4):921–6.
105. Sarrafian SK. Biomechanics of the subtalar joint complex. Clin Orthop Relat Res. 1993;290:17–26.
106. Kamada K, Watanabe S, Yamamoto H. Chronic subtalar instability due to insufficiency of the calcaneofibular ligament: a case report. Foot Ankle Int. 2002;23(12):1135–7.
107. Kjaersgaard-Andersen P, Wethelund JO, Helmig P, Nielsen S. Effect of the calcaneofibular ligament on hindfoot rotation in amputation specimens. Acta Orthop Scand. 1987;58(2):135–8.
108. Leonard MH. Injuries of the lateral ligaments of the ankle; a clinical and experimental study. J Bone Joint Surg Am. 1949;31a(2):373–7.
109. Martin LP, Wayne JS, Owen JR, Smith RT, Martin SN, Adelaar RS. Elongation behavior of calcaneofibular and cervical ligaments in a closed kinetic chain: pathomechanics of lateral hindfoot instability. Foot Ankle Int. 2002;23(6):515–20.
110. Michelson J, Hamel A, Buczek F, Sharkey N. The effect of ankle injury on subtalar motion. Foot Ankle Int. 2004;25(9):639–46.
111. Ruth CJ. The surgical treatment of injuries of the fibular collateral ligaments of the ankle. J Bone Joint Surg Am. 1961;43:229–39.
112. Bonnel F, Toullec E, Mabit C, Tourne Y. Chronic ankle instability: biomechanics and pathomechanics of ligaments injury and associated lesions. Orthop Traumatol Surg Res. 2010;96(4):424–32.
113. Ringleb SI, Dhakal A, Anderson CD, Bawab S, Paranjape R. Effects of lateral ligament sectioning on the stability of the ankle and subtalar joint. J Orthop Res. 2011;29(10):1459–64.
114. Tochigi Y. Effect of arch supports on ankle-subtalar complex instability: a biomechanical experimental study. Foot Ankle Int. 2003;24(8):634–9.
115. Tochigi Y, Amendola A, Rudert MJ, Baer TE, Brown TD, Hillis SL, et al. The role of the interosseous talocalcaneal ligament in subtalar joint stability. Foot Ankle Int. 2004;25(8):588–96.
116. Tochigi Y, Takahashi K, Yamagata M, Tamaki T. Influence of the interosseous talocalcaneal ligament injury on stability of the ankle-subtalar joint complex--a cadaveric experimental study. Foot Ankle Int. 2000;21(6):486–91.
117. Iglesias-Durán E, Guerra-Pinto F, García-Esteo F, Vilá-Rico J. Anatomic arthroscopic graft reconstruction of the interosseous talocalcaneal ligament for subtalar instability. Arthrosc Tech. 2020;9(12):e1903–e6.
118. Kato T. The diagnosis and treatment of instability of the subtalar joint. J Bone Joint Surg. 1995;77(3):400–6.
119. Liu C, Jiao C, Hu Y, Guo QW, Wand C, Ao Y. Interosseous talocalcaneal ligament reconstruction with hamstring autograft under subtalar arthroscopy: case report. Foot Ankle Int. 2011;32(11):1089–94.
120. Liu C, Zhu JX, Hu YL, Jiao C, Guo QW, Ao YF. Secondary effects of the rupture and reconstruction of the interosseous talocalcaneal ligament on the peritalar joints. Med Sci Monit. 2021;27:e925292.

8 Lateral Ankle Instability: The Modified Brostrom

Lorraine Boakye, Cortez Brown, Nia James, and MaCalus V. Hogan

Introduction

Ankle injuries are among the most common orthopedic injuries both in the general and athletic populations. A 1-year nationwide emergency department surveillance study reported an incidence of 3.29 per 1000 person-years for ankle sprains [1]. In comparison, the incidence rate for lateral ankle sprains among 25 National Collegiate Athletic Association (NCAA) sports was 4.95 per 10,000 athlete exposures (AE) [2]. The authors defined AE as one student-athlete participating in one NCAA-sanctioned practice or competition in which he or she was exposed to the possibility of an athletic injury regardless of the time associated with that participation. Clinicians dichotomize lateral ankle sprains into mechanical and functional pathologies. Patients with a mechanical injury have ligamentous damage, while patients with functional pathology sense their ankle as being weak or unstable. The lateral ankle ligamentous complex is comprised of the anterior talofibular ligament (ATFL), calcaneofibular ligament (CFL), and posterior talofibular ligament (PTFL). Of those three ligaments, the ATFL is most commonly injured first due to its decreased strength. Lateral ankle sprains range in severity from overstretching and microtears (grade I) to complete ligament rupture (grade III) [3]. In grade III sprains, the ATFL is oftentimes torn at its midpoint or avulsed from the talus.

Diagnosis

To diagnose a patient with lateral ankle instability (LAI), several steps should be taken in order to gather sufficient information to confirm the pathological process in question. To begin the process of making this diagnosis, a thorough history and physical examination should be completed first. It is important to ask patients what they were doing at the time of injury and how the injury specifically occurred. Knowing the mechanism of injury allows the examiner to formulate an idea regarding which ligamentous complex

L. Boakye · N. James
Department of Orthopaedic Surgery, University of Pittsburgh Medical Center, Pittsburgh, PA, USA
e-mail: boakyela@upmc.edu; jamesn2@upmc.edu

C. Brown
Department of Orthopaedic Surgery, University of Pittsburgh Medical Center, Pittsburgh, PA, USA

Florida State University College of Medicine, Tallahassee, FL, USA
e-mail: cortezbl@upmc.edu

M. V. Hogan (✉)
Department of Orthopaedic Surgery, University of Pittsburgh Medical Center, Pittsburgh, PA, USA

The Foot and Ankle Injury Research [F.A.I.R.] Group, University of Pittsburgh Medical Center, Pittsburgh, PA, USA
e-mail: hoganmv@upmc.edu

P. D'Hooghe et al. (eds.), *Ligamentous Injuries of the Foot and Ankle*,
https://doi.org/10.1007/978-3-031-08682-3_8

was potentially stressed, if any, as it could be a non-ligamentous injury altogether. The most common mechanism of injury for lateral ankle instability is inversion of a plantar-flexed foot [4]. Therefore, if a patient describes a plantar-flexed inversion movement at the time of injury, LAI may be moved higher on the differential diagnosis. A patient's ability to bear weight following the injury and whether or not they heard an audible pop are also helpful pieces of information to gather during history taking. The time frame in which the patient has been dealing with this issue also plays a role because if it has been at least 12 months since the original injury, it may be considered a chronic issue. Patients may also report experiencing recurrent ankle sprains, feeling as if their ankle is giving way, pain, swelling, limited range of motion, weakness, and decreased function overall [5]. If weakness is present, it can be helpful to clarify if it is subjectively secondary to pain or the pure inability to fire the necessary muscles. Depending on the response, it may potentially be due to a mechanical or neurologic deficit, respectively. When first assessing a patient, the history alone can strongly suggest a diagnosis of lateral ankle instability, but a detailed physical examination should be done to further characterize the working diagnosis.

When approaching the physical examination with a diagnosis of lateral ankle instability in mind, special attention should be paid to the lateral ligamentous complex. This complex includes the anterior talofibular ligament (ATFL), posterior talofibular ligament (PTFL), and calcaneofibular ligament (CFL) [4]. The examiner should begin by inspecting the lower extremities bilaterally, noting any visual deformities or other discrepancies between the patient's lower legs, ankles, and feet. In the acute setting, edema and ecchymosis would still be expected to be present. However, in a patient with a more chronic injury pattern, edema and ecchymosis may not be appreciated on examination. It is important to note that this does not mean the patient does not experience these symptoms intermittently. Palpation should be done to grade both the dorsalis pedis and posterior tibial pulses, illicit areas of tenderness, and determine the severity of active edema if present. Additionally, his or her ability to passively and actively rotate about the joint should be established. The patient's strength should be tested against resistance, and any report of lack of sensation, numbness, or tingling should be noted as well. Performing special tests such as the anterior drawer test and talar tilt test can assist in diagnosing ATFL and CFL pathologies, respectively [6]. It is vital to compare the contralateral side to ensure that any laxity detected cannot be contributed to a patient's baseline anatomy. Additionally, with a sensitivity approaching 100%, the Ottawa ankle rules should be applied to further work up the patient's ankle pain [7]. This set of well-established guidelines is very useful in excluding ankle fractures, especially in the emergent setting. However, if ligamentous laxity or a fracture is suspected after the history and examination are completed, the next step in diagnosis should be to order detailed imaging.

Stress radiographs and magnetic resonance imaging (MRI) allow for the opportunity to closely look for clues that may help with the diagnosis that cannot be appreciated on gross examination. Stress radiographs assist in diagnostic decision-making by providing an image with force applied so the amount of separation at the joint can be quantified [8]. Excessive translation in any direction should be noted and compared to the contralateral side. Furthermore, if a fracture is involved, that will be seen on plain imaging as well. An MRI will contribute more insight as to what is going on with the surrounding soft tissue and the ligaments themselves. Edema and partial or complete tears may be appreciated using this method.

Management

The primary goal of the clinician is to determine the patient's ankle stability. If they are stable and experiencing minimal pain with weight-bearing, the clinician is less worried about a completely torn ligament. The majority of these lateral ankle sprains are managed conservatively. Patients with grade I or II sprains typically do not have severe pain while weight-bearing and are functionally stable. Current treatments involve proprioceptive training, peroneal tendon strengthening, semi-rigid ankle bracing plus taping, and shoe modifications [9, 10]. A recent systematic review reported good outcomes with all of these methods [11]. Failed conservative management of these sprains is an indication for surgical management. While grade III sprains oftentimes require surgical management, there are some conservative options clinicians consider: short leg cast for 3 weeks followed by 12 weeks of physical therapy and functional management via rest, ice, compression, elevation (RICE), and rehabilitation. If the patient is an elite athlete, current recommendations are to consider surgical management and accelerated postoperative rehabilitation [12]. Additionally, if a patient fails conservative management and has persistent signs of instability, surgical management is the next step.

There are various surgical management options to consider for chronic ankle instability. These options can be divided into nonanatomic and anatomic techniques. In 1932, Nilsonne described the first nonanatomic technique. He transferred the peroneus brevis muscle to the fibula [13]. In 1941, Watson-Jones introduced another nonanatomic technique where he weaved the peroneus brevis through drilled holes in the fibula to reconstruct the ATFL [14]. Although the nonanatomic techniques mentioned above and others (e.g., Evans [15] and Chrisman-Snook [16]) reported good outcomes, several complications were reported also (i.e., peroneal muscle fatigue, persistent instability, decreased range of motion, and ankle tightness) [17–21]. In 1966, Dr. Brostrom introduced the initial version of today's standard of care for chronic ankle instability [22]. Fourteen years later, Dr. Gould modified this approach by suturing the lateral portion of the inferior retinaculum onto the distal fibula for increased ATFL reinforcement and subtalar stability [23]. Recently, Hattori et al. reported performing an ultrasound-guided anatomic reduction of the ATFL with minimal iatrogenic damage [24]. Musculoskeletal ultrasound is cost-effective, readily available, and both diagnostic and interventional. As such, the authors believe that this paradigm is a valuable adjunct to the modified Brostrom procedure. The authors also discuss reduced surgical time, decreased iatrogenic neurovascular damage, and direct visualization of anatomic landmarks needed to improve surgical accuracy. However, the Brostrom-Gould (modified Brostrom) is considered the standard of care for lateral ligament injuries and has a record of persistent good and excellent outcome data [25, 26].

Modified Brostrom Surgical Technique

We place the patient in a lateral decubitus position and pad all bony prominences. We make note to appropriately pad the thigh prior to applying the tourniquet. The lead author prefers an anterior J incision over the posterior curvilinear option because of his training. It should be the surgeon's preference. The incision is made about the distal fibula, superior and inferior to ATFL origin. In doing so, we ensure to avoid superficial peroneal and sural nerves. We dissect down to the fibular periosteum and mobilize the flaps anteriorly and posteriorly. We stop to identify the anterolateral capsule, peroneal tendons, and inferior extensor retinaculum. We then open the peroneal sheath proximally and distally while preserving the superior peroneal retinaculum. After addressing the peroneal tendon pathology, we make an anterior J-shaped incision along the anterior and distal aspect of the fibula. When doing so, we make sure to avoid branches of the superficial peroneal nerve. In the distal aspect of our incision, we locate the inferior extensor retinaculum. As mentioned, this will be used later for the Gould modification. We retract the retinaculum with a tag suture and proceed to our next steps. We then identify and divide the joint capsule. When doing so, we leave tissue on the distal fibula for the Gould modification.

When completing the arthrotomy from the tibiotalar joint to peroneal tendons, we take note of protecting said tendons. This arthrotomy will divide both the ATFL and CFL. After resecting scar tissue, we imbricate the ligaments in a pants-over-vest fashion with 0 Vicryl sutures. We do not set our sutures until placing the patient's ankle in dorsiflexion and eversion. We also avoid anterior subluxation of the talus. After placing the sutures, we test the ankle's range of motion to verify appropriate ankle excursion and fixation. We progress to the Gould modification by securing the inferior extensor retinaculum onto the distal fibular periosteum. After undergoing a final range of motion testing, we irrigate and close the subcutaneous and skin layers. Intraoperatively, we place the patient in a short leg plaster posterior and stirrup splint until their first postoperative visit.

Rehabilitation

Early rehabilitation following a diagnosis of lateral ankle instability is crucial for adequate regain of ankle function. If possible, as soon as the injury occurs, the patient should begin rehabilitation within that same week for best outcomes [27]. This can be achieved through many different exercises that target the surrounding muscle groups that provide support to the ankle. A study done by Lee et al. [28] demonstrated that a rehabilitation course as little as 4 weeks in duration can prevent functional foot and ankle deficits. Although 4 weeks of rehabilitation has been proven to be effective, there are patients who will require a longer course to recover. Some patients may opt for a conservative approach only. However, others may proceed with surgical management in conjunction with rehabilitation. Either way, the ultimate goal of rehabilitation is to restore function and strength and to prevent reinjury in the future [6].

References

1. Shah S, Thomas AC, Noone JM, Blanchette CM, Wikstrom EA. Incidence and cost of ankle sprains in United States Emergency Departments. Sports Health. 2016;8(6):547–52. https://doi.org/10.1177/1941738116659639.
2. Roos KG, Kerr ZY, Mauntel TC, Djoko A, Dompier TP, Wikstrom EA. The epidemiology of lateral ligament complex ankle sprains in National Collegiate Athletic Association Sports. Am J Sports Med. 2017;45(1):201–9. https://doi.org/10.1177/0363546516660980.
3. Dias LS. The lateral ankle sprain: an experimental study. J Trauma. 1979;19(4):266–9. https://doi.org/10.1097/00005373-197904000-00009.
4. Chan KW, Ding BC, Mroczek KJ. Acute and chronic lateral ankle instability in the athlete. Bull NYU Hosp Jt Dis. 2011;69(1):17–26.
5. Hertel J, Corbett RO. An updated model of chronic ankle instability. J Athl Train. 2019;54(6):572–88. https://doi.org/10.4085/1062-6050-344-18.
6. Czajka CM, Tran E, Cai AN, DiPreta JA. Ankle sprains and instability. Med Clin North Am. 2014;98(2):313–29. https://doi.org/10.1016/j.mcna.2013.11.003.
7. Bachmann LM, Kolb E, Koller MT, Steurer J, ter Riet G. Accuracy of Ottawa ankle rules to exclude fractures of the ankle and mid-foot: systematic review. BMJ. 2003;326(7386):417. https://doi.org/10.1136/bmj.326.7386.417.
8. Gribble PA. Evaluating and differentiating ankle instability. J Athl Train. 2019;54(6):617–27. https://doi.org/10.4085/1062-6050-484-17.
9. Stephenson D, Charlton T, Thordarson D. Ankle instability. In: Saxena A, editor. International advances in foot and ankle surgery. London: Springer London; 2012. p. 169–78.
10. Beynnon BD, Renström PA, Haugh L, Uh BS, Barker H. A prospective, randomized clinical investigation of the treatment of first-time ankle sprains. Am J Sports Med. 2006;34(9):1401–12. https://doi.org/10.1177/0363546506288676.
11. Petersen W, Rembitzki IV, Koppenburg AG, Ellermann A, Liebau C, Brüggemann GP, et al. Treatment of acute ankle ligament injuries: a systematic review. Arch Orthop Trauma Surg. 2013;133(8):1129–41. https://doi.org/10.1007/s00402-013-1742-5.
12. van den Bekerom MP, Kerkhoffs GM, McCollum GA, Calder JD, van Dijk CN. Management of acute lateral ankle ligament injury in the athlete. Knee Surg Sports Traumatol Arthrosc. 2013;21(6):1390–5. https://doi.org/10.1007/s00167-012-2252-7.
13. Nilsonne H. Making a new ligament in ankle sprain. J Bone Joint Surg. 1932;14(2):380–1.
14. Watson-Jones R. Fractures and other bone and joint injuries. 2nd ed. Baltimore: Williams & Wilkins; 1941.
15. Evans D. Recurrent instability of the ankle; a method of surgical treatment. Proc R Soc Med. 1953;46(5):343–4.
16. Chrisman OD, Snook GA. Reconstruction of lateral ligament tears of the ankle. An experimental study and clinical evaluation of seven patients treated by a new modification of the Elmslie procedure. J Bone Joint Surg Am. 1969;51(5):904–12.
17. Sugimoto K, Takakura Y, Akiyama K, Kamei S, Kitada C, Kumai T. Long-term results of Watson-Jones tenodesis of the ankle. Clinical and radiographic

findings after ten to eighteen years of follow-up. J Bone Joint Surg Am. 1998;80(11):1587–96. https://doi.org/10.2106/00004623-199811000-00004.
18. van der Rijt AJ, Evans GA. The long-term results of Watson-Jones tenodesis. J Bone Joint Surg Br. 1984;66(3):371–5. https://doi.org/10.1302/0301-620X.66B3.6725348.
19. Karlsson J, Bergsten T, Lansinger O, Peterson L. Lateral instability of the ankle treated by the Evans procedure. A long-term clinical and radiological follow-up. J Bone Joint Surg Br. 1988;70(3):476–80. https://doi.org/10.1302/0301-620X.70B3.3372575.
20. Kaikkonen A, Lehtonen H, Kannus P, Järvinen M. Long-term functional outcome after surgery of chronic ankle instability. A 5-year follow-up study of the modified Evans procedure. Scand J Med Sci Sports. 1999;9(4):239–44. https://doi.org/10.1111/j.1600-0838.1999.tb00240.x.
21. Snook GA, Chrisman OD, Wilson TC. Long-term results of the Chrisman-Snook operation for reconstruction of the lateral ligaments of the ankle. J Bone Joint Surg Am. 1985;67(1):1–7.
22. Broström L, Sprained ankles. VI. Surgical treatment of "chronic" ligament ruptures. Acta Chir Scand. 1966;132(5):551–65.
23. Gould N, Seligson D, Gassman J. Early and late repair of lateral ligament of the ankle. Foot Ankle. 1980;1(2):84–9. https://doi.org/10.1177/107110078000100206.
24. Hattori S, Alvarez CAD, Canton S, Hogan MV, Onishi K. Ultrasound-guided ankle lateral ligament stabilization. Curr Rev Musculoskelet Med. 2019;12(4):497–508. https://doi.org/10.1007/s12178-019-09592-0.
25. Bell SJ, Mologne TS, Sitler DF, Cox JS. Twenty-six-year results after Broström procedure for chronic lateral ankle instability. Am J Sports Med. 2006;34(6):975–8. https://doi.org/10.1177/0363546505282616.
26. Broström L, Sprained ankles. V. Treatment and prognosis in recent ligament ruptures. Acta Chir Scand. 1966;132(5):537–50.
27. Bleakley CM, O'Connor SR, Tully MA, Rocke LG, Macauley DC, Bradbury I, et al. Effect of accelerated rehabilitation on function after ankle sprain: randomised controlled trial. BMJ. 2010;340:c1964. https://doi.org/10.1136/bmj.c1964.
28. Lee KY, Lee HJ, Kim SE, Choi PB, Song SH, Jee YS. Short term rehabilitation and ankle instability. Int J Sports Med. 2012;33(6):485–96. https://doi.org/10.1055/s-0032-1301933.

9 Lateral Ankle Instability: Arthroscopic Broström and Minimally Invasive Techniques

Kenneth J. Hunt and Francisco Rodriguez-Fontan

Introduction

Ankle sprains are the most common musculoskeletal injury in physically active people and account for approximately 25% of sports injuries [1, 2]. An estimated 85% percent of ankle sprains include injury to the lateral ankle ligaments with the majority of ankle sprains causing injury to the anterior talofibular ligament (ATFL) and about half causing injury to the calcaneofibular ligament (CFL) [1, 3]. The most common mechanism of injury is foot inversion [4]. Chronic ankle instability (CAI) can occur in up to 40% of the cases, especially in higher-grade ankle ligament injuries [1]. CAI can lead to chronic dysfunction, pain with physical activity, and restrictions in participation in competitive or recreational sports and physical activities and eventually can lead to post-traumatic osteoarthritis [2, 5, 6]. For patients who do not improve with conservative treatment, surgical options and postoperative rehabilitation have evolved considerably over the last 50 years, particularly with the advent and utilization of arthroscopy [3].

K. J. Hunt (✉)
Department of Orthopedic Surgery, University of Colorado School of Medicine, Aurora, CO, USA
e-mail: Kenneth.j.hunt@cuanschutz.edu

F. Rodriguez-Fontan
Department of Orthopedics, University of Colorado Anschutz Medical Campus, Aurora, CO, USA
e-mail: francisco.rodriguezfontan@cuanschutz.edu

In 1966, Broström described an anatomical procedure to imbricate and primarily repair the ATFL and CFL ligaments in patients with chronic instability. While the Broström procedure remains the gold standard upon which modifications of the procedure have emerged [7], the availability of small joint arthroscopy and the success of arthroscopic repair techniques in the other major joints have led to the development of arthroscopic and minimally invasive lateral ankle ligament repair techniques that have been described with promising results [3, 8]. The key purported advantage of these techniques is significantly less soft tissue dissection, less postoperative swelling, shorter operative times, and more rapid rehabilitation. Current literature focuses primarily on the safety of these techniques and their effectiveness as compared to open repair techniques [3, 9]. The arthroscopic technique has been shown to be biomechanically similar to the open repair technique [10, 11].

Arthroscopic surgical techniques for lateral ankle ligament repair have been generally categorized into arthroscopic-assisted, all-arthroscopic, and all-inside techniques [9]. Besides the aforementioned benefits of arthroscopy, additional advantages include the ability to diagnose and address concurrent pathology which are identified in 50% or more of unstable ankles and can contribute to overall patient symptomatology (common examples include soft tissue or degenerative impingement, synovitis, loose bodies, and osteochondral lesions) [12–14].

P. D'Hooghe et al. (eds.), *Ligamentous Injuries of the Foot and Ankle*,
https://doi.org/10.1007/978-3-031-08682-3_9

The purpose of this chapter is to review current techniques and published outcomes of arthroscopic and minimally invasive repair of the lateral ligamentous complex.

Arthroscopy in Lateral Ligament Repair

Ankle arthroscopy gained popularity in the 1990s because it allowed a better understanding of chronic ankle pain and allowed better identification of, and access to, intra-articular injuries and conditions [15]. In 1987, Hawkins pioneered on arthroscopic ankle stabilization with use of a staple for lateral ankle ligaments plication [16]. Despite advocating for minimal discomfort, shorter recovery and disability periods, and promising results, the studies lacked adequate long-term follow-up or outcomes [16]. In the mid-1990s, Kashuk et al. [17, 18] implemented an arthroscopic suture anchor-based repair with adequate gain in stability, yet they advocated that injury to the CFL may require an open procedure [17]. Multiple recent studies support isolated ATFL repair, leaving the CFL repair at surgeons' discretion [7].

The purported benefit of arthroscopic techniques includes shorter operative time, more rapid recovery, and a single approach that allows for the treatment of other conditions as mentioned [19]. Rates of complication are reported with wide range (0–35%), similar to open procedures (0–29.6%) [3]. Complications of the arthroscopic technique include nerve pain (e.g., superficial peroneal nerve [SPN], sural nerve), delayed wound healing, and deep vein thrombosis [1, 3]. Reported clinical outcomes from arthroscopic lateral ligament repair procedures are promising despite reported complication rates [3]. We explore both arthroscopic and percutaneous ligament repair techniques, including the value of including these techniques in your treatment arsenal for ankle instability.

Lateral Ligamentous Complex Anatomy

The lateral ligamentous complex can be defined by three ligamentous structures from anterior to posterior: ATFL, CFL, and posterior talofibular ligament (PTFL). The ATFL of quadrilateral shape, composed mostly of 1–2 bands, spans in a 45-degree angle from the lateral malleolus at approximately 10–14 mm from the distal aspect of the fibula to the lateral aspect of the talar body. The ATFL prevents anterior translation of the talocrural joint and resists inversion with the ankle plantarflexed. It is the most commonly injured ligament (~75% rate) in a plantar flexion inversion mode, likely due to its lower maximal load to failure as compared to the CFL and PFTL [1, 4, 20].

The CFL originates just distal to the ATFL, at approximately 5 mm from the distal aspect of the fibula, coursing roughly at a 130-degree antero-posterior angle deep to the peroneal tendons to insert on the lateral aspect of the calcaneus. This ligament also stabilizes the subtalar joint. It is the second most frequently injured ligament (~20–41% rate) in a dorsiflexion and inversion mode and rarely occurs in isolation [1, 4, 20].

The PTFL is a broad horizontal spanning ligament that originates from the posteromedial fibula and inserts at the posterior aspect of the talus. It restrains the ankle from inversion and internal rotation. It is rarely injured but more frequently injured in high-energy sprains (5–10% rate) [7, 20].

Besides the abovementioned ligaments, the inferior extensor retinaculum (IER) has been reported to perform a similar function to the CFL for subtalar joint stabilization [21]. In addition, and with this in mind, the Broström-Gould modification implicates using this structure to reinforce the ATFL repair, with proven functional outcomes [22]. Often, the crural fascia is inadvertently used instead of the IER [23], but this can be improved with accurate positioning of an accessory portal [24]. Interestingly, both open and arthroscopically assisted use of IER reinforcement showed no significant functional or radiographic benefit compared to repairing ligaments alone, and inclusion of IER in the repair can lead to stiffness of the posterior subtalar joint [25, 26]. When incorporating IER in the repair, one must also use caution to protect the SPN to mitigate risk of injury [1, 24].

Arthroscopic Lateral Ligament Repair Technique

The following stepwise operative technique is the senior author's preferred technique. We will review anesthesia, positioning, landmarks, portal placement, arthroscopic diagnostics, and procedure.

1. *Anesthesia*. General anesthesia is most frequently used although regional block and monitored anesthesia can be utilized based on patient preference or risk factors. It is important to have an experienced provider administer the regional anesthetic.
2. *Manual examination* of the ankle is performed under anesthesia to assess the ankle ligamentous complex by an anterior drawer test and talar tilt test in comparison to the contralateral ankle. Live fluoroscopy can be helpful, particularly to differentiate ankle and subtalar instability at the outset (Fig. 9.1).
3. *Positioning*. The patient is positioned supine with an ipsilateral bump under the hip, a nonsterile thigh tourniquet, and an ankle distractor on the operative side. Antibiotics are administered. The operative leg is exsanguinated. The peroneal tendons are marked inferior and lateral to the lateral malleolus. The SPN is traced and marked lateral to peroneus tertius and medial to the lateral malleolus (Fig. 9.2).
4. *Portal placement*. A needle is used to localize the medial arthroscopic portal, and the joint is insufflated with 10 cc of sterile saline solution. Standard anteromedial and anterolateral portals are created with small incisions and "nick and spread" technique to enter the joint prior to insertion of the arthroscopic cannula. The anteromedial portal aids in visualizing the SPN over the lateral aspect of the ankle by transillumination to avoid its injury prior to making the anterolateral portal.
5. *Diagnostic arthroscopy*. Standard diagnostic arthroscopy is performed, and intra-articular pathology is addressed and treated as indicated. An accessory portal can be utilized if necessary for thorough debridement of synovitis or removal of loose bodies. The lateral gutter must be debrided extensively to allow for visualization of the distal fibula and for removal of scar tissue.

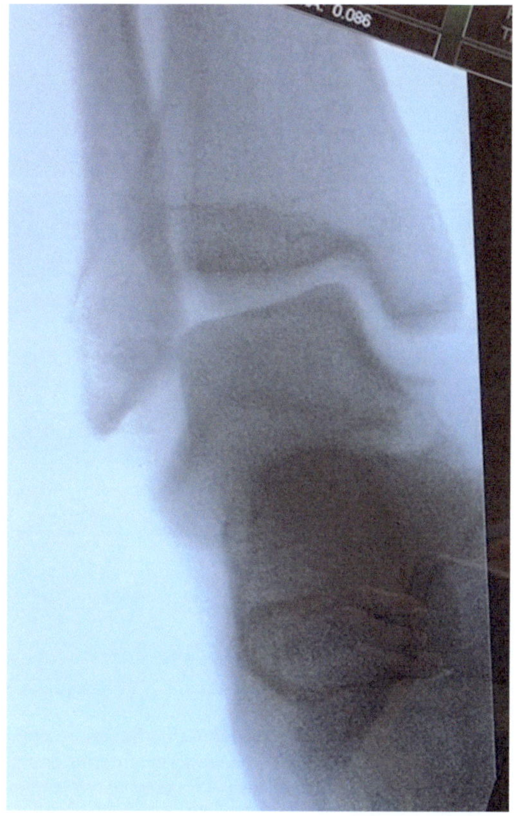

Fig. 9.1 Fluoroscopic image showing ankle under eversion stress. Note tilt of the talus relative to the ankle mortise (suggesting tibiotalar instability) and medial translation of the subtalar joint (suggesting subtalar instability)

6. *Anchor placement*. The distal fibula is identified with a probe (Fig. 9.3). The ATFL fibular footprint is debrided and burred to healthy bone (Fig. 9.4). Using an arthroscopic cannula, one suture anchor is placed in the fibular footprint (starting ~1 cm proximal to the fibular tip) with a second anchor placed 1.5 cm above this if indicated. The anchors can typically be placed through the anterolateral arthroscopic portal; thus, the sutures are readily accessible (Fig. 9.2).

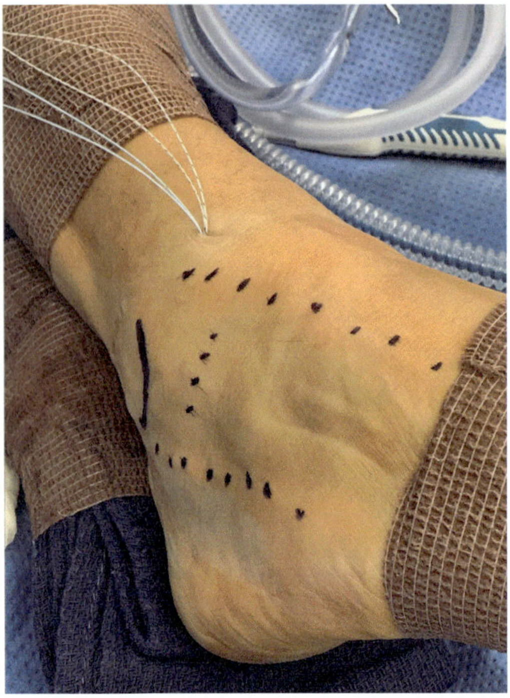

Fig. 9.2 Photographs of skin landmarks. Superior dotted line represents superficial peroneal nerve. Inferior dotted line represents peroneal tendons. The sural nerve is inferior to the peroneal tendons at this level. Note that sutures are retrieved in the "safe zone" between these two landmarks

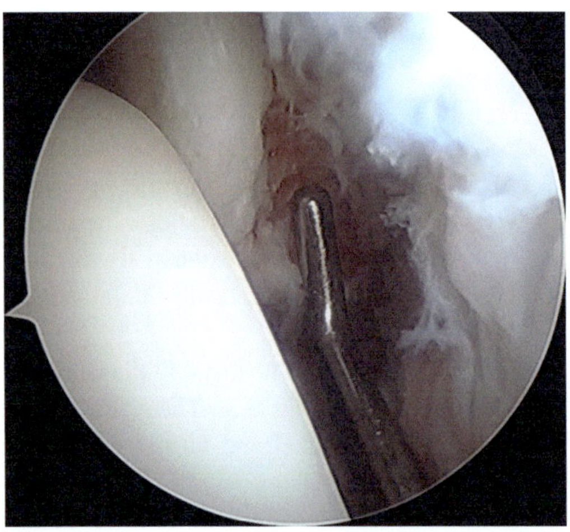

Fig. 9.3 Arthroscopic image of distal fibula. The probe is positioned where the ATFL fibular footprint has been burred to healthy-appearing bone for anchor positioning

7. *Passing sutures*. The sutures are passed in sequence with a sharp-tipped suture passer, penetrating the ATFL and inferior extensor retinaculum and exiting the skin 2–3 cm inferior to the distal tip of the fibula. It is imperative that the sutures exit between the sural and lateral branch SPN to avoid nerve injury. The first suture limb is passed immediately superior to the peroneal tendon margin. The second suture limb is passed 1 cm anterior/dorsal to the first suture. The ankle is held in neutral dorsiflexion, allowing capture of the IER.

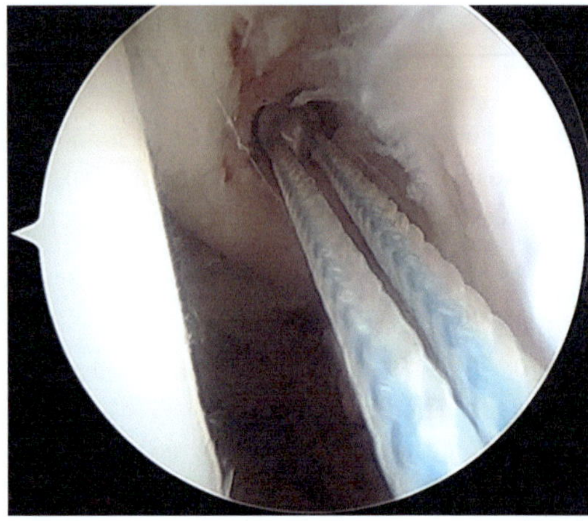

Fig. 9.4 Arthroscopic image of first suture anchor in place at the distal fibula

8. The suture strands from the second anchor are then passed in a similar manner with a sharp-tipped suture passer, each about 5 mm separated from the last (Fig. 9.5).
9. A small longitudinal incision (about 3–4 mm) is then made between the two sets of sutures. Subcutaneous passage of the sutures through this incision is facilitated with a small arthroscopic hook/probe (Fig. 9.6). If there is any concern about nerve entrapment, it is important to gently retract the tissues anteriorly through this incision to confirm that the sutures are passing deep to the superficial peroneal nerve. If the sutures remain in the safe zone [27] between the two nerves (see Fig. 9.2), nerve injury is unlikely.
10. *Repair*. Once all suture strands have passed through the central incision, arthroscopic knots are tied using a knot pusher (Fig. 9.7). When tightening the suture knots, the ankle

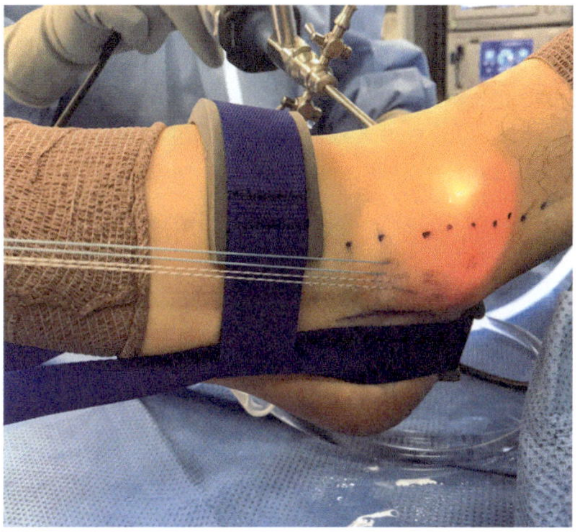

Fig. 9.5 Photograph of insufflated joint and transillumination through anteromedial portal aiding in SPN visualization. Note sutures retrieved inferiorly. The sutures are advanced through both the ATFL and extensor retinaculum before exiting the skin in sequence

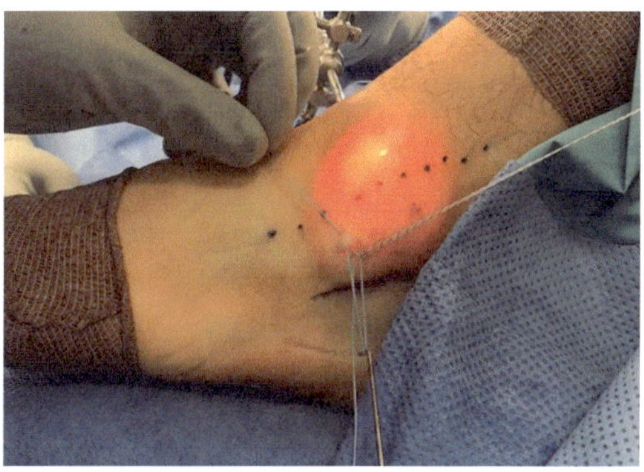

Fig. 9.6 Photograph demonstrating capture of the suture strands with a small probe. Each suture strand is advanced subcutaneously to exit the small central incision

should be held in neutral with the foot in eversion. Direct visualization from the anteromedial portal provides optimal feedback. Skin is then closed with interrupted nylon suture.

11. *Rehabilitation.* Postoperative rehabilitation is covered elsewhere in this text. The authors begin with a 7- to 10-day period of non-weight-bearing splint immobilization with the ankle in neutral. The patient then transitions to progressive weight-bearing and range of motion following a standard Broström rehabilitation protocol.

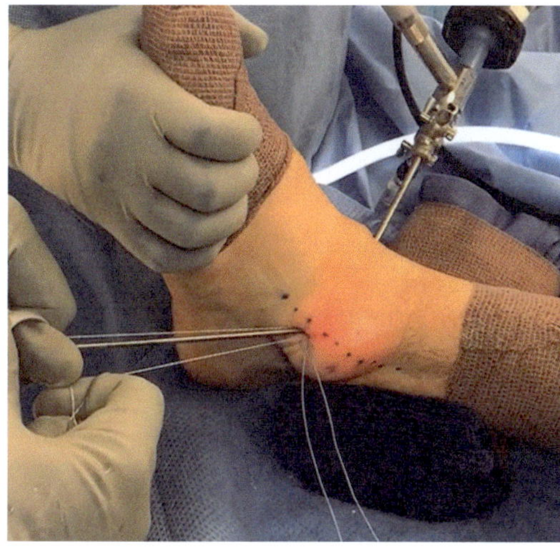

Fig. 9.7 Photograph depicting placement of suture knots through small incision inferiorly within the safe zone using an arthroscopic knot device

Minimally Invasive and Percutaneous Techniques

Arthroscopic Reconstruction

Guillo et al. [28] and others have described an arthroscopic repair with reconstruction of the lateral ligaments using tendon allograft or autograft (e.g., gracilis). In this technique, the endoscopic or arthroscopic visualization allows confirmation of drill hole location and graft anatomy while facilitating percutaneous placement and fixation of the graft. This technique provides the mechanical and physiologic advantages of ligament reconstruction while maintaining the advantages of the arthroscopic technique. It has been shown to be effective, resulting in good outcomes in terms of maintenance of stability and patient return to activities [29]. However, it is associated with a 10% rate of neurologic complications [29]. The challenge is to determine when reconstruction with graft or suture tape material is necessary and how to mitigate risk of nerve injury. In most primary cases where there is sufficient ligamentous tissue and reasonable foot posture, a primary arthroscopic ligament repair is typically sufficient. However, in a revision setting, when local tissue is sparse, with generalized tissue laxity, or in the presence of mild cavovarus alignment, the addition of graft material to reconstruct the ligaments can optimize clinical outcomes.

Percutaneous Anti-ROLL

A similar percutaneous technique was described by a group led by Glazebrook and Takao [30, 31]. A complete description of this procedure is available in their published work [30, 31]. Briefly, the Percutaneous Ankle Reconstruction of the Lateral Ligaments (ANTI-ROLL) stems from the initially proposed open procedure that utilizes gracilis tendon graft in a Y-graft fashion to reconstruct the ATFL and CFL with an inside-out suture technique. The authors describe a percutaneous repair technique following the same principles as Guillo et al., utilizing fluoroscopic guidance for drill hole and anchor placement. Arthroscopy is still used to address any concomitant intra-articular pathology [32]. Overall, the authors believe that this procedure is an effective salvage procedure for severe and recurrent CAI, particularly when soft tissue quality is limited.

Outcomes

In general, both arthroscopic and percutaneous techniques are associated with good treatment outcomes and low recurrence rates. Acevedo and McWilliams [33] treated 42 patients with arthroscopic Broström repair augmented with suture tape and evaluated them at an average of 33 months follow-up. They showed encouraging results with improved AOFAS and FAAM scores with averaging return to activity of 18 weeks. There were no recurrences of instability [33]. Similarly, Vega et al. [34] published a case series of 15 patients who underwent arthroscopic all-inside lateral ligament reconstruction with suture augmentation with a median follow-up of 18 months. They showed an AOFAS score of 95 at final follow-up. The patients underwent an early rehabilitation protocol, and there were no patients with recurrence of instability and no major complications reported.

Oliva et al., in a systematic review, found arthroscopic procedures to have higher American Orthopaedic Foot and Ankle Society (AOFAS) scores (92.5 vs 90.3) and high satisfaction rate as compared to open technique [3]. In their analysis, the complication rate was 15% for arthroscopic versus 7.9% for open procedures. However, the arthroscopic group maintained a patient satisfaction rate of 96.4% [3]. Kennedy et al. [14] used the PEARL DIVER database to compare reoperation rates for arthroscopic versus open lateral ligament repairs in more than 8000 patients. They found equivalent rates of revision in each group (5.9% vs 5.9%, respectively) with a significantly lower wound complication rate in arthroscopic repairs. Interestingly, the authors found a 4.9% rate of ankle arthrodesis in the open group compared to none in the arthroscopic group [14].

As an alternative or supplement to tendon grafts, suture tape devices can be utilized in arthroscopic and percutaneous repairs with good success [35]. A recent randomized study by Cho et al. [36] compared outcomes for arthroscopic modified Broström repair with and without suture tape internal bracing (28 vs 27 patients). The postoperative rehabilitation protocol was the same for both groups with a more conservative approach (e.g., 3 weeks non-weight-bearing) relative to other studies [34, 35, 37]. They found no differences in clinical outcomes (FAOS, FAAM, recurrent instability, stress radiographs) comparing the two procedures. The authors also described higher costs in the suture tape group despite shorter operative times [36].

Conclusions

Advancement in arthroscopic techniques and instrumentation have led to more efficient and less invasive ankle ligament repair techniques. While these techniques continue to undergo iterative improvement and better understanding of risks, outcomes, and return to sport implications, they are already proven approaches with some advantages over open techniques such as smaller incisions, less wound complications, overall rehabilitation time, simultaneous intra-articular assessment, and treatment of concomitant pathology. As with all advanced arthroscopic and endoscopic techniques, there is an associated learning curve to the surgical techniques. Long-term outcomes data will continue to refine the role of these techniques in treating lateral ankle ligamentous instability.

References

1. Acevedo JI, Mangone PG. Arthroscopic surgical technique for lateral ankle ligament instability. Foot Ankle Clin. 2021;26(1):65–85.
2. Golditz T, Steib S, Pfeifer K, Uder M, Gelse K, Janka R, et al. Functional ankle instability as a risk factor for osteoarthritis: using T2-mapping to analyze early cartilage degeneration in the ankle joint of young athletes. Osteoarthr Cartil. 2014;22(10):1377–85.
3. Guelfi M, Zamperetti M, Pantalone A, Usuelli FG, Salini V, Oliva XM. Open and arthroscopic lateral ligament repair for treatment of chronic ankle instability: a systematic review. Foot Ankle Surg. 2018;24(1):11–8.
4. Golanó P, Vega J, de Leeuw PAJ, Malagelada F, Manzanares MC, Götzens V, et al. Anatomy of the ankle ligaments: a pictorial essay. Knee Surg Sport Traumatol Arthrosc. 2016;24(4):944–56.
5. Delco ML, Kennedy JG, Bonassar LJ, Fortier LA. Post-traumatic osteoarthritis of the ankle: a distinct clinical entity requiring new research approaches. J Orthop Res. 2017 Mar;35(3):440–53.
6. Gribble PA, Bleakley CM, Caulfield BM, Docherty CL, Fourchet F, Fong DT-P, et al. 2016 consensus statement of the international ankle consortium: prevalence, impact and long-term consequences of lateral ankle sprains. Br J Sports Med. 2016 Dec;50(24):1493–5.
7. Hunt KJ, Griffith R. Open Brostrom for lateral ligament stabilization. Curr Rev Musculoskelet Med. 2020;13(6):788–96.
8. Nuno MC-R, Moreira RM. Arthroscopic repair of chronic lateral ankle instability. Foot Ankle Int. 2009;30(3):213–7.
9. Acevedo JI, Palmer RC, Mangone PG. Arthroscopic treatment of ankle instability. Foot Ankle Clin. 2018 Dec;23(4):555–70.
10. Giza E, Shin EC, Wong SE, Acevedo JI, Mangone PG, Olson K, et al. Arthroscopic suture anchor repair of the lateral ligament ankle complex. Am J Sports Med. 2013;41(11):2567–72.
11. Giza E, Whitlow SR, Williams BT, Acevedo JI, Mangone PG, Haytmanek CT, et al. Biomechanical analysis of an arthroscopic Broström ankle ligament repair and a suture anchor–augmented repair. Foot Ankle Int. 2015;36(7):836–41.
12. Ahn B-H, Cho B-K. Persistent pain after operative treatment for chronic lateral ankle instability. Orthop Res Rev. 2021;13:47–56.
13. Hua Y, Chen S, Li Y, Chen J, Li H. Combination of modified Broström procedure with ankle arthroscopy for chronic ankle instability accompanied by intra-articular symptoms. Arthroscopy. 2010;26(4):524–8.
14. Yasui Y, Murawski CD, Wollstein A, Kennedy JG. Reoperation rates following ankle ligament procedures performed with and without concomitant arthroscopic procedures. Knee Surg Sport Traumatol Arthrosc. 2017;25(6):1908–15.
15. Ferkel RD, Fischer SP. Progress in ankle arthroscopy. Clin Orthop Relat Res. 1989;240:210–20.
16. Hawkins RB. Arthroscopic stapling repair for chronic lateral instability. Clin Podiatr Med Surg. 1987;4(4):875–83.
17. Kashuk KB, Landsman AS, Werd MB, Hanft JR, Roberts M. Arthroscopic lateral ankle stabilization. Clin Podiatr Med Surg. 1994;11(3):407–23.
18. Kashuk KB, Carbonell JA, Blum JA. Arthroscopic stabilization of the ankle. Clin Podiatr Med Surg. 1997;14(3):459–78.
19. Treuting R. Minimally invasive orthopedic surgery: arthroscopy. Ochsner J. 2000;2(3):158–63.
20. Hertel J. Functional anatomy, pathomechanics, and pathophysiology of lateral ankle instability. J Athl Train. 2002;37(4):364–75.
21. Weindel S, Schmidt R, Rammelt S, Claes L, Campe A, v., Rein S. Subtalar instability: a biomechanical cadaver study. Arch Orthop Trauma Surg. 2010;130(3):313–9.
22. Gould N, Seligson D, Gassman J. Early and late repair of lateral ligament of the ankle. Foot Ankle. 1980;1(2):84–9.
23. Dalmau-Pastor M, Malagelada F, Kerkhoffs GMMJ, Manzanares MC, Vega J. X-shaped inferior extensor retinaculum and its doubtful use in the Bröstrom–Gould procedure. Knee Surg Sport Traumatol Arthrosc. 2018;26(7):2171–6.
24. Jorge JT, Gomes TM, Oliva XM. An anatomical study about the arthroscopic repair of the lateral ligament of the ankle. Foot Ankle Surg. 2018;24(2):143–8.
25. Jeong BO, Kim MS, Song WJ, SooHoo NF. Feasibility and outcome of inferior extensor retinaculum reinforcement in modified Broström procedures. Foot Ankle Int. 2014;35(11):1137–42.
26. Jo J, Lee JW, Kim HJ, Suh DH, Kim WS, Choi GW. Arthroscopic all-inside anterior Talofibular ligament repair with and without inferior extensor retinacular reinforcement. J Bone Jt Surg. 2021;103(17):1578–87.
27. Flores Santos F, Santos NR. Arthroscopic treatment of lateral ankle instability. Is there a safe zone? An anatomic study. Foot Ankle Surg. 2020;26(1):61–5.
28. Guillo S, Archbold P, Perera A, Bauer T, Sonnery-Cottet B. Arthroscopic anatomic reconstruction of the lateral ligaments of the ankle with Gracilis autograft. Arthrosc Tech. 2014;3(5):e593–8.

29. Lopes R, Andrieu M, Cordier G, Molinier F, Benoist J, Colin F, et al. Arthroscopic treatment of chronic ankle instability: prospective study of outcomes in 286 patients. Orthop Traumatol Surg Res. 2018;104(8):S199–205.
30. Glazebrook M, Eid M, Alhadhoud M, Stone J, Matsui K, Takao M. Percutaneous ankle reconstruction of lateral ligaments. Foot Ankle Clin. 2018;23(4):581–92.
31. Glazebrook M, Stone J, Matsui K, Guillo S, Takao M, Batista J, et al. Percutaneous ankle reconstruction of lateral ligaments (perc-anti RoLL). Foot Ankle Int. 2016;37(6):659–64.
32. Iwashita K, Jujo Y, Inokuchi R, Glazebrook M, Stone J, Takao M. Hybrid ankle reconstruction of lateral ligaments. Arthrosc Tech. 2021;10(3):e931–9.
33. Acevedo J, McWilliams J. Results of Arthroscopic internal brace augmentation Presentation. J Japanese Soc Surg Foot. 2018;39 Supplem(5th Ankle Instability Group Annual Meeting): Kisarazu, November 3.
34. Vega J, Montesinos E, Malagelada F, Baduell A, Guelfi M, Dalmau-Pastor M. Arthroscopic all-inside anterior talo-fibular ligament repair with suture augmentation gives excellent results in case of poor ligament tissue remnant quality. Knee Surg Sport Traumatol Arthrosc. 2020;28(1):100–7.
35. Ulku TK, Kocaoglu B, Tok O, Irgit K, Nalbantoglu U. Arthroscopic suture-tape internal bracing is safe as arthroscopic modified Broström repair in the treatment of chronic ankle instability. Knee Surg Sport Traumatol Arthrosc. 2020;28(1):227–32.
36. Cho B-K, Park J-K, Choi S-M, SooHoo NF. A randomized comparison between lateral ligaments augmentation using suture-tape and modified Broström repair in young female patients with chronic ankle instability. Foot Ankle Surg. 2019;25(2):137–42.
37. Yoo J-S, Yang E-A. Clinical results of an arthroscopic modified Brostrom operation with and without an internal brace. J Orthop Traumatol. 2016;17(4):353–60.

10 Lateral Ankle Instability: Tendon Transfers and Grafts

Marissa D. Jamieson and Thomas O. Clanton

Introduction

Over 50 surgical techniques have been described to treat chronic lateral ankle instability [1], and the preferred treatment has changed significantly over the years. In the pre-antibiotic era, bracing was the preferred treatment; in the pre-anatomic era (1940–1985), tenodesis was the preferred stabilization technique; and since the late 1980s, anatomic repair or reconstruction has become the preferred surgical option.

Tendon grafts and transfers for lateral ankle instability were first described and utilized by Elmsie in 1934 who reported using a fascia lata v for reconstruction of the lateral ankle ligaments [2]. Secondary repair of a torn ATFL was first popularized by Lennart Broström in 1966 [3] and then modified by Karlsson to involve shortening, imbricating, and reinserting the torn ligaments onto the fibula [4]. The Broström repair was further modified with the "Gould modification," which involves reinforcing the repair with inferior extensor retinaculum [5]. This procedure has been accepted by many as the standard for surgical treatment of chronic ankle instability [6]. More recently, augmentation of a standard Broström repair with suture tape has gained traction with good short-term clinical results [7].

Tenodesis or transfer procedures were popularized by Watson-Jones (1940), Evans (1952), and Chrisman-Snook (1969) and were used extensively. These surgeries typically involved harvesting all or part of the peroneal tendons and routing the tendon through bone tunnels in the fibula and/or calcaneus. The tendon grafts were typically placed perpendicular to the line of instability in order to restore stability of the ankle and subtalar joints through restraint of inversion and anterior translation [8]. In general, tendon transfers have fallen out of favor due to basic science and clinical outcomes research that have shown restricted ankle and subtalar motion and arthritic changes associated with these procedures [9, 10].

In 2002, Coughlin et al. described a technique for anatomic reconstruction of the lateral ligaments in chronic instability with a gracilis autograft through drill holes in the talus, fibula, and calcaneus [1, 8]. The technique was modified by Jeys and Harris in 2003 with the use of interference fit screws to anchor the hamstring autograft which avoided the need for trans-osseous tensioning [11]. Since then, numerous types of autografts and allografts have been described and used successfully to treat chronic lateral ankle instability [8].

M. D. Jamieson (✉)
Orthopedic Surgery Division of Foot and Ankle, University of Colorado, Denver, CO, USA
e-mail: marissa.jamieson@ucdenver.edu

T. O. Clanton
Orthopedic Surgery Foot and Ankle, Steadman Clinic, Vail, CO, USA
e-mail: tclanton@thesteadmanclinic.com

P. D'Hooghe et al. (eds.), *Ligamentous Injuries of the Foot and Ankle*,
https://doi.org/10.1007/978-3-031-08682-3_10

Methods of fixation of grafts have also evolved from suturing the tendon to itself to cortical onlay with suture anchors or staples and endobuttons and more recently to interference fit screws in bone tunnels or tension-slide methods. Recent literature supports these latter techniques over other techniques [12, 13].

Diagnosis: Patients with chronic lateral ankle instability typically present with recurrent ankle sprains and a sense of ankle insecurity and "giving way" that may or may not be associated with pain [14]. Physical examination typically reveals positive anterior drawer and/or positive talar tilt tests. Tenderness on exam is often associated with concomitant pathology such as osteochondral lesions, synovitis, bony or soft tissue impingement, and/or peroneal tendon pathology. Instability can be confirmed under live fluoroscopy or stress radiographs with an anterior drawer greater than 1 cm or side-to-side difference greater than 3 mm and/or a talar tilt greater than 15° or side-to-side difference of greater than 10° [14]. These parameters should be used as general guidelines, but clinical signs and symptoms are typically more important. Advanced imaging with magnetic resonance imaging (MRI) is frequently indicated to document the extent of ligamentous injury and quality of residual ligamentous tissue and to evaluate for other pathology [15].

Management: Initially, patients should be treated with a comprehensive physical therapy program to improve proprioception, strength, and flexibility. Activity modification, shoe-wear modification (lower or wider heel, stiffer soles, lateral wedge), and various degrees of immobilization with ankle taping or bracing can also help relieve symptoms; however, 10–40% of patients who sustain an ankle sprain may develop symptoms of chronic ankle instability and long-term morbidity [16]. Surgical intervention should be considered only after the patient has failed extensive conservative management. However, nonoperative management may not be an acceptable long-term solution for some athletes, so surgical stabilization is often the preferred treatment [14]. This can also be the situation for certain "consequence athletes" in which the consequence from an instability episode would be worse in comparison to the risk of surgical stabilization. For example, a mountain climber or firefighter falling from a height is a result of ankle instability.

There are limited indications for a tendon transfer based on the current literature. The authors believe that whenever possible, the surgeon should avoid sacrificing or weakening the peroneal tendons that provide eversion stability and should aim to preserve subtalar and ankle motion during a lateral ankle stabilization surgery. This is particularly important for athletes that require subtalar motion and peroneal strength, such as dancers [8]. However, there are some with expertise in the Broström-Evans procedure in which secondary repair of the lateral ligaments is augmented with a small slip of the peroneus brevis tendon and have shown good intermediate and long-term results in specific patients [6, 17].

While most patients can be managed with a modified Broström or direct repair of the lateral ligaments, some require a graft reconstruction. Relative indications for reconstruction with an autograft or allograft include patients with insufficient native tissue for repair, long-standing instability, obese patients or heavy laborers, as a salvage procedure for failed repair or Broström procedure, subtalar or combined instability, patients with generalized ligamentous laxity, cavovarus deformity, larger high-demand athletes (weighing over 250 pounds), or athletes with hyperflexibility [6, 13, 16].

Relative contraindications for surgery include tarsal coalitions, hindfoot arthritis, neuromuscular disease, collagen disorders, vascular compromise, the presence of active infection, inadequate bone stock in the distal fibula, lateral ankle pain without documented instability, complex regional pain syndrome, sedentary patients, and comorbidities that make general anesthesia and surgery too medically risky [14]. Every patient is different and individual factors must be considered before choosing the best surgical option.

Associated foot and ankle conditions such as hindfoot varus, peroneal tendon pathology, tarsal coalitions, ankle or subtalar arthritis, osteochondral lesions, and osteophytes should be identified and worked up appropriately prior to surgical intervention for ankle stability. This allows for appropriate preoperative planning and decision-making regarding whether or not to address additional pathology simultaneously or as a staged procedure [8].

Operative Treatment

It is easiest to separate ankle-stabilizing surgical procedures into two different categories: nonanatomic tenodesis procedures and anatomic reconstruction with a graft. Detailed surgical technique will focus on anatomic reconstruction as this is most widely used and accepted for surgical stabilization of the lateral ankle.

Nonanatomic Reconstruction

Due to the well-documented inherent problems associated with nonanatomic tenodesis procedures, we consider these procedures primarily of historical value, but the techniques will be briefly described here [14]. The most commonly described transfer or tenodesis procedures utilize the peroneus brevis tendon to replace or supplement insufficient lateral ligaments in a dynamic or static fashion.

The original Evans procedure anchors the fibula to the base of the fifth metatarsal using the entire peroneus brevis tendon, acting as a vector sum of the ATFL and CFL. There is no direct connection to the talus or calcaneus. The Watson-Jones procedure reconstructs the ATFL by anchoring the peroneus brevis tendon from the base of the fifth metatarsal to the fibula and to the talar neck. In the Chrisman-Snook reconstruction, the ATFL and CFL are reconstructed with half of the peroneus brevis routed from the base of the fifth metatarsal through a transverse fibula tunnel into the calcaneus. There is no direct connection to the talus [18]. A more anatomic reconstruction patterned after the Chrisman-Snook method was championed by Colville in the 1990s based primarily on research involving lateral ankle ligament strain measurements leading to more anatomic location of the bone tunnels for both the ATFL and CFL portions of the graft [19].

The Larsen procedure was developed in order to provide more subtalar stability, which was thought to be lacking in the Evans and Watson-Jones procedures. The distal peroneus brevis tendon was left attached to the base of the fifth metatarsal, and the entire tendon was pulled through two converging bone tunnels in the lateral malleolus aiming from the native origin of the ATFL to the origin of the CFL and then fixed to a tunnel in the calcaneus by two sutures or a staple [20]. There are numerous variations to the above procedures, which will not be discussed in detail in this chapter.

Additionally, several hybrid techniques involving direct tissue repair in combination with tenodesis have been described. Girard et al. [6] reinforced a modified Broström procedure with the anterior third of the peroneus brevis through a distal fibular drill tunnel named the modified Broström-Evan procedure. This has been described as a "poor man's internal brace" that provides a supplemental lateral static restraint while allowing for biological healing. The technique describes placing the fibular tunnel halfway between the CFL and ATFL origin [17].

Anatomic Reconstruction

Various types of grafts, both autograft and allograft, have been used to reconstruct the ATFL and CFL by recreating the anatomy of the native ligaments through appropriately placed bone tunnels with various fixation methods. Graft options include bone patellar tendon, free gracilis tendon, plantaris, extensor digitorum longus, fascia lata, palmaris, semitendinosus, and a strip of the Achilles [14].

Multiple options for fixation of a graft exist, but the authors prefer bioabsorbable interference fit screws for several different reasons. Biomechanical studies have shown a clear advantage of bioabsorbable interference screws over suture anchors in load to failure and resistance to graft elongation [12]. Additionally, screws allow for a shorter bone tunnel and less graft length, provide adequate fixation strength, are easy to use and efficient in the operating room, do not require removal, and will not distort any repeat imaging (MRI, CT) [8].

Perhaps the most important principal for lateral ankle ligament reconstruction is anatomic placement of the graft. This avoids the problems with nonanatomical placement, which will either "capture" the joint and restrict motion in the subtalar and/or tibiotalar joints or will stretch out over time. Therefore, knowledge of anatomical landmarks and ligament anatomy is essential (see the previous chapter for details). Other key principals for successful reconstruction include appropriate tension, strong enough fixation in the bone, avoidance of any stress risers by addressing any bone spurs or varus heel/ankle alignment, and incorporation of an appropriate rehabilitation program.

The authors' preferred procedure is reconstruction with a free graft using either a semitendinosus or gracilis allograft. In our opinion, this has multiple advantages including avoidance of comorbidities associated with harvesting a tendon, a smaller incision and exposure, faster recovery, low incidence of arthrofibrosis, easy anatomic placement, adequate tendon length independent of incision length, and availability of appropriately sized grafts (typically 4.5–5.0 mm). Disadvantages of allograft include increased cost, very rare risk of disease transmission, slower graft incorporation, and possible immune response [8, 16].

Surgical Technique [8]

1. A semitendinosus or gracilis allograft that is 4.5–5.0 mm in diameter is preferred (a smaller graft and smaller tunnels should be considered in a small individual). The size of the graft determines the size of the bone tunnels and the interference screws. The graft should be tensioned on the back table at 89 N (20 lbs) for 15 min to remove crimp in the collagen fibers. Both ends of the graft are sutured with a FiberLoop® (Arthrex, Inc., Naples, Florida) or Krackow stitch.
2. The lateral ankle is exposed through one of two incisions depending on the underlying pathology. When the problem is limited to the lateral ligamentous complex, a small curvilinear incision paralleling the anterior and distal border of the fibula is used as described by Broström [21]. For cases in which other structures need to be addressed (peroneal tendons, anterior tibial or talar osteophytes, subtalar joint, etc.), an extensile longitudinal incision is made over the posterior border of the fibula curving distally toward the sinus tarsi. In both approaches, the ankle joint and the anterolateral capsule are exposed while preserving as much potentially useful tissue as possible. The lateral capsule is opened leaving the fibular periosteum intact, and the origin and insertion sites of the ATFL and CFL are defined.
3. For a 4.5- to 5.0-mm graft, a 5.5-mm tunnel is made in the talus to a depth of 25–30 mm at the insertion site of the ATFL, approximately 62% of the distance between the lateral process of the talus and the distal articular border of the talus [22], aiming approximately 20° posterior into the body of the talus (toward the medial malleolus tip). The graft is inserted into the bone tunnel and secured with a 5.5-mm interference screw. We have found that the Arthrex Bio-Tenodesis System® (Arthrex, Inc., Naples, Florida) facilitates this technique.
4. Drill holes are made in the distal fibula to create a V-shaped tunnel from anterior to posterior. The first drill hole is made with a 5-mm cannulated reamer from the origin of the ATFL on the distal anterior fibula directed 30° superior and posterior. When using the smaller Broström approach, a small incision is made at the posterior border of the fibula where the guide pin and reamer will exit in order to protect the peroneal tendons. The second drill hole is made at the origin of the CFL, approximately 5 mm anterior to the distal tip of the fibula [22], and aims proximal and posterior to exit the fibula in the same posterior hole in the fibula. There should be at least 1 cm of a bone bridge between the two tunnels on the anterior distal fibula. (Note: This method may not be suitable for very small individuals or those with osteoporotic bone. In such cases, the tension-slide method can be used with an endobutton

holding the looped graft within the fibula and bringing one limb of the graft into the talus and the other into the calcaneus. Tunnel placement on the anterior fibula can be moved 1–2 mm inferior to the normal placement for this tunnel and no interference screw is necessary.)

5. The last tunnel is drilled in the lateral calcaneus at the anatomical site of insertion of the CFL. Normally, there is a small tuberosity on the calcaneus that helps define this location. Other helpful reference information include [1] the CFL is 2–3 cm in length, [2] the CFL angles are 10–45° posterior to the line of the fibula (we prefer to use 15–20° in most cases), and [3] the CFL makes an angle of 104–132° with the ATFL [23]. The Beath pin is placed across the calcaneus and out the medial cortex being careful to avoid the medial neurovascular structures. A 6.0-mm cannulated reamer then makes a 25- to 30-mm tunnel without penetrating the far cortex of the calcaneus.
6. The tendon graft is passed from anterior to posterior through the first more anterior drill hole in the fibula using a suture passer or a looped suture. With tension of approximately 20 pounds placed on the suture pulling the graft through this tunnel, a 4.75 nonmetallic interference screw is used to fix the graft while the ankle is held in relaxed plantar flexion, neutral inversion/eversion, and a slight posterior drawer. We recommend having a bump placed proximal to heel during this step (see Fig. 10.1).
7. The graft is then passed through the fibula out the more distal fibular tunnel (at the site of the CFL origin). The graft is marked where it will enter the calcaneal tunnel and again 25 mm distal to that. An absorbable Krackow stitch is placed in the tendon just proximal to the distal mark, and the excess tendon is cut distal to the suture.
8. The graft sutures are passed through the eyelet of the Beath pin, and the pin is pulled out the medial side of the calcaneus with sutures in tow. We have found that oscillating the pin helps with this step. The graft is pulled completely into the calcaneal tunnel and tensioned while holding the ankle in neutral dorsiflexion, neutral inversion/eversion, and a slight posterior drawer. A 5.5- or 6.25-mm interference fit screw (based on bone density) is used to secure the graft into the calcaneal bone tunnel (see Fig. 10.2).
9. The ankle is tested for stability and range of motion, and stress radiographs are performed under fluoroscopy to confirm that the talar

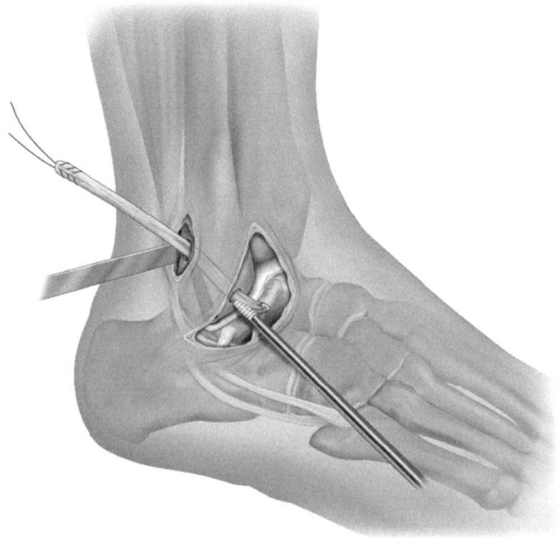

Fig. 10.1 Illustration of the tendon graft being secured to the distal fibula at the ATFL origin with an interference screw. (Illustration courtesy of Thomas O. Clanton, MD)

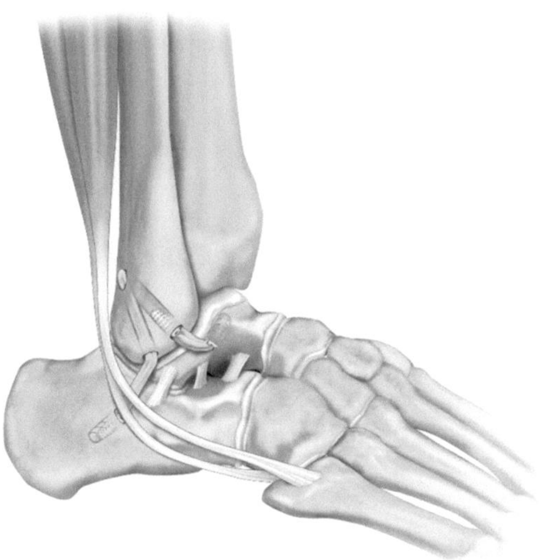

Fig. 10.2 Illustration of completed reconstruction of the ATFL and CFL with interference screws in the talus, fibula, and calcaneus. (Illustration courtesy of Thomas O. Clanton, MD)

tilt and anterior drawer have been restored to normal.

10. The inferior extensor retinaculum or other local tissue can be used for augmentation if further stability is desired. Closure is performed in standard fashion, and a dressing is applied followed by a splint or a walking boot with the ankle in a neutral position.

A percutaneous approach for this procedure has also been described and used successfully [16, 24].

Rehabilitation

Along with evolving surgical techniques for lateral ankle instability, the rehabilitation process has also evolved to allow earlier weight-bearing and less restrictions on range of motion. This is the authors' standard rehabilitation protocol for the above-described allograft anatomic reconstruction. For the first 2 weeks, the ankle is protected in a splint, and the patient remains non-weight-bearing. After suture removal at 2 weeks, the patient is placed in a walking boot, and progressive weight-bearing is allowed over the next 2 weeks. At 4 weeks, the patient is full weight-bearing in the boot and allowed to transition to regular shoes over the following 2 weeks.

The typical ankle rehabilitation program for range of motion, strength, Achilles stretching, and proprioceptive training begins at 3–4 weeks postoperatively and progresses as tolerated (see Table 10.1). Other pathology in the ankle will dictate any alterations that need to be made to this general protocol.

Determination of readiness for return to play is always an important decision following rehabilitation after an injury or surgery. There are no clear evidence-based guidelines for clearing an athlete to return to their sport and competition, particularly for foot and ankle injuries and surgery. Currently, our preferred method for determining return to play involves the athlete's ability to perform sport-specific tests, such as single hop for distance, box hop, or figure-of-eight hop. These factors along with the athlete's psychological state are critical elements in determining that the athlete/patient has completed the rehabilitation process to the degree that they are ready to resume sport-specific training and return to play. Working closely with a physical therapist, athletic trainer, and at times with a sport or position coach is essential to help manage and recommend load progression and advancement to pre-injury training schedule and finally return to play. See the chapter on rehabilitation and return to sport for further details.

Outcomes

Despite initial reports of good clinical outcomes with nonanatomic tenodesis procedures for lateral ankle instability [20], the past five decades of literature have demonstrated poor long-term functional outcomes, high rates of complications, recurrence of instability, ankle and subtalar stiffness and arthritis, and weak eversion [10, 14, 25]. In a large, long-term follow-up, multicenter outcomes study by Krips et al. comparing Evans tenodesis to anatomic reconstruction, patients who underwent tenodesis had more revision procedures and demonstrated more instability, osteoarthritis, chronic pain, and limited dorsiflexion. Good to excellent results were found in 80% of patients after anatomic reconstruction versus only 33% after Evans tenodesis [10]. A prospective randomized comparison of the Chrisman-Snook procedure and modified Broström found significantly more complications in the tenodesis group including sural nerve injuries, wound complications, a sensation that the ankle was "too tight," and iatrogenic flatfoot [26]. Biomechanical studies also support anatomic reconstruction or augmentation because these procedures restore force patterns more closely than nonanatomic tenodesis or tendon transfers [8, 9].

The hybrid technique as described by Girard et al. [6], the Broström-Evans, was created based on the concern that local tissue repair would eventually fail in specific patients, such as those that are overweight, ligamentously lax, or involved in strenuous work or sport. In a 5-year clinical outcomes study by Hsu et al. [17] that

Table 10.1 Lateral ankle ligament reconstruction rehabilitation protocol, ROM = range of motion. Courtesy of Anastasia Robinson, DPT

Postoperative timeline	Precautions	Weight-bearing orders	Footwear	Rehabilitation recommendations
0–2 weeks	No inversion × 6 weeks	Non-weight-bearing	Splint or boot	
2–6 weeks ROM/muscle initiation	No inversion × 6 weeks	Wean off crutches over 2-week period. Wean out of boot over 2 weeks after walking without pain in the boot Full weight-bearing	Boot and supportive shoe	• Swelling modalities • Restore active ROM. • Begin resisted strengthening with therabands. • Strengthen within limits of weight-bearing orders. • Intrinsic strengthening • Gait training • Pool program—Deep water program • Stationary bike—Start no resistance
6–12 weeks Endurance	No restrictions *Never work to gain inversion mobility beyond functional demand		Supportive shoe	• Restore functional dorsiflexion • Gait training • Resisted strengthening—Pilates reformer, shuttle, and leg press • Pool program—Can gait train and begin closed chain strength in shallow end • Begin closed chain strength progression—Squats, heel raises, and dead lifts • Begin balance progression
3–5 months Strength	Full ROM		Most desired footwear (check with your therapist if you want to wear heels and feel ready to wear heels)	• Pool program—Cardio; can perform future exercises in pool first • Continue closed chain strength program—Transition to single leg strength and add weight depending on patient goals • Restore double and single leg heel raise strength • Continue with balance progression on dynamic surfaces without visual dependence and with upper extremity challenges as able • Build patient's training plan to resume desired cardiovascular training
4–6+ months Agility Return to sport	Full ROM		All desired athletic footwear (running shoes, ski boots, etc.)	• Continue to progress strength and balance • Continue adding volume to desired cardiovascular training • Progress agility and power training specific to sport • Initiate absorption and landing strategies

included 19 patients undergoing a modified Broström-Evan procedure for chronic ankle instability, they reported minimal loss of peroneal strength, no recurrent instability, and no progressive symptomatic subtalar arthritis requiring reoperation. However, they did note 41% decreased inversion range of motion. This technique may be warranted in specific patient populations, but they should be counseled on possible loss of inversion.

Current clinical literature on the use of allograft or autograft tendons in the surgical management of chronic ankle instability is limited primarily to retrospective reviews and case series with limited length of follow-up and number of patients. However, good to excellent outcomes have been reported in 85–100% of patients in short- to medium-term follow-up. In general, the studies show retained motion at the ankle and subtalar joints, low complication rates, no cases of graft rejection, small rates of recurrent instability, and high rates of return to sport [16]. Reported complications with anatomic reconstruction include arthrofibrosis, sural and superficial peroneal nerve neuropraxia or neuralgia, incisional swelling, delayed wound healing, complex regional pain syndrome, and irritation of the peroneal tendons [27–29]. See Table 10.2 for details on the findings in the most recent literature.

Table 10.2 Results of lateral ankle ligament reconstruction

Author (year)	No. of patients	Surgical details	Mean age of patient (years)	Mean follow-up in months (range)	Success rate	Results
Miller et al. (2013) [28]	28	Semitendinosus allograft, 12 requiring concomitant correction of varus		32 (12–79)	89% good to excellent patient satisfaction	– VAS improved from 8 to 1 – No subtalar arthritis or pain – 3 patient with mild persistent instability – 1 patient without varus correction – 1 patient with CRPS
Xu et al. (2014) [24]	68	Minimally invasive approach, semitendinosus autograft (32 patients) or allograft (36 patients)	33 ± 3.2	33.5 ± 6.5 autograft, 28.5 ± 6.5 allograft		– AOFAS score increased from 60 to 85 in allograft group – 5 patients (7%) with recurrent instability – No significant difference in outcomes between two groups – Talar tilt decreased from 13° to 3.6° degrees in allograft group
Hong-Geun Jung et al. (2015) [29]	66	Semitendinosus allograft, bioabsorbable tenodesis screws	30 (16–59)	22 (12–68)	89% patients very satisfied or satisfied	– VAS improved from 5.5 to 1.3 – AOFAS score improved from 71 to 91 – Talar tilt decreased from 14.8° to 3.8° – 8 cases (12%) of postoperative neuralgia – 4 cases (6%) with wound problems – 1 case of subtalar stiffness

Table 10.2 (continued)

Author (year)	No. of patients	Surgical details	Mean age of patient (years)	Mean follow-up in months (range)	Success rate	Results
Dierckman et al. (2015) [30]	38	Semitendinosus allograft	28 (16–74)	38 (24–107)	– 85% good to excellent results – 100% patients satisfied	– VAS improved from 7.3 to 1.9 – Talar tilt decreased from 14.3° to 3.1° – 71% patients at or 1 level below preoperative activity level – No arthritis beyond grade 1 on x-rays
Matheny et al. (2016) [27]	86	Broström-Gould repair (61 patients), semitendinosus allograft (25 patients)	38 (19–68)	36 (24–64)	– no patients in either group had revision surgery	– No significant difference in outcome measures or patient satisfaction – Four patients (19%) in reconstruction group had arthrofibrosis requiring debridement
Wang et al. (2017) [31]	19	Semitendinosus allograft	28 (19–41)	30 (24–40)	– all patients returned to activity without instability, pain, or limited motion	– AOFAS score improved from 64 to 90 – Mean talar tilt 17° to 4° – Ultrasound showed ligaments in good continuity and excellent tension
Cordier et al. (2020) [32]	53	Endoscopic approach with gracilis autograft	38 (21–58)	31.5 ± 7	– 92% patients satisfied or very satisfied	– VAS improved from 1.9 to 0.8 – AOFAS score improved from 76 to 95 – 85% returned to sports at the same level – Two patients had recurrent instability

AOFAS American Orthopaedic Foot and Ankle Society, *VAS* visual analog scale, *CRPS* complex regional pain syndrome

Additionally, a biomechanical cadaveric study showed that reconstruction of the ATFL with a semitendinosus allograft fixed with interference screws demonstrated similar strength and stiffness to an intact model at time zero [13].

Although long-term clinical outcome studies and randomized prospective studies are lacking with regard to anatomic allograft reconstruction of the lateral ligaments, the authors' opinion is that this technique reliably restores ankle instability in patients with insufficient native tissue, failed prior repair, and global ligamentous laxity.

References

1. Coughlin MJ, Schenck RC, Grebing BR, Treme G. Comprehensive reconstruction of the lateral ankle for chronic instability using a free gracilis graft. Foot Ankle Int. 2004;25(4):231–41.
2. Elmslie RC. Recurrent subluxation of the ankle-joint. Ann Surg. 1934;100(2):364–7.
3. Broström L. Sprained ankles. V. Treatment and prognosis in recent ligament ruptures. Acta Chir Scand. 1966;132(5):537–50.
4. Karlsson J, Bergsten T, Lansinger O, Peterson L. Surgical treatment of chronic lateral instability of the ankle joint. A new procedure. Am J Sports Med. 1989;17(2):268–73; discussion 73–4

5. Gould N, Seligson D, Gassman J. Early and late repair of lateral ligament of the ankle. Foot Ankle. 1980;1(2):84–9.
6. Girard P, Anderson RB, Davis WH, Isear JA, Kiebzak GM. Clinical evaluation of the modified Brostrom-Evans procedure to restore ankle stability. Foot Ankle Int. 1999;20(4):246–52.
7. Coetzee JC, Ellington JK, Ronan JA, Stone RM. Functional results of open Broström ankle ligament repair augmented with a suture tape. Foot Ankle Int. 2018;39(3):304–10.
8. Clanton T, Waldrup NI. Athletic injuries to the soft tissues of the foot and ankle. In: Coughlin M, Saltzman C, Anderson R, editors. Mann's surgery of the foot and ankle. 9th ed. Philadelphia, PA: Saunders/Elsevier; 2013. p. 1531–687.
9. Bahr R, Pena F, Shine J, Lew WD, Tyrdal S, Engebretsen L. Biomechanics of ankle ligament reconstruction. An in vitro comparison of the Broström repair, Watson-Jones reconstruction, and a new anatomic reconstruction technique. Am J Sports Med. 1997;25(4):424–32.
10. Krips R, Brandsson S, Swensson C, van Dijk CN, Karlsson J. Anatomical reconstruction and Evans tenodesis of the lateral ligaments of the ankle. Clinical and radiological findings after follow-up for 15 to 30 years. J Bone Joint Surg Br. 2002;84(2):232–6.
11. Jeys LM, Harris NJ. Ankle stabilization with hamstring autograft: a new technique using interference screws. Foot Ankle Int. 2003;24(9):677–9.
12. Jeys L, Korrosis S, Stewart T, Harris NJ. Bone anchors or interference screws? A biomechanical evaluation for autograft ankle stabilization. Am J Sports Med. 2004;32(7):1651–9.
13. Clanton TO, Viens NA, Campbell KJ, Laprade RF, Wijdicks CA. Anterior talofibular ligament ruptures, part 2: biomechanical comparison of anterior talofibular ligament reconstruction using semitendinosus allografts with the intact ligament. Am J Sports Med. 2014;42(2):412–6.
14. Clanton TO. Ankle sprains, ankle instability, and syndesmosis injuries. In: Porter D, Schon L, editors. Baxter's the foot and ankle in sport. 3rd ed. Philadelphia: Elsevier; 2020. p. 255–75.
15. Schneck CD, Mesgarzadeh M, Bonakdarpour A. MR imaging of the most commonly injured ankle ligaments. Part II. Ligament injuries. Radiology. 1992;184(2):507–12.
16. Espinosa N, Bluman E. Lateral ankle ligament reconstruction using allograft. In: Alexander I, Bluman E, Greisberg J, editors. Advanced reconstruction: foot and ankle 2. Rosemont, IL: American Academy of Orthopaedic Surgeons; 2015. p. 349–55.
17. Hsu AR, Ardoin GT, Davis WH, Anderson RB. Intermediate and long-term outcomes of the modified Brostrom-Evans procedure for lateral ankle ligament reconstruction. Foot Ankle Spec. 2016;9(2):131–9.
18. Hollis JM, Blasier RD, Flahiff CM, Hofmann OE. Biomechanical comparison of reconstruction techniques in simulated lateral ankle ligament injury. Am J Sports Med. 1995;23(6):678–82.
19. Colville MR, Grondel RJ. Anatomic reconstruction of the lateral ankle ligaments using a split peroneus brevis tendon graft. Am J Sports Med. 1995;23(2):210–3.
20. Larsen E. Tendon transfer for lateral ankle and subtalar joint instability. Acta Orthop Scand. 1988;59(2):168–72.
21. Broström L, Sprained ankles. VI. Surgical treatment of "chronic" ligament ruptures. Acta Chir Scand. 1966;132(5):551–65.
22. Clanton TO, Campbell KJ, Wilson KJ, Michalski MP, Goldsmith MT, Wijdicks CA, et al. Qualitative and quantitative anatomic investigation of the lateral ankle ligaments for surgical reconstruction procedures. J Bone Joint Surg Am. 2014;96(12):e98.
23. Kelikian AS, Sarrafian SK. Syndesmology. In: Kelikian AS, Sarrafian SK, editors. Sarrafian's anatomy of the foot and ankle: descriptive, topographic, functional. 3rd ed. Philadelphia: Wolters Kluwer Health/Lippincott Williams & Wilkins; 2011. p. 163–75.
24. Xu X, Hu M, Liu J, Zhu Y, Wang B. Minimally invasive reconstruction of the lateral ankle ligaments using semitendinosus autograft or tendon allograft. Foot Ankle Int. 2014;35(10):1015–21.
25. Krips R, van Dijk CN, Halasi PT, Lehtonen H, Corradini C, Moyen B, et al. Long-term outcome of anatomical reconstruction versus tenodesis for the treatment of chronic anterolateral instability of the ankle joint: a multicenter study. Foot Ankle Int. 2001;22(5):415–21.
26. Hennrikus WL, Mapes RC, Lyons PM, Lapoint JM. Outcomes of the Chrisman-Snook and modified-Broström procedures for chronic lateral ankle instability. A prospective, randomized comparison. Am J Sports Med. 1996;24(4):400–4.
27. Matheny LM, Johnson NS, Liechti DJ, Clanton TO. Activity level and function after lateral ankle ligament repair versus reconstruction. Am J Sports Med. 2016;44(5):1301–8.
28. Miller AG, Raikin SM, Ahmad J. Near-anatomic allograft tenodesis of chronic lateral ankle instability. Foot Ankle Int. 2013;34(11):1501–7.
29. Jung HG, Shin MH, Park JT, Eom JS, Lee DO, Lee SH. Anatomical reconstruction of lateral ankle ligaments using free tendon allografts and Biotenodesis screws. Foot Ankle Int. 2015;36(9):1064–71.
30. Dierckman BD, Ferkel RD. Anatomic reconstruction with a semitendinosus allograft for chronic lateral ankle instability. Am J Sports Med. 2015;43(8):1941–50.
31. Wang W, Xu GH. Allograft tendon reconstruction of the anterior talofibular ligament and calcaneofibular ligament in the treatment of chronic ankle instability. BMC Musculoskelet Disord. 2017;18(1):150.
32. Cordier G, Ovigue J, Dalmau-Pastor M, Michels F. Endoscopic anatomic ligament reconstruction is a reliable option to treat chronic lateral ankle instability. Knee Surg Sports Traumatol Arthrosc. 2020;28(1):86–92.

Lateral Ankle Instability: The Role of Synthetic Ligament Augmentation

11

Richard J. Lamour and Troy S. Watson

Introduction

Chronic lateral ankle instability (CLAI) is the late sequelae of an ankle sprain, secondary to lateral ligaments that allow a pathologic increase in motion. Initial conservative management is typically recommended for an ankle sprain. The RICE formula is advocated: rest, ice, compression, and elevation. However, 34–70% of patients have been reported to experience persistent pain, swelling, or a feeling of instability [1]. CLAI is defined by recurrent instability and subsequent symptoms, reported in 20–30% of patients after the index ankle sprain.

The lateral ligament complex of the ankle is comprised of the anterior talofibular ligament (ATFL), calcaneofibular ligament (CFL), and posterior talofibular ligament (PTFL). The ATFL is the weakest of the lateral ligaments and most injured. It functions as the primary restraint to inversion with the ankle in plantar flexion and resists anterolateral translation of the talus in the ankle mortise. The ligament is located at the anteroinferior fibular border, 10 mm proximal to the lateral malleolar tip, and extends to just beyond the talus' lateral process articular margin where it meets the talar neck. Its course runs 45–90° to the longitudinal axis of the tibia [2].

The CFL is the primary restraint to inversion with the ankle in the neutral or dorsiflexed position. It restrains subtalar inversion, thereby limiting talar tilt within the mortise. It courses from the fibula's anterior border approximately 9 mm proximal to the distal tip and inserts on the calcaneus 13 mm distal to the subtalar joint and deep to the peroneal tendon sheaths [2].

The PTFL is the strongest of the lateral ligaments. Though the lateral ligament complex is intact, its role is supplementary and limits posterior talar displacement in ankle dorsiflexion. However, when ATFL and CFL are functionally incompetent, the PTFL resists internal and external rotation, talar tilt, and dorsiflexion. It courses from the fibula's posterior border to the posterolateral tubercle of the talus running perpendicular to the longitudinal axis of the tibia [2].

CLAI Assessment

As with many diagnoses, assessment of CLAI begins with a thorough history that typically includes a history of multiple inversion sprain injuries. Often patients will specify instability on uneven surfaces and an overall lack of confidence

R. J. Lamour (✉)
Olympia Orthopaedic Associates,
Olympia, WA, USA
e-mail: rlamour@olyortho.com

T. S. Watson
Las Vegas Orthopaedic Foot and Ankle Fellowship,
Desert Orthopaedic Center, Las Vegas, NV, USA

Orthopaedic Surgery Residency, Valley Hospital
Medical Center/OPTI West, Las Vegas, NV, USA
e-mail: twatson@doclv.com

P. D'Hooghe et al. (eds.), *Ligamentous Injuries of the Foot and Ankle*,
https://doi.org/10.1007/978-3-031-08682-3_11

with the ankle with activity. With further investigation, hypermobility syndrome should be ruled out with questioning regarding hyperextension, subluxation, or dislocation of other joints, i.e., shoulder, elbow, wrist, hand, hip, and knee. The identification of hypermobility syndromes can have drastic implications on the selection of surgical stabilization procedures. The patient should be asked about mechanical symptoms at the ankle, i.e., snapping, popping, or locking. These symptoms can result from CLAI-associated pathologies, such as peroneal instability and osteochondral lesions. Finally, prior treatment history should be reviewed to help determine future management plans.

Next, a systematic physical exam of the ankle and foot is performed, including alignment, ankle/subtalar joint range of motion, motor strength, and provocative stability testing. Shoes and socks should be removed for appropriate visualization and testing. For alignment, the ankle's resting posture in the non-weight-bearing position may be varus from lax lateral ligaments and weakness of the peroneal tendons. The weight-bearing alignment of the ankle and heel must be noted to determine if increased varus alignment contributes to lateral ankle instability. Standard range-of-motion testing of the ankle documenting coronal and sagittal plane motion is performed. In addition, subtalar joints flexibility can be appreciated with traditional Coleman block testing, eliminating forefoot varus effects on hindfoot motion and alignment. Correction of heel varus helps make decisions on types of corrective orthoses or surgical stabilization procedures. Traditional motor strength testing of the major ankle muscle groups is important, particularly the peroneal brevis and longus muscles. Often with CLAI, the peroneal muscles are weakened, resulting in poor dynamic stability. Provocative testing of the ATFL and CFL, with the anterior drawer and lateral tilt test, assesses functional stability. Anterior drawer maneuver is done with the ankle in approximately 20–30° of plantar flexion to appreciate the amount of translation in millimeters and whether there is a soft or firm endpoint. The talar tilt test is done with the ankle in a neutral position with a varus stress applied. Resisted dorsiflexion eversion test can reproduce peroneal subluxation or dislocation that can occur concomitantly with ankle sprains. If hypermobility syndrome is suspected, the Beighton scoring system should be utilized to identify excessive laxity. Generalized ligamentous laxity may affect outcomes of the lateral ligament complex surgical repair [3].

Diagnostic Imaging

Further evaluation of CLAI and concomitant pathologies is performed with diagnostic imaging such as plain radiographs, stress radiographs, ultrasound, and MR imaging. Weight-bearing plain radiographs are used to look for overall alignment of the ankle and hindfoot, joint space, presence of acute or chronic fracture, and osteochondral lesions. Stress radiography is done using talar tilt and anterior drawer testing maneuvers to demonstrate instability. Typically, a difference of 10° on talar tilt with the ankle held in a neutral position under varus stress determines a pathologic talar tilt through CFL failure [4]. For anterior drawer testing, 10 mm of increased anterior translation compared with that of the opposite side is used as a guide to detect an incompetent ATFL [4]. The subtalar opening is compared with that of the normal stable subtalar joint. However, it is still not well defined what degree of radiographic abnormality in subtalar opening confirms subtalar instability. The authors do not routinely obtain stress radiographs in the workup of patients with CLAI and prefer to diagnose with history and physical examination.

Ultrasound has been described as a point-of-care tool to visualize the lateral ligament complex for tears and under stress to identify pathologic instability of the lateral ankle. This is operator dependent, and thorough training is required for appropriate utilization.

Magnetic resonance imaging (MRI) may provide useful information regarding ligamentous injury around the ankle. However, ligamentous functional capacity is best determined by patient history and clinical examination. MRI is critical for evaluating associated osteochondral lesions, peroneal tendon pathology, and deltoid ligament tears. MRI is also useful in determining the quality of the lateral ligamentous tissues for surgical repair. Thus, an MRI is frequently used in the evaluation of ankle instability but should be used in combination with other imaging and the history and physical examination [4].

Nonsurgical Treatment

Typical nonsurgical treatment after an ankle sprain should focus on functional rehabilitation with rest, brief immobilization, and physical therapy or the RICE formula. Bracing and boot immobilization allow for the torn lateral ligament complex to heal without excessive elongation. Physical therapy focuses particularly on proprioceptive training, peroneal muscle strengthening, and range of motion restoration. Nonsurgical treatment is typically recommended for a minimum of 3–6 months before considering surgical intervention [1].

Consequences of long-term ankle instability are focal cartilage defects, peroneal tendon tears, global ankle arthritis, and ankle deformity. Surgical treatment for CLAI is preferred when nonsurgical treatment options have failed to improve a patients' symptoms and prevent these late complications.

Historical Surgical Options

The surgical treatment for CLAI began with a nonanatomic reconstruction by Nilsonne in 1932, followed by other nonanatomic operations such as the Watson-Jones, Evans, and Chrisman-Snook procedures. Despite excellent short-term results, nonanatomic reconstruction has been implicated in altering the ankle and subtalar joint kinematics and associated with subsequent posterior facet arthritis of the subtalar joint, laxity of the graft, and poor postoperative functional recovery [1]. Therefore, anatomical repair was proposed by Brostrom in 1966 [5] and modified by Gould (MB) in 1980 [6]. Since that time, this combination has been regarded as the gold standard with which all other techniques are compared [1]. Anatomic ligament repair restores near-normal anatomic characteristics and joint mechanics by repairing the ligament remnants.

Despite promising results with the Brostrom repair, there are reported deficiencies in the procedure. Brostrom reports that 10% of CLAI patients have insufficient tissue quality from recurrent tissue damage. The patients with generalized joint hypermobility tend to have increased failure secondary to an inherent connective tissue disorder. These concerns result in a lack of surgeon confidence in primary repair alone in certain situations. In addition, Maffulli reported 16% of recurrent instability in a 9-year case series follow-up study of Brostrom repairs [7]. The Brostrom repair has been studied for its biomechanical properties, and the native ATFL strength is 154 N (load to failure) compared to the traditional modified Brostrom repair at 68 N [8]. These findings highlight the inherent weakness of the Brostrom repair construct at time zero, which is concerning for repair failure, especially if early motion postoperatively is advocated. Kirk et al. reported in a cadaveric biomechanical study statistically significant ATFL elongation with early unprotected mobilization [9]. Since elongation of the ligament and possible failure of the repair are concerns of the MB procedure, surgeons have searched for alternatives to reduce postoperative casting and facilitate a more functional rehabilitation.

To this end, a significant effort has been dedicated to optimizing and strengthening repairs, developing a Brostrom variation that would provide superior repair strength, facilitating early and aggressive postoperative rehabilitation, and ultimately accelerating return to preinjury activity levels [10].

Brostrom Procedure Modifications and Augmentations

Brostrom with Gould Modification

Incorporating the inferior extensor retinaculum (IER) in the Gould modification of a traditional

Brostrom procedure has been used for more than 30 years, and the results of this modification to the anatomical repair have been well reported [11]. In the absence of suitable tissue to repair, the IER provides an excellent tissue source to facilitate lateral ligament repair.

However, the use of the IER in all cases of lateral ankle stability surgery may not be indicated as the IER crosses the subtalar joint. Overtightening this structure may cause stiffness in the posterior subtalar joint, which may cause functional impairment, especially in the athlete. Recent biomechanical testing has also questioned the role of the IER in direct anatomical repair using a time zero cadaveric model. This study found that incorporating the IER in the traditional Brostrom repair had no mechanical advantage compared with the mechanical testing of those specimens in which the IER was not employed [12].

In addition, the actual incorporation of the IER with the Brostrom repair has been questioned considering the significant anatomical variation of the IER. This is particularly evident when the Brostrom repair is done through a limited incision where it is often difficult to differentiate the anterior part of the sural fascia from the IER. Typically, the IER is a Y-shaped structure composed of the stem or frondiform ligament, an oblique superomedial band, and an oblique inferomedial band. The stem or frondiform ligament has three roots that arise from the sinus tarsi and divide into the oblique superomedial band, which inserts on the anterior aspect of the tibial malleolus, and into the oblique inferomedial band, which splits to insert on the abductor hallucis muscle and the navicular and medial cuneiform [11]. In 25% of cases, an X-shaped morphology is present with an additional superolateral band, which inserts into the lateral surface of the lateral malleolus; subsequently, there is limited incorporation of IER into the MB construct.

Neoligament Augmentation

Tourne et al. have described the anatomic Brostrom repair augmentation with a formal harvest of the IER superomedial and frondiform bands as a neoligament [13]. This technique appears to have similar advantages of the Gould modification by mobilizing neighboring autologous tissue without concerns of over-constraining the extensor tendons. However, the described surgical technique can be more technically challenging and require more invasive exposure as it mobilizes autogenous tissue similar to the non-anatomic tenodesis techniques.

Additional Suture Anchor Repair Augmentation

Brostrom repair by shortening the lateral ligament capsular sleeve from the insertion at the fibula with two suture anchors is a well-described version of the anatomical repair. Giza et al. added a more proximal anchor incorporating the suture limbs from the repair anchors in suture-bridge fashion to augment the biomechanical construct strength [10]. In this cadaveric study, the standard Brostrom repair and augmented Brostrom repair was done arthroscopically and not significantly different in load to failure.

Synthetic Augmentation

In a continued effort to improve the original Brostrom repair's strength, synthetic augments have been applied for decades. These devices have the intended benefits of avoiding donor site morbidity from autograft harvest, providing a strong stabilizing construct, and allowing aggressive rehabilitation and a faster return to work/sporting activity without the risk of disease transmission from allografts. These augmentation devices are meant to act as a "safety belt" to protect the primary repair from elongation and failure.

Ligament Augmentation Reconstruction System (LARS)

The LARS is a synthetic ligament augmentation device made of polyethylene terephthalate (PET).

This device developed popularity initially with cruciate ligament reconstruction surgery; however, intra-articular polyethylene synovitis has been reported. The LARS AC 30 DB (LARS, Surgical Implants and Devices, Arc-sur-Tille, France) implant was used in a 5-year randomized controlled trial comparing the modified Brostrom-Gould repair group with primary lateral ligament repair with LARS augmentation group [14]. The LARS group had a significantly better improvement in the total FAOS at 1-year, 2-year, and 5-year post surgery. This was also seen within each of the subscales of the FAOS. The 5-year Tegner activity scores were significantly better in the LARS group as well. The complication rates were low, and none were related to the LARS device material.

Leeds-Keio Artificial Ligament

Leeds-Keio artificial ligament or Leeds-Keio device (Xiros [formerly Neoligaments], Leeds, England) is another synthetic device initially used in the knee with increased complications secondary to the intra-articular placement. The later versions of the polyester mesh device have improved biocompatibility properties. Its application is not well described in the ankle. However, there are few isolated reports of use as an augment to ankle ligament repair. Kakarala et al. published a case report describing a novel technique in a revision setting where the extensor digitorum brevis (EDB) tendinous flap was used to reconstruct the lateral ligaments with the Leeds-Keio polyester mesh as an augment [15]. The single patient in this case report did well without any early complication. There are no additional reports of the Leeds-Keio artificial ligament for lateral ankle instability.

Mersilene® Suture-Tape

Sarhan et al. reported in their prospective study investigating a polyester suture-tape as the augmentation device to the primary lateral ligament repair [16]. In this particular cohort of 30 patients, a 5-mm Mersilene® tape (Ethicon, Inc., Somerville, NJ, USA) was passed through transosseous tunnels to augment an anatomic lateral ligament transosseous repair. There was a significant improvement in 1-year American Orthopaedic Foot and Ankle Society (AOFAS) and Foot and Ankle Ability Measure (FAAM) scores with no complications related to polyester material.

Arthrex® Suture-Tape (InternalBrace™)

Watson et al. described the surgical technique using the Arthrex® *Internal*Brace™ (IB) (Arthrex Inc., Naples, FL, USA) to augment the MB [17]. This device system is an ultra-high molecular weight polyethylene (UHMWPE) collagen-coated, 2-mm-wide suture-tape (FiberTape®) secured to the bone with SwiveLock® suture anchors to complete the knotless construct. Biomechanically, this construct, paired with the MB, has demonstrated superior strength compared to MB repair and even to the native ATFL at time zero [8]. The increased repair strength has translated to markedly improved clinical results, detailed in the following section. Additionally, the added strength at time zero allows surgeons to mobilize patients quickly in the postoperative period without concern for failure of the repair or elongation of the construct.

The Biomechanical Evidence

Despite the well-validated effectiveness, safety, and durability of the Brostrom procedure, sufficient evidence indicates the procedure is not a panacea. Biomechanical investigations have provided sufficient evidence to indicate that suture-tape augmentation (STA) confers superior strength to the native ATFL and MB: ATFL ligament repair [18] and ATFL STA [19] were at least as strong and stiff as the native ATFL, MB STA demonstrated superior resistance to failure [20], and ATFL reconstruction with STA restored sagittal plane stability to an ankle with anterolateral instability [21].

ATFL repair with STA was at least as strong and stiff as the native ATFL in a laboratory study of 18 cadaveric specimens. ATFL STA without a Brostrom demonstrated approximately 50% higher mean load to failure and stiffness than the intact ATFL [18]. The importance of this data is readily appreciable when compared to data showing the MB fails at less than half the load to failure of the native ligament or about 68 N [8].

ATFL ligament reconstruction with STA was not significantly different from native ATFL in a controlled laboratory study of 12 randomized cadaveric specimens [19]. This study showed that STA for lateral ligament reconstruction demonstrated similar biomechanical stability and torque and angle at failure to the native ligament. Failure angle and torque at failure were used as a surrogate measure of stability. Similarly, there was a 94% increase in the angle at failure of suture anchor fixation with STA compared to the MB in a study of 18 cadaveric specimens [20]. Ankle stability following ATFL STA did not significantly differ from the native ankle stability, measured on a validated ankle arthrometer during anterior drawer exam [21]. Serial dissection of ankle support structures increased arthrometer readings on anterior talar drawer exam, whereas STA reduced translation.

Collectively, STA confers superior strength to the construct at time zero. Biomechanical investigations do not study healing and cannot incorporate change over time, so there are notable limitations in translating biomechanical findings to clinical practice.

The Clinical Evidence

The laboratory data demonstrated superior construct strength with STA, which may enable earlier and more aggressive rehab during healing and more rapid return to sport without concern for recurrent instability. Though early data indicate favorable surgical outcomes, patient satisfaction, and pain resolution, STA's efficacy has been demonstrated in publications with levels of evidence I–IV and limited to specific patient populations.

The first prospective study to report clinical outcomes of ligament STA without concomitant MB [22] reported the clinical and patient-reported outcomes of 34 patients. Their patient cohort had significantly improved FAOS and FAAM scores at final follow-up, and their radiographic measurements, including talar tilt angle (TTA) and anterior talar translation (ATT), significantly improved ($P < 0.001$). Subsequently, the senior author published the first comparative prospective study of minimally invasive ligament STA and MB [23], which established the procedure as a viable alternative that obviated the need for free tendon graft nonanatomic ligament reconstruction. The methodological strengths of a priori power analysis and randomization were tempered by strict inclusion and exclusion criteria. Nevertheless, the reported instruments (FAOS, FAAM) are well validated, and radiographic outcomes were consistent with the current literature.

Further, the senior author introduced STA to resolve the challenging problem of recurrent instability following a failed index MB procedure [24]. Contraindications to the MB procedure are unclear, and the mechanism of failure has been attributed to trauma, poor compliance, poor tissue quality, and poor technique. Consequently, the study reported short-term clinical and operative findings in 30 patients. The mean FAOS and FAAM scores and radiographic measurements (TTA and ATT) improved significantly at the final follow-up ($P < 0.001$). One patient failed the revision procedure and required revision using allograft tendon.

Evidence of safety and durability in a high-demand military population has been reported [25, 26]. MB was compared to MB STA, which demonstrated a significant difference in American Orthopaedic Foot and Ankle Society (AOFAS) scores at six weeks and 12 weeks after surgery ($P = 0.001$) in 85 patients. Further, the rate of return to sport at 12 weeks after surgery showed a significant difference ($P < 0.001$) in favor of the STA group (18 patients, 81.8%) compared to the group without STA (17 patients, 27%). The authors suggested the additional strength may act as a secondary stabilizer to repair and may help resist injury recurrence to enable the return to sport [25]. The safety of the MB STA with accelerated rehabilitation was reported in a retrospective case series of 93 military patients [26]. Patients returned to agility drills 4 weeks sooner than their previous institution protocols, with 82 (96%) performing single-leg hop and single-leg heel raise at 6 weeks postop. Only one patient required revision surgery.

To determine if STA would enable accelerated rehab and protect the repair, one group investigated the clinical results of immediate weight-bearing and early range of motion after MB STA [27]. The observational study reported on 81 patients with an average follow-up of 11.5 months. Mean return to sport (68, 84%) was 84.1 days, and no significant ankle joint mechanical differences were noted between the operative and contralateral side. Similarly, a randomized controlled trial compared return to preoperative activity level in MB to MB STA [28]. Notably, the previously published rehab protocol [27] was utilized for all patients, except those transitioned to standard protocols due to intolerance. The MB STA cohort returned 4.2 weeks earlier than the MB cohort ($P < 0.001$). There was no significant difference in return to preinjury activity at 26 weeks postoperatively or transition out of accelerated rehab. The authors concluded that both accelerated rehabilitation and STA are safe and improved return to preoperative activity.

The publications comparing clinical outcomes of STA repair and MB were analyzed in a systematic review and meta-analysis [29]. The review included four studies and 254 patients (105 STA repair compared to 149 Brostrom). The authors concluded that both repair techniques were effective management options for chronic ankle instability, with no significant difference in instability incidence, functional outcomes, or complication rate. Notably, there were significant differences in the cohorts studied, and the follow-up duration was short. Considering the data-collated findings from a male-only cohort [25] and a female-only cohort [22], the findings should be interpreted cautiously.

Modified Brostrom-Gould Repair with *Internal*Brace™ Augmentation

Surgical Technique

The authors' preferred surgical technique has been previously reported [17]. An MB STA is performed using a linear incision across the distal fibula, approximately 1 cm proximal to the distal terminus (Fig. 11.1), with two all-suture anchors.

1. Drilling for the talus anchor (Fig. 11.2): Initially, the provided talar offset guide is positioned firmly within the sinus tarsi, so it is approximately 2 cm from the tip of the lateral process of the talus. The guide is angled into the talar body at a 45-degree angle to avoid articular violation of the ankle and subtalar joints. A solid 3.4-mm drill bit is used to drill through the guide into the talus' nonarticular surface.
2. Placement of the talus anchor (Fig. 11.3): Through the guide, the drill tunnel is tapped to the laser line on the 4.75-mm tap (green handle) with a mallet. The 4.75-mm SwiveLock® anchor loaded with FiberTape® suture is placed into the talar hole. As the square green paddle on the driver is held stationary, the pear-shaped driver is turned clockwise, which advances the threaded suture anchor into the tunnel with the FiberTape®. When the laser line in the window of the driver appears, the screw is flush, and when it is line to line, the screw is 2 mm countersunk.

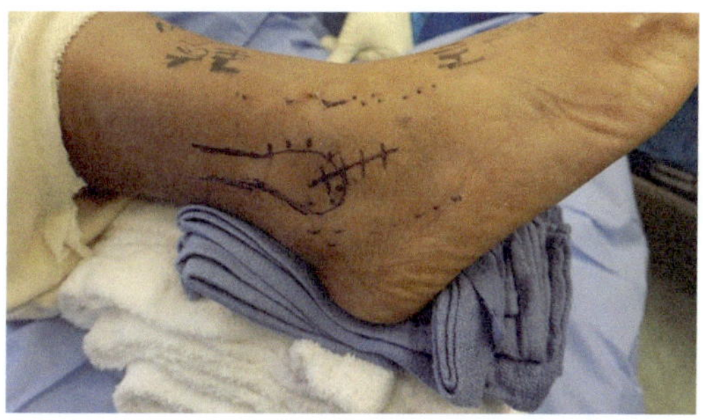

Fig. 11.1 Pertinent landmarks are identified, and the surgical incision is planned

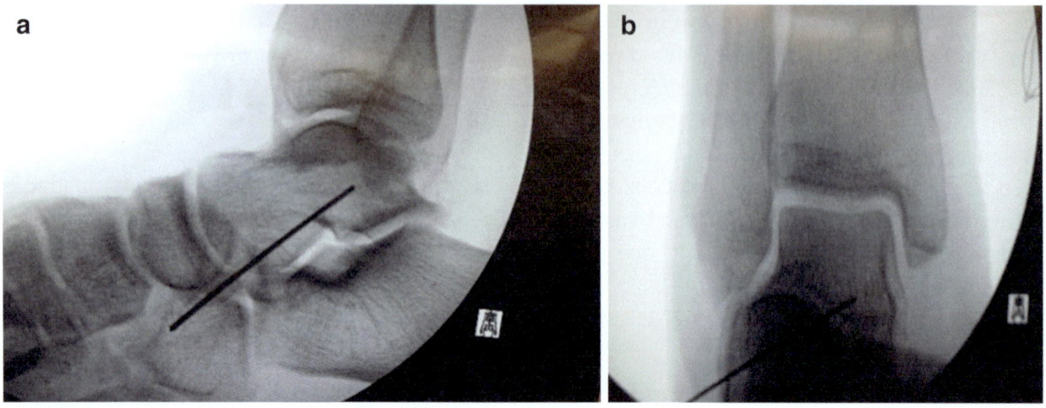

Fig. 11.2 (**a–b**) Guidewire confirmation of anchor tunnel on fluoroscopy

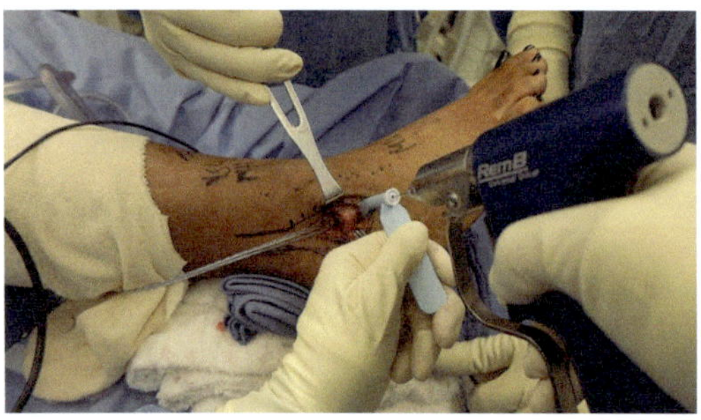

Fig. 11.3 Drilling for the talus anchor

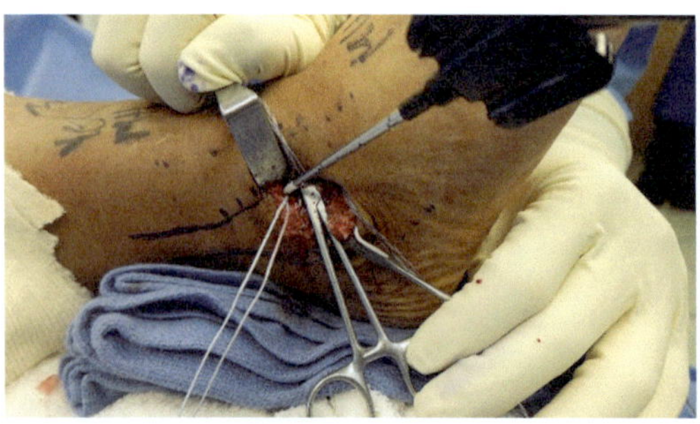

Fig. 11.4 Fibula anchor

3. Completed MB (Fig. 11.4): At this time, the MB is completed by securing the ATFL/capsular sleeve to the fibula with the previously placed suture anchors. The ankle is typically placed in a neutral position with a posterior drawer maneuver performed.
4. Drilling for the fibular anchor: The fibular tunnel is drilled approximately 1.5 cm proximal from the distal fibula's tip, splitting the difference of the insertion points of the all-suture anchors. This is done with the 3.4-mm drill bit and without tapping for this tunnel.
5. Tensioning/placement of fibular anchor: Both limbs of the FiberTape suture are passed through the eyelet of the 3.5-mm SwiveLock anchor. With the ankle placed in the desired position, which is neutral in coronal and sagittal planes, the eyelet is placed at the drill hole, and the FiberTape sutures are marked at the laser line. The eyelet is slid down to the line on the FiberTape, and the anchor is inserted into the drilled hole in the same sequence as the previous anchor.
6. Release excess FiberTape/additional repair sutures (Fig. 11.5): After final anchor placement is inserted, the remnant FiberTape® tails with FiberWire® scissors. Suture the inferior extensor retinaculum to the fibula or capsule as desired.

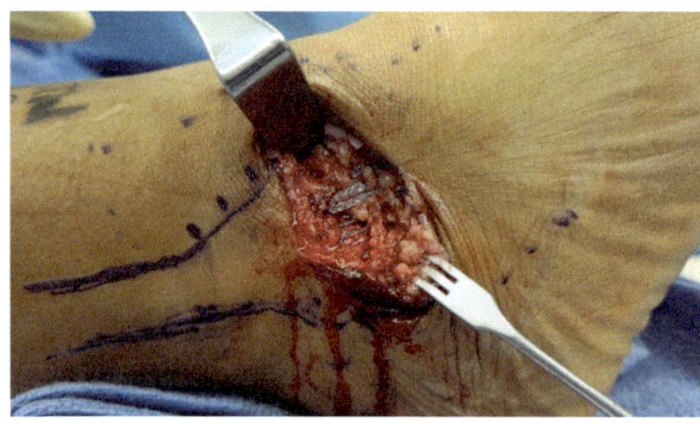

Fig. 11.5 Final modified Brostrom repair with suture-tape augmentation

A variety of anchor configurations and order of anchor placement are possible to complete the IB construct. The authors prefer to place the 4.75-mm SwiveLock® first in the talus and then place the 3.5 SwiveLock® in the fibula second. This configuration has been shown in a biomechanical study to have superior construct strength to the native ATFL [30].

Acknowledgments The authors would like to give special thanks to John P. Walsh, DO for his assistance with the preparation of this chapter.

References

1. Song Y, Li H, Sun C, Zhang J, Gui J, Guo Q, et al. Clinical guidelines for the surgical management of chronic lateral ankle instability: a consensus reached by systematic review of the available data. Orthop J Sports Med. 2019;7(9):2325967119873852. https://doi.org/10.1177/2325967119873852.
2. Golano P, Fariñas O, Sáenz I. The anatomy of the navicular and periarticular structures. Foot Ankle Clin. 2004;9(1):1–23.
3. Folci M, Capsoni F. Arthralgias, fatigue, paresthesias and visceral pain: can joint hypermobility solve the puzzle? A case report. BMC Musculoskelet Disord. 2016;17:58. https://doi.org/10.1186/s12891-016-0905-2.
4. Schenck RC, Coughlin MJ. Lateral ankle instability and revision surgery alternatives in the athlete. Foot Ankle Clin. 2009;14(2):205–14.
5. Broström L. Sprained ankles. V. Treatment and prognosis in recent ligament ruptures. Acta Chir Scand. 1966;132(5):537–50.
6. Gould N, Seligson D, Gassman J. Early and late repair of lateral ligament of the ankle. Foot Ankle. 1980;1(2):84–9.
7. Maffulli N, Del Buono A, Maffulli GD, Oliva F, Testa V, Capasso G, et al. Isolated anterior talofibular ligament Broström repair for chronic lateral ankle instability: 9-year follow-up. Am J Sports Med. 2013;41(4):858–64.
8. Waldrop NE, Wijdicks CA, Jansson KS, LaPrade RF, Clanton TO. Anatomic suture anchor versus the Broström technique for anterior talofibular ligament repair: a biomechanical comparison. Am J Sports Med. 2012;40(11):2590–6.
9. Kirk KL, Campbell JT, Guyton GP, Parks BG, Schon LC. ATFL elongation after Brostrom procedure: a biomechanical investigation. Foot Ankle Int. 2008;29(11):1126–30.
10. Giza E, Whitlow SR, Williams BT, Acevedo JI, Mangone PG, Haytmanek CT, et al. Biomechanical analysis of an arthroscopic Broström ankle ligament repair and a suture anchor-augmented repair. Foot Ankle Int. 2015;36(7):836–41.
11. Cordier G, Lebecque J, Vega J, Dalmau-Pastor M. Arthroscopic ankle lateral ligament repair with biological augmentation gives excellent results in case of chronic ankle instability. Knee Surg Sports Traumatol Arthrosc. 2020;28(1):108–15.
12. Behrens SB, Drakos M, Lee BJ, Paller D, Hoffman E, Koruprolu S, et al. Biomechanical analysis of Brostrom versus Brostrom-Gould lateral ankle instability repairs. Foot Ankle Int. 2013;34(4):587–92.
13. Tourné Y, Peruzzi M. Lateral collateral ligament repair: anatomical ligament reinsertion with augmentation using inferior extensor retinaculum flaps. Oper Orthop Traumatol. 2019;31(3):169–79.
14. Porter M, Shadbolt B, Ye X, Stuart R. Ankle lateral ligament augmentation versus the modified Broström-Gould procedure: a 5-year randomized controlled trial. Am J Sports Med. 2019;47(3):659–66.
15. Kakarala G, Rajan DT. Anterior talo-fibular ligament reconstruction using synthetic ligament and the extensor digitorum brevis. Clin J Sport Med. 2006;16(4):366–8.
16. Sarhan I, Mubark I, Waly A. Chronic lateral ankle instability: results of anatomic repair with polyester tape augmentation. Ortop Traumatol Rehabil. 2020;22(1):25–31.
17. Watson TS, Lamour RJ. Open modified Broström ankle reconstruction with internal brace augmentation: a novel approach. 2015 [cited 2020 Oct 16]. https://www.healio.com/news/orthopedics/20150811/open-modified-brostrm-ankle-reconstruction-with-internal-brace-augmentation-a-novel-approach
18. Viens NA, Wijdicks CA, Campbell KJ, LaPrade RF, Clanton TO. Anterior talofibular ligament ruptures, part 1: biomechanical comparison of augmented Broström repair techniques with the intact anterior talofibular ligament. Am J Sports Med. 2014;42(2):405–11.
19. Willegger M, Benca E, Hirtler L, Hradecky K, Holinka J, Windhager R, et al. Biomechanical stability of tape augmentation for anterior talofibular ligament (ATFL) repair compared to the native ATFL. Knee Surg Sports Traumatol Arthrosc. 2016;24(4):1015–21.
20. Schuh R, Benca E, Willegger M, Hirtler L, Zandieh S, Holinka J, et al. Comparison of Broström technique, suture anchor repair, and tape augmentation for reconstruction of the anterior talofibular ligament. Knee Surg Sports Traumatol Arthrosc. 2016;24(4):1101–7.
21. Lohrer H, Bonsignore G, Dorn-Lange N, Li L, Gollhofer A, Gehring D. Stabilizing lateral ankle instability by suture tape – a cadaver study. J Orthop Surg. 2019;14(1):175.
22. Cho B-K, Park K-J, Kim S-W, Lee H-J, Choi S-M. Minimal invasive suture-tape augmentation for chronic ankle instability. Foot Ankle Int. 2015;36(11):1330–8.
23. Cho B-K, Park J-K, Choi S-M, SooHoo NF. A randomized comparison between lateral ligaments augmentation using suture-tape and modified Broström

repair in young female patients with chronic ankle instability. Foot Ankle Surg. 2019;25(2):137–42.
24. Cho BK, Kim YM, Choi SM, Park HW, SooHoo NF. Revision anatomical reconstruction of the lateral ligaments of the ankle augmented with suture tape for patients with a failed Broström procedure. Bone Joint J. 2017;99-B(9):1183–9.
25. Yoo J-S, Yang E-A. Clinical results of an arthroscopic modified Brostrom operation with and without an internal brace. J Orthop Traumatol. 2016;17(4):353–60.
26. Martin KD, Andres NN, Robinson WH. Suture tape augmented Broström procedure and early accelerated rehabilitation. Foot Ankle Int. 2020;42(2):145–50.
27. Coetzee JC, Ellington JK, Ronan JA, Stone RM. Functional results of open Broström ankle ligament repair augmented with a suture tape. Foot Ankle Int. 2018;39(3):304–10.
28. Kulwin R, Watson T, Rigby R, Coetzee JC, Vora A. Traditional modified Broström versus suture tape ligament augmentation. Foot Ankl Int. 2021;42(5):554–61.
29. Li H, Zhao Y, Chen W, Li H, Hua Y. No differences in clinical outcomes of suture tape augmented repair versus Broström repair surgery for chronic lateral ankle instability. Orthop J Sports Med. 2020;8(9):2325967120948491. https://doi.org/10.1177/2325967120948491.
30. Gates N. InternalBrace™ ligament augmentation. Arthrex Research and Development; 2014.

12 Lateral Ankle Instability: Rehab and Return to Sport

Christopher Neville, Erin Haggerty, Jeannie Park, Robert Carrier, and Eric Giza

Background

Ankle sprains are a common sports-related injury with a reported incidence of 2.15 per 1000 person-years in the United States [1]. An ankle sprain typically results from an inversion force on a plantarflexed foot resulting in lateral ankle ligament injury. While the majority of patients recover from an ankle sprain with minimal residual dysfunction, approximately 10–30% of patients with an ankle sprain develop chronic symptoms of giving way of the ankle, mechanical instability, pain and swelling, loss of strength, recurrent sprain, and functional instability [2]. These chronic symptoms characterize a condition called chronic ankle instability (CAI) [3].

In this chapter, CAI is defined as recurrent ankle instability episodes occurring for a minimum of 1 year after an initial injury [4]. Persistent symptoms of CAI can result from multiple factors, including:

1. Primary tissue injury.
   (a) ATFL and CFL.
2. Pathomechanical impairments.
   (a) Pathological laxity, range of motion restrictions, secondary tissue injury, and tissue adaptation.
3. Sensory-perceptual impairments.
   (a) Pain, diminished somatosensation, perceived instability, kinesiophobia, lower reported function, and reduced HRQL.
4. Motor-behavioral impairments.
   (a) Altered reflexes, neuromuscular inhibition, muscle weakness, balance deficits, altered movement patterns, and reduced physical activity.
5. Personal factors.
   (a) Demographics, medical history, physical attributes, and psychological profile.
6. Environmental factors.
   (a) Physical activity and sport demands, home and work demands, social support, and access to health care.
7. Component interactions.
   (a) Interactions among the factors listed above.
8. Clinical outcomes.
   (a) Range of clinical outcome presentation from ongoing signs of CAI to full recovery.

Overall, these components result in functional and/or mechanical instability. Functional insta-

C. Neville · R. Carrier
Department of Physical Therapy Education, Upstate Medical University, Rochester, NY, USA
e-mail: nevillec@upstate.edu; CarrierR@upstate.edu

E. Haggerty · J. Park · E. Giza (✉)
Department of Orthopedics, University of California, Davis, Sacramento, CA, USA
e-mail: jeapark@ucdavis.edu; egiza@ucdavis.edu

P. D'Hooghe et al. (eds.), *Ligamentous Injuries of the Foot and Ankle*,
https://doi.org/10.1007/978-3-031-08682-3_12

bility has been described as "the occurrence of recurrent joint instability and the sensation of joint instability due to the contributions of any neuromuscular deficit" [5]. Functional instability can also be thought of as persistent instability despite absence of pathological laxity on exam. The primary cause of such functional instability is injury to the joint mechanoreceptors and afferent nerves resulting in impaired balance, reduced joint position sense, slowed firing of the peroneal muscles in response to inversion stress, slowed nerve conduction velocity, impaired cutaneous sensation, strength deficits, and decreased ankle dorsiflexion. Functional instability typically responds well to a thoughtful rehabilitation program. Mechanical instability, on the other hand, may occur as a result of adverse anatomical changes due to structural damage of the ligamentous tissues resulting in laxity. Mechanical instability can lead to altered joint kinematics and arthritic changes, which often require surgical intervention [6]. Mechanical and functional instability can occur concurrently in a patient making treatment more complex.

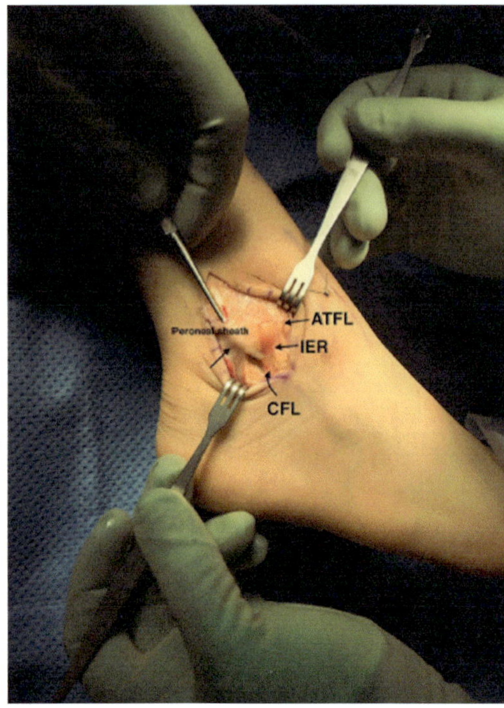

Fig. 12.1 Intraoperative view of the lateral ankle ligaments (CFL and ATFL) along with the peroneal sheath and inferior extensor retinaculum (IER)

Anatomy and Biomechanics

To understand the pathology of CAI, one must first understand the anatomy and biomechanics of ankle stability. Ankle stability is a function of extrinsic elements, such as ligaments and tendons, and intrinsic elements, such as the geometry of the articular surface. The contribution of each element varies with the load level, the direction in which force is applied, and the integrity of the ligaments [7]. In general, the ankle is most stable when dorsiflexed and loaded and least stable when plantarflexed and unloaded. The unloaded ankle relies on ligaments for stability.

The three lateral ligaments of the ankle include the anterior talofibular ligament (ATFL), the calcaneofibular ligament (CFL), and the posterior talofibular ligament (PTFL) (Fig. 12.1). Ankle stability is conferred by passive ligamentous restraints, articular surface congruity, and active musculotendinous units. The ATFL, CFL, and PTFL provide static restraint to the lateral aspect of the ankle.

The ATFL is continuous with the joint capsule and can have a variable number of bands [8]. Clanton et al.'s cadaveric study of lateral ankle ligaments found 50% (7 out of 14) of specimens had a single-banded ATFL, while the remaining 50% had two bands. They localized the origin of the ATFL on the anterior fibula as 13.8 mm from the lateral malleolus' inferior tip and the insertion on the talus just anterior to the lateral articular surface. The ATFL is taut in plantarflexion and prevents anterior talar translation and excessive plantarflexion. The ATFL is the weakest of the three lateral ligaments and most at risk of rupture following an inversion injury on a plantarflexed foot [9]. As the force increases and progresses laterally, the CFL tends to be injured next.

The CFL originates approximately 5.3 mm anterior to the inferior tip of the lateral malleolus [9]. Importantly, the CFL not only crosses the ankle joint but also spans the subtalar joint, coursing posteroinferiorly underneath the peroneal tendons to insert onto the lateral aspect of the calcaneal body. In contrast to the ATFL, the CFL is taut when the ankle is dorsiflexed. It prevents excessive tibiotalar and subtalar inversion.

The PTFL is the largest of the three lateral ligaments and originates approximately 4.8 mm superior to the lateral malleolus' inferior tip along the medial aspect of the lateral malleolus, and its fibers spread onto the posterolateral aspect of the talus [9]. The PTFL is also taut in dorsiflexion and helps to prevent excessive ankle inversion and internal rotation [10]. Given its size and strength, the PTFL is rarely affected and usually ruptures only after severe injuries [11].

Working together with the static stabilizers of the ankle, the musculotendinous units provide dynamic stability to the ankle via muscular contractions [10]. The most important active stabilizers of the lateral ankle are the peroneal muscles. During a sprain, the peroneal muscles help to counteract the inversion force [12]. Delayed peroneal reaction time has been found to be associated with CAI.

History and Physical Exam

Patients with CAI typically present complaining of their ankle "giving way" without warning and a sensation of instability while ambulating, especially on uneven ground. Most report a history of prior or recurrent lateral ankle sprains in the past. Traditionally, a history of a prior ankle sprain has been considered a more consistent risk factor for recurrent sprains [13]. In a recent meta-analysis, a prior history of ankle sprain conferred a nonsignificant relative risk of 1.44 [4]. However, most patients with a history of ankle sprain do not go on to develop CAI. This inconsistency can be explained by a few factors that could potentially influence clinical outcomes after a sprain: successful rehabilitation, type of rehab protocol, treatment compliance, and presence/type of associated injuries [14].

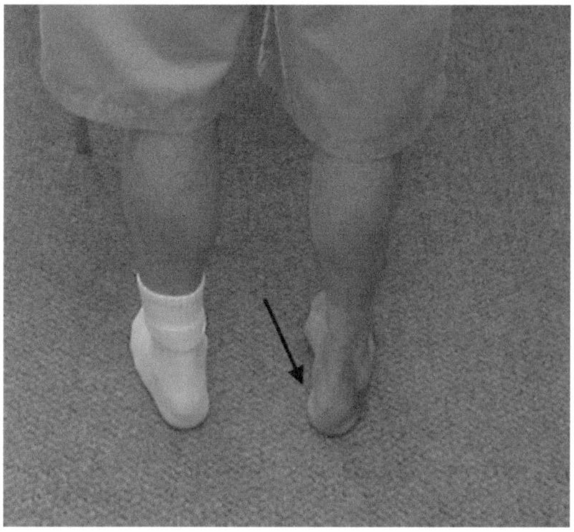

Fig. 12.2 Clinical photo demonstrating hindfoot varus malalignment

After obtaining a complete history, a thorough yet focused physical exam can help aid in diagnosis. Inspection for alignment is important as both tibia vara and hindfoot varus can predispose one to CAI (Fig. 12.2). Hindfoot alignment is best assessed with the patient standing and the practitioner standing behind the patient. A normal hindfoot typically has 5–10° of valgus; therefore, any amount of hindfoot varus should raise suspicion.

In addition to inspection of alignment, neurovascular status should also be evaluated. Occasionally, the superficial peroneal nerve (SPN) can suffer traction damage after a severe inversion injury [15]. Additionally, in a patient with injury to the ATFL, an abnormal increase in the ankle's motion can place the SPN under a greater amount of excursion and strain. This can lead to a loss of normal nerve function and potentially a loss of protective reflexes.

Both the ATFL and CFL should be palpated for tenderness. Laxity of these ligaments should also be assessed and compared to laxity of the contralateral side. The anterior drawer test (ADT) specifically assesses for ATFL laxity. The ADT is performed with the patient seated and the knee flexed approximately 90°. The ankle is placed in 20° of plantarflexion, and the practitio-

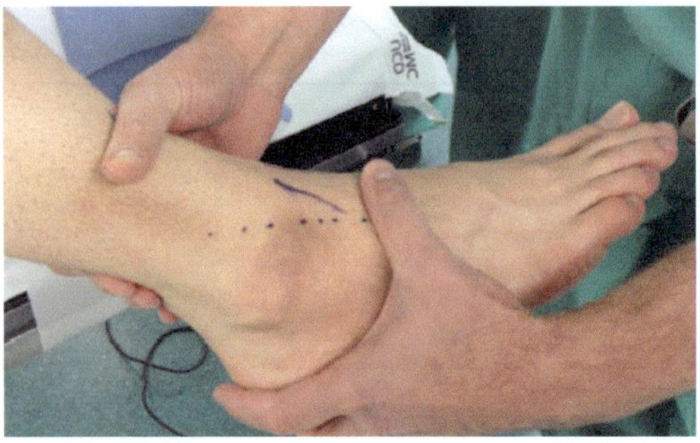

Fig. 12.3 Image demonstrating the anterior drawer test (ADT) to evaluate for anterior talar displacement relative to the tibia

ner translates the talus anteriorly against a fixed tibia (Fig. 12.3). Accuracy of the ADT may be enhanced if performed in conjunction with palpation for ligament tenderness and compared to the contralateral side. The competency of the CFL is assessed via the talar tilt (TT) or inversion test. The test is performed with the ankle dorsiflexed and the hindfoot inverted. Having the patient lay prone on the exam table with the midshaft of the tibia positioned at the edge of the table and repeating the TT test can be helpful as the excursion of the hindfoot compared to the lateral fibula is easier to visualize with the patient prone. Like the ADT, the TT test should not be used in isolation and should be used cautiously as mechanical laxity is not always present in patients with CAI. Both the ADT and TT have variable interobserver reliability and are also practitioner dependent.

It is important to evaluate the motor strength of the peroneal muscles as weakness can lead to functional instability. A single leg balance test can be performed and is especially useful for predicting future ankle sprains in the athletic population [16]. To perform this test, the patient is asked to balance on one leg with their eyes opened and then closed. A test is positive if the patient complains of imbalance.

Imaging

Bilateral weight-bearing radiographs of the ankle should first be obtained. Bilaterality allows for direct comparison to the contralateral side and can be especially helpful in more subtle malalignment [17]. The Saltzman view can be helpful to supplement clinical examination of hindfoot alignment in the coronal plane. Plain radiography may also reveal osteoarthritis, osteophytes, and possible subtalar joint pathology.

Occasionally, stress radiography may be employed when diagnosing CAI. With stress radiography, imaging is obtained while a clinical laxity test such as the ADT or TT test is performed. The ADT is evaluated in the lateral view, and anterior talar displacement is measured and compared to static imaging and/or the contralateral side under stress. The TT test is performed in the anteroposterior view, and the angle between the dome of the talus and the tibial plafond is measured after performing the inversion stress. Traditionally, an ADT greater than 10 mm or 5 mm side-to-side difference, or a TT greater than 10° or 5° side-to-side difference, has been considered diagnostic of ankle instability [18]. Controversies and criticisms remain surrounding stress radiography and include underestimating the anterior talar displacement and the TT angles, variable reference ranges, and whether manual stress versus mechanical devices should be applied to assess laxity [19].

Ultrasound (US) and magnetic resonance imaging (MRI) are other helpful imaging modalities. One meta-analysis evaluating the efficacy of varying imaging methods for diagnosis of CAI found US to be more sensitive than MRI in detecting both chronic ATFL and CFL injuries [20]. The accuracy of MRI was mostly limited to diagnosing chronic ATFL injuries. Such findings highlight the fact that imaging alone is insufficient in diagnosing CAI and that accurate diagnosis must be coupled with history and physical examination. Despite this, MRI can still be quite helpful to assess for associated pathology such as talar or tibial osteochondral damage or peroneal tendon tearing.

Concomitant Pathology

Pathologies associated with CAI can include bony and soft tissue ankle impingement, osteochondral lesions of the talus (OLT), loose bodies, and peroneal tenosynovitis and tearing. The senior authors routinely perform ankle arthroscopy at the time of ligamentous stabilization due to the high rate of intra-articular lesions in this patent population, including OLTs and soft tissue or bony impingement.

Subtalar joint instability (STJI) is another condition commonly associated with CAI and can occur in approximately 10–30% of patient who have CAI. Although an ATFL and CFL injury primarily compromise stability of the tibiotalar joint, a CFL injury can also present as STJI given that the CFL crosses both the tibiotalar and subtalar joints. As a result, STJI and CAI present similarly with patients complaining of instability in the setting of recurrent sprains [3]. CAI and STJI can be differentiated via stress radiography. The Broden projection is a popular subtalar stress view, and nonparallelity between the talus and calcaneus is suggestive of STJI. Even this projection may not fully evaluate the subtalar joint, and therefore, differentiating between CAI and STJI remains complicated.

A potential sequela of CAI is osteoarthritis and hindfoot varus or valgus malalignment. In a case series evaluating posttraumatic ankle osteoarthritis, Valderrabano et al. found 13% was attributed to a ligamentous lesion with the majority involving the lateral ligaments [21]. Interestingly, they found that the time span for developing arthritis was shorter in those with a single severe sprain compared to those with chronic lesions. The authors also found that approximately 67% of patients with chronic lateral ankle instability had varus malalignment. This varus malalignment was attributed to progressive degeneration of the medial ankle as a result of peroneal muscle dysfunction and abnormal ankle kinematics.

Nonoperative Management

Manual Therapy

High-level evidence has pointed to the benefit of manual therapy including joint mobilizations, manipulations, and mobilizations with movement to improve ankle dorsiflexion ROM and ankle proprioception. Lack of dorsiflexion ROM has been identified to increase ankle sprain risk by five times compared to those with average weight-bearing dorsiflexion of 45° [22]. Programs between 2 and 4 weeks that include mobilization of the talocrural joint have shown to improve ankle dorsiflexion ROM in a series of systematic reviews and controlled trials [23–26]. With evidence supporting mobilization in CAI, focus on dosage and patient compliance remains an interest of current and future studies. A recent study included both clinician-applied mobilizations and a self-mobilization home program with findings that the self-mobilization may be as effective and improve patient compliance with the program [27]. Studies now also support longer treatment durations (higher dosage), which impart even greater improvements in ankle motion and dynamic postural control [28, 29]. More recently, rehabilitation strategies have added a focus on the sensory deficits observed in patients with CAI. Joint mobilizations and plantar massage have both shown promise in improving balance and patient-reported outcomes with effects seen at a 1-month follow-up [30]. Although higher-level evidence supports manual therapy techniques in the management of CAI, long-term outcomes and incidence of reinjury remain areas of future study.

Exercise Interventions

Rehabilitation programs have addressed the impairments identified in CAI with a focus on strengthening and balance impairment. The evidence clearly demonstrates that balance programs for those with CAI not only improves postural control but also reduces recurrent ankle sprains [31] and the prevalence of functional ankle instability. Exercise also is associated with a quicker time to recovery and enhanced outcomes. A majority of intervention studies have focused on interventions that target one or more of the aforementioned impairments. For example, joint mobilization interventions have primarily improved dorsiflexion ROM as well as postural control [32, 33]. Balance training programs have improved static and dynamic postural control [34]. Ankle-strengthening programs have improved ankle strength [35]. Many of these interventions have also demonstrated the ability to enhance ankle-specific patient-reported outcomes (PROs) [36]. A focus of the balance interventions has been improving balance with weight-bearing exercise on unstable surfaces. In a systematic review of studies involving functional (weight-bearing) rehabilitation strategies and outcomes measurements, a wobble board was the most common training strategy. It was concluded that functional exercises and activities, especially utilizing unstable surfaces, promote improvement in dynamic postural control [37]. This is consistent with a predominance of evidence supporting improvements in measures of postural sway for individuals with CAI who undergo progressive balance retraining programs [34, 38–41]. Controlled trials that have combined balance exercise and manual therapy have shown improvements across clinician and patient-focused outcomes, but the follow-up time remains limited [36]. Current and future studies are beginning to identify those most likely to benefit from rehabilitation; however, this has currently only identified specific characteristics linked to interventions. For example, those with >3 balance test errors had a 73% probability of treatment success following ankle mobilization, and participants that reported between limb differences <16.07% and who made >2.5 errors had a 99% probability of treatment success with plantar massage [42]. In summary, exercise programs that incorporate balance and strengthening have positive effects on improving balance and patient-reported clinical outcomes in those with CAI. However, the clinical endpoint from these programs has not been investigated over longer-term follow-ups. The potential for these rehabilitation programs to reduce risk for further injury, return to sport, and improve overall outcomes after 1 year remains an area of ongoing study.

Ankle Supportive Devices and Taping

CAI rehabilitation programs focus on the use of taping and/or bracing as a method of targeting both mechanical and functional ankle instability and preventing further ankle sprains. With the risk of re-sprain within 3 years after initial ankle sprain ranging from 3% to 34% and re-sprain rate within a lifetime of 56% to 74%, the prevention of the development of CAI remains a focus [43, 44]. The goals of taping and bracing are to restrict the range of motion of the ankle and increase the sensory stimulation of the ankle and surrounding tissues. With regard to restricting range of motion, a meta-analysis compared tape, lace-up bracing, and semirigid bracing in their ability to restrict motion before and after exercise. All three supports were found significantly more restrictive than no support. When comparing all three supports, semirigid was more restrictive in both inversion and eversion than lace-up and tape, and only the semirigid bracing increased restriction with exercise [45]. A decrease in restriction following exercise is important because fatigue increases during exercise and results in a decrease in proprioception and balance that increases the risk of ankle sprains [22].

With regard to increasing sensory stimulation, a recent meta-analysis showed that soft, lace-up, and semirigid braces all resulted in a weak increase in dynamic balance in individuals with CAI while decreasing dynamic balance in healthy individuals. The conclusion was braces promoted sensorimotor feedback typically lost in people with CAI that still remains in people with healthy ankles [46]. A randomized controlled trial found similar results with improvements in balance using soft ankle orthosis, semirigid orthosis, and ankle kinesiotape. After 4 weeks, all treatment groups showed significant improvements in both static and dynamic balance, with no between-group differences in the outcomes [47]. However, there are contrasting perspectives on the effectiveness of kinesiotaping in improving balance with another controlled study finding no performance difference between taping [48]. In another study, Shields et al. found minor but not clinically meaningful balance improvements with the use of kinesiotaping [49]. One factor that may explain differences between studies is the time (dosage) the tape is left on. While Bicici evaluated the immediate effect of kinesiotape on balance, Shield left the tape on for 24 h, and

Jackson et al. concluded that kinesiotape application for 48 h improved balance, which was the same duration intervals that Hadidi used [47–50].

In summary, the use of taping and bracing has resulted in reduced risk of ankle sprains. In a recent systematic review, two of the three studies reviewed found that groups receiving lace-up-style bracing reported significantly lower incidence and risk of ankle sprains during athletic activity. From the 3581 combined subjects from the bracing group and control group, 432/1753 athletes sustained an ankle sprain when wearing a brace, compared to 529/1828 athletes spraining their ankle not wearing a brace [51]. Overall, athletes wearing ankle braces had a significantly lower incidence of ankle sprains ($p = 0.0037$) and a 64% reduced risk of ankle sprains (RR = 0.36) compared to no-treatment control [52, 53]. The use of brace or tape reduces the risk of both recurrent (RR 0.30, 95%CI 0.21–0.43) and first-time ankle sprains (RR 0.69, 95%CI 0.49–0.96), especially in those who participate in sports [54–57]. From this information, the *Journal of Sport Rehabilitation* consensus recommendation is taping and bracing can be used early during a comprehensive rehabilitation program to help prompt proper gait biomechanics and reduce ankle sprain risk [58]. Whether being used in a rehabilitative or preventive way, the use of taping and bracing promotes a reduction in risk of ankle sprains in individuals with CAI.

Recommendations for Return to Activity and Sports with CAI

Despite an abundance of studies focused on identifying the impairments present in CAI, and how these can be addressed with interventions, there remains little consensus on specific cutoffs that can be used to determine return-to-sport decisions [59]. There is a lack of criterion-based cutoffs that might help with return-to-sport decisions. Since up to 40% of individuals who incur a first-time LAS injury will develop CAI within a 1-year time frame, it is important for clinicians to identify possible prognostic factors for developing CAI. Suggestions for objective measures include reduced ankle dorsiflexion range of motion, decreased proprioception, reduced static and dynamic postural balance, poor neuromuscular control and running technique, reduced ankle muscle strength, reduced cardiorespiratory endurance, and delayed peroneus brevis reaction time. These intrinsic modifiable risk factors should be targeted by the appropriate prescription of exercises. Regarding extrinsic risk factors, clinicians should be cognizant of type of sport (e.g., basketball, volleyball), position played (e.g., center in basketball), athlete exposure, and playing surface [60]. In summary, the current evidence leaves clinical decisions about return to sports to an assessment of current impairments and an evaluation of the risk potential when returning to activity. Future work should focus on specific criterion comparing to an uninvolved side, or healthy norms, to inform decision-making and reducing risk of reinjury.

Operative Management

If patients do not respond to nonoperative rehabilitation, there are several surgical options available to address mechanical instability. Surgical techniques are broadly categorized into nonanatomic versus anatomic approaches. Nonanatomic approaches do not recreate the ligaments' native anatomic insertion points and rely on local grafts to reconstruct the strained ligaments [61]. Disadvantages to the nonanatomic approach include impaired ankle range of motion, sacrifice of a normal tendon to use as a graft, and long-term degenerative changes [62, 63]. Anatomic approaches are generally preferred because they attempt to recreate the normal ankle's biomechanics. However, studies determining which anatomic procedure is most appropriate for CAI are limited [20].

The open Broström-Gould anatomic repair is one of the most common anatomic techniques for lateral ankle instability. It combines the Broström technique, which directly repairs the ATFL and CFL by sewing over and tightening the attenuated ligaments using continuous sutures, with the Gould technique, which reinforces the repair by

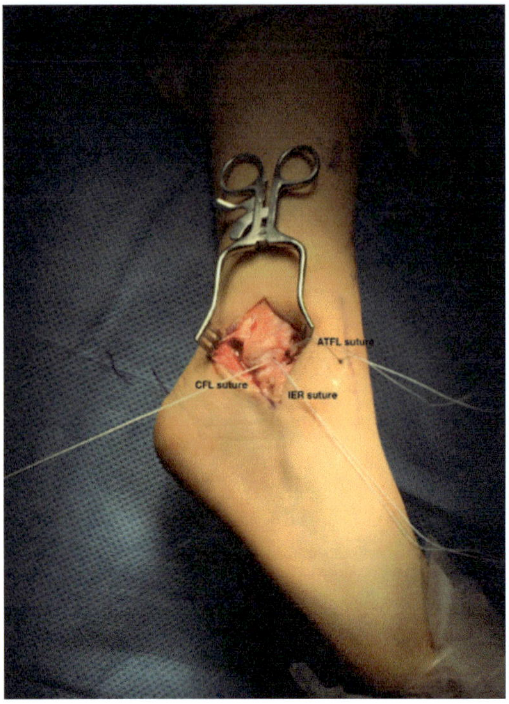

Fig. 12.4 Intraoperative view of the open Broström-Gould anatomic repair in which suture anchors have been placed for repair of the lateral ligaments (ATFL and CFL) and IER

suturing the inferior extensor retinaculum (IER) to the fibula [64–68] (Fig. 12.4). Occasionally, the use of an autograft or allograft is necessary, especially in the setting of revision surgery, long-standing instability, and generalized ligamentous laxity [68, 69]. A comparative study found that patients who received reconstruction with allograft tendons had similar function and activity levels at minimum 2-year follow-up as patients who received standard anatomic repair only [68]. Suture tape and/or suture anchor augmentation has also been found to be biomechanically superior to the traditional Broström repair and is especially useful in cases where the Broström repair may fail [70]. A prospective case series of patients treated with suture tape augmentation had significantly improved Foot and Ankle Outcome Scores and Foot and Ankle Ability Measure Scores from baseline, with only one subject experiencing recurrence of CAI [71]. This suggests that suture tape augmentation is also an effective adjuvant to the Broström repair.

Minimally invasive approaches like arthroscopic surgery have also increased in usage in the past decade due to their potential to decrease patient recovery time and morbidity [72]. Arthroscopic repair also has the advantage of allowing the surgeon to concurrently diagnose and treat intra-articular pathologies [72]. In a randomized control study, there was no difference in clinical or radiologic outcomes at 1 year post-op between the "all-inside" arthroscopic modified Broström and the open technique [73]. In a separate study, there was no observable difference between the arthroscopic and open techniques with respect to pain, American Orthopaedic Foot and Ankle Score (AOFAS), and Karlsson-Peterson scores [74]. In addition, the arthroscopic group had earlier time to ambulation (12 versus 22 days) compared to the open group [74]. Finally, in a case series of patients treated with an "all-inside" arthroscopic knotless suture anchor technique, the patients similarly reported subjective improvement in ankle stability and ability to return to normal activities, with the added benefit of avoiding the suture knot prominence often associated with postoperative neuritis [75]. Arthroscopic techniques, however, are not without their disadvantages, including risk for entrapment of nearby structures such as extensor tendons, superficial peroneal nerve, and peroneus tertius by the suture anchors' knots [72, 76].

Conclusion

CAI results from recurrent lateral ankle sprains. Such recurrent sprains compromise the static stabilizers of the ankle joint: the lateral ligaments. Adverse anatomical and/or neuromuscular changes can occur following a sprain. A comprehensive evaluation is important in order to accurately diagnose and appropriately address any associated pathology such as STJI or OLTs. The preferred initial treatment includes pain control, activity restriction, bracing, and functional rehabilitation. Physical therapy includes proprioceptive training with balance and postural control exercises. When conservative measures fail to improve symptoms of CAI, surgery becomes necessary. The open modified Broström anatomic repair is one of the most commonly performed repair techniques with good results reported in the literature.

References

1. Waterman BROB, Davey S, Zacchilli MA, Belmont PJ. The epidemiology of ankle sprains in the United States. J Joint Bone Surg Am. 2010;92(13):2279–89.
2. Hintermann B. Biomechanics of the unstable ankle joint and clinical implications. Med Sci Sports Exerc. 1999;31(7):459–69.
3. Renstrom PA, Lynch SA. Ankle ligament injuries. Rev Bras Med Esporte. 1998;4(3):71–80.
4. Vuurberg G, Hoorntje A, Wink LM, et al. Diagnosis, treatment and prevention of ankle sprains: update of an evidence-based clinical guideline. Br J Sports Med. 2018;52(15):956. https://doi.org/10.1136/bjsports-2017-098106.
5. Hertel J. Functional instability following lateral ankle sprain. Sports Med. 2000;29(5):361–71.
6. Caputo AM, Lee JY, Spritzer CE, et al. In vivo kinematics of the tibiotalar joint after lateral ankle instability. Am J Sports Med. 2009;37(11):2241–8.
7. Clanton T, Waldrop N, Johnson N, Whitlow S. Ankle and foot injuries and other disorders. Orthopaedic knowledge update: sports medicine, Chapter 22. 5th ed. Rosemont, IL: American Academy of Orthopaedic Surgeons; 2016.
8. Clanton TO, Campbell KJ, Wilson KJ, et al. Qualitative and quantitative anatomic investigation of the lateral ankle ligaments for surgical reconstruction procedures. J Bone Joint Surg Am. 2014;96(12):e98. https://doi.org/10.2106/JBJS.M.00798.
9. Golano P, Vega J, de Leeuw PA, et al. Anatomy of the ankle ligaments: a pictorial essay. Knee Surg Sports Traumatol Arthrosc. 2010;18(5):557–69. https://doi.org/10.1007/s00167-010-1100-x.
10. Hertel J. Functional anatomy, pathomechanics, and pathophysiology of lateral ankle instability. J Athl Train. 2002;37(4):364–75.
11. Polzer H, Kanz KG, Prall WC, et al. Diagnosis and treatment of acute ankle injuries: development of an evidence-based algorithm. Orthop Rev (Pavia). 2012;4(1):e5. https://doi.org/10.4081/or.2012.e5.
12. Hoch MC, McKeon PO. Peroneal reaction time after ankle sprain: a systematic review and meta-analysis. Med Sci Sports Exerc. 2014;46(3):546–56. https://doi.org/10.1249/MSS.0b013e3182a6a93b.
13. de Noronha M, Franca LC, Haupenthal A, Nunes GS. Intrinsic predictive factors for ankle sprain in active university students: a prospective study. Scand J Med Sci Sports. 2013;23(5):541–7. https://doi.org/10.1111/j.1600-0838.2011.01434.x.
14. Beynnon BD, Murphy DF, Alosa DM. Predictive factors for lateral ankle sprains: a literature review. J Athl Train. 2002;37(4):376–80.
15. O'Neill PJ, Parks BG, Walsh R, Simmons LM, Miller SD. Excursion and strain of the superficial peroneal nerve during inversion ankle sprain. J Bone Joint Surg Am. 2007;89(5):979–86. https://doi.org/10.2106/JBJS.F.00440.
16. Trojian TH, McKeag DB. Single leg balance test to identify risk of ankle sprains. Br J Sports Med. 2006;40(7):610–3; discussion 13. https://doi.org/10.1136/bjsm.2005.024356.
17. Krause F, Seidel A. Malalignment and lateral ankle instability: causes of failure from the Varus tibia to the cavovarus foot. Foot Ankle Clin. 2018;23(4):593–603. https://doi.org/10.1016/j.fcl.2018.07.005.
18. Hoffman E, Paller D, Koruprolu S, et al. Accuracy of plain radiographs versus3D analysis of ankle stress test. Foot Ankle Int. 2011;32(10):994–9. https://doi.org/10.3113/FAI.2011.0994.
19. Dowling LB, Giakoumis M, Ryan JD. Narrowing the normal range for lateral ankle ligament stability with stress radiography. J Foot Ankle Surg. 2014;53(3):269–73. https://doi.org/10.1053/j.jfas.2013.12.014.
20. Cao Y, Hong Y, Xu Y, Zhu Y, Xu X. Surgical management of chronic lateral ankle instability: a meta-analysis. J Orthop Surg Res. 2018;13(1):159. https://doi.org/10.1186/s13018-018-0870-6.
21. Valderrabano V, Hintermann B, Horisberger M, Fung TS. Ligamentous posttraumatic ankle osteoarthritis. Am J Sports Med. 2006;34(4):612–20. https://doi.org/10.1177/0363546505281813.
22. de Noronha M, Refshauge KM, Herbert RD, Kilbreath SL, Hertel J. Do voluntary strength, proprioception, range of motion, or postural sway predict occurrence of lateral ankle sprain? Br J Sports Med. 2006;40(10):824–8; discussion 828
23. Collins N, Teys P, Vicenzino B. The initial effects of a Mulligan's mobilization with movement technique on dorsiflexion and pain in subacute ankle sprains. Man Ther. 2004;9(2):77–82.
24. van der Wees PJ, Lenssen AF, Hendriks EJ, Stomp DJ, Dekker J, de Bie RA. Effectiveness of exercise therapy and manual mobilisation in ankle sprain and functional instability: a systematic review. Aust J Physiother. 2006;52(1):27–37.
25. Vicenzino B, Branjerdporn M, Teys P, Jordan K. Initial changes in posterior talar glide and dorsiflexion of the ankle after mobilization with movement in individuals with recurrent ankle sprain. J Orthop Sports Phys Ther. 2006;36(7):464–71.
26. Whitman JM, Cleland JA, Mintken PE, Keirns M, Bieniek ML, Albin SR, Magel J, McPoil TG. Predicting short-term response to thrust and nonthrust manipulation and exercise in patients post inversion ankle sprain. J Orthop Sports Phys Ther. 2009;39(3):188–200.
27. Burton CA, Arthur RJ, Rivera MJ, Powden CJ. The examination of repeated self-mobilizations with movement and joint mobilizations on individuals with chronic ankle instability. J Sport Rehabil. 2020;30(3):458–66.

28. Shi X, Han J, Witchalls J, Waddington G, Adams R. Does treatment duration of manual therapy influence functional outcomes for individuals with chronic ankle instability: a systematic review with meta-analysis? Musculoskelet Sci Pract. 2019;40:87–95.
29. Holland CJ, Hughes JD, De Ste Croix MBA. Acute effects of increased joint mobilization treatment duration on ankle function and dynamic postural control in female athletes with chronic ankle instability. Orthop J Sports Med. 2020;8(6):2325967120927371.
30. McKeon PO, Wikstrom EA. Sensory-targeted ankle rehabilitation strategies for chronic ankle instability. Med Sci Sports Exerc. 2016;48(5):776–84.
31. McGuine TA, Keene JS. The effect of a balance training program on the risk of ankle sprains in high school athletes. Am J Sports Med. 2006;34(7):1103–11.
32. Hoch MC, McKeon PO. Joint mobilization improves spatiotemporal postural control and range of motion in those with chronic ankle instability. J Orthop Res. 2011;29(3):326–32.
33. Cruz-Diaz D, Lomas Vega R, Osuna-Perez MC, Hita-Contreras F, Martinez-Amat A. Effects of joint mobilization on chronic ankle instability: a randomized controlled trial. Disabil Rehabil. 2015;37(7):601–10.
34. McKeon PO, Hertel J. Systematic review of postural control and lateral ankle instability, part II: is balance training clinically effective? J Athl Train. 2008;43(3):305–15.
35. Hall EA, Docherty CL, Simon J, Kingma JJ, Klossner JC. Strength-training protocols to improve deficits in participants with chronic ankle instability: a randomized controlled trial. J Athl Train. 2015;50(1):36–44.
36. Powden CJ, Hoch JM, Hoch MC. Rehabilitation and improvement of health-related quality-of-life detriments in individuals with chronic ankle instability: a meta-analysis. J Athl Train. 2017;52(8):753–65.
37. Webster KA, Gribble PA. Functional rehabilitation interventions for chronic ankle instability: a systematic review. J Sport Rehabil. 2010;19(1):98–114.
38. Rozzi SL, Lephart SM, Sterner R, Kuligowski L. Balance training for persons with functionally unstable ankles. J Orthop Sports Phys Ther. 1999;29(8):478–86.
39. Kidgell DJ, Horvath DM, Jackson BM, Seymour PJ. Effect of six weeks of dura disc and mini-trampoline balance training on postural sway in athletes with functional ankle instability. J Strength Cond Res. 2007;21(2):466–9.
40. Han K, Ricard MD, Fellingham GW. Effects of a 4-week exercise program on balance using elastic tubing as a perturbation force for individuals with a history of ankle sprains. J Orthop Sports Phys Ther. 2009;39(4):246–55.
41. Wright CJ, Arnold BL, Ross SE, Linens SW. Recalibration and validation of the Cumberland ankle instability tool cutoff score for individuals with chronic ankle instability. Arch Phys Med Rehabil. 2014;95(10):1853–9.
42. Wikstrom EA, McKeon PO. Predicting manual therapy treatment success in patients with chronic ankle instability: improving self-reported function. J Athl Train. 2017;52(4):325–31.
43. van Rijn RM, van Os AG, Bernsen RM, Luijsterburg PA, Koes BW, Bierma-Zeinstra SM. What is the clinical course of acute ankle sprains? A systematic literature review. Am J Med. 2008;121(4):324–31. e326
44. Kobayashi T, Takabayashi T, Kudo S, Edama M. The prevalence of chronic ankle instability and its relationship to foot arch characteristics in female collegiate athletes. Phys Ther Sport. 2020;46:162–8.
45. Cordova ML, Sefton JM, Hubbard TJ. Mechanical joint laxity associated with chronic ankle instability: a systematic review. Sports Health. 2010;2(6):452–9.
46. Raymond J, Nicholson LL, Hiller CE, Refshauge KM. The effect of ankle taping or bracing on proprioception in functional ankle instability: a systematic review and meta-analysis. J Sci Med Sport. 2012;15(5):386–92.
47. Hadadi M, Haghighat F, Mohammadpour N, Sobhani S. Effects of kinesiotape vs soft and semirigid ankle orthoses on balance in patients with chronic ankle instability: a randomized controlled trial. Foot Ankle Int. 2020;41(7):793–802.
48. Bicici S, Karatas N, Baltaci G. Effect of athletic taping and kinesiotaping(R) on measurements of functional performance in basketball players with chronic inversion ankle sprains. Int J Sports Phys Ther. 2012;7(2):154–66.
49. Shields CA, Needle AR, Rose WC, Swanik CB, Kaminski TW. Effect of elastic taping on postural control deficits in subjects with healthy ankles, copers, and individuals with functional ankle instability. Foot Ankle Int. 2013;34(10):1427–35.
50. Jackson K, Simon JE, Docherty CL. Extended use of kinesiology tape and balance in participants with chronic ankle instability. J Athl Train. 2016;51(1):16–21.
51. Bellows R, Wong CK. The effect of bracing and balance training on ankle sprain incidence among athletes: a systematic review with meta-analysis. Int J Sports Phys Ther. 2018;13(3):379–88.
52. McGuine TA, Brooks A, Hetzel S. The effect of lace-up ankle braces on injury rates in high school basketball players. Am J Sports Med. 2011;39(9):1840–8.
53. McGuine TA, Hetzel S, Wilson J, Brooks A. The effect of lace-up ankle braces on injury rates in high school football players. Am J Sports Med. 2012;40(1):49–57.
54. Verhagen EA, van Mechelen W, de Vente W. The effect of preventive measures on the incidence of ankle sprains. Clin J Sport Med. 2000;10(4):291–6.
55. Handoll HH, Rowe BH, Quinn KM, de Bie R. Interventions for preventing ankle ligament injuries. Cochrane Database Syst Rev. 2001;(3):CD000018.
56. Kerkhoffs GM, Struijs PA, Marti RK, Assendelft WJ, Blankevoort L, van Dijk CN. Different functional treatment strategies for acute lateral ankle ligament injuries in adults. Cochrane Database Syst Rev. 2002;(3):CD002938.
57. Wilson B, Bialocerkowski A. The effects of kinesiotape applied to the lateral aspect of the ankle: rel-

evance to ankle sprains--a systematic review. PLoS One. 2015;10(6):e0124214.
58. Migel K, Wikstrom E. Gait biomechanics following taping and bracing in patients with chronic ankle instability: a critically appraised topic. J Sport Rehabil. 2019;29(3):373–6.
59. Tassignon B, Verschueren J, Delahunt E, Smith M, Vicenzino B, Verhagen E, Meeusen R. Criteria-based return to sport decision-making following lateral ankle sprain injury: a systematic review and narrative synthesis. Sports Med. 2019;49(4):601–19.
60. Wikstrom EA, Cain MS, Chandran A, Song K, Regan T, Migel K, Kerr ZY. Lateral ankle sprain increases subsequent ankle sprain risk: a systematic review. J Athl Train. 2020.
61. Baumhauer JF, O'Brien T. Surgical considerations in the treatment of ankle instability. J Athl Train. 2002;37(4):458–62.
62. Bahr R, Pena F, Shine J, Lew WD, Tyrdal S, Engebretsen L. Biomechanics of ankle ligament reconstruction. An in vitro comparison of the Brostrom repair, Watson-Jones reconstruction, and a new anatomic reconstruction technique. Am J Sports Med. 1997;25(4):424–32.
63. Bell SJ, Mologne TS, Sitler DF, Cox JS. Twenty-six-year results after Brostrom procedure for chronic lateral ankle instability. Am J Sports Med. 2006;34(6):975–8. https://doi.org/10.1177/0363546505282616.
64. Brostrom L. Sprained ankles. V. Treatment and prognosis in recent ligament ruptures. Acta Chir Scand. 1966;132(5):537–50.
65. Brostrom L. Sprained ankles. VI. Surgical treatment of "chronic" ligament ruptures. Acta Chir Scand. 1966;132(5):551–65.
66. Gould N. Repair of lateral ligament of ankle. Foot Ankle. 1987;8(1):55–8.
67. Gould N, Seligson D, Gassman J. Early and late repair of lateral ligament of the ankle. Foot Ankle. 1980;1(2):84–9. https://doi.org/10.1177/107110078000100206.
68. Matheny LM, Johnson NS, Liechti DJ, Clanton TO. Activity level and function after lateral ankle ligament repair versus reconstruction. Am J Sports Med. 2016;44(5):1301–8. https://doi.org/10.1177/0363546515627817.
69. Coughlin MJ, Schenck RC Jr, Grebing BR, Treme G. Comprehensive reconstruction of the lateral ankle for chronic instability using a free gracilis graft. Foot Ankle Int. 2004;25(4):231–41. https://doi.org/10.1177/107110070402500407.
70. Schuh R, Benca E, Willegger M, et al. Comparison of Brostrom technique, suture anchor repair, and tape augmentation for reconstruction of the anterior talofibular ligament. Knee Surg Sports Traumatol Arthrosc. 2016;24(4):1101–7. https://doi.org/10.1007/s00167-015-3631-7.
71. Cho BK, Park KJ, Park JK, SooHoo NF. Outcomes of the modified Brostrom procedure augmented with suture-tape for ankle instability in patients with generalized ligamentous laxity. Foot Ankle Int. 2017;38(4):405–11. https://doi.org/10.1177/1071100716683348.
72. Drakos MC, Behrens SB, Paller D, Murphy C, DiGiovanni CW. Biomechanical comparison of an open vs arthroscopic approach for lateral ankle instability. Foot Ankle Int. 2014;35(8):809–15. https://doi.org/10.1177/1071100714535765.
73. Yeo ED, Lee KT, Sung IH, Lee SG, Lee YK. Comparison of all-inside arthroscopic and open techniques for the modified Brostrom procedure for ankle instability. Foot Ankle Int. 2016;37(10):1037–45. https://doi.org/10.1177/1071100716666508.
74. Rigby RB, Cottom JM. A comparison of the "all-inside" arthroscopic Brostrom procedure with the traditional open modified Brostrom-Gould technique: a review of 62 patients. Foot Ankle Surg. 2018. https://doi.org/10.1016/j.fas.2017.07.642.
75. Vega J, Golano P, Pellegrino A, Rabat E, Pena F. All-inside arthroscopic lateral collateral ligament repair for ankle instability with a knotless suture anchor technique. Foot Ankle Int. 2013;34(12):1701–9. https://doi.org/10.1177/1071100713502322.
76. Guelfi M, Zamperetti M, Pantalone A, Usuelli FG, Salini V, Oliva XM. Open and arthroscopic lateral ligament repair for treatment of chronic ankle instability: a systematic review. Foot Ankle Surg. 2018;24(1):11–8. https://doi.org/10.1016/j.fas.2016.05.315.

Syndesmosis Injury: Classification, Evaluation, and Prevention

13

Umile Giuseppe Longo, Giovanna Stelitano, Bart Lubberts, Christopher W. Di Giovanni, Niek van Dijk, and Vincenzo Denaro

Introduction

Syndesmosis injuries usually derive from high-energy trauma, especially as consequences of stress during boot-immobilized sport such as skiing and ice hockey [1, 2] or collision sport such as American football, wrestling, and rugby [3]. They can arise as isolated ligamentous damage or be associated with ankle fracture. Both presentations represent a diagnostic and therapeutic challenge for the orthopedic surgeon. Though knowledge about injury mechanism and treatment has significantly increased in recent years, several controversies concerning the diagnosis of joint instability, injury classification, surgical procedures, and postoperative protocols remain. Below is an overview of what is currently known about the joint biomechanics, diagnostic methods, and management [4].

Anatomy

The tibiofibular syndesmosis is a complex joint made of fibrous connective tissue which connects the medial surface of distal fibula to the lateral surface of tibia. The latter is characterized by the presence of the fibular notch, bordered by an anterior tubercle referred to as the "tubercle of Chaput" or "Tillaux-Chaput" and a posterior tubercle, also known as Volkmann's tubercle. These structures, when shallow, increase the risk of recurrent ankle sprain or syndesmosis injury with fracture. At the base of the joint, the tibia and fibula are connected by a small contact region made of hyaline cartilage and thick about 0.5–1 mm [5]. A synovial membrane is almost always present among the two bones. With a width of about 2 mm, this synovial

U. G. Longo (✉) · G. Stelitano · V. Denaro
Research Unit of Orthopaedic and Trauma Surgery, Fondazione Policlinico Universitario Campus Bio-Medico, Roma, Italy

Research Unit of Orthopaedic and Trauma Surgery, Department of Medicine and Surgery, Università Campus Bio-Medico di Roma, Roma, Italy
e-mail: g.longo@policlinicocampus.it; g.stelitano@unicampus.it; denaro@policlinicocampus.it

B. Lubberts
Foot & Ankle Research and Innovation Laboratory, Massachusetts General Hospital/Harvard Medical School, Boston, MA, USA

C. W. Di Giovanni
Massachusetts General Hospital, Harvard Medical School, Boston, MA, USA
e-mail: cwdigiovanni@mgh.harvard.edu

N. van Dijk
Department of Orthopedic Surgery, University of Amsterdam, Amsterdam, The Netherlands

FIFA Medical Centre of Excellence Ripoll-De Prado Sport Clinic, Madrid, Spain

FIFA Medical Centre of Excellence Clínica do Dragão, Porto, Portugal
e-mail: c.niekvandijk@jisakos.com

P. D'Hooghe et al. (eds.), *Ligamentous Injuries of the Foot and Ankle*,
https://doi.org/10.1007/978-3-031-08682-3_13

membrane can be observed during arthroscopy, especially when syndesmosis recess injuries occur [5]. Three ligaments stabilize the ankle syndesmosis: the anterior inferior tibiofibular ligament (AITFL), the posterior inferior tibiofibular ligament (PITFL), and the tibiofibular interosseous ligament (IOL). The AITFL extends from the anterolateral tibial tubercle to the longitudinal tubercle located on the anterior border of the lateral malleolus. It is the most vulnerable structure of the syndesmosis complex and is commonly the first to be injured during external rotation movement through the foot with the ankle in dorsiflexion and the foot pronated—the most common mechanism of syndesmosis injury. The PITFL consists of both a superficial and deep component. The superficial portion extends obliquely from the lateral malleolus to the posterolateral tibial tubercle. The deep structure, referred to as the inferior transverse tibiofibular ligament (TTFL), extends transversely across the back of the ankle joint, from the lateral malleolus to the posterior border of the tibial articular surface. The IOL originates from the distal expansion of the tibiofibular interosseous membrane and terminates superior to the AITFL and PITFL. It is made of small fibers which connect the tibia and fibula at the level of the fibular notch. On the medial side of the ankle, the deltoid ligaments (DL) also contribute to the ankle mortise stability by holding the talus medially and preventing lateral translation of the talus.

Biomechanics

Although the syndesmosis ligaments provide stabilization to the ankle joint during physical load, they also allow for slight multiplanar fibular motion [6]. Physiologically, the fibula rotates about 2° with respect to the tibia and translates approximately 1–3 mm posteriorly in the axial plane [7, 8]. In healthy ankles, translation of the distal tibiofibular joint does not exceed beyond 1 mm in the coronal plane during plantar and dorsal flexion of the foot. Ligament contribution to joint stability seems to be partitioned as follows:

- AITFL is responsible for 35% of stability.
- TTFL for 33%.
- IOL for 22%.
- PITFL only for 9% [9].

These biomechanical considerations suggest that isolated injury to the PITFL, which is the most robust syndesmosis ligament, should not be expected to significantly compromise joint stability [10].

Due to its resistant structure, the syndesmosis can contemporaneously sustain the strengths generated during weight-bearing and unload the tibial plafond articular surface. These forces are distributed partially to the IOL and the fibula, although the latter lacks direct contact with the weight-bearing surface of the trochlea of the talus. When syndesmosis injuries occur, the talar trochlea usually moves laterally, causing a reduction of the contact zone among the articular surface of the talus and tibia. In cases of syndesmosis instability, reduction of the contact area may reach up to 40%, inducing a redistribution of the force on the remaining articular surface.

Espinosa et al. found that the AITFL primarily limits internal rotation of ankle mortise, the PITFL generally blocks posterior dislocation and translation, and the IOL helps prevent lateral fibular translation. These findings can be explained by the anatomic position of each ligament relative to the anatomic planes. Finally, it is important to consider the role of the superficial and deep deltoid ligaments, which are essential in the stabilization of the syndesmosis joint through the limitation of the external rotation and lateral translation of the talus [11].

Mechanism of Injury

Syndesmosis injuries of the ankle are present in approximately 18% of all ankle sprains and up to 23% of all ankle fractures, although it is important to differentiate that this represents a continuum of injury severity because injury does not always predicate instability. Syndesmosis trauma may cause tears or ruptures to one or more of the syndesmosis ligaments, which in turn may result in syndesmosis instability. In more severe cases, injury to the medial deltoid ligaments is not unusual. In the majority of patients, the mechanism of injury is characterized by an exceeding external rotation of the foot with the ankle in dorsiflexion and the foot pronated, causing the distal fibula to move away from the tibia [5, 12]. This condition is supported by the talar trochlea posterior dislocation and its external rotation. Other mechanisms of injury have been described, including excessive dorsiflexion, internal rotation (or inversion), and plantar flexion of the foot. Moreover, syndesmosis injuries can occur as the result of a more complex pattern of high fibular fracture known as a Maisonneuve fracture, secondary to external rotation of the foot and ankle. The radiographic identification of these fractures should be led to the exclusion of concomitant syndesmosis ligament injuries. Syndesmosis ligamentous tears are involved in about 50% of Weber B fractures and in the majority of Weber C fractures [13]. It remains incompletely clear, however, how often the deep and superficial deltoid components are involved with this injury constellation nor how much they independently contribute to it – beyond the fact that it has become clear in recent years that the deltoid complex plays an important role in ankle instability and requires further study.

Stable Versus Unstable Syndesmosis Injuries

Studies highlight the clinical significance of high ankle sprains [14] with a longer recovery and higher predisposition to residual symptoms than isolated lateral ankle sprains. Critical to the successful treatment of syndesmosis injuries lies the ability to separate stable from unstable injuries. Not all ligamentous syndesmosis injuries destabilize the distal tibiofibular articulation. Syndesmosis instability is a condition of abnormal, multiplanar distal fibular motion relative to the incisura that [15], if inappropriately managed, not only delays a return to athletic play but, critically, can lead to degenerative changes of the ankle joint. Grading systems such as the West Point Ankle Grading System [16] underscore that a spectrum of injuries exist (Grades I, II, and III) and provide some clinical and imaging guidelines to differentiate stable from unstable. These include the proximity of syndesmosis tenderness (0, $\leq$4, and $\geq$ 4 cm relative to the ankle joint line) and the presence of radiographic mortise widening (Grade III) but have not been validated and are generally more useful at the extremes of stability vs. instability [2].

The Deltoid Ligament Dilemma

The deltoid ligament represents a separate anatomic entity from the syndesmosis, but it plays a crucial role in maintaining ankle mortise stability. Its mechanism of injury appears interestingly overlapping with that of the syndesmosis, characterized by an excessive external rotation and hyperdorsiflexion of the ankle. At the same time, the majority of the isolated injuries of the syndesmosis have shown the involvement of the deltoid ligament. Therefore, the assessment of its integrity is essential to accurately evaluate and define stable and unstable injuries and to choose their optimal management. The medial ligament of the ankle is made of two distinct structures (the superficial layer and the deep layer) which differentially provide deltoid ligament biomechanical function. The deltoid complex mainly contributes to the limitation of talar abduction, pronation, and external rotation, even if foot inversion-eversion and the physiologic gait pattern would be impaired after the isolated rupture of the medial ligament. The evidence of the deltoid ligament impairment in the unstable lesions of the syndesmosis derives from different studies that have investigated the specific contribution of ankle ligaments on its joint stability.

In the current literature, the role of the deltoid ligament has been widely confirmed [17]. Hunt et al. have defined, through a cadaveric model, three different types of syndesmosis injuries: mild lesion (involving the AITFL and superficial layer deltoid disruption), moderate lesion (including AITFL, IOL, PITFL, and the superficial deltoid disruption), and severe lesion (characterized by both complete syndesmosis disruption and disruption of both superficial and deep layers of the deltoid ligament). Moreover, they have described a significant increase in average contact pressure, a concomitant decrease in the average contact area, and a shift in the location of the center of pressure from mild to moderate and severe injuries, employing axial load with external rotation forces rather of axial load alone. In agreement, a cadaveric study, performed on 20 fresh-frozen leg specimens, subjected to different simulated syndesmosis ligament lesions, has shown that lesions of the deep deltoid ligament considerably impair the stability of the ankle in both the sagittal and coronal planes as well as in external rotation, while the singular involvement of the superficial deltoid ligament, AITFL, PITFL, and distal IOL up to 5 cm does not alter the stability of the ankle joint. A separate consideration must be made concerning lesions >5 cm which, in each case, determine joint instability. The study above has defined the articular instability with a tibiofibular diastasis greater than 4 mm in the coronal or sagittal plane and an ankle external rotation greater than 20°. In support of these considerations, the action of the deltoid ligament as the primary restraint to external rotation in both the neutral and dorsiflexed positions has been proved by another biomechanical research, through the evaluation of the effects of serial ankle ligament sectioning.

Clinical Evaluation

Patients affected by syndesmosis ligamentous injuries normally report a previous history of ankle injury, as described above. Clinicians must maintain a high index of suspicion, as clinical presentation may vary widely. Often patients complain about pain in the involved ankle region during weight-bearing, located in the anterior part proximal to the ankle joint. Pain typically surges during external rotation and dorsiflexion of the foot [18]. Other clinical symptoms include the feeling of the ankle giving away, tenderness, swelling, difficulty in dorsiflexion of the foot, and repeated effusions within the ankle joint. Chronic injuries are characterized by a specific clinical triad, including pain in the anterolateral region of the ankle, repeated effusions, and sensation of instability. Sometimes, ankle stiffness is present [19].

During physical examination of the injured side, comparison to the contralateral side as an internal control is essential. Several clinical tests have been described to assess syndesmosis injuries, although still today a singular test with equally high specificity and sensitivity eludes us.

The external rotation test is one of the most commonly used tests. It is performed with the patient in a sitting position, with the limb flexed at 90°, free over the ground. The examinator stabilizes the shin with one hand, forcing foot external rotation and concomitant dorsiflexion with the other. The test is considered positive if the patient complains of pain in the syndesmosis region. When a painful sensation occurs around the medial malleolus, the test suggests injury to one or more of the deltoid medial ankle ligaments.

- *The squeeze test* consists in exercising a strong medial to lateral compression in the middle of the shin, and it is positive if the action produces pain around the AITFL zone.
- *The Cotton test* is executed with the patient in a sitting position. The examinator stabilizes with one hand the distal tibiofibular joint while applying a lateral translation to the foot with the other. Lateral ankle translation greater than 3–5 mm, or wider than the healthy side, and the occurrence of pain over the syndesmosis are indicative for syndesmosis or deltoid ligament injuries.
- The *fibular translation test* is less frequently used because it can cause severe pain in the involved ankle. The patient is placed in

sideline position. The examiner blocks the syndesmosis with one hand while moving lateral malleolus anteriorly and posteriorly with the other. The test is positive if the patient complains about pain in the lateral malleolus region or if the fibular translation is greater than the contralateral one.

The efforts to identify the best method for the evaluation of syndesmosis injury and instability have not yet led to definitive results. For this reason, an accurate ankle and syndesmosis examination should be not based on the execution of a single test.

Imaging

Assessment of syndesmosis injuries can be challenging, especially in cases of subtle instability. Misdiagnosing unstable injuries can lead to inadequate conservative treatment, causing prolonged time to return to play and degenerative changes of the ankle joint over time. Therefore, distinguishing between stable and unstable syndesmosis injuries is crucial.

X-Rays

When the patient is able to do so, bilateral weight-bearing radiographs of the ankle should be taken in order to compare the injured to the uninjured side. The radiological evaluation should include at least three images in standard projections: AP, lateral, and ankle mortise views (10–20° of foot internal rotation). AP and lateral x-ray of the entire leg should be required if Maisonneuve fracture is suspected. X-ray parameters to evaluate are:

- The distal tibiofibular clear space measured 1 cm above the ankle joint line; normal values are less than 6 mm on both AP and mortise views.
- The tibiofibular overlap measured 1 cm above the ankle joint line; normal values are less than 6 mm on AP view and more than 1 mm on mortise view.
- The medial clear space measured as the distance between the medial border of the talus and the lateral border of the medial malleolus on a line parallel to and 5 mm below the talar dome. A gap of less than or equal to 4 mm on mortise view is considered normal [20].

Several indirect radiological findings are indicative of syndesmosis damages [20, 21]. Among these, the avulsion fractures and heterotopic calcifications around the tibiofibular joint have to be included. Avulsion fractures usually are secondary to AITFL or PITFL rupture. The first case can present as the Chaput-Tillaux fracture, fibular fragment fracture, or, infrequently, both. When the PITFL is the ligament involved, the avulsion affects almost exclusively the posterior tibial tubercle. Thanks to its anatomical reposition, this kind of injury rarely requires the introduction of a syndesmosis screw, unless concomitant ligament injuries occur. Radiological findings are marked by low accuracy of detecting syndesmosis instability, caused by imperfect execution of AP and mortise views or the presence of anatomical tibiofibular variations [20, 22, 23]. For this reason, additional diagnostic modalities should be considered.

Ultrasound

Ultrasound affords an exciting new means of evaluating subtle syndesmosis instability by virtue of being a dynamic test available at the point of clinical care with the ability to readily compare to the contralateral side as an internal control. Recent research by Hagemeijer et al. has highlighted its utility in assessing sagittal translation of the distal fibula [24]. The average anterior to posterior fibular sagittal translation was 0.89 ± 0.6 mm, and posterior to anterior fibular sagittal translation was 0.49 ± 1.1 mm in healthy individuals. Future cadaveric or in vivo research is needed to evaluate the use of ultrasound for distinguishing stable and unstable injuries.

Weight-Bearing Computed Tomography

Weight-bearing computed tomography (WBCT) scans may play a role in diagnosing more subtle cases of syndesmosis instability. WBCT allows cross-sectional visualization of the ankle while under physiologic load [25–31]. Furthermore, its ability to evaluate both the injured and uninjured sides is critical given the variable anatomy of the incisura across individuals [26–28]. Syndesmosis instability is a three-dimensional problem, with destabilization of the distal tibiofibular articulation expressing itself to individualized degrees and in varying combinations of the coronal, sagittal, and/or rotational planes; for adequate diagnosis, therefore, it should also be evaluated as such. Correspondingly, a recent study found that volumetric measurement of the syndesmosis on bilateral ankle WBCT scan effectively diagnoses syndesmosis instability among patients with arthroscopically confirmed instability [32]. Given currently available data, the volumetric boundaries of this measurement should ideally extend from the tibial plafond to a height 5 cm proximal to the joint line. Widespread adoption of WBCT to evaluate syndesmosis instability depends on the incorporation of artificial intelligence algorithms that allow volume measurement into the viewing programs currently employed in clinical practice. Despite the considerations above, the use of bilateral CT still requires further investigations and insights for the choice of radiological parameters to be used in the identification of malreduction and/or instability of the syndesmosis. The most recent study published in 2021 shows that a specific radiological distinction between mild inherent anatomical asymmetry and malreduction of the syndesmosis does not still establish and that current radiological parameters are inadequate to define it. In the cited study, 213 bilateral lower limb CT scans of uninjured ankles have been analyzed through multiple measurements recorded on the axial CT 1 cm above the plafond. The parameters employed have been anterior, posterior, and central syndesmosis distance, fibular rotation, and sagittal fibular translation. Previously studied malreduction criteria were assessed on bilateral CT, including differences in anterior, central, and posterior syndesmosis distance; mean syndesmosis distance; fibular rotation; sagittal translational distance; and syndesmosis area. Unilateral CT was used to compare the anterior to posterior syndesmosis distances. The results have shown that 35% of native, uninjured syndesmoses would be classified as malreduced by current diagnostic standards on bilateral CT and that 89% of the ankles had an asymmetric incisura on unilateral CT [33].

Magnetic Resonance Imaging

Magnetic resonance imaging (MRI) is a crucial radiological tool for the assessment of specific ligament injuries in both acute and chronic cases. It is characterized by high sensitivity and specificity and is able to show injuries localized inside the ankle joint, such as bone marrow edema of the calcaneal trochlea, cartilaginous defects, bony injuries, tibiofibular incongruence, or degenerative variations in chronic damages. However, as well as the investigations above described, it remains a static exam, which does not provide clear identification of syndesmosis instability. To overcome this problem, orthopedic surgeons need to appeal to functional tests, usually practiced under anesthesia to control the painful feeling around the ankle involved. Among these, the gravitation test is one of the most performed. It consists of the execution of x-ray projections with a horizontal beam of the ankle joint which protrudes outside the board, moving freely with the leg at 90° of external rotation. Subsequently, the obtained image of the injured side should be compared to the contralateral uninjured side [22].

Functional Intraoperative Tests

If instability is suspected but imaging is inconclusive, several intraoperative procedures for evaluating syndesmosis injuries can be performed. Among these, the modified Cotton test and external rotational stress test are the main intraoperative fluoroscopic tests described. The modified Cotton test, also known as the bone hook stress test, is performed by making a 5 mm small incision laterally 5 cm proximal to ankle joint. It consists of the intraoperative lateral abduction of the lateral malleolus, performed with a bone hook, to stretch the tibiofibular joint, while intraoperative fluoroscopic mortise view of the ankle is obtained. A width greater than 3 mm of the tibiofibular space in the coronal plane, or more than 2 mm translation in the sagittal plane [34], suggests unstable syndesmosis damages. The external rotational stress test is particularly necessary for assessment of deltoid ligament damage. It is executed intraoperatively, as above explained, after lateral fibular fixation. The test is considered positive in case of a medial clear space greater than or equal to 5 mm. Both of these intraoperative tests are characterized by high intra-observer security but low sensitivity.

Arthroscopy

In the setting of subtle or chronic syndesmosis instability, ankle arthroscopy has been proposed as an invasive diagnostic tool that currently represents the gold standard for diagnosis of subtle instability given the ability to directly visualize the distal tibiofibular articulation [35]. The direct intra-articular investigation allows evaluation of syndesmosis ligamentous injury, as well as related syndesmosis instability. It is relevant to remember that the anteromedial and anterolateral port are used for the visualization of the AITFL and PITFL and that tibiofibular translation of more than 2 mm is suggestive of instability. Stoffel et al. suggested that the modified Cotton test should be performed with a 100 N of force applied 5 cm above the ankle joint [36]. In addition, for optimal assessment of joint instability, arthroscopy should be performed without ankle distraction [37].

Classification Systems

Still today a worldwide shared classification system of syndesmosis injuries does not exist. Current models employ several different parameters to subdivide the injury. Below, we describe the most relevant classification systems.

First of all, a temporal classification distinguishes tibiofibular injuries into three categories considering the time between trauma and the presentation or definitive diagnosis: acute injuries, up to 3 weeks; subacute, from 3 weeks to 3 months; and chronic, over 3 months.

On the basis of the ligaments affected, three grades of severity are identified. Grade I includes stable syndesmosis injury with no diastasis. Grade II is characterized by occult instability with the ankle regularly aligned on standard plain x-rays. Grade III includes ligamentous injuries associated with fractures of the proximal fibula, marked by frank instability on clinical examination and a tibiofibular diastasis on standard radiographs.

The West Point Ankle Grading System [16] is one of the most commonly used classification systems. It subdivides syndesmosis lesions into three grades of severity in relation to clinical findings. Grade I holds damages that do not produce ankle instability. Grade II includes injuries with a slight instability elicited in external rotation and characterized by a squeeze test positive and negative x-rays. Grade III comprises damages with frank instability of the ankle.

Various other systems have been developed according to radiological signs. The most common of these divides syndesmosis injuries into three grades based on plain x-rays which include stable ankle sprain, latent diastasis, and frank diastasis [38]. In latent diastasis, the instability is observable only through stress radiographs; in the frank diastasis, instability signs are directly evident on standard plain radiographs. The frank diastasis is moreover classified into four categories: type I, marked by lateral subluxation of the fibula without plastic deformation, type II in which plastic deformation occurs, type III characterized by posterior subluxation of the fibula, and type IV defined by talar wedging in absence of fractures. Finally, MRI-based classification systems have been proposed but their use remains limited.

Treatment

Conservative Treatment

Treatment choice for syndesmosis injury depends on the degree of stability that remains. Stable injuries should be managed with conservative treatment, which includes PRICEM protocol (protection, rest, ice, compression, evaluation, and medications), ankle in unloading, severe restriction of physical activity (for about 6 weeks), limb elevation, immobilization (employing orthosis which limits external foot rotation), and early rehabilitation [39]. During rehabilitation, the patient is allowed to bear weight as tolerated in a boot while allowing ankle range of motion to minimize long-term stiffness. This is followed by resistance and proprioception exercises. If adequately diagnosed, clinical outcomes for stable injuries following conservative management have shown to be satisfying. Calder et al. found that the mean time to return to sports after conservative treatment was 45 days [40].

Surgical Treatment

Unstable injuries require surgical management to avoid long-term morbidity and degenerative changes of the ankle joint [17]. The aims of surgical fixation include (1) reduction of the distal fibula into the tibiofibular incisura and (2) stabilization of syndesmosis in order to allow the ligaments to heal and restore their function and strength. Surgical treatment is indicated for both acute and chronic syndesmosis instabilities [41]. Discussion regarding specific surgical techniques and fixation options are beyond the scope of this chapter.

Conclusion

With any history of ankle trauma, awareness for potential occult or overt syndesmosis injury is critical. Syndesmosis ankle injuries require accurate clinical and radiological evaluation as well as specific management associated with the injury being stable or unstable. The main element in achieving excellent clinical outcomes is maintaining the anatomic reduction of the syndesmosis, anatomic reestablishment of normal syndesmosis ligament anatomy, and anatomic fixation of ankle fractures when they exist. In the unstable syndesmosis, surgical intervention will be required. The specifics on surgical intervention for syndesmosis stabilization will be covered in subsequent chapters.

References

1. Fritschy D. An unusual ankle injury in top skiers. Am J Sports Med. 1989;17(2):282–5; discussion 285-6
2. Wright RW, et al. Ankle syndesmosis sprains in national hockey league players. Am J Sports Med. 2004;32(8):1941–5.
3. Kaplan LD, et al. Incidence and variance of foot and ankle injuries in elite college football players. Am J Orthop (Belle Mead NJ). 2011;40(1):40–4.
4. Błasiak A, Sadlik B, Brzóska R. Injuries of the distal tibio-fibular syndesmosis. Pol Orthop Traumatol. 2013;78:139–50.
5. Lin CF, Gross ML, Weinhold P. Ankle syndesmosis injuries: anatomy, biomechanics, mechanism of injury, and clinical guidelines for diagnosis and intervention. J Orthop Sports Phys Ther. 2006;36(6):372–84.
6. Ogilvie-Harris DJ, Reed SC, Hedman TP. Disruption of the ankle syndesmosis: biomechanical study of the ligamentous restraints. Arthroscopy. 1994;10(5):558–60.
7. Clanton TO, et al. Biomechanical analysis of the individual ligament contributions to syndesmotic stability. Foot Ankle Int. 2017;38(1):66–75.
8. Massri-Pugin J, et al. Role of the deltoid ligament in syndesmotic instability. Foot Ankle Int. 2018;39(5):598–603.
9. Fort NM, et al. Management of acute injuries of the tibiofibular syndesmosis. Eur J Orthop Surg Traumatol. 2017;27(4):449–59.
10. van Dijk CN, et al. Conservative and surgical management of acute isolated syndesmotic injuries: ESSKA-AFAS consensus and guidelines. Knee Surg Sports Traumatol Arthrosc. 2016;24(4):1217–27.

11. Espinosa N, Smerek JP, Myerson MS. Acute and chronic syndesmosis injuries: pathomechanisms, diagnosis and management. Foot Ankle Clin. 2006;11(3):639–57.
12. Jones MH, Amendola A. Syndesmosis sprains of the ankle: a systematic review. Clin Orthop Relat Res. 2007;455:173–5.
13. Merrill KD. The Maisonneuve fracture of the fibula. Clin Orthop Relat Res. 1993;287:218–23.
14. Gerber JP, et al. Persistent disability associated with ankle sprains: a prospective examination of an athletic population. Foot Ankle Int. 1998;19(10):653–60.
15. Lubberts B, et al. The arthroscopic syndesmotic assessment tool can differentiate between stable and unstable ankle syndesmoses. Knee Surg Sports Traumatol Arthrosc. 2018;28(1):193–201.
16. Del Buono A, et al. Syndesmosis injuries of the ankle. Curr Rev Musculoskelet Med. 2013;6(4):313–9.
17. Longo UG, et al. Deep deltoid ligament injury is related to rotational instability of the ankle joint: a biomechanical study. Knee Surg Sports Traumatol Arthrosc. 2021;29(5):1577–83.
18. Beumer A, Swierstra BA, Mulder PG. Clinical diagnosis of syndesmotic ankle instability: evaluation of stress tests behind the curtains. Acta Orthop Scand. 2002;73(6):667–9.
19. Alonso A, Khoury L, Adams R. Clinical tests for ankle syndesmosis injury: reliability and prediction of return to function. J Orthop Sports Phys Ther. 1998;27(4):276–84.
20. Beumer A, et al. Radiographic measurement of the distal tibiofibular syndesmosis has limited use. Clin Orthop Relat Res. 2004;423:227–34.
21. Jiang KN, et al. Comparison of radiographic stress tests for syndesmotic instability of supination-external rotation ankle fractures: a cadaveric study. J Orthop Trauma. 2014;28(6):e123–7.
22. Pneumaticos SG, et al. The effects of rotation on radiographic evaluation of the tibiofibular syndesmosis. Foot Ankle Int. 2002;23(2):107–11.
23. Shah AS, et al. Radiographic evaluation of the normal distal tibiofibular syndesmosis. Foot Ankle Int. 2012;33(10):870–6.
24. Hagemeijer NC, et al. Diagnosing syndesmotic instability with dynamic ultrasound - establishing the natural variations in normal motion. Injury. 2020;51(11):2703–9.
25. Burssens A, et al. Templating of syndesmotic ankle lesions by use of 3D analysis in Weightbearing and classical CT. Foot Ankle Orthop. 2018;3(3):2473011418S00173.
26. Dikos GD, et al. Normal tibiofibular relationships at the syndesmosis on axial CT imaging. J Orthop Trauma. 2012;26(7):433–8.
27. Hagemeijer NC, et al. Range of Normal and abnormal syndesmotic measurements using Weightbearing CT. Foot Ankle Int. 2019;40(12):1430–7.
28. Lepojärvi S, et al. Rotational dynamics of the normal distal tibiofibular joint with weight-bearing computed tomography. Foot Ankle Int. 2016;37(6):627–35.
29. Malhotra G, Cameron J, Toolan BC. Diagnosing chronic diastasis of the syndesmosis: a novel measurement using computed tomography. Foot Ankle Int. 2014;35(5):483–8.
30. Warner SJ, et al. The measurement and clinical importance of syndesmotic reduction after operative fixation of rotational ankle fractures. JBJS. 2015;97(23):1935–44.
31. Abdelaziz ME, et al. Evaluation of syndesmosis reduction on CT scan. Foot Ankle Int. 2019;40(9):1087–93. https://doi.org/10.1177/1071100719849850.
32. Bhimani R, et al. Utility of volumetric measurement via weight-bearing computed tomography scan to diagnose syndesmotic instability. Foot Ankle Int. 2020;41(7):859–65.
33. Kubik JF, et al. Assessment of malreduction standards for the syndesmosis in bilateral CT scans of uninjured ankles. Bone Joint J. 2021;103-B(1):178–83.
34. Lubberts B, et al. The arthroscopic syndesmotic assessment tool can differentiate between stable and unstable ankle syndesmoses. Knee Surg Sports Traumatol Arthrosc. 2020;28(1):193–201.
35. Mei-Dan O, et al. A dynamic ultrasound examination for the diagnosis of ankle syndesmotic injury in professional athletes: a preliminary study. Am J Sports Med. 2009;37(5):1009–16.
36. Stoffel K, et al. Comparison of two intraoperative assessment methods for injuries to the ankle syndesmosis. A cadaveric study. J Bone Joint Surg Am. 2009;91(11):2646–52.
37. Lubberts B, et al. The effect of ankle distraction on arthroscopic evaluation of syndesmotic instability: a cadaveric study. Clin Biomech (Bristol, Avon). 2017;50:16–20.
38. van Dijk CN, et al. Classification and diagnosis of acute isolated syndesmotic injuries: ESSKA-AFAS consensus and guidelines. Knee Surg Sports Traumatol Arthrosc. 2016;24(4):1200–16.
39. Hunt KJ. Syndesmosis injuries. Curr Rev Musculoskelet Med. 2013;6(4):304–12.
40. Calder JD, et al. Stable versus unstable grade II high ankle sprains: a prospective study predicting the need for surgical stabilization and time to return to sports. Arthroscopy. 2016;32(4):634–42.
41. Lemmers DHL, et al. Factors associated with adverse events after distal tibiofibular syndesmosis fixation. Injury. 2020;51(2):542–7.

14 Syndesmosis Injuries: Surgical Indications, Techniques, and Outcomes

Kenneth J. Hunt and Stephen Blake Wallace

Introduction

Over the past two decades, injuries to the ankle syndesmosis have demonstrated increased prevalence among athletes of all levels. Impact and collision sports such as soccer, skiing, football, ice hockey, wrestling, and rugby exhibit the highest prevalence of injury [1]. It is also widely recognized that ligamentous syndesmosis injuries result in substantially longer times missed from sport compared to other ankle ligament injuries, are much more likely to require surgical stabilization, and are associated with more long-term functional sequelae. Increased recognition and higher prevalence of these injuries have intensified the focus in recent years on diagnosis, surgical constructs, and postoperative management of syndesmosis injuries in the orthopedics and sports medicine communities.

Most athletes who suffer complete disruptions of the ankle syndesmosis also have fractures of the fibula and/or medial malleolus. Thus, most of the surgical outcome data available are related to fractures with associated syndesmosis injuries. Since this text places focus on ligamentous injuries, we will focus on the surgical indications and management of purely ligamentous injury to the syndesmosis. Meanwhile, most of the principles discussed herein are also applicable to syndesmosis fixation during fracture repair.

Indications for Surgical Treatment

Ligamentous injuries to the ankle syndesmosis are commonly referred to as "high ankle sprains" because they occur to the ligaments (e.g., AITFL, PITFL, IOL) proximal to those that are more commonly injured during lateral inversion sprains (e.g., ATFL, CFL). More severe (i.e., complete) ligamentous injuries can occur and typically require surgical stabilization [2], but these are uncommon without an associated fracture. High ankle sprains, which are less common than inversion ankle sprains, comprise up to 12% of all ankle sprains [3] but represent up to 25% of ankle sprains in collision sports such as American football [2, 3]. Due to the potential long-term consequences of these injuries, careful diagnosis and treatment decision-making are warranted.

Chapter 13 summarizes the available classification systems that have been created to help guide treatment and outcomes. Briefly, surgical stabilization of the syndesmosis should be considered in the presence of an athlete with an unstable ligamentous injury. Grade III injuries are generally easy to identify as unstable, and grade I injuries are easy to identify as stable. The former should be indicated for surgery, and the latter should not. The challenge, and therefore

K. J. Hunt (✉) · S. B. Wallace
Department of Orthopaedic Surgery, University of Colorado School of Medicine, Aurora, CO, USA
e-mail: Kenneth.j.hunt@cuanschutz.edu

P. D'Hooghe et al. (eds.), *Ligamentous Injuries of the Foot and Ankle*,
https://doi.org/10.1007/978-3-031-08682-3_14

recent attention in the literature, is to differentiate grade IIa (stable) from grade IIb (unstable) injuries. In these cases, instability can be very difficult to detect with plain radiography. Stress radiography, MRI, weight-bearing CT, and arthroscopy can be used to help confirm the injury pattern and the presence of instability, but these findings are not included in all current classification schemes. The functional kinematics of the syndesmosis in athletes consist of considerable rotation of the fibula and talus and posterior translation of the fibula, which are difficult to assess even with stress radiography [4]. When routine and stress radiographs are normal in patients with grade II injuries, serial physical examination, advanced imaging, and possibly arthroscopic evaluation need to be considered to determine whether there is instability.

In the authors' practice, unstable ligamentous syndesmosis injuries in athletes meet indication requirements for surgery. This includes all grade III injuries, grade II injuries with widening of the syndesmosis or medial clear space on stress radiography, or disruption of the PITFL, deltoid, and interosseous ligaments on MRI (Fig. 14.1 MRI). A new classification recently described by van Dijk et al. [5] highlights the diagnostic advantage of the magnetic resonance imaging (MRI) scan over two-dimensional radiography. This classification scheme separates ligament involvement into four different groups instead of three based on MRI findings. Grade I injuries involve an isolated injury to the AITFL, with grade II including further involvement of the IOL/IOM. Grade III syndesmosis injury adds injury to the PITFL, and grade IV encompasses injury to all ligaments and rupture of the deltoid ligament [5]. While not a perfect tool, we consider MRI an essential aid in the diagnosis of moderately unstable syndesmosis injuries because it can identify the extent of injury to specific ligamentous structures, has excellent interobserver agreement, and can identify important secondary MRI findings such as bone bruises, osteochondral lesions, and joint incongruity (Fig. 14.1) [5]. In addition, arthroscopy is incorporated in all syndesmosis repair

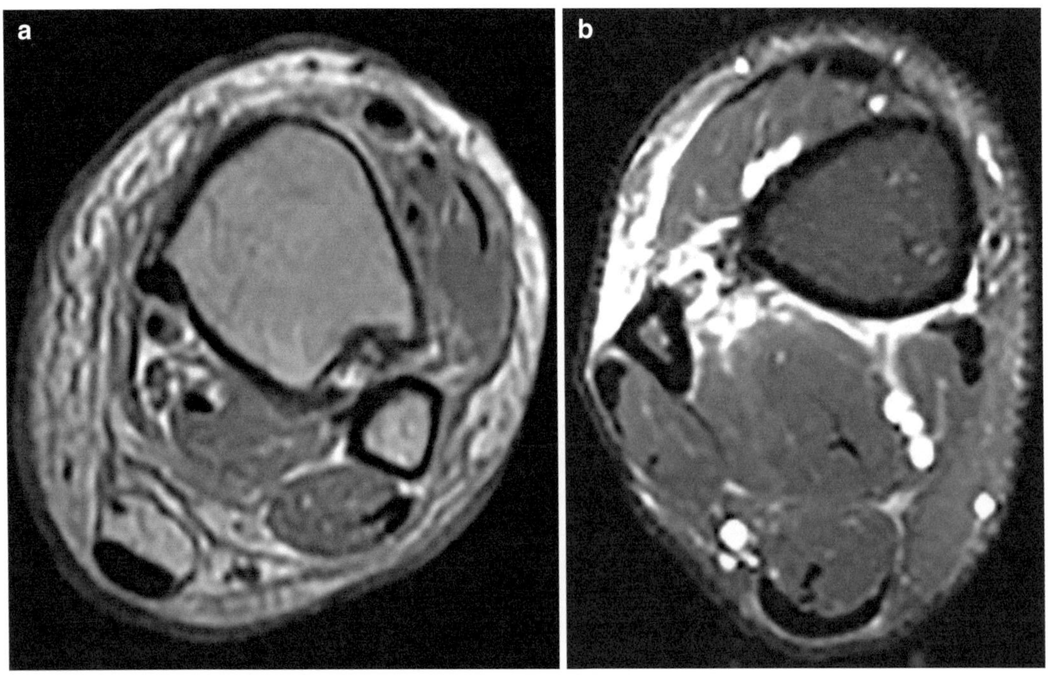

Fig. 14.1 MRI findings. (**a**) T1-weighted axial MRI at the level of the tibiofibular syndesmosis demonstrating discontinuity of the AITFL (red arrow) and PITFL (blue arrow) fibers. (**b**) T2-weighted axial MRI proximal to the syndesmosis demonstrating discontinuity of the IOM (red arrow) and surrounding edema

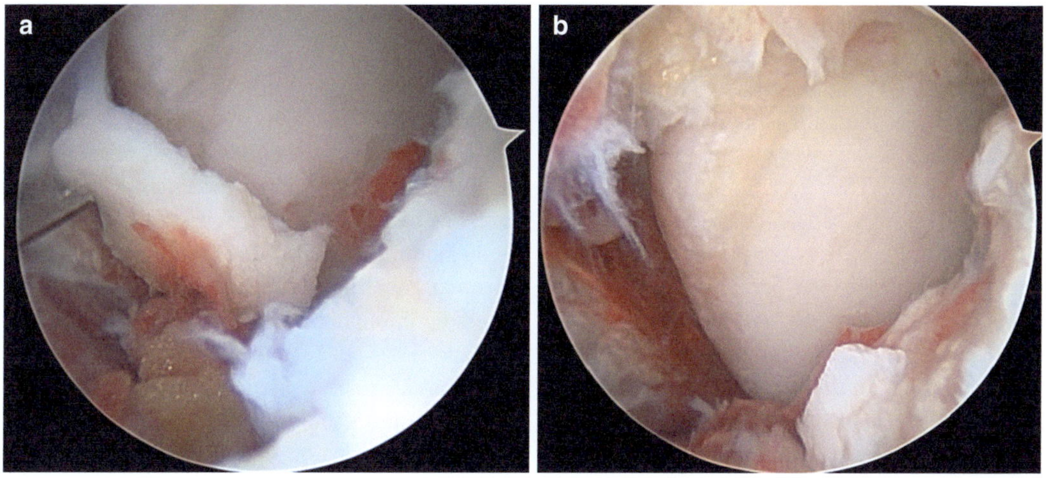

Fig. 14.2 Intraoperative arthroscopic images during fixation of syndesmosis injury. (**a**) View of the medial gutter of a left ankle from the anterolateral portal demonstrating loose osteochondral defect fragments (*) and (**b**) showing defect (*) after removal of loose fragment

cases to confirm anatomic reduction and identify actionable intraoperative findings such as loose bodies or osteochondral injuries which are often not seen on MRI scan (Fig. 14.2). Ankle fractures with syndesmosis disruption should undergo careful evaluation of syndesmosis instability (we use arthroscopy to confirm) following fracture fixation and syndesmosis stabilization as outlined in the next section.

Surgical Techniques

The goals of surgical treatment are (1) anatomic reduction of the syndesmosis and (2) stable fixation restoring kinematics. A variety of techniques exist to accomplish both goals, which are discussed separately. The authors' preferred methods will be detailed, and outcome studies for the various alternative techniques will be discussed in the following section.

Reduction Techniques

Reduction of the fibula in the incisura is paramount to ensure optimal function of the ankle after surgery. The authors' preferred method is to

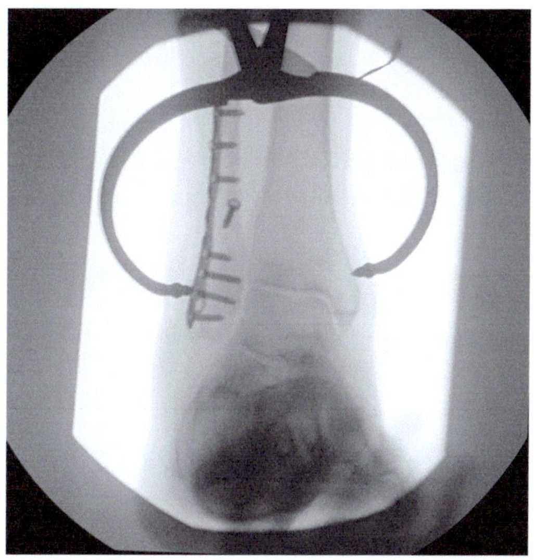

Fig. 14.3 Intraoperative fluoroscopic image demonstrating clamp application to reduce the tibiofibular syndesmosis

use a large point-to-point clamp from the posterolateral fibula to the anteromedial tibia at or just proximal to the ankle joint line (Fig. 14.3). Careful review of the incisura on axial cuts of preoperative cross-sectional imaging, if available, can guide the trajectory of the clamp. The surgeon should ensure that the clamp is large enough to avoid crushing the adjacent soft tissues. The assistant holds the ankle in a neutral position as the clamp is tightened to avoid over-compression as the talus is narrower posteriorly, but the potential for over-compression has been questioned [6]. The reduction can be visually confirmed through an open lateral surgical wound if present. Alignment is confirmed with fluoroscopy—AP, mortise, and lateral views. Attention is paid to the tibiofibular overlap on the AP and mortise and sagittal alignment of the fibula relative to the tibia on the lateral view, which varies widely between patients. Preoperative radiographs of the contralateral ankle are routinely obtained for comparison, particularly in the setting of severe diastasis or comminuted fibula fractures or if percutaneous reduction and fixation are planned.

After fixation is achieved, a cotton test and external rotation stress exam are performed under live fluoroscopy on the mortise view (Fig. 14.4). Attention is paid to the tibiofibular overlap and the medial gutter. If medial ankle instability persists, we routinely repair the deltoid ligament, which will be detailed in a separate chapter. If arthroscopy equipment is available, the reduction can be confirmed by direct visualization.

Alternatively, the fibula can be reduced in the incisura by manual pressure, which some have claimed prevents over-compression and allows the fibula to "settle" within the incisura [7]. The authors believe that this is less reliable as the reduction must be held throughout the process of fixation. An elastic wrap can be used to apply even pressure throughout the entire leg [8, 9], but this technique has not been well studied clinically.

If an adequate reduction cannot be achieved, several issues should be considered. The appropriate length, rotation, and alignment of the fibula must be ensured in the setting of a fibula fracture. In skeletally immature patients, plastic deformation of the fibula can occur, which should be recognized and may be addressed with an osteotomy to achieve syndesmosis reduction if needed [10]. The incisura, lateral gutter, and medial gutter should be evaluated for soft tissue blocking the reduction. The authors routinely perform arthroscopy of the ankle to clear debris from the ankle joint and incisura prior to reduction/fixation of the syndesmosis.

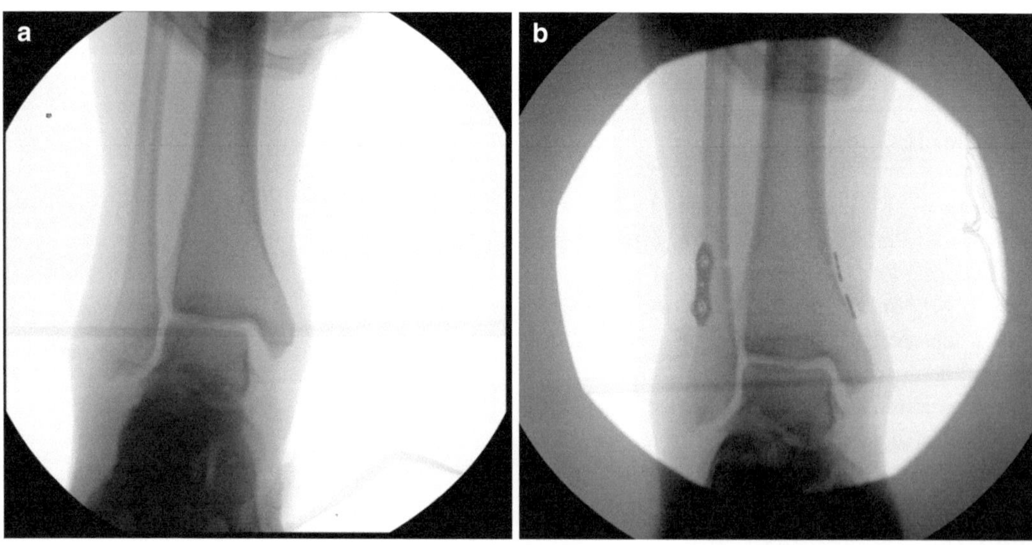

Fig. 14.4 Intraoperative fluoroscopic stress views. (**a**) Widening of the syndesmosis (tibiofibular overlap) and medial clear space with external rotation stress. (**b**) Eversion/lateral translation stress test after flexible fixation was performed. The tibiofibular overlap and medial clear space are restored to their anatomic relationships

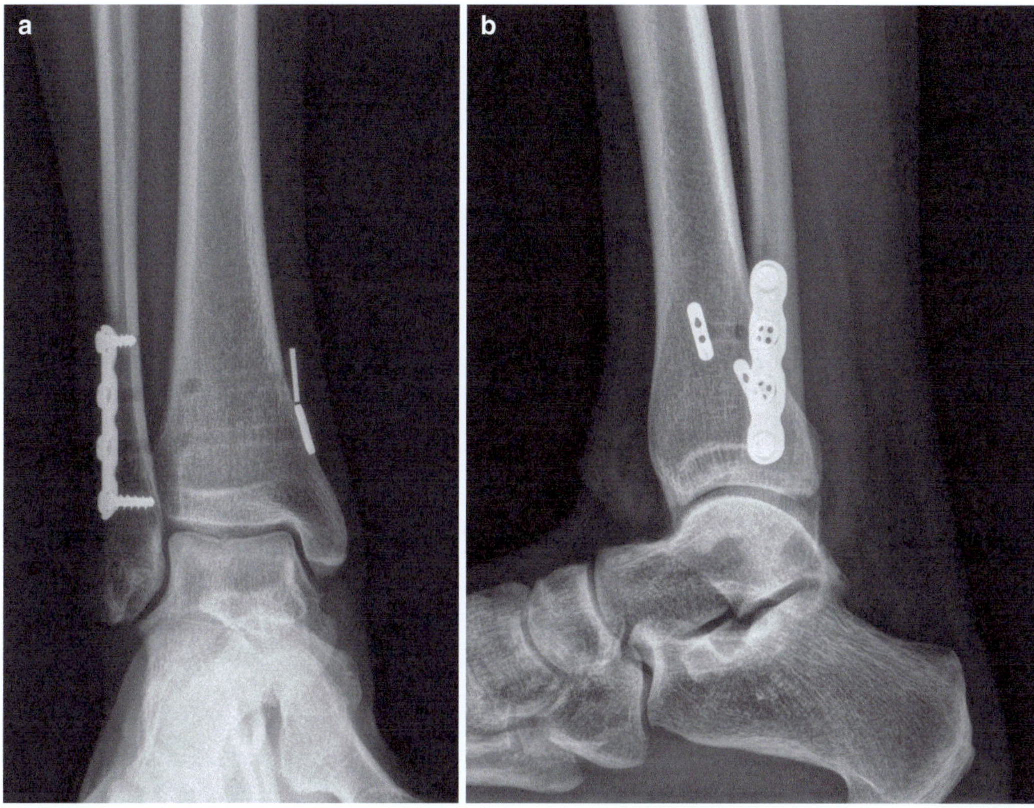

Fig. 14.5 Postoperative weight-bearing mortise (**a**) and lateral (**b**) radiographs of flexible fixation construct for a professional soccer player. A four-hole plate with bicortical screws placed proximally and distally and divergent suture button orientation maximizes stability to allow more rapid rehabilitation and mitigate the risk of fracture through the flexible fixation drill holes

Fixation Techniques

Flexible Fixation

The authors' preferred method for the majority of syndesmosis injuries is two knotless suture buttons in divergent planes (Fig. 14.5). The flexibility of the sutures allows for micromotion of the tibiofibular articulation which is optimal for healing and expedient rehabilitation. After reduction of the syndesmosis, a drill hole is made 2 cm above the ankle joint from the posterolateral fibula to the anteromedial tibia. More distal placement risks injury to the articular surface and a perforating branch of the peroneal artery [11]. The suture button is passed and tightened, and reduction is confirmed. The second button is placed 1–2 cm proximally and aimed divergently, either more anterior or posterior depending on the patient's anatomy. In the setting of a distal fibula fracture, an attempt is made to place the suture buttons through the existing plate. In the absence of a distal fibula fracture, we routinely place the buttons through a two-hole plate on the fibula. For larger patients or if rapid return to activity is desired, a four-hole plate can be used with screws in the most distal and most proximal holes to mitigate the risk of fracture through the drill holes (Fig. 14.5).

Screw Fixation

In the setting of a length-unstable fracture or diabetic patients, more rigid fixation is preferred in the form of screws (Fig. 14.6). These are also placed 2–5 cm above the ankle joint from the posterolateral fibula to the anteromedial tibia. We recommend 3.5 mm or 4.5 mm screws through

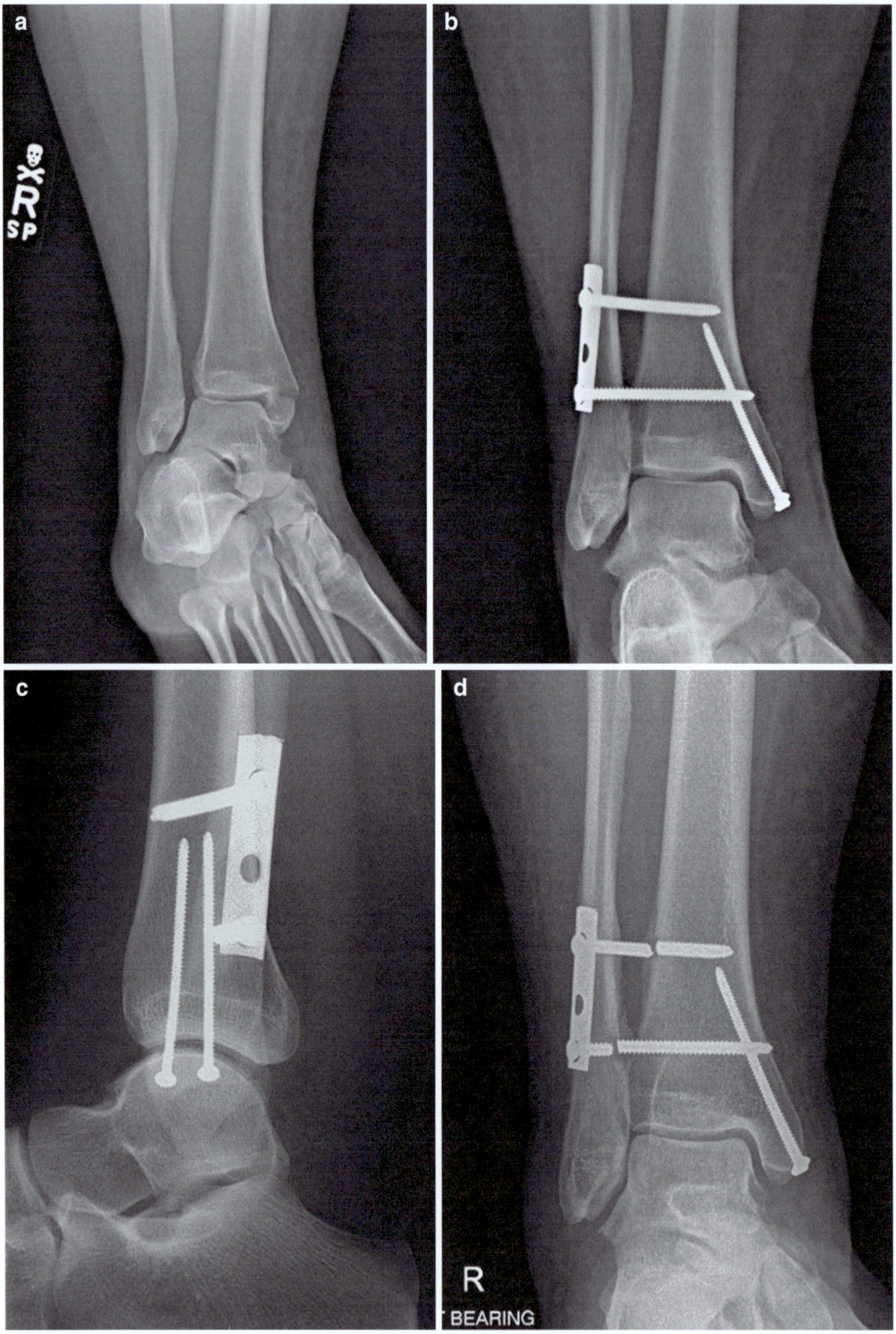

Fig. 14.6 (**a**) Mortise radiograph of a Maisonneuve fracture with syndesmosis disruption. Postoperative anteroposterior (**b**) and lateral (**c**) radiographs showing ORIF of the medial malleolus and dual divergent quadricortical screw fixation of the syndesmosis with a plate. Six months postoperative radiograph (**d**) demonstrating broken screws. The patient was back to her full, pain-free activities and did not desire screw removal. Radiographs courtesy of Daniel Moon, MD

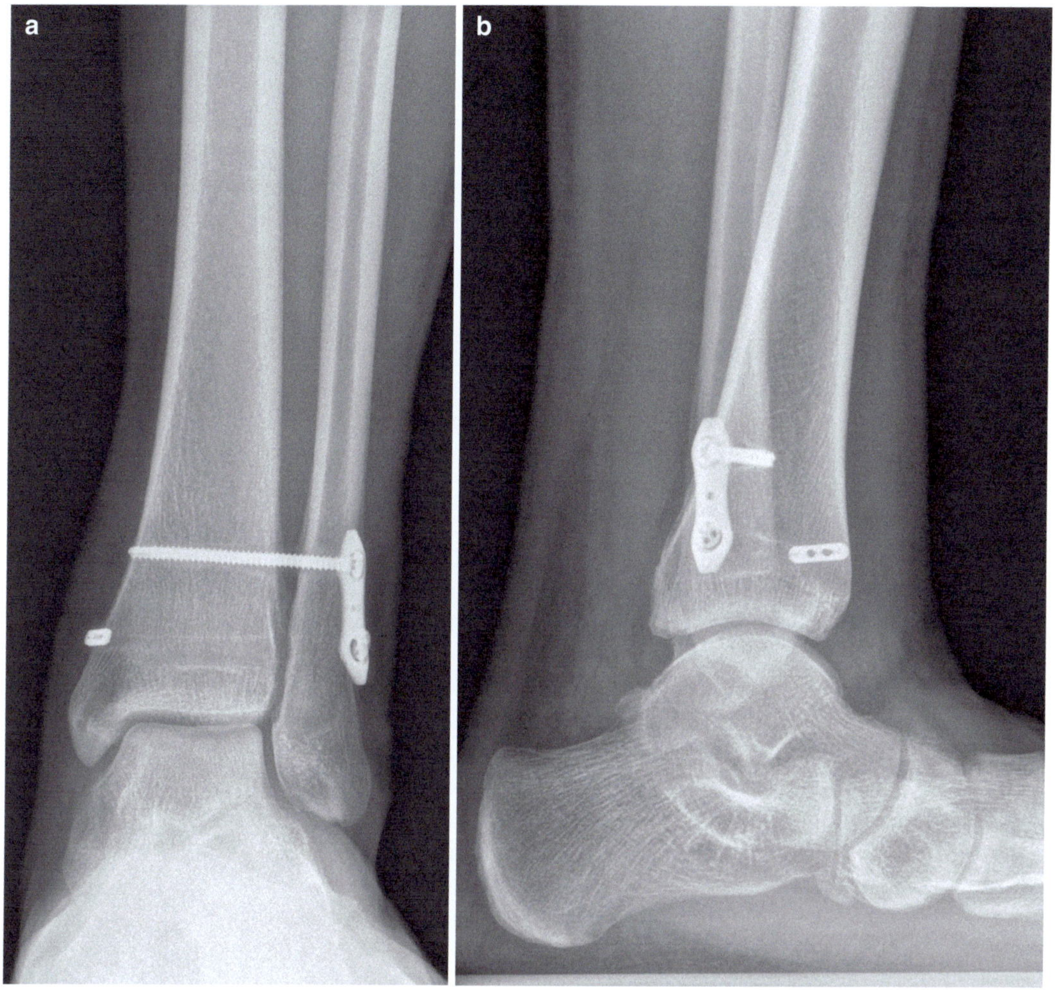

Fig. 14.7 (**a**) Anteroposterior and (**b**) lateral radiographs of syndesmosis fixation with hybrid construct

four cortices, which allows for easier removal if broken. If syndesmosis screw removal is anticipated after several months, a bridging four-hole plate can be placed with bicortical screws proximally and distally to protect the bone after the hardware removal. To avoid potential malreductions with rigid screw fixation, a hybrid construct can be used (Fig. 14.7). A suture button is placed first which allows the fibula to settle within the incisura, and then a screw is placed more proximally to provide more rigid fixation.

Anatomic Reconstruction

Anatomic reconstruction of the AITFL and/or PITFL may be useful in certain circumstances, but the indications for anatomic reconstruction versus trans-syndesmosis fixation have not been delineated. If a bony avulsion of the ligamentous attachments is present, this can be reduced and fixed with screws or suture anchors through an open approach. If inadequate soft tissue is present (after recurrent ligamentous injuries or with systemic ligamentous laxity), the AITFL and/or PITFL can be reconstructed with allograft and/or suture tape [12, 13].

Syndesmosis Fusion

If significant arthritic changes are present in the syndesmosis and causing significant pain, for example, after chronic injury and instability, a fusion of the syndesmosis can be performed. Through an open approach, the incisura is debrided of any remaining cartilage, and the bony edges are prepared with a surgeon's preferred technique. Multiple trans-syndesmosis screws are placed to provide compression. Care must still be taken to maintain a reduced position of the distal fibula to optimize the biomechanics of the remaining ankle joint.

Surgical Outcomes

The topic of syndesmosis injuries has been heavily studied, with over 1100 studies available on PubMed published from 2010 to 2020. The majority of literature reports on syndesmosis injuries associated with fibula fractures, and high-quality outcome studies on isolated syndesmosis injuries are lacking. Recent high-quality literature will be highlighted for several topics: reduction, fixation, management of postoperative complications, and return to activity/sport.

Reduction Techniques

Syndesmosis malreduction has been suggested as the primary predictor of poor clinical outcomes [14–16]. Equivocal outcomes have been reported on the use of clamp vs. manual pressure for reduction [7]. The highly variable anatomy, depth, and inclination of the incisura have been implicated in malreductions [17]. When using a clamp, placing it in the neutral intermalleolar axis may help avoid anterior or posterior displacement of the fibula [18]. Regarding the potential for over-compression during fixation and the position of the ankle during fixation, there is no consensus, and conflicting literature has been reported [6, 19, 20]. The authors prefer to reduce the syndesmosis with the ankle held in a neutral position, using a large clamp. Sufficient force is necessary to apply mild compression, but it is important not to over-tension the joint prior to or during fixation placement. An elastic wrap technique has been described which provides circumferential pressure and could allow for percutaneous reduction and fixation. Promising results have been reported in cadaver models [8, 9], but further research is needed to reproduce these results clinically.

The optimal method of intraoperative confirmation of reduction has yet to be established. Miller et al. reported a lower rate of postoperative malreductions on CT scan with open reduction of the syndesmosis with direct visualization than closed reduction with fluoroscopy (16% vs. 52%) [21]. Summers et al. reported their method of fluoroscopic comparison to the normal ankle, which yielded an anatomic reduction in 17 of 18 patients based on subsequent intraoperative CT [22]. Increasing prevalence of intraoperative cross-sectional imaging offers a new option for confirmation of reduction, but the increased radiation exposure, device availability, and increased cost must be considered. The authors prefer arthroscopic evaluation to confirm syndesmosis reduction as this allows for debridement of intra-articular debris, impingement lesions, and evaluation for osteochondral lesions [23].

Postoperative loss of reduction can also portend a poor outcome. Mendelsohn et al. found that obese patients were more likely to have a loss of reduction postoperatively, but diabetes mellitus, smoking, and the type of fixation were not predictors of loss of reduction [24].

Fixation Techniques: Outcomes

For screw fixation, no consensus exists on the size of screws necessary [25], material, number of screws (1 vs. 2), or cortices involved (3 vs. 4) [26]. Suture button fixation allows for micromotion between the distal tibia and fibula, which more closely matches the normal physiologic relationship [27, 28]. Multiple studies report good results with suture button fixation for both isolated syndesmosis injuries and those with rotational ankle fractures [15, 29–31]. Naqvi et al. found that there were fewer malreductions in patients treated with suture button than screws, 0% vs. 21.7%, respectively [32].

Shimozono et al. performed a meta-analysis of five randomized controlled trials comparing suture buttons versus screws for syndesmosis injuries [33]. With 285 patients included, they reported improved AOFAS scores at an average of 20.8 months for patients treated with suture button versus screws (95.3 vs. 86.7, $p < 0.001$). The patients treated with suture button also had lower incidence of implant removal (6.0% vs. 22.4%, $p = 0.01$), broken implants (0.0% vs. 25.4%, $p < 0.001$), and joint malreduction (0.8% vs. 11.5%) compared to the group treated with screws.

Anatomic reconstruction of the syndesmosis ligaments has been reported to provide similar biomechanical strength as screws or suture buttons [13]. Zhan et al. reported a randomized controlled trial of 53 patients with external rotational ankle fractures with posterior malleolus fractures, randomized to screw fixation versus AITFL reconstruction and suture button fixation [12]. They found a higher complication rate in the group treated with a screw (26.9% vs. 3.7%) and a longer time to return to work (7.2 months vs. 5.3 months).

Management of Complications

Screw breakage is the most common complication following screw placement (Fig. 14.6d). However, a broken screw does not necessarily mean that screws must be removed. Schepers et al. performed a systematic review of seven studies and found that screw retention vs. removal did not impact clinical outcomes [34]. They also found similar outcomes between patients with broken screws and intact screws. Hardware removal for intact screws is recommended after 4–6 months if dorsiflexion is limited or hardware is irritating. If planovalgus alignment is present, a suture button can be placed at the time of screw removal as this alignment places extra stress on the syndesmosis. The authors recommend patient counseling on the potential for broken screws at the time of initial surgery. In cases where patients desire avoidance of broken screws, these can be removed at a minimum of 12 weeks post-op. The authors prefer 16 weeks before screw removal, reassessing instability and being prepared to place flexible devices during the removal procedure if indicated.

Early versions of the suture button device had large knots that were often prominent, and a complication rate of 8% was reported [35]. However, newer devices are knotless and may reduce the incidence of soft tissue irritation. The failure rate for suture button devices is unknown since the suture material is radiolucent making it difficult to assess stretching or failure radiographically.

Postoperative Rehabilitation

Postoperative Protocol

The paradigm shift in fixation constructs over the past 15 years has been paralleled by a trend toward more rapid rehabilitation timelines. For isolated ligament injuries (i.e., no rotational ankle fracture component) treated with a flexible fixation construct, the authors favor 5–7 days in a splint, non-weight-bearing, followed by weight-bearing as tolerated in a CAM walker boot with initiation of range of motion and swelling reduction modalities. Transition from a boot to a lace-up brace generally occurs 3–4 weeks post-up, running 5–6 weeks post-op, and return to sport at 8 weeks post-op. This protocol can certainly be adjusted based on the needs of the athlete as demands on the ankle vary by sport, position, and time of season. See Chapter 24 for an overview of metrics guiding return to sport.

Return to Sport

There is currently no consensus on a return to sport protocol or anticipated timing for athletes to return to play following surgical repair for a grade IIb or III syndesmosis injury. Anderson et al. reported on 14 professional American football players treated with suture button fixation and open deltoid repair for pronation-external rotational ankle injuries, with 86% of players returning to play at 6 months [36]. D'Hooghe et al. recently reported data from a large injury database of professional soccer players with grade IIb and III syndesmosis injuries [37]. They reported that the mean time to begin on-field/sport-specific rehabilitation was 37 ± 12 days, with a mean time of 103 ± 28 days to the first match after syndesmosis stabilization. Out of 110 professional soccer players with high-grade syndesmosis injuries, none had participated in an official match at 4 weeks status postoperatively and only 4% of athletes returned to an official game within 8 weeks after surgery [38]. Some American football programs have introduced vastly accelerated return to sport protocols for syndesmosis injuries [39]. Given the heterogeneity of concomitant injuries with syndesmosis injuries, a case-by-case approach is warranted.

Hunt et al. [40] recently reported on the results of a survey of 742 orthopedic surgeons specializing in ankle injuries from across the globe through major orthopedic sports medicine societies. They identified that flexible devices were the preferred fixation construct (48%), followed by screws (27%), hybrid fixation (19%), and others (6%). There was a higher preference for flexible devices among sports medicine-trained providers (58%) relative to non-sports medicine-trained providers (44%). Sixty-two percent of respondents noted that their rehabilitation protocols would not change for larger athletes or higher-grade injuries that included disruption of the deltoid ligament. Of note, there was considerable variability in anticipated full return to sport, ranging from immediately following injury to 6 months post-op. This highlights a huge discrepancy in current return to sport protocols for syndesmosis injuries and indicates a need for careful outcome tracking to identify the best and safest return to sport practices.

Conclusion

Injuries to the tibiofibular syndesmosis are increasingly common in athletes participating in field and court sports. Our understanding of the pathomechanics of these injuries, as well as optimal treatment, has evolved considerably in recent years. Treatment trends are toward flexible fixation devices and accelerated rehabilitation, allowing safe return to sport. The development of anatomic ligament reconstruction techniques may lead to restoration of joint mechanics that are more similar to normal anatomy than current fixation constructs.

References

1. Lubberts B, D'Hooghe P, Bengtsson H, DiGiovanni CW, Calder J, Ekstrand J. Epidemiology and return to play following isolated syndesmotic injuries of the ankle: a prospective cohort study of 3677 male professional footballers in the UEFA elite Club injury study. Br J Sports Med. 2019;53(15):959–64.
2. Hunt KJ, George E, Harris AH, Dragoo JL. Epidemiology of syndesmosis injuries in intercollegiate football: incidence and risk factors from National Collegiate Athletic Association injury surveillance system data from 2004-2005 to 2008-2009. Clin J Sport Med. 2013;23(4):278–82.
3. Waterman BR, Belmont PJ Jr, Cameron KL, Svoboda SJ, Alitz CJ, Owens BD. Risk factors for syndesmotic and medial ankle sprain: role of sex, sport, and level of competition. Am J Sports Med. 2011;39(5):992–8.
4. Hogg-Cornejo VHK, Bartolomei J, Rullkoetter PJ, Myers C, Shelburne KB. Normal kinematics of the syndesmosis and ankle mortise during dynamic movements. Foot Ankle Orthop. 2020;5(3):2473011420933007. https://doi.org/10.1177/2473011420933007.
5. van Dijk CN, Longo UG, Loppini M, et al. Classification and diagnosis of acute isolated syndesmotic injuries: ESSKA-AFAS consensus and guidelines. Knee Surg Sports Traumatol Arthrosc. 2016;24(4):1200–16.
6. Tornetta P 3rd, Spoo JE, Reynolds FA, Lee C. Overtightening of the ankle syndesmosis: is it really possible? J Bone Joint Surg Am. 2001;83(4):489–92.
7. Park YH, Ahn JH, Choi GW, Kim HJ. Comparison of clamp reduction and manual reduction of syndesmosis in rotational ankle fractures: a prospective randomized trial. J Foot Ankle Surg. 2018;57(1):19–22.
8. Schlatterer D, Ramirez M, Deshpande C. Eliminating syndesmotic reduction variability: a novel elastic wrap reduction tool. Orthopedic Trauma Association Meeting 2018; Scientific Poster #17; 2018.
9. Schlatterer D, Despande C, Morgenstein A. A novel elastic wrap for syndesmotic reduction with postoperative CT scan analysis. Foot Ankle Orthop. 2019;4:2473011419S2473010037.
10. Edwards GS Jr, DeLee JC. Ankle diastasis without fracture. Foot Ankle. 1984;4(6):305–12.
11. McKeon KE, Wright RW, Johnson JE, McCormick JJ, Klein SE. Vascular anatomy of the tibiofibular syndesmosis. J Bone Joint Surg Am. 2012;94(10):931–8.

12. Zhan Y, Yan X, Xia R, Cheng T, Luo C. Anterior-inferior tibiofibular ligament anatomical repair and augmentation versus trans-syndesmosis screw fixation for the syndesmotic instability in external-rotation type ankle fracture with posterior malleolus involvement: a prospective and comparative study. Injury. 2016;47(7):1574–80.
13. Akoh CC, Phisitkul P. Anatomic ligament repairs of syndesmotic injuries. Orthop Clin North Am. 2019;50(3):401–14.
14. Sagi HC, Shah AR, Sanders RW. The functional consequence of syndesmotic joint malreduction at a minimum 2-year follow-up. J Orthop Trauma. 2012;26(7):439–43.
15. Naqvi GA, Shafqat A, Awan N. Tightrope fixation of ankle syndesmosis injuries: clinical outcome, complications and technique modification. Injury. 2012;43(6):838–42.
16. Weening B, Bhandari M. Predictors of functional outcome following transsyndesmotic screw fixation of ankle fractures. J Orthop Trauma. 2005;19(2):102–8.
17. Boszczyk A, Kwapisz S, Krummel M, Grass R, Rammelt S. Correlation of incisura anatomy with syndesmotic malreduction. Foot Ankle Int. 2018;39(3):369–75.
18. Phisitkul P, Ebinger T, Goetz J, Vaseenon T, Marsh JL. Forceps reduction of the syndesmosis in rotational ankle fractures: a cadaveric study. J Bone Joint Surg Am. 2012;94(24):2256–61.
19. Darwish HH, Glisson RR, DeOrio JK. Compression screw fixation of the syndesmosis. Foot Ankle Int. 2012;33(10):893–9.
20. Michelson JD. Ankle fractures resulting from rotational injuries. J Am Acad Orthop Surg. 2003;11(6):403–12.
21. Miller AN, Carroll EA, Parker RJ, Boraiah S, Helfet DL, Lorich DG. Direct visualization for syndesmotic stabilization of ankle fractures. Foot Ankle Int. 2009;30(5):419–26.
22. Summers HD, Sinclair MK, Stover MD. A reliable method for intraoperative evaluation of syndesmotic reduction. J Orthop Trauma. 2013;27(4): 196–200.
23. Wake J, Martin KD. Syndesmosis injury from diagnosis to repair: physical examination, diagnosis, and arthroscopic-assisted reduction. J Am Acad Orthop Surg. 2020;28(13):517–27.
24. Mendelsohn ES, Hoshino CM, Harris TG, Zinar DM. The effect of obesity on early failure after operative syndesmosis injuries. J Orthop Trauma. 2013;27(4):201–6.
25. Thompson MC, Gesink DS. Biomechanical comparison of syndesmosis fixation with 3.5- and 4.5-millimeter stainless steel screws. Foot Ankle Int. 2000;21(9):736–41.
26. Moore JA Jr, Shank JR, Morgan SJ, Smith WR. Syndesmosis fixation: a comparison of three and four cortices of screw fixation without hardware removal. Foot Ankle Int. 2006;27(8):567–72.
27. Forsythe K, Freedman KB, Stover MD, Patwardhan AG. Comparison of a novel FiberWire-button construct versus metallic screw fixation in a syndesmotic injury model. Foot Ankle Int. 2008;29(1):49–54.
28. Klitzman R, Zhao H, Zhang LQ, Strohmeyer G, Vora A. Suture-button versus screw fixation of the syndesmosis: a biomechanical analysis. Foot Ankle Int. 2010;31(1):69–75.
29. Qamar F, Kadakia A, Venkateswaran B. An anatomical way of treating ankle syndesmotic injuries. J Foot Ankle Surg. 2011;50(6):762–5.
30. Degroot H, Al-Omari AA, El Ghazaly SA. Outcomes of suture button repair of the distal tibiofibular syndesmosis. Foot Ankle Int. 2011;32(3):250–6.
31. Willmott HJ, Singh B, David LA. Outcome and complications of treatment of ankle diastasis with tightrope fixation. Injury. 2009;40(11):1204–6.
32. Naqvi GA, Cunningham P, Lynch B, Galvin R, Awan N. Fixation of ankle syndesmotic injuries: comparison of tightrope fixation and syndesmotic screw fixation for accuracy of syndesmotic reduction. Am J Sports Med. 2012;40(12):2828–35.
33. Shimozono Y, Hurley ET, Myerson CL, Murawski CD, Kennedy JG. Suture button versus syndesmotic screw for syndesmosis injuries: a meta-analysis of randomized controlled trials. Am J Sports Med. 2019;47(11):2764–71.
34. Schepers T. To retain or remove the syndesmotic screw: a review of literature. Arch Orthop Trauma Surg. 2011;131(7):879–83.
35. Storey P, Gadd RJ, Blundell C, Davies MB. Complications of suture button ankle syndesmosis stabilization with modifications of surgical technique. Foot Ankle Int. 2012;33(9):717–21.
36. Hsu AR, Lareau CR, Anderson RB. Repair of acute superficial deltoid complex avulsion during ankle fracture fixation in National Football League players. Foot Ankle Int. 2015;36(11):1272–8.
37. D'Hooghe P, Grassi A, Alkhelaifi K, et al. Return to play after surgery for isolated unstable syndesmotic ankle injuries (west point grade IIB and III) in 110 male professional football players: a retrospective cohort study. Br J Sports Med. 2020;54(19):1168–73.
38. D'Hooghe P, Grassi A, Alkhelaifi K, et al. Return to play after surgery for isolated unstable syndesmotic ankle injuries (west point grade IIB and III) in 110 male professional football players: a retrospective cohort study. Br J Sports Med. 2020;54(19):1168–73. https://doi.org/10.1136/bjsports-2018-100298.
39. Dellenger R. Tua Tagovailoa's ankle injury pins Alabama in familiar territory. https://www.si.com/college/2019/10/20/tua-tagovailoa-ankle-injury-alabama-lsu-outlook. Published 2019. Accessed 7 Dec 2020.
40. Hunt KJ, Bartolomei J, Challa S, Tuffiash M, Annunziato A, ISAKOS LAF. Significant variations in surgical construct and return to sport protocols with syndesmotic injuries: an ISAKOS global perspective. J ISAKOS. 2022;7(1):13–8.

Syndesmotic Injuries in Athletes: Return to Play and Rehabilitation

15

Pieter D'Hooghe, Frederique Neys, Jonathan Bartolomei-Aguillar, and Kenneth J. Hunt

Introduction

Injuries to the ankle syndesmosis have demonstrated increased prevalence among athletes of all levels. Syndesmotic injuries occur in athletes at an estimated incidence of 0.05 injuries per 1000 h of exposure [1]. Impact and collision sports such as soccer, skiing, football, ice hockey, wrestling, and rugby exhibit a higher prevalence of injury [1]. It is also widely recognized that ligamentous syndesmotic injuries result in substantially longer times missed from sport compared to other ankle ligament injuries, are much more likely to require surgical stabilization (Fig. 15.1), and are

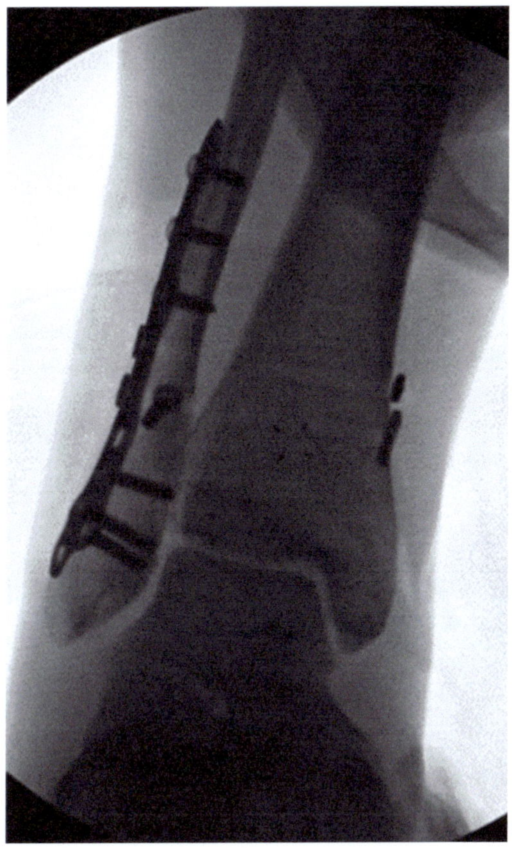

Fig. 15.1 Intraoperative fluoroscopic images of stress test of syndesmosis following fixation of a fibular fracture with flexible fixation devices. Note restoration of the ankle mortise and talus relative to the plafond. Anteroposterior fluoroscopic image with applied stress demonstrating stable syndesmosis following flexible fixation device application

P. D'Hooghe (✉)
Department of Orthopaedic Surgery,
Aspetar Orthopaedic and Sports Medicine Hospital,
Doha, Qatar
e-mail: pieter.dhooghe@aspetar.com

F. Neys
Department of Orthopaedic Surgery,
UC Health Anschutz Medical Campus,
Aurora, CO, USA
e-mail:
JONATHAN.BARTOLOMEIAGUILAR@cuanschutz.edu

J. Bartolomei-Aguillar
Department of Physiotherapy, Move to Cure,
Antwerpen, Belgium

K. J. Hunt
Department of Orthopaedic Surgery, University of Colorado School of Medicine, Aurora, CO, USA
e-mail: Kenneth.j.hunt@cuanschutz.edu

P. D'Hooghe et al. (eds.), *Ligamentous Injuries of the Foot and Ankle*,
https://doi.org/10.1007/978-3-031-08682-3_15

associated with more long-term functional sequelae. Increasing prevalence of a higher risk injury has intensified the focus in recent years on diagnosis and management of syndesmotic injuries in sports medicine and athletic training circles [2–5].

The goal of this chapter is to present meaningful advances and innovative expert-opinion suggestions on the return to play protocols and rehabilitation criteria after syndesmotic ankle injury.

Return to Play Protocol/Survey Results

Return to Play

There is no current consensus on a return to sport protocol for athletes to return to play following syndesmotic injury. D'Hooghe et al. reported on a large professional soccer registry to study players with Grade IIb and III syndesmotic injuries and collect information on rehabilitation, the time to return to sport-specific rehabilitation, and the time to first official soccer match after injury [6]. They found that out of 110 professional soccer players in the registry, none had participated in an official match at 1 month after surgery [6]. Additionally, only 4% of the athletes returned to an official game within 2 months after surgery [6]. Their data also revealed that the mean time to begin on-field/sport-specific rehabilitation was 37 ± 12 days, with a mean time of 103 ± 28 days to the first match after syndesmotic stabilization [6].

Global Perspective

The Leg, Ankle and Foot (LAF) Committee of the International Society of Arthroscopy, Knee Surgery and Orthopaedic Sports Medicine (ISAKOS) recently surveyed 742 orthopedic surgeons specializing in ankle injuries from across the globe through ISAKOS and all major orthopedic sports medicine societies. Survey participants answered questions focused on their indications for the treatment of syndesmotic injuries and the information that was used during their decision-making process. Each respondent's preferred technique, either suture buttons, syndesmotic screws, or hybrid constructs for operative repair of indicated syndesmotic injuries, was also queried. Six hypothetical athlete scenarios were constructed to assess the preferred duration of rehabilitation and graduation to activity in each variation of syndesmotic injury. Flexible devices were the preferred fixation construct (47.1%), followed by screws (29.6%), hybrid fixation (18%), and others (5.3%) (Fig. 15.2). There was a higher preference for flexible devices among sports medicine-trained providers (58%) relative to non-sports medicine-trained providers (44%). In total, 63.7% of respondents noted that their rehabilitation protocols would not change for each athlete scenario. Considerable variability was present in an anticipated full return to sport, ranging from immediately following an injury to 6 months post-op. From our survey collection, we were able to infer that regardless of the severity of the injury to the syndesmosis, device choice and return to play protocol were not consistent internationally. Thus, no consensus has been made among providers that treat syndesmotic injuries.

Recent anecdotal reports (NCAA) have questioned the dogma of immobilization for syndesmotic ankle injuries in athletes. These considerations have ignited a renewed discussion

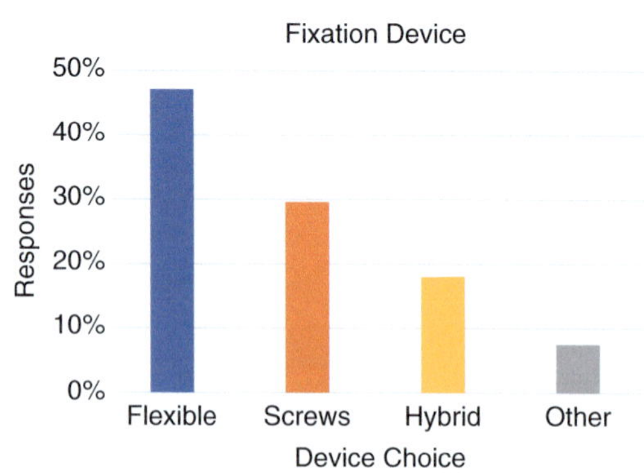

Fig. 15.2 Graph illustrating percentage of surveyed surgeons that would choose one of the four techniques (flexible fixation, surgical screws, hybrid construct, or others)

on accelerated rehabilitation and consequently brought more awareness to the flexible device techniques. The ISAKOS Leg, Ankle and Foot Committee survey suggests that there is substantial variability in return to sport protocols, although the mean values of survey responses and those in D'Hooghe et al.'s 2019 study are strikingly similar.

Rehabilitation

Background on Guidelines

Although there are clear differences in etiology, mechanism of injury, and treatment options/RTP between lateral ligament ankle injuries and syndesmotic injuries, most syndesmotic ankle sprains are still treated by "classic" ankle sprain rehabilitation protocols. In order to improve our understanding in syndesmotic ankle sprain rehabilitation, there is a need for validated rehabilitation protocols and post-injury discharge criteria.

In this chapter section, a new rehabilitation plan is presented which focuses on a rapid and flexible post-injury approach that more closely mimics the function of the syndesmosis together with a special attention to the intrinsic foot flexors and tibialis anterior/posterior, especially in the early stages of rehabilitation.

This plan evidently also incorporates the whole lower limb alignment and movement chain focus, implements the newest available technology (instant feedback alignment, integration of frontal lobe to facilitate new movement pattern, virtual reality), and integrates the required changes in speed, direction, and rhythm, especially in the last phases of rehabilitation.

The presented criteria-based rehabilitation plan is considered expert-opinion and is based on clinical experience and the highlighted need to tackle some specific biomechanical properties of the syndesmotic ankle injury.

First Phase (0–2 Weeks)

- Brace/walker boot: progressive increase in weight-bearing, guided by pain and swelling.
- Gentle manual mobilizations (sagittal plane).
- Maintaining ROM of the ankle, no force on dorsiflexion.
- Non-weight-bearing exercises.
- Activation and facilitation of the proximal global movement chain.
- Improve hip mobility: hip extension and external rotation.
- Correct movement pattern and gait facilitation.
- Implementation of the brain: frontal lobe activation.
- Isometric activation of (deep) calf musculature and intrinsic foot musculature.

Gold standard: pain is your guide.

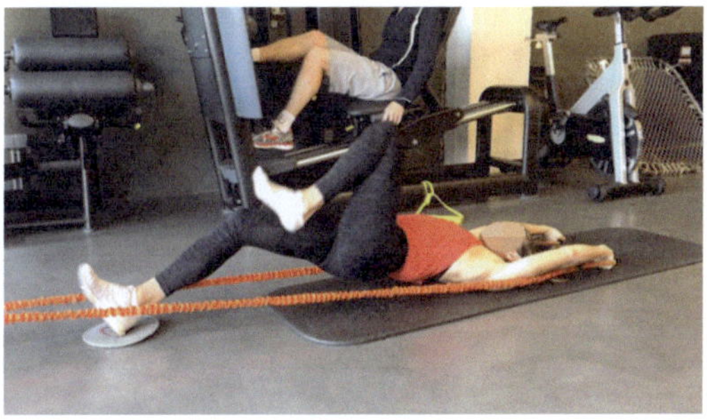

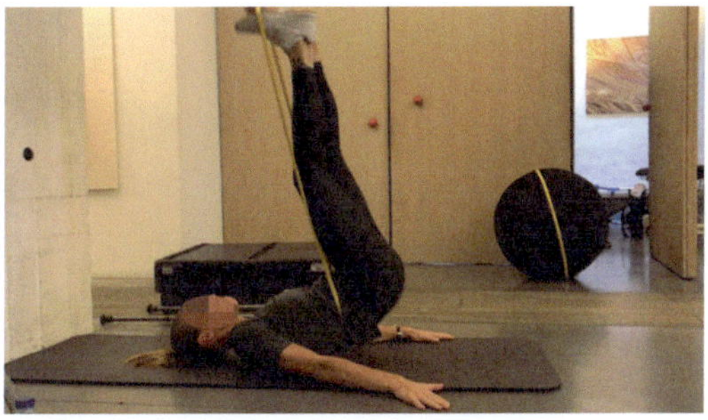

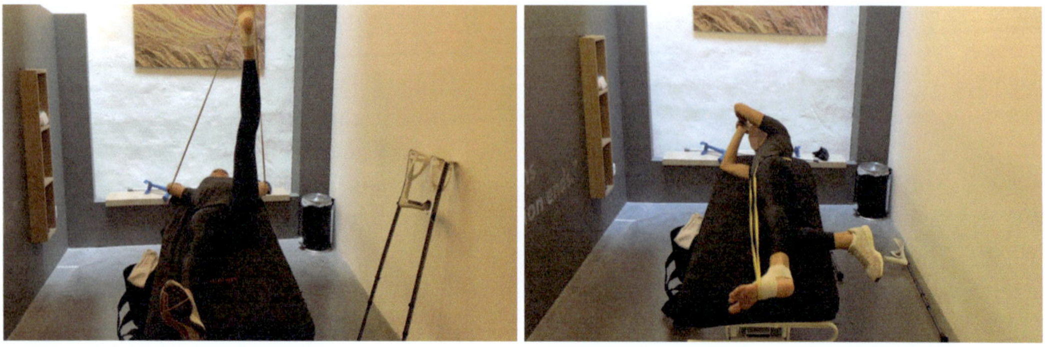

Second Phase (2–3 Weeks)

- Full weight-bearing.
- Active mobilization + passive ROM of the ankle.
- Improve proximal control with body weight exercises.
- Intrinsic foot and calf muscle activation with weight-bearing.
- Correct movement pattern and gait facilitation with video feedback: alignment corrections over shoulder-hip-knee-ankle.
- Corrective frontal and sagittal weight transfer exercises.
- Implementation of the brain feedback: frontal lobe activation (movements toward targets).
- Eventually start with neurostimulation of the motor cortex. However, no solid evidence yet presented in sports (optional).

Gold standard: no syndesmotic stress exercises with weight-bearing exercises.

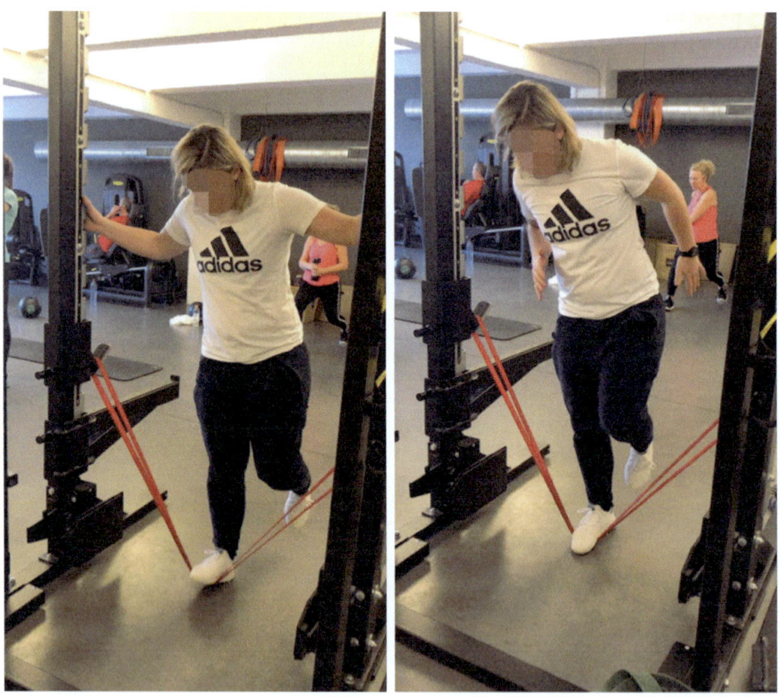

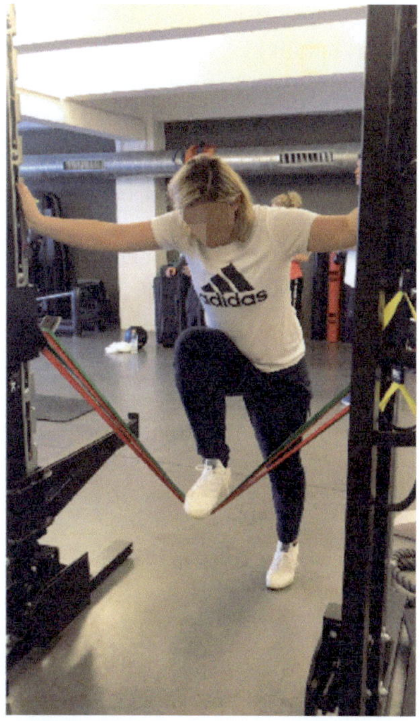

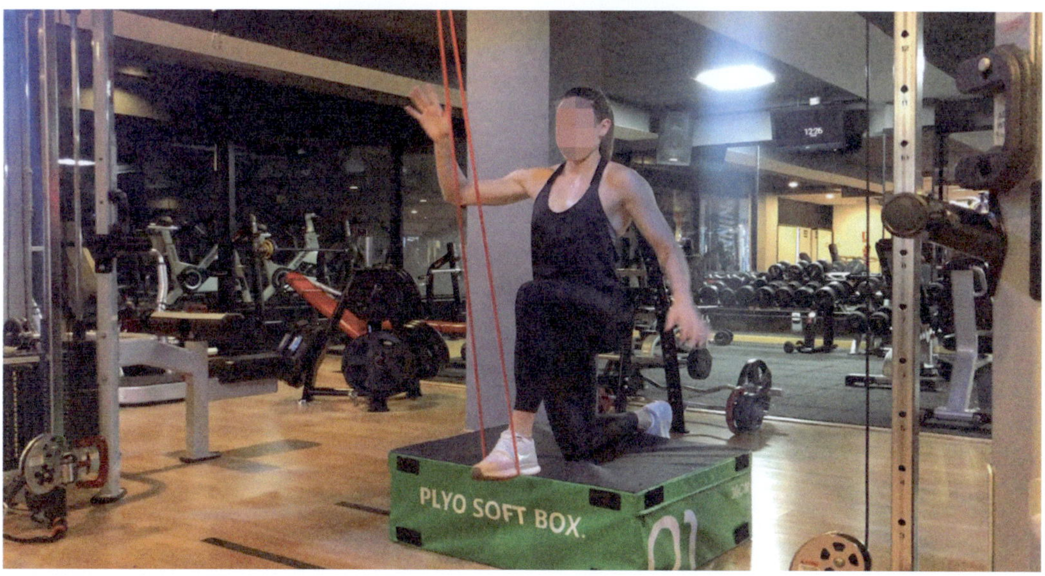

Third Phase (3–5 Weeks)

- Integrate rotations and variations with a fixed talus: forefoot to mid-foot.
- If a good movement pattern and ROM is in place: start running drills and include gradual impact. Meanwhile ongoing focus on a proper alignment and ROM ankle dorsiflexion (left–right).
- Active mobilization exercises and integration of ankle rotation with progressive resistance.
- Passive ROM with mobilization toward full ankle ROM.
- Improving proximal control in impact situations.
- Intrinsic muscle activation with eccentric exercise (e.g., backward walking/jumping/running).

- Implementation of the brain: frontal lobe activation (e.g., virtual reality, cognitive skills).

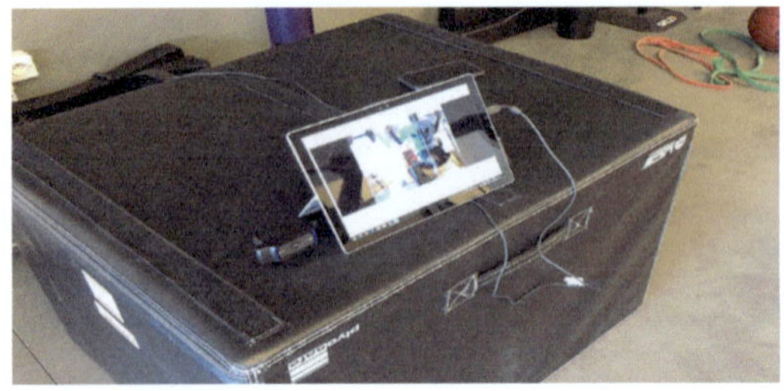

> *Gold standard: Correct frontal and sagittal and rotational weight transfer with higher impact.*

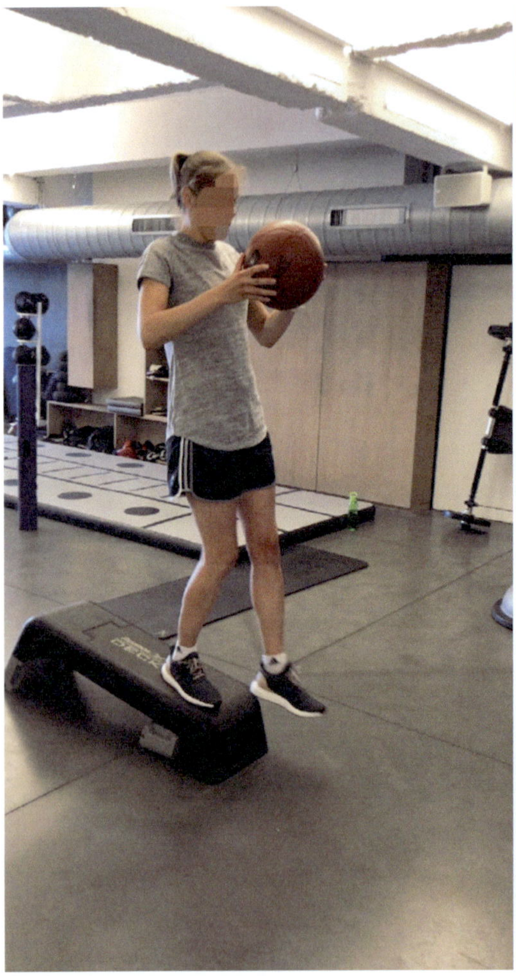

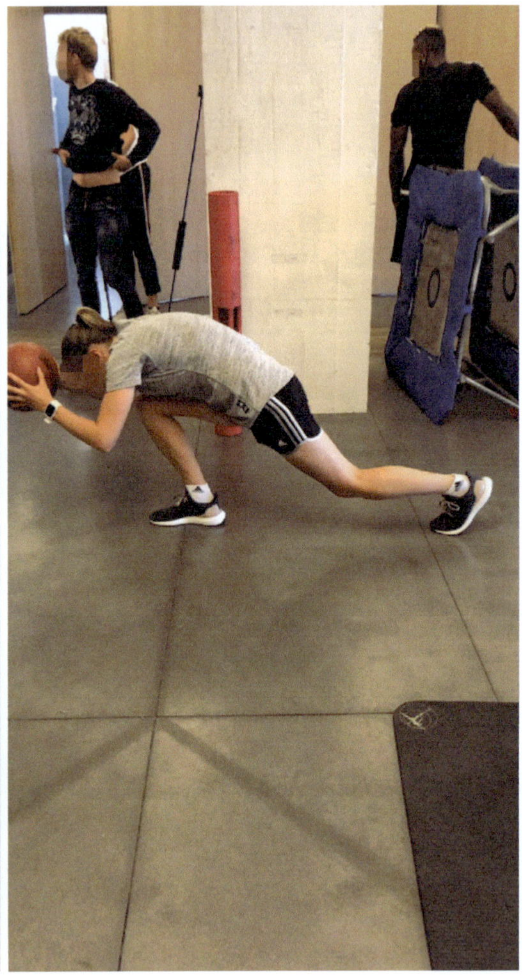

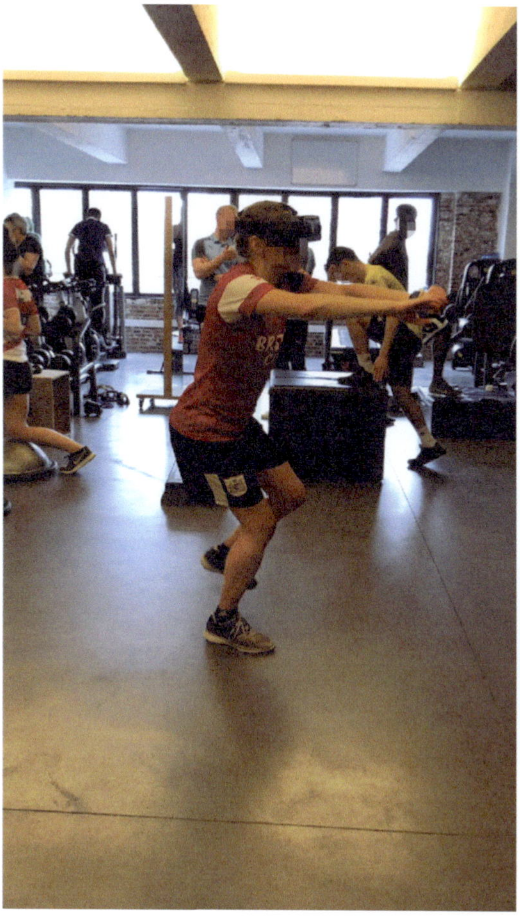

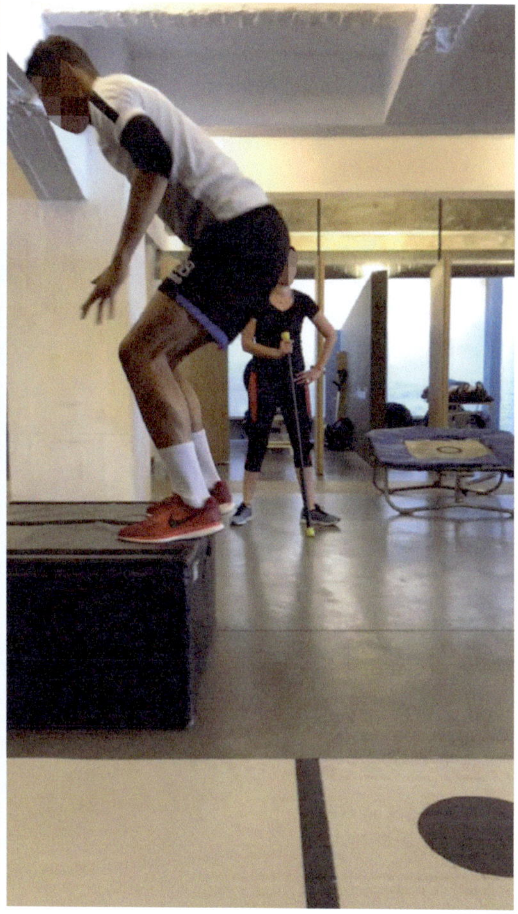

Last Phase (5 Weeks +)

- Focus toward RTP and changes in shoe/boot and surfaces.
- High-impact movements (multidimensional).
- Rotation exercises with resistance.
- Start from eversion ankle position and then implement stress and rotation exercises from this position.
- Increase slowly the load (ligaments are adaptive to load and impact).
- Implement deceleration exercises and forces (with and without impact).
- Implement full-impact strength exercises.
- Implementation of multi-coordination exercises.

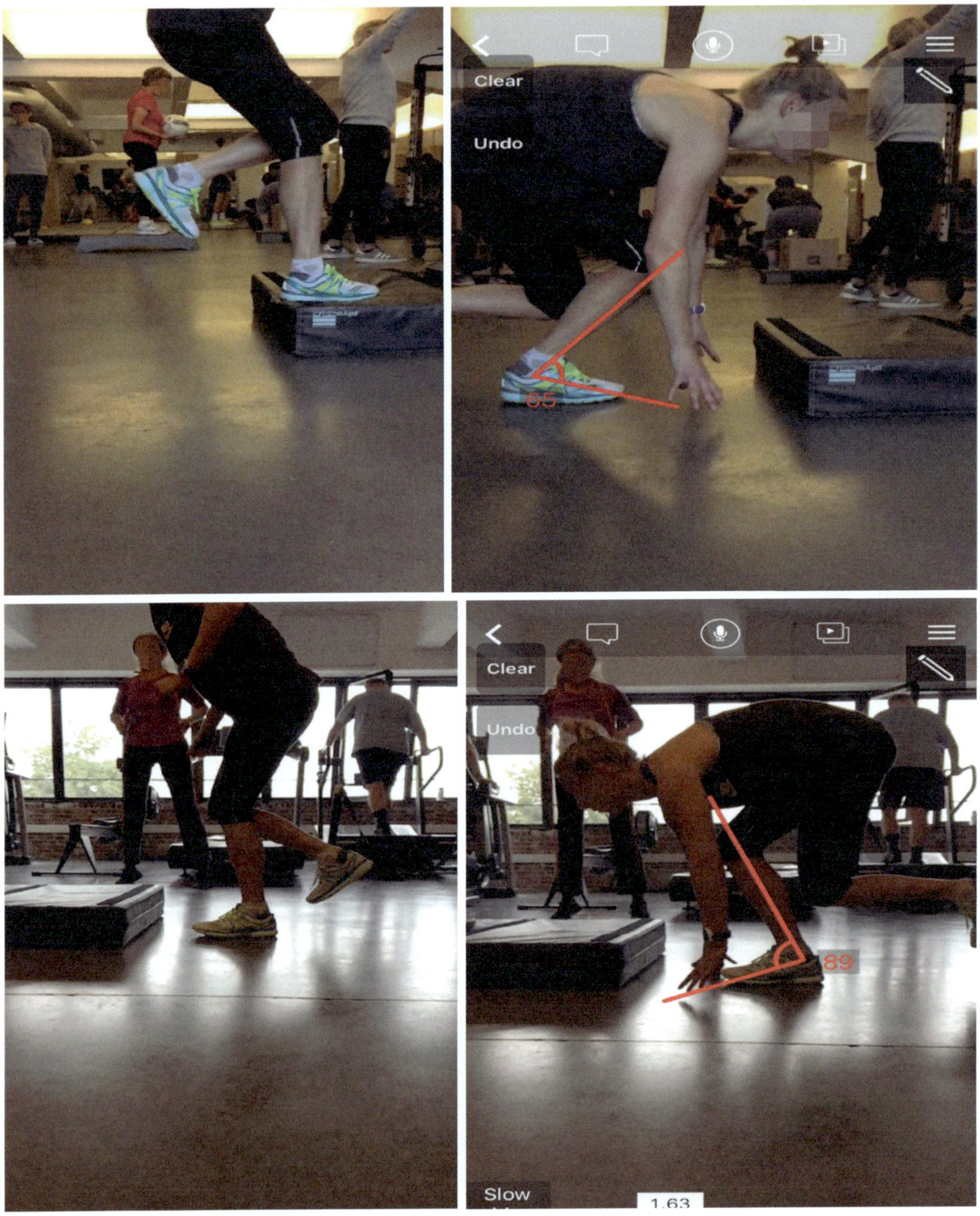
Clear
Undo
65
Clear
Undo
89
Slow
1.63

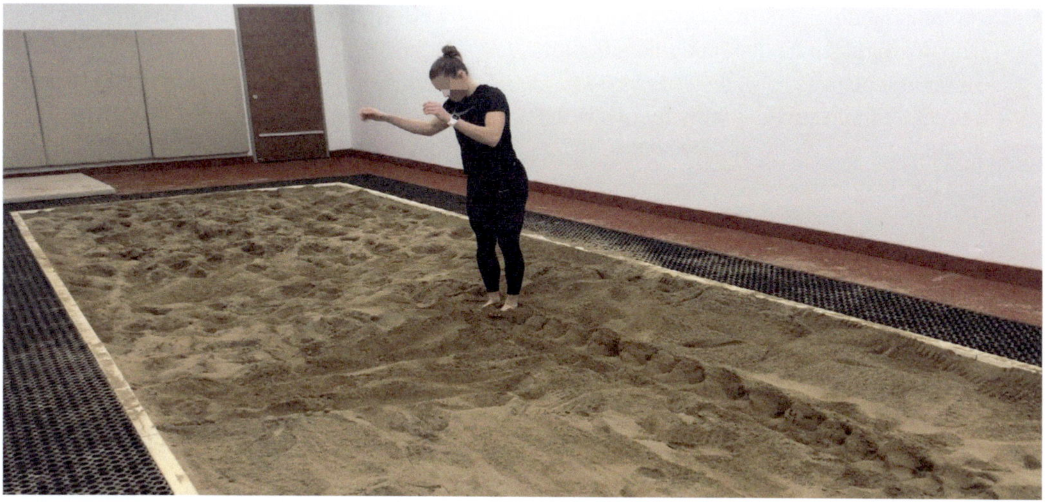

Tests to Include Prior to RTP

- Body weight: increased BMI has a higher risk (Waterman et al. 2011).
- Mobility testing.
  - Lack of hip external rotation/more external rotation in the ankle: this foot position plays a key role in the mechanism of (re-) injury.
  - Lack of hip extension.
  - Dorsiflexion: left–right difference testing.
  - End-range extension mobilizations (active + passive) of the first toe.
- Single-leg step-down.
  - Hip flexion/knee flexion/ankle dorsiflexion in the sagittal plane.
  - Alignment adjustments with focus on the frontal plane.

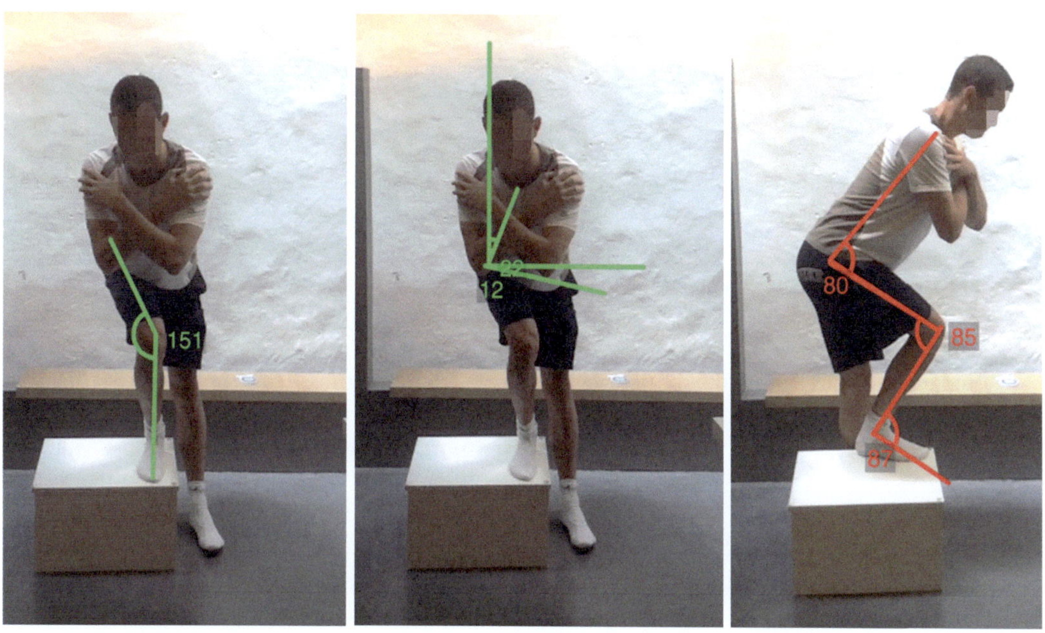

- Drop-jump landing pattern.
  - Hip flexion/knee flexion/ankle dorsiflexion in sagittal plane.
  - Alignment adjustments with focus on the frontal plane.
- Single hop test.
  - Exclude a potential stiff knee pattern.
  - Left–right difference measurement and adjustment.
  - Ankle dorsiflexion angle analysis by landing: left versus right.
- Force decks.
  - Jump height.
  - Reaction time.

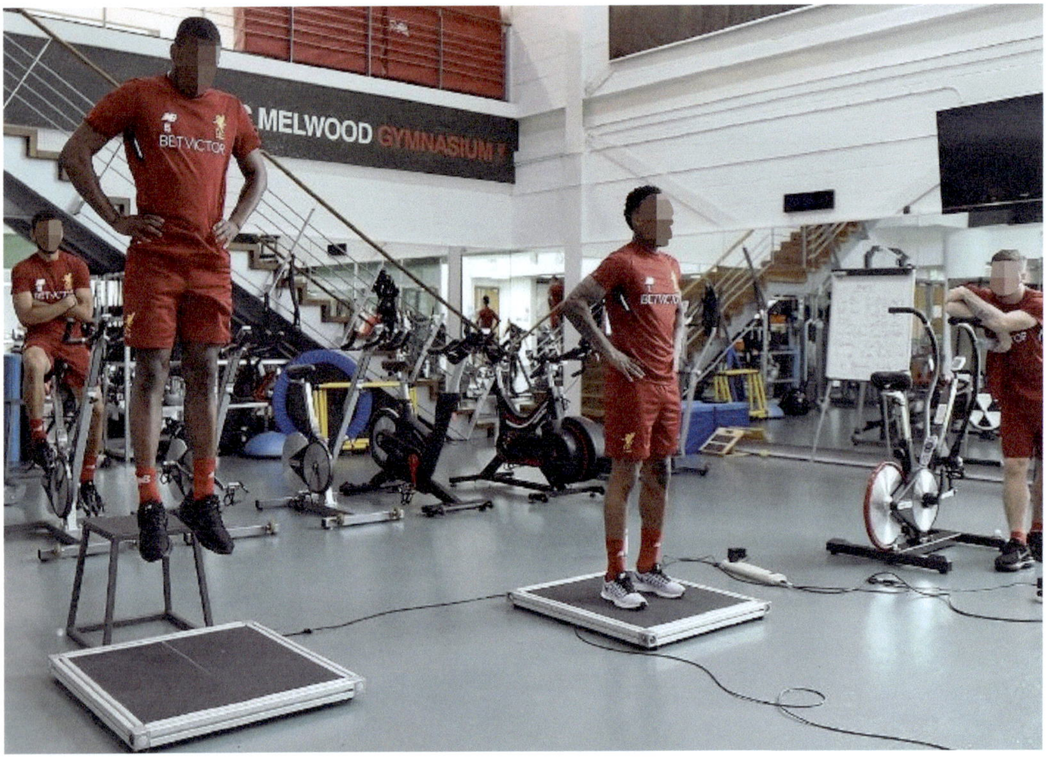

- T-running test: rotation time analysis left versus right.
- Rotation stress exercise.
  - Smooth knee flexion to achieve.
  - Pain-free ankle/knee rotation stress to achieve.
  - Symmetrical ankle dorsiflexion left versus right to achieve.

Conclusion

Syndesmotic injuries are increasingly common in the field and court sports. Injury severity, nuanced diagnosis, and long-term functional risk have led to significant advances in diagnosis and management protocols. Indeed, our approach to these athletes has changed considerably, even in the last decade. While there is an ongoing need for additional science to support new surgical stabilization constructs and accelerated return to sport protocols, the current management ethos has evolved toward flexible fixation device constructs and accelerated return to sport protocols. Perhaps the most valuable tools to inform our understanding of the results of evolving treatment strategies are sport registries which offer guidance for treatment protocols for athletes. Until data from such registries is evaluated and is broadly available, we rely on reports of outcomes from a rapidly evolving treatment landscape.

References

1. Lubberts B, D'Hooghe P, Bengtsson H, DiGiovanni CW, Calder J, Ekstrand J. Epidemiology and return to play following isolated syndesmotic injuries of the ankle: a prospective cohort study of 3677 male professional footballers in the UEFA elite Club injury study. Br J Sports Med. 2019;53(15):959–64.
2. van Dijk CN, Longo UG, Loppini M, et al. Classification and diagnosis of acute isolated syndesmotic injuries: ESSKA-AFAS consensus and guidelines. Knee Surg Sports Traumatol Arthrosc. 2016;24(4):1200–16.
3. Soin SP, Knight TA, Dinah AF, Mears SC, Swierstra BA, Belkoff SM. Suture-button versus screw fixation in a syndesmosis rupture model: a biomechanical comparison. Foot Ankle Int. 2009;30(4):346–52.
4. Shimozono Y, Hurley ET, Myerson CL, Murawski CD, Kennedy JG. Suture button versus syndesmotic screw for syndesmosis injuries: a meta-analysis of randomized controlled trials. Am J Sports Med. 2018;47(11):2764–71.
5. Grassi A, Samuelsson K, D'Hooghe P, Romagnoli M, Mosca M, Zaffagnini S, Amendola A. Dynamic stabilization of syndesmosis injuries reduces complications and reoperations as compared with screw fixation. Am J Sports Med. 2020;48(4):1000–13.
6. D'Hooghe P, Grassi A, Alkhelaifi K, et al. Return to play after surgery for isolated unstable syndesmotic ankle injuries (west point grade IIB and III) in 110 male professional football players: a retrospective cohort study. Br J Sports Med. 2019;54(19):1168–73. https://doi.org/10.1136/bjsports-2018-100298.

Deltoid Ligament Injury: When to Repair, Reconstruct, or Let It Heal

16

Matteo Guelfi and Jordi Vega

Introduction

The deltoid ligament (DL) can be affected by different pathological conditions, and acute or chronic DL injury is usually the result of an ankle sprain or chronic overload, as the case of a longstanding posterior tibialis dysfunction [1]. Injury of DL can result in medial ankle instability (MAI) or in rotational ankle instability (RAI).

MAI is defined as a medial giving way when walking or during sports, and typically, an asymmetric hindfoot valgus can be seen in relaxed position with weight bearing. Otherwise, RAI is defined as an abnormal talar rotation within the tibiofibular mortise. RAI is usually associated with chronic lateral collateral ligament injury with subsequently increased internal talar rotation, which may stretch out the anterior DL fascicles that have become overloaded [2].

Acute DL injuries usually involve pronation-external rotation or less common supination-external rotation sprains [3]. According to the trauma mechanism, the sprain may lead to lateral and/or medial malleolus fracture, syndesmosis injury, DL injury, or a combination of them. However, isolated DL injury is an uncommon observation [4, 5]. Surgical repair after acute DL injury is controversial, and usually a conservative therapy is proposed [6, 7]. When conservative therapy fails, patient can develop a MAI [8, 9].

Ankle inversion is the most common mechanism of injury [10], and injury to the lateral ligaments is observed as a result. Chronic ankle instability (CAI) as classically described is observed in 15–20% of patients after an acute ankle inversion sprain [11]. In CAI, an incompetent anterior talofibular ligament (ATFL) causes an increased anterolateral extrusion of talus out of the mortise, internal rotation of the talus, and superior translation [12]. These biomechanical changes may cause several intra-articular pathologies and degenerative arthritis. Injury of DL has been observed in as much as 40% of patients with CAI [13, 14]. It is estimated that 10% to 15% of patients with CAI will develop a RAI, although

M. Guelfi
Casa di Cura Villa Montallegro, Genoa, Italy

Department of Orthopaedic Surgery "Gruppo Policlinico di Monza", Clinica Salus, Alessandria, Italy

Human Anatomy and Embryology Unit, Department of Morphological Sciences, Universitat Autònoma de Barcelona, Barcelona, Spain

J. Vega (✉)
Laboratory of Arthroscopic and Surgical anatomy, Department of Pathology and Experimental Therapeutics (Human Anatomy Unit), University of Barcelona, Barcelona, Spain

Foot and Ankle Unit, iMove Traumatology-Clinica Tres Torres, and Hospital Quirón Barcelona, Barcelona, Spain

MIFAS by GRECMIP, Merignac, France

Clinique Montchoisi, Lausanne, Switzerland
e-mail: jordivega@ub.edu

P. D'Hooghe et al. (eds.), *Ligamentous Injuries of the Foot and Ankle*,
https://doi.org/10.1007/978-3-031-08682-3_16

in the authors' experience, this percentage may be underestimated [2, 15].

Clinical Presentation

Patients with both MAI and RAI may report a history of ankle sprain. As the underlying pathology involving the DL is different between MAI and RAI, they will be discussed separately through the chapter.

Patients with MAI may indicate medial and lateral ankle symptoms of pain, swelling, and tenderness or a combination of them. Several physical tests ranging from talar tilt test, valgus test, or external rotation test have been proposed to evaluate mechanical competence of the DL [8, 16, 17]. Frequently, no signs are observed in most patients, and these physical tests have been reported inadequate when evaluating MAI [18]. An asymmetric hindfoot valgus and pronation deformity can be typically seen with the weight bearing, whereas the patient is usually able to correct the deformity when asked to activate the posterior tibial tendon.

Patients with RAI report chronic symptoms of lateral ankle instability and medial ankle pain and tenderness located at the anterior area of the medial malleolus. Usually, medial symptoms appear after many years of lateral ankle symptoms. However, about 25% of patients never report medial ankle symptoms, and thus, the MAI remains neglected [2]. With loss of anterior DL restraint, the talus can anteriorly translate and externally rotate within the ankle mortise, which may result in a RAI.

With no intermediate DL fascicle injury, no valgus or pronation deformity is observed.

Deltoid Ligament Injury and Ankle Arthroscopy

In the last two decades, ankle arthroscopy has significantly evolved [19]. The usefulness of arthroscopy has been established for both the acute and chronic DL injury [2]. Arthroscopic assessment of DL injury is helpful when imaging studies are unable to observe ligament tear [19].

When DL injury is suspected, the arthroscopic examination should be completed with the camera introduced through the anterolateral portal and the probe through the anteromedial portal. Intra-articular fatty tissue generally occupies the central and medial aspect of the anterior ankle compartment, and it may be resected with a shaver to allow for full arthroscopic visualization of the anterior ankle compartment and gutters.

The medial gutter arthroscopic examination may include the medial malleolus and the DL. A thin fringe of cartilage covers the medial malleolus. This cartilage articulates with the medial wall of the talus. Next, a central fringe of the cortical bone and the insertion of the deep DL fascicles are observed from lateral to medial. In dorsiflexion, the deep DL fascicles can be seen on the floor of the medial gutter as a hammock between the medial wall of the talus and the medial malleolus. The anterior fascicles, the anterior tibiotalar and tibionavicular ligament, are attached to the anterior aspect of the anterior colliculus of the medial malleolus, while the tibiospring and tibiocalcaneal ligament are attached to the tip of the anterior colliculus of the medial malleolus. The DL posterior fascicle, composed of the posterior tibiotalar ligament, is not visible by anterior arthroscopy.

These anatomic features are crucial for DL injury recognition. Any arthroscopic vision that differs from the normally described on the medial gutter should raise the suspicion of a DL tear.

According to observations during open surgery, a specific classification of medial instability has been proposed by Hintermann et al. [8] This divided medial instability into proximal, intermediate, and distal injury of the DL.

Recently, an arthroscopic classification of medial ankle instability has been proposed [19]. According to DL injury location observed during arthroscopic procedure, DL injury can be divided into injury affecting the anterior fascicles (tibiotalar and tibionavicular ligaments) or the intermediate fascicles (tibiospring and tibiocalcaneal ligaments).

Injury affecting the anterior fascicle is described as the open-book lesion and it describes a RAI [13]. Open-book injury is only observed when talar internal rotation or the instruments

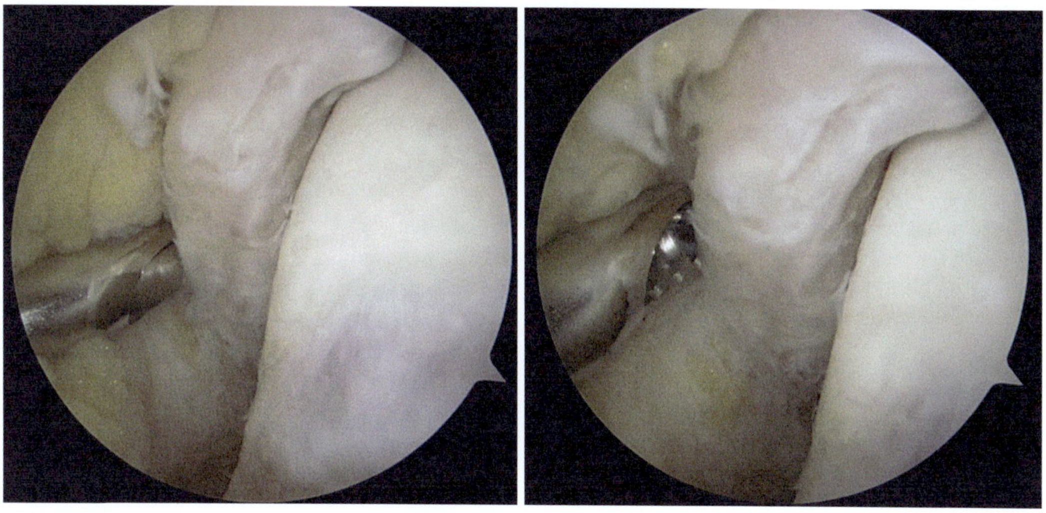

Fig. 16.1 Arthroscopic vision of a deltoid ligament "open-book" injury in a rotational ankle instability (left ankle). The instruments can separate the deltoid ligament from the medial malleolus at the anterior level

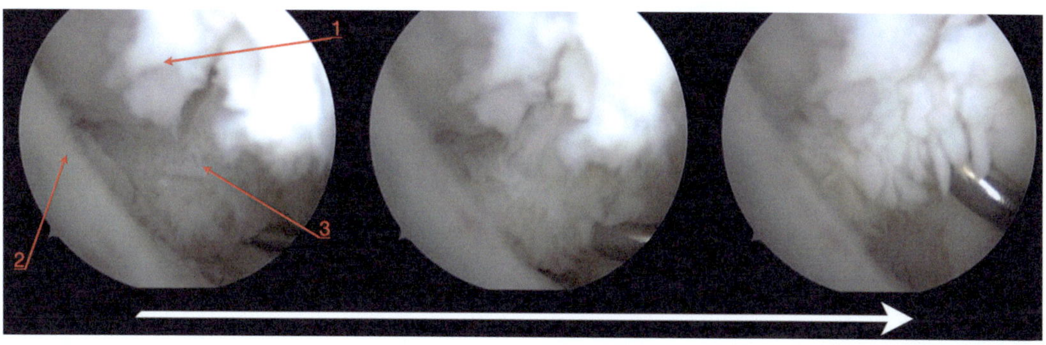

Fig. 16.2 Arthroscopic vision of a deltoid ligament injury in a medial ankle instability (right ankle) (1). Medial malleolus (anterior colliculus) (2). Medial wall of the talus (3). Deltoid ligament detached from the medial malleolus. With the help of a probe, deltoid ligament can be placed in contact with malleolus

push the ligament to medial. Then, the DL anterior fascicle is observed separated from the medial malleolus (Fig. 16.1). Open book can be graded into two types according to instruments passed through the space between the medial malleolus and the DL anterior fascicle.

Injury affecting the DL intermediate fascicle is observed in patients with MAI. As the deep DL fascicles are shorter than that from the superficial fascicles, deep DL fascicles are more prone to injury after an eversion ankle trauma. Although the DL deep fascicle can probably be injured along its length, the ligament injury has always been arthroscopically observed at the level of the medial malleolus attachment (in its anterior colliculus) and never at the midportion or talar attachment (Fig. 16.2). DL intermediate fascicle injury can be partial or complete [19].

Treatment of Deltoid Ligament Injury

Conservative Treatment

Acute injuries of DL are usually treated non-surgically using functional treatment with the goal of providing optimal healing circumstances by decreasing pain, swelling, and hematoma and to prevent further damage.

In patients of chronic DL injury, conservative treatment with the aim to improve ankle stability should be attempted before surgery [8]. This may include neuromuscular coordination training and muscular strengthening in particular of posterior tibial and peroneal muscles. Orthotics with a medial support or bracing may be used additionally to provide mechanical support.

When conservative treatment fails, a surgical procedure should be proposed in order to treat the ligament injury.

Open Treatment

Open DL repair is the current gold standard treatment when surgical treatment. It is usually performed through a slightly curved skin incision, starting 2 cm proximal to the medial malleolar tip and toward the navicular bone (Fig. 16.3). After blunt dissection, both the deltoid ligament and the posterior tibialis tendon are exposed. The posterior tibialis tendon, the DL, and the spring ligament are carefully explored. In most cases, the DL is injured at its proximal part, and the quality of the remnant allows for anatomical repair. In these cases, the tibial footprint of the DL is exposed and roughened. Then, with the ankle in neutral position, the ligament is reattached to the medial malleolus with the help of 3.5 mm or 4 mm suture anchors. The anchor should be placed in the anterior edge of the medial malleolus and 0.5 cm proximal to the tip of the malleolus (Fig. 16.4).

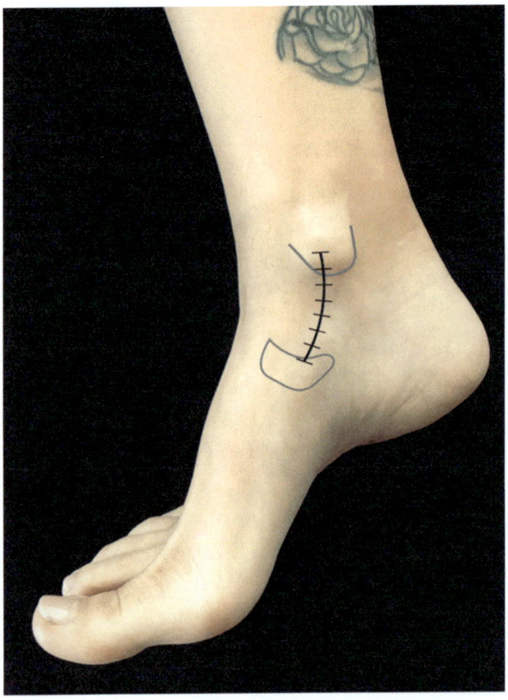

Fig. 16.3 Medial view of the ankle to show the skin incision to approach the deltoid ligament. Medial malleolus and navicular are highlighted

In patients where the ligament remnant has poor quality, direct repair of the DL may not be possible. In these cases, a DL reconstruction with a tendon graft should be considered.

Arthroscopic Treatment

The role of arthroscopy in treatment of ankle instability has increased during the last years. Given the success of arthroscopic lateral ankle ligament repair or reconstruction [20–22], some authors have evolved techniques for repairing the DL through an arthroscopic approach with the aim to decrease the postoperative recovery time and to facilitate an earlier return to full function [2, 23, 24].

Ankle arthroscopy is performed with the patient positioned in supine. A tight tourniquet is recommended and inflated. After highlighting cutaneous landmarks, two portals are used, anteromedial and anterolateral. The anteromedial portal is created first and placed at the ankle joint line just medial to the tibialis anterior tendon. The anterolateral portal is placed just lateral to the peroneus tertius tendon, paying attention not to injure the intermediate dorsocutaneous nerve, a branch of the superficial peroneal nerve (Fig. 16.5).

The arthroscope is first introduced through the anteromedial portal. It is recommended to use a protocolized arthroscopic evaluation of the ankle joint in order to detect all possible intra-articular pathologies. A non-distraction and ankle dorsi-

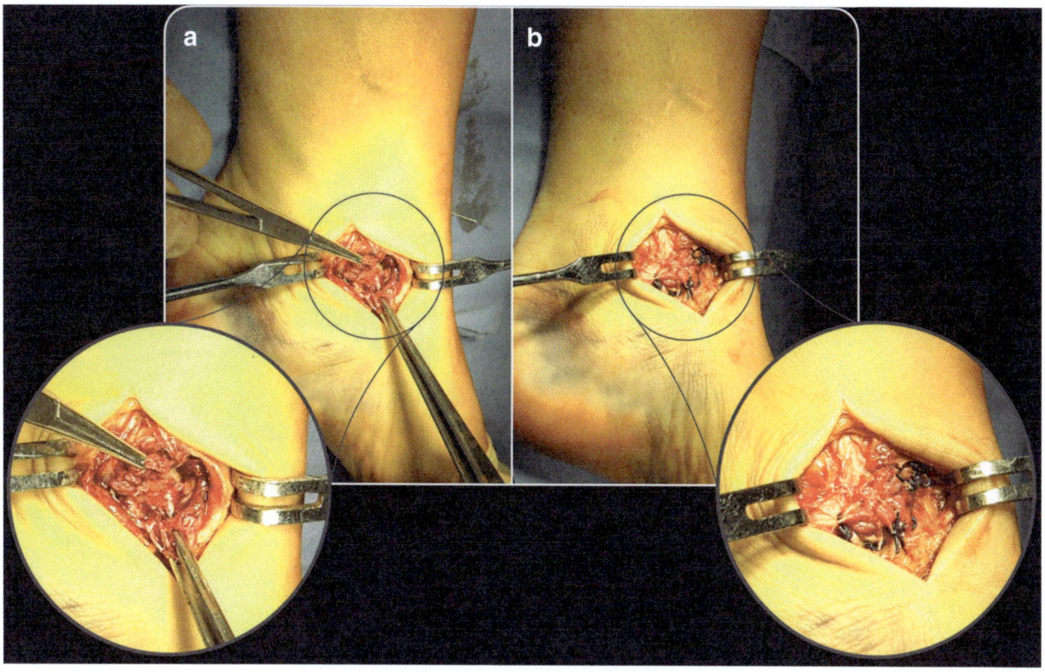

Fig. 16.4 Open approach to repair a deltoid ligament injury. Deltoid ligament injury is grasped with a mosquito clamp (**a**) and reattached to the medial malleolus with suture anchors (**b**)

flexion arthroscopic technique is recommended when gutters need to be explored [25]. Arthroscopic examination of the anterior ankle compartment when non-distraction and ankle dorsiflexion technique includes seven points [25]: (1) AITFL's distal fascicle, (2) ATFL's superior fascicle (lateral gutter), (3) lateral talar neck, (4) medial talar neck, (5) deep layer of DL and tip of the medial malleolus (medial gutter), (6) medial tibial angle (notch of Henry), and (7) anterior tibial rim.

After arthroscopic examination, concomitant intra-articular pathologies are addressed. Next, DL injury needs to be treated.

An arthroscopic-assisted technique treating DL injury has been described [23, 22]. Under arthroscopic view, suture anchors are inserted into the medial malleolus. Then, the ligament is percutaneously penetrated with sutures. It has been described as a safe procedure [23].

The arthroscopic all-inside DL repair with a knotless suture anchor technique was the first all-arthroscopic method treating DL injury [2]. With this procedure and without any percutaneous step, DL is repaired under direct arthroscopic view. The authors' preferred arthroscopic procedure utilized an ankle dorsiflexion technique without distraction and the anteromedial and anterolateral portals. After full arthroscopic examination and treatment of the secondary intra-articular injuries, the deltoid ligament is repaired under arthroscopic vision. The arthroscope is introduced through the anterolateral portal and directed toward the medial gutter. The medial malleolus footprint for the attachment of the deltoid ligament is debrided with a shaver introduced through the anteromedial portal. Under direct arthroscopic visualization, the area of the ligament detached is penetrated with a suture passer clamp, and the sutures subsequently grasp the ligament (Fig. 16.6). Next, the drill guide is placed through the anteromedial portal and centered over the medial malleolus (Fig. 16.7). The hole is drilled, and the bone anchor charged with the suture is introduced by impaction. As a knotless suture anchor technique, tensioning of the suture is adjusted before introduction of the anchor. The deltoid ligament is

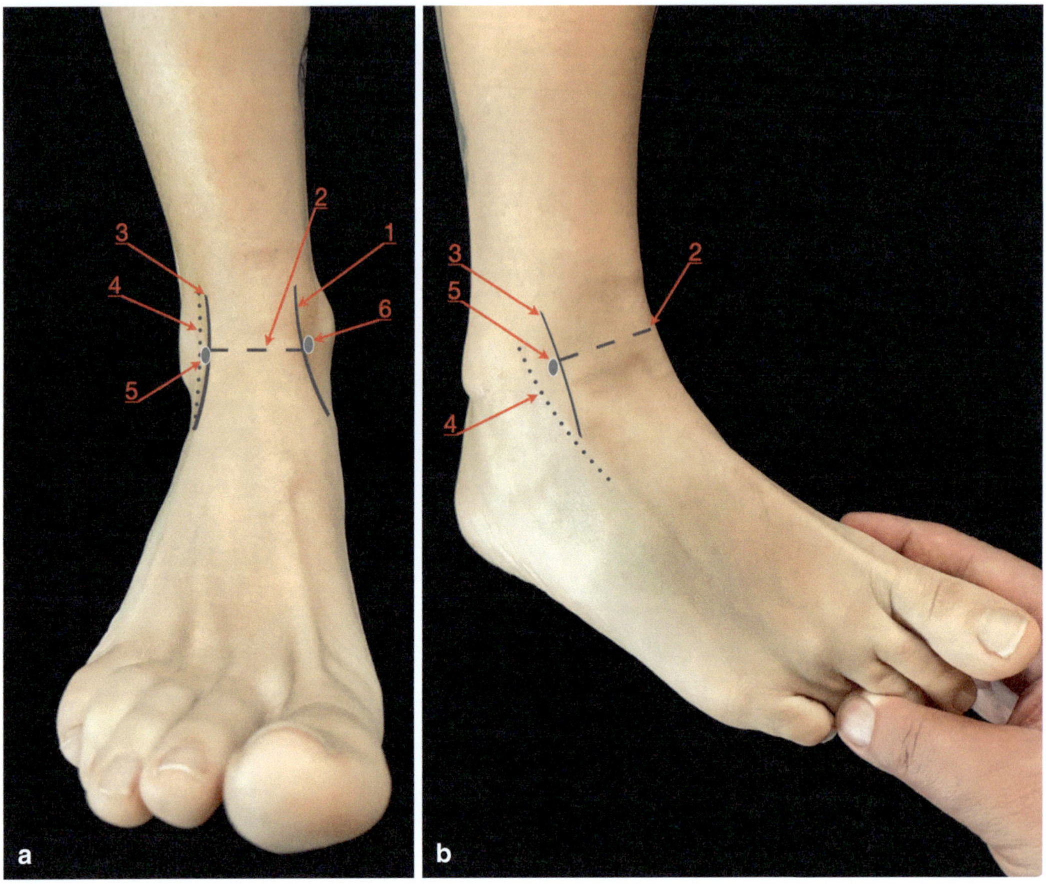

Fig. 16.5 Anterior (**a**) and anterolateral (**b**) view of the ankle to show the arthroscopic approaches to treat deltoid ligament injury. Cutaneous landmarks are highlighted: (1) anterior tibialis tendon (2). Joint line (3). Peroneus tertius tendon (4). Superficial peroneal nerve (dotted line) (5). Anterolateral portal (6). Anteromedial portal. (**b**) The anterolateral portal (5) is placed between the peroneus tertius (3) and the superficial peroneal nerve (4)

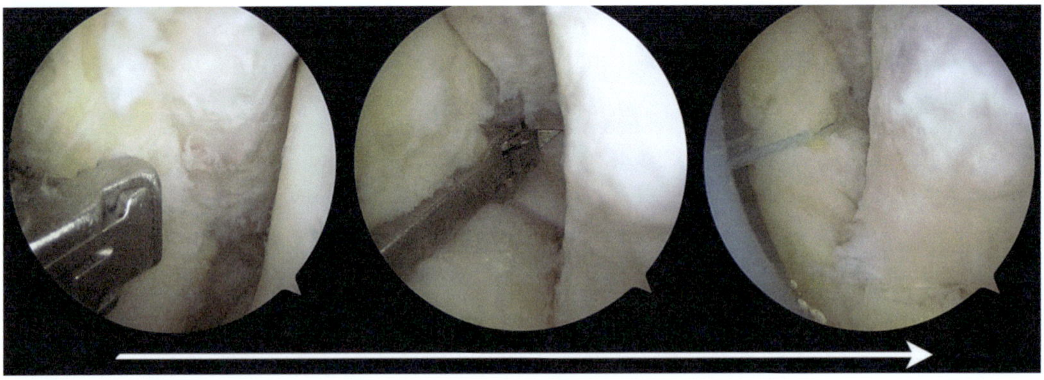

Fig. 16.6 Arthroscopic deltoid ligament repair. The deltoid ligament injury is grasped with the help of a suture passer

reattached with the ankle positioned in dorsiflexion and neutral rotation and varus-valgus (Fig. 16.8). Although excellent preliminary results with low rates of minor complications have been reported to treat RAI [2], it also can be used to treat MAI. In the author's experience, the

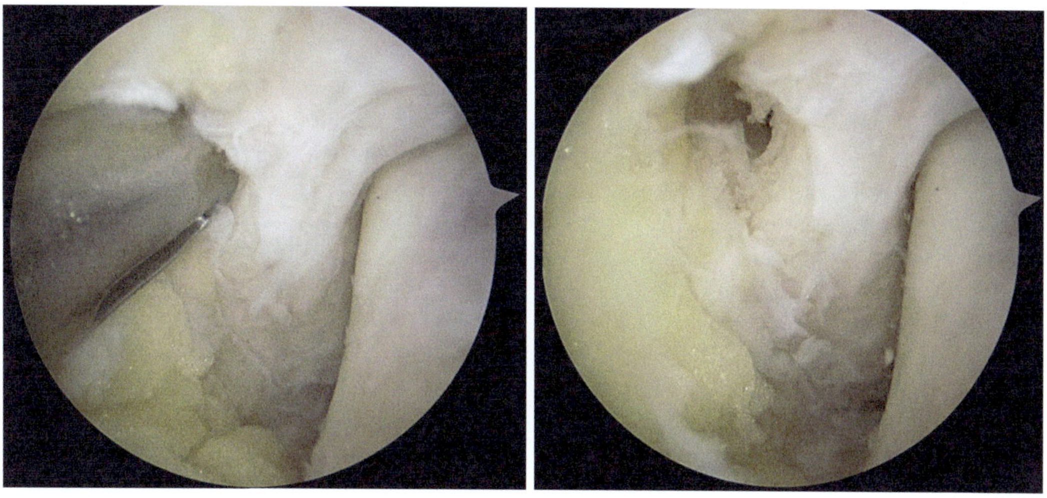

Fig. 16.7 Once the deltoid ligament is grasped, a tunnel for the bone anchor is performed at the anterior medial malleolus

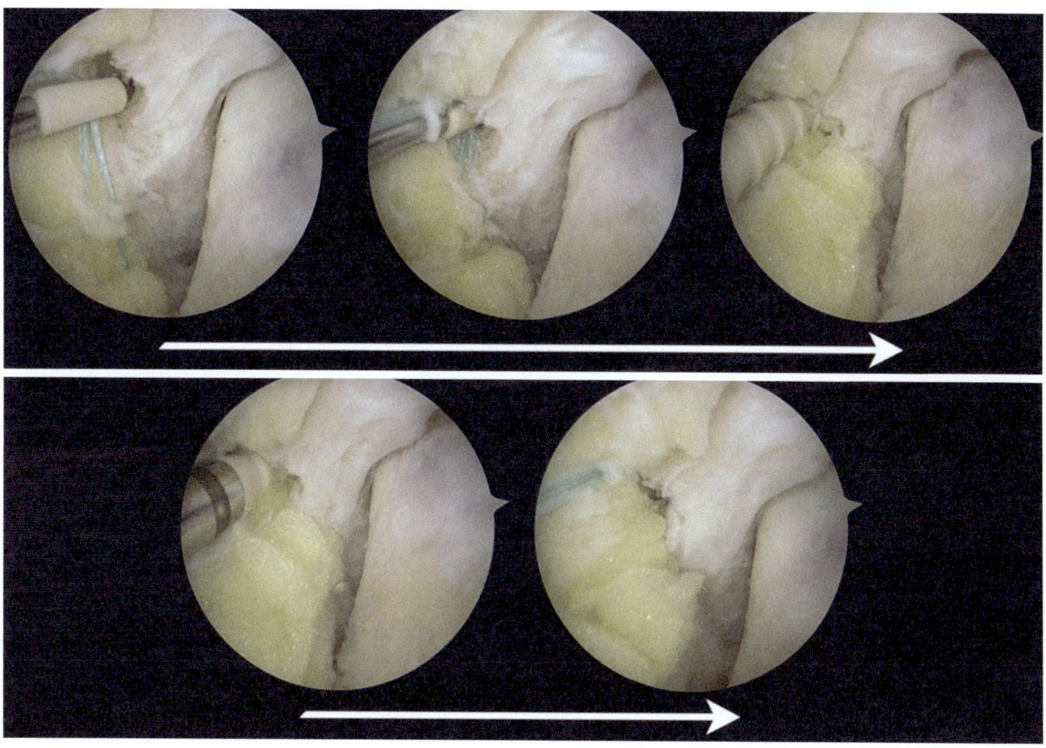

Fig. 16.8 The deltoid ligament is repaired after introduction of the knotless bone anchor charged with the sutures. The bone anchor is introduced by impaction

arthroscopic all-inside DL repair yields excellent results treating both RAI and MAI.

If associated with lateral collateral ligament injury, that should be addressed after completing the DL repair. The arthroscopic all-inside repair technique as previously reported is the authors' technique of choice [26–28].

As a general postoperative protocol, a removable walker boot is maintained for 3–4 weeks postoperatively at all times. Weight bearing as tolerated with the aid of crutches is encouraged when RAI; however, if MAI is treated, weight bearing is allowed after 3 weeks postoperatively. In cases of chondral or osteochondral injuries, no weight bearing is allowed for 4–6 weeks. Antithrombotic prophylaxis is indicated minimally for the first 15 days postoperatively. Once the walking boot is removed, active and passive range of motion exercises and gait training are encouraged. Two weeks later, strengthening in ankle dorsiflexion, plantar flexion, eversion, and inversion and proprioceptive training with weight bearing are initiated. Non-contact sports (swimming or cycling) are allowed 2 months postoperatively, and unrestricted sports, including contact sports, can be expected at 3 months depending on muscle conditioning.

To authors' knowledge, only a few studies are available in the literature reporting on arthroscopic treatment of DL injury [2, 23]. The arthroscopic-assisted DL repair associated with a percutaneous passage reported a 90% satisfaction rate in a group of 87 patients [23]. However, only 30 patients presented with MAI not associated with an ankle fracture. Of these 30 patients, only 6 reported a persistent ankle pain at final follow-up.

A combined arthroscopic all-inside repair of both lateral and medial ankle ligaments in 13 patients with the diagnosis of RAI was recently published [2]. All patients reported subjective improvement in ankle stability and returned to their daily activities without difficulties, except one patient who continued to experience medial ankle pain. Patients who had engaged in sports returned to their preinjury activity without limitations. The median AOFAS score increased from 70 (range 44–77) preoperatively to 100 (range 77–100) at the time of final follow-up. In all patients, the anterior drawer test and talar tilt test were negative on clinical examination. Five patients (38.5%) experienced ankle plantar flexion deficit compared to the contralateral side; the deficit was less than 10° in all cases. Two patients (15.4%) had a deficit of 5° or less in ankle dorsiflexion, reporting mild discomfort when squatting or kneeling. Deficit in range of motion was not considered a complication but as a consequence of the arthroscopic ankle stabilization. No major complications were reported.

Conclusion

According to damage location, DL injury can result in a MAI or in a RAI. MAI is the result of a DL intermediate fascicle injury secondary to an eversion giving way of the ankle. On the other hand, RAI is the result of a chronic lateral ankle instability that as a consequence of an increased internal talar rotation causes an open-book DL injury.

When conservative treatment fails, surgical treatment of the DL injury should be performed by an open or arthroscopic procedure. Open treatment allows to perform a DL repair with suture anchors or a reconstruction with tendon graft, depending on the quality of the ligament remnant. In the last years, given the success of arthroscopic treatment for lateral ankle instability, new arthroscopic techniques to address the DL injury were proposed with the aim to decrease the postoperative recovery time and to facilitate an earlier return to full function. Despite few studies are available in the literature about arthroscopic treatment of DL injury, preliminary results have showed promising clinical results. However, further clinical studies are needed to evaluate the clinical outcomes of arthroscopic treatment of DL injury.

References

1. Deland JT, de Asla RJ, Sung IH, et al. Posterior tibial tendon insufficiency: which ligaments are involved? Foot Ankle Int. 2005;26(6):427–35.
2. Vega J, Allmendinger J, Malagelada F, et al. Combined arthroscopic all-inside repair of lateral and medial ankle ligaments is an effective treatment for rotational ankle instability. Knee Surg Sports Traumatol Arthrosc. 2020;28(1):132–40.
3. Lauge-Hansen N. Fractures of the ankle. III. Genetic roentgenologic diagnosis of fractures of the ankle. Am J Roentgenol Radium Ther Nucl Med. 1954;71(3):456–71.

4. Ribbans WJ, Garde A. Tibialis posterior tendon and deltoid and spring ligament injuries in the elite athlete. Foot Ankle Clin. 2013;18(2):255–91.
5. Gerber JP, Williams GN, Scoville CR, et al. Persistent disability associated with ankle sprains: a prospective examination of an athletic population. Foot Ankle Int. 1998;19(10):653–60.
6. Lee TH, Jang KS, Choi GW, et al. The contribution of anterior deltoid ligament to ankle stability in isolated lateral malleolar fractures. Injury. 2016;47(7):1581–5.
7. Strömsöe K, Höqevold HE, Skjeldal S, et al. The repair of a ruptured deltoid ligament is not necessary in ankle fractures. J Bone Joint Surg Br. 1995;77(6):920–1.
8. Hintermann B. Medial ankle instability. Foot Ankle Clin. 2003;8(4):723–38.
9. Knupp M, Horn Lang T, Zwicky L, et al. Chronic ankle instability (medial and lateral). Clin Sports Med. 2015;34(4):679–88.
10. Ferran NA, Maffulli N. Epidemiology of sprains of the lateral ankle ligament complex. Foot Ankle Clin. 2006;11:659–62.
11. DiGiovanni BF, Partal G, Baumhauer JF. Acute ankle injury and chronic lateral instability in the athlete. Clin Sports Med. 2004;23(1):1–19.
12. Caputo AM, Lee JY, Spritzer CE, et al. In vivo kinematics of the tibiotalar joint after lateral ankle instability. Am J Sports Med. 2009;37(11):2241–8.
13. Hintermann B, Boss A, Schäfer D. Arthroscopic findings in patients with chronic ankle instability. Am J Sports Med. 2002;30(3):402–9.
14. Schäfer D, Hintermann B. Arthroscopic assessment of the chronic unstable ankle joint. Knee Surg Sports Traumatol Arthrosc. 1996;4(1):48–52.
15. Buchhorn T, Sabeti-Aschraf M, Dlaska CE, et al. Combined medial and lateral anatomic ligament reconstruction for chronic rotational instability of the ankle. Foot Ankle Int. 2011;32(12):1122–6.
16. Richardson DR. Ankle injuries. In: Canale ST, Beaty JH, editors. Campbell's operative orthopaedics. 11th ed. Philadelphia: Mosby Elsevier; 2007. p. 2353–89.
17. Beals TC, Crim J, Nickisch F. Deltoid ligament injuries in athletes: techniques of repair and reconstruction. Oper Tech Sports Med. 2010;18(1):11–7.
18. Van den Bekerom MP, Mutsaerts EL, Van Dijk CN. Evaluation of the integrity of the deltoid ligament in supination external rotation ankle fractures: a systematic review of the literature. Arch Orthop Trauma Surg. 2009;129(2):227–35.
19. Vega J, Guelfi M. Arthroscopic assessment and treatment of medial collateral ligament complex. Foot Ankle Clin. 2021;26(2):305–13. https://doi.org/10.1016/j.fcl.2021.03.005.
20. Vega J, Dalmau-Pastor M, Malagelada F, et al. Ankle arthroscopy: an update. J Bone Joint Surg Am. 2017;99(16):1395–407.
21. Acevedo JI, Palmer RC, Mangone PG. Arthroscopic treatment of ankle instability: Brostrom. Foot Ankle Clin. 2018;23(4):555–70.
22. Glazebrook M, Eid M, Alhadhoud M, et al. Percutaneous ankle reconstruction of lateral ligaments. Foot Ankle Clin. 2018;23(4):581–92.
23. Acevedo JI, Kreulen C, Cedeno AA, et al. Technique for arthroscopic deltoid ligament repair with description of safe zones. Foot Ankle Int. 2020;41(5):605–11.
24. Kim JG, Gwak HC, Lee MJ, et al. Arthroscopic deltoid repair: a technical tip. J Foot Ankle Surg. 2017;56(6):1253–6.
25. Dalmau-Pastor M, Malagelada F, Kerkhoffs GMMJ, et al. Redefining anterior ankle arthroscopic anatomy: medial and lateral ankle collateral ligaments are visible through dorsiflexion and non-distraction anterior ankle arthroscopy. Knee Surg Sports Traumatol Arthrosc. 2020;28(1):18–23.
26. Vega J, Guelfi M, Heyrani N, et al. Ankle microinstability. Tech Foot Ankle Surg. 2019;18(2):73–9.
27. Vega J, Golanó P, Pellegrino A, et al. All-inside arthroscopic lateral collateral ligament repair for ankle instability with a knotless suture anchor technique. Foot Ankle Int. 2013;34(12):1701–9.
28. Vega J, Guelfi M, Malagelada F, et al. Arthroscopic all-inside anterior talofibular ligament repair through a three-portal and no-ankle-distraction technique. JBJS Essent Surg Tech. 2018;8(3):1–11.

17 Spring Ligament Injuries and Instability: Repair/Reconstruction Indications and Techniques

Gordon Mackay and William Ribbans

Introduction

The spring (or calcaneonavicular) ligament is an important static stabiliser of the medial foot column. Following damage, its role in the development of foot deformity has been discussed over the last few decades.

Its precise anatomy has been debated, and only since the advent of MRI scanning has its structure (and pathology) been clearly imaged. Clinical signs pathognomonic of its failure are few and not validated. Its frequent involvement with other adjacent damaged structures has clouded our understanding of its contribution to the patient's symptoms and observed disability. Even at surgery, inspection of the entire ligament complex is restricted.

However, clinicians have increasingly recognised that a functioning spring ligament (or its substitute) enhances the restoration of normal foot posture and post-operative patient outcomes.

G. Mackay (✉)
University of Stirling, Stirling, UK
e-mail: office@mackayclinic.co.uk

W. Ribbans
University of Northampton, Northampton, UK
e-mail: billribbans@billribbans.com

Anatomy of the Spring Ligament

Chopart's level of the foot contains two articulations. It links the hindfoot to the midfoot. Its lateral column, involving the calcaneocuboid joint, is relatively rigid and stable. The medial column is more flexible and contains the talocalcaneonavicular joint.

Talocalcaneonavicular Joint Complex (Fig. 17.1)

The talocalcaneonavicular joint comprises an articulation between:

- Talar head.
- *Acetabulum pedis*. This was first described by Sarrafian [1] and includes a combination of:
  - Anterior and middle articular facets of the calcaneum.
  - Talar articular surface of the navicular.
  - Spring ligament.

Talocalcaneonavicular joint flexibility requires adequate ligamentous support from:

P. D'Hooghe et al. (eds.), *Ligamentous Injuries of the Foot and Ankle*,
https://doi.org/10.1007/978-3-031-08682-3_17

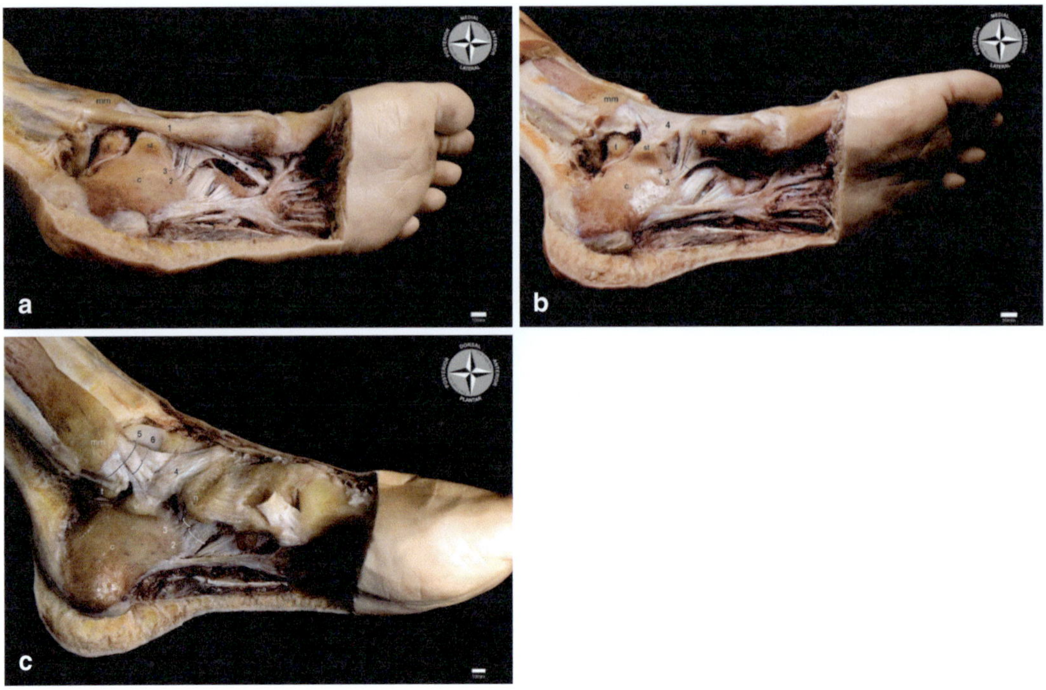

Fig. 17.1 Spring ligament anatomy. *mm* medial malleolus, *n* navicular, *c* calcaneus, *st* sustentaculum tali, ** tibialis posterior projections into the midfoot. (1) Tibialis posterior tendon, (2) Inferior calcaneonavicular ligament (ICNL), (3) Third ligament, or medioplantar oblique ligament (TCNL), (4) Superomedial calcaneonavicular ligament (SMCNL), (5) Deltoid ligament-tibiotalar ligament, (6) Deltoid ligament-tibiocalcaneal part. (Courtesy of Associate Professor Quentin Fogg, University of Melbourne)

- Talonavicular ligament.
- Spring ligament.
- Tibionavicular part of the superficial component of the deltoid ligament.

Components of the Spring Ligament

The extent and number of components of the spring ligament varies in different publications, but four elements have been described [2–8].

- **Superomedial calcaneonavicular ligament (SMCNL)**
- SMCNL is the most medial and largest of the spring ligament components. It is twice as strong as the ICNL [4]. It is described variously as triangular, quadrangular and hammock shaped.

Its origin is the entire anterior margin of the subtalar joint middle facet (sustentaculum tali). It inserts onto the superior, medial and inferior margins of the medial side of the navicular articular margin. Its most medial and superficial fibres are intimately connected to the distal part of the tibialis posterior tendon (TPT) which runs inferior to it. With the TPT, it acts as a load-bearing sling for the talar head.

Part of the deep surface of the SMCNL is covered with articular fibrocartilage forming an articulation with the inferior aspect of the medial side of the talus. This is termed the *spring ligament fibrocartilaginous complex* and is thought to have formed in response to the repetitive loads to which it is subjected.

- **Inferoplantar longitudinal calcaneonavicular ligament (ICNL)**

ICNL is the most lateral of the spring ligament components. It is short, broad and described as trapezoidal with two distinct fascicles [9]. It arises from a concavity (coronoid fossa) between the anterior and middle facets of the subtalar joint and passes to the lateral navicular beak. ICNL displays histologically longitudinal fibres laid down in the line of tensile stresses to which it is primarily subjected [4]. ICNL is separated from the TCNL and SMCNL by fat close to their respective navicular insertions.

- **Third (medioplantar oblique) calcaneonavicular ligament (TCNL)**

  The third ligament lies between the SMCNL and ICNL and first described in 2003 [7]. It is strip-like and originates from the anterior and middle facets of the calcaneum medial to the ICNL. It attaches to the navicular tuberosity.
- **Tibiospring ligament**

  The tibiospring ligament is one of the four parts of the superficial deltoid (medial) ligament of the ankle joint [10]. It arises from the anterior colliculus of the medial malleolus posterior to the tibionavicular ligament and anterior to the tibiocalcaneal ligament.

  It has no distal bony insertion but instead attaches to the proximal fibres of SMCNL. It becomes taut in ankle eversion and plantar flexion and influences tension within SMCNL. This function emphasises the combined activity of the deltoid and spring ligaments (in conjunction with TPT) in stabilising the medial structures of the ankle and hind- and midfoot.

  The spring ligament's blood supply is derived from intra-osseous sources at its different components' origins and insertions and from penetrating branches from the medial plantar and calcaneal arteries [4]. The mid-portion of the ligament is relatively avascular.

Functions of the Spring Ligament

TPT is the most important dynamic stabiliser of the medial longitudinal arch, but research has established that isolated TPT insufficiency does not necessarily result in AAFD [11, 12].

The spring ligament helps maintain arch height and stability and resist forefoot abduction. It resists the tendency for the talar head to displace medially and inferiorly as commonly observed in AAFD.

Several ligaments appear important in maintaining arch height [13]:

- Plantar fascia.
- Long and short plantar ligaments.
- Spring ligament.
- Medial talocalcaneal ligament.
- Talocalcaneal interosseous ligament.
- Tibionavicular part of the deltoid ligament.

The spring ligament has been reported to be less important than other structures, especially the plantar fascia, in maintaining arch height. One computational model reported the spring ligament contributed only 8% of the total ligament contribution to arch stability – the plantar fascia contributing 79.5% [14]. A cadaveric model, involving sequential division of ligaments, revealed that the plantar fascia was the most important contributor to medial arch stiffness [15].

Conversely, others have regarded the spring ligament as important in maintaining medial arch stability and acting as a sling for the talar head [4, 16]. SMCNL has properties suggestive of a significant load-bearing function, while ICNL has more of a pure tensile load function.

Pasapula [17] reported that spring ligament division increased translation on applying a lateral force to the foot. Surgical repair of the ligament or reconstruction of the TPT with the flexor digitorum longus (FDL) tendon failed to arrest this deformity commonly seen in AAFD. However, spring ligament augmentation utilising the *Internal*Brace with FibreTape (*Arthrex,* Naples, Florida) returned the biomechanics to normal. Jennings [12] found that division of the spring ligament in cadavers produced instability which was uncompensated for by active tibialis posterior contraction. They considered that the spring ligament was the main stabiliser of the arch during midstance.

Conversely, Deland [18] found that spring ligament sectioning alone in a cadaver did not produce immediate major deformity. However, subsequent cyclical loading of the foot, deprived of an intact spring ligament, caused progressive deformity.

Injury to the Spring Ligament

The overwhelming majority of spring ligament injuries occur in conjunction with TPT dysfunction. The combination has been reported in 70–92% of patients at surgery and on MR imaging [19–21]. The most common element of the spring ligament injured is the SMCNL [18, 20]. ICNL injury is rarer [18].

Traditionally, it was believed that isolated spring ligament ruptures were incapable of producing the planovalgus deformity observed in AAFD. Instead weakening of the TPT produces increasing spring ligament strain leading to progressive failure of the latter [18, 22]. This concept has been challenged by some recent researchers who have emphasised the importance of spring ligament disease in the initial development of AAFD [12, 17, 23–25].

Isolated injuries to the spring ligament have been occasionally reported in the literature but not with great frequency [18, 26–33]. Whereas the SMCNL is most commonly implicated in isolated injuries, a complete rupture of the spring ligament complex can occur in traumatic talonavicular dislocations [34].

Explosive athletic events [26] place significant strain upon the ligament. Repetition can produce microtrauma and degenerative change and, rarely, sudden catastrophic rupture.

Most spring ligament tears occur in the distal part of the SMCNL [22]. Spring ligament tears vary in orientation and position. Most appear as transverse tears of SMCNL on MR imaging [35, 36] and at surgery [18, 37]. Hintermann [37] noted that the ligament tears at surgery were usually larger than expected, often distally placed with several patterns, including longitudinal L-shaped tears. Hintermann recorded combined injuries of the spring ligament with the deltoid tibionavicular ligament and in association with TPT lengthening.

Clinical Features of Spring Ligament/Instability

In an isolated injury, the patient frequently identifies the injury mechanism. Acute injury is usually caused by a pronatory force producing initial medial swelling and bruising. Tenderness persists on the medial and plantar aspects of the foot in line with the SMCNL.

A more chronic, but isolated, progressive weakening of the spring ligament can occur when subjected to high stresses often in association with an excessive BMI [29]. Additionally, high loading of the ligament complex during repetitive high-impact sports, e.g. triple jumping, can produce similar injuries.

In cases of isolated injury, the patient retains normal TPT strength. Hintermann demonstrated how TPT activation corrects the medial arch height in the standing patient (Fig. 17.2). Pasapula described the 'neutral heel lateral push test' per-

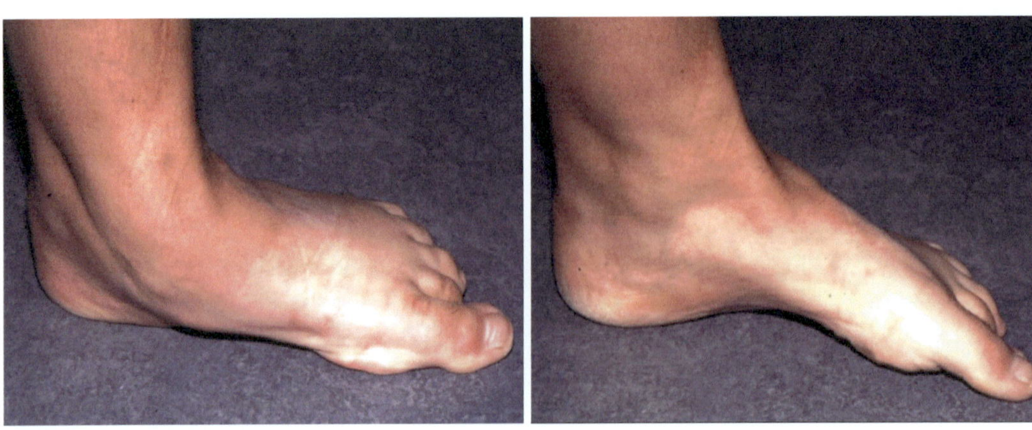

Fig. 17.2 TPT activation correcting flatfoot deformity. (Courtesy Professor Hintermann)

formed with the patient seated and the heel held in neutral while an abduction force is applied to the forefoot. A deficient spring ligament will allow excessive lateral translation [38]. The test is yet to be validated.

Unrecognised and extensive spring ligament tears are capable of producing progressive medial arch collapse, hindfoot valgus deformity and forefoot abduction.

Borton's case report [26] could not perform repetitive single heel raises or actively invert the heel. Tryfonidis [29] described nine patients with isolated spring ligament injuries retaining the ability to both single-stance tiptoe and correct their medial arch height but without correction of the heel valgus translation or any persistent forefoot abduction.

In association with TPT dysfunction, individual assessment of spring ligament function is more difficult and usually reliant on imaging and operative findings.

Classification of Spring Ligament Injuries

Gazdag [20] classified spring ligament injuries based upon surgical observations during TPT reconstruction with concomitant spring ligament injury (Table 17.1).

Pasapula reclassified conventional staging systems for AAFD incorporating the theory that the spring ligament is the primary pathology in this condition [17, 25] (Table 17.2).

Hintermann [37] included spring ligament injury combined with deltoid tibionavicular ligament injury as a Type III (distal) lesion in his classification of medial ankle instability.

Table 17.2 Pasapula's biomechanical staging system for AAFD incorporating spring ligament failure

Stage	Pathology	Test
Stage 0	Spring ligament failure	Lateral push positive
Stage 1	Spring ligament failure and tibialis synovitis	Lateral push positive and retromalleolar tenderness
Stage 2	1st TMT plantar ligament failure causing and driving hindfoot valgus and hence planovalgus	Positive Dynamic Hicks test Positive Klaue test
Stage 2b	First TMT failure and fixed dorsiflexed first ray or fixed supination deformity with hindfoot reduced	Hintermann's positive metatarsal rise sign
Stage 3	Fixed hindfoot valgus	Hindfoot Rigid non-correctible
Stage 3b	Fixed hindfoot valgus with degeneration	Hindfoot rigid Tender and non-correctible
Stage 4	Deltoid failure	Excess valgus

From: Pasapula C, Shariff S, Cutts S, West J, Kobezda T. Adult Acquired Flat Foot: A New Biomechanical Classification for the Deformity Based on two Point Failure of the Medial Column. Clinical Research on Foot and Ankle. 2018;6(2):1–7

Table 17.1 Gazdag classification of spring ligament injury

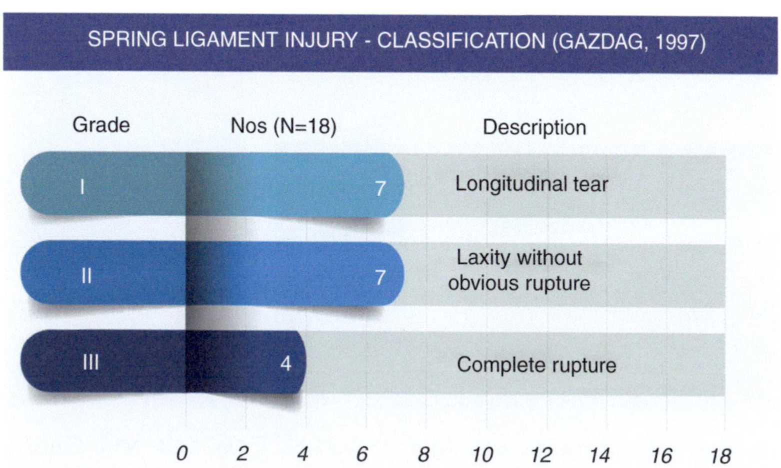

Imaging of the Spring Ligament

Plain X-Ray

X-rays should be the initial imaging for suspected spring ligament injury either in isolation or associated with TPT pathology. Weight-bearing AP and lateral views of the foot and ankle combined with oblique foot images are routine. Additional Saltzmann views [39] for hindfoot alignment provide a comprehensive assessment for alignment, deformity and degenerative change.

Plain radiography in the chronic situation, especially in relation to TPT dysfunction, may demonstrate midfoot sag, hindfoot valgus and midfoot abduction. Angles >5° for the first metatarsal-talus angle on weight-bearing anteroposterior (AP) and lateral radiographs (Meary's angle; Fig. 17.3) and more than 30% of talar head uncovering on AP weight-bearing X-rays are strongly associated with spring ligament disease [23].

Further imaging of the spring ligament requires MRI and/or ultrasound.

Ultrasound

Ultrasound has a limited role in spring ligament pathology assessment particularly in visualisation of ICNL. However, SMCNL is more readily identifiable with a 94% concordance between ultrasound and MRI for spring ligament injury [40, 41].

Ultrasound can simultaneously examine the TPT for any pathology.

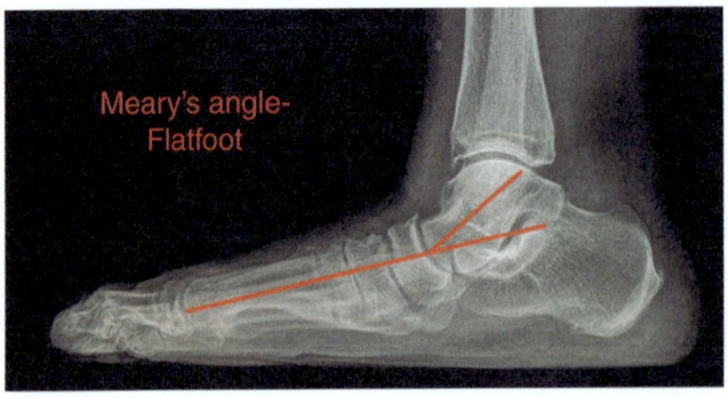

Fig. 17.3 Weight-bearing lateral X-ray of the foot illustrating Meary's angle in flatfoot. Image Library

MRI

MRI is the imaging modality of choice for visualising the spring ligament [35, 36, 42–44].

Like ultrasound, MRI is more reliable for SMCNL assessment than other components and well visualised on axial and coronal views. Normal SMCNL thickness is 2–4 mm. Acute SMCNL injuries are associated with ligament gapping and soft-tissue and osseous oedema with haematoma formation (Fig. 17.4).

Chronic injuries occur most commonly in conjunction with TPT abnormalities. Disorders of SMCNL on MRI evaluation were reported as having 54–77% sensitivity and 100% specificity in detecting pathology [35]. SMCNL may be thinned (<2 mm) and thickened (>5 mm) by disease [35, 36]. As well as demonstrating partial or complete tears, disruptions between the tibiospring and SMCNL have been reported. 'Normal' patients may show apparent spring ligament abnormalities (17–28%) on MRI [35, 36].

ICNL is smaller with a thickness of 2–6 mm. It is less easily visualised on MRI, but specific sequences have been described to examine this component [45]. The proximal ICNL may exhibit lack of homogeneity on MRI, and this should not be interpreted as necessarily pathological [36]. The TCNL has a thickness of between 1 and 5 mm and separated from the ICNL by fat [36, 43].

MRI is excellent at demonstrating associated TPT pathology and deltoid ligament pathology.

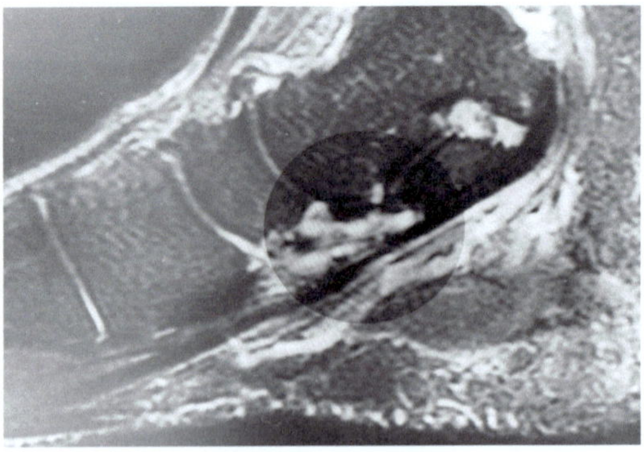

Fig. 17.4 MRI Partial tear of the spring ligament. Courtesy Mackay Clinic

In AAFD cases, it has been reported that MRI reveals TPT pathology in 100%, spring ligament problems in 87% and deltoid damage in 33% [46]. Additionally, it reveals problems in adjacent structures including degenerative joint damage, tarsal tunnel anomalies and congenital tarsal coalitions.

Conservative Treatment for Spring Ligament Injury and Instability

For acute partial spring ligament injury, it is reasonable to rest the foot in a non-weight-bearing cast for up to 6 weeks followed by progressive rehabilitation. Subsequently any biomechanical issues need to be addressed, full strength and proprioception restored and required orthotic supports provided.

Tryfonidis [29] treated six out of nine patients with acute partial SMCNL tears with orthotics. These patients had evidence of surrounding soft-tissue oedema and bleeding but no clinical or plain imaging deformity.

There is little place for conservative treatment for acute complete tears or chronic injury with progressive deformity in active younger patients. Older more sedentary patients and those with significant co-morbidities may be treated in a similar fashion to acute partial spring ligament pathology.

Surgical Treatment for Spring Ligament Injury and Instability

Surgical management options for spring ligament damage depend upon the scope of pathology being addressed. Is it being repaired or reconstructed as part of a more extensive procedure to correct a flexible (Stage IIB) flatfoot deformity (secondary to TPT dysfunction) or as an isolated injury?

It is in combination with TPT dysfunction where most surgical experience has been gained. However, the value of a specific spring ligament repair in such circumstances has been a matter of controversy.

Mann [47] reported no difference in outcomes between 49 patients receiving no spring ligament repair and 26 repaired during TPT reconstruction. Zanolli reported no improvement in deformity correction when a spring ligament reconstruction was added to conventional procedures (FDL transfer and various calcaneal osteotomies in cadaver models) [48].

Others report that a spring ligament reconstruction in IIB flexible AAFD may spare additional osseous (e.g. osteotomies) or articular procedures (fusions) [49]. A 2002 review of surgical practice revealed that 53% of American orthopaedic surgeons repair the SMCNL as part of routine reconstruction for AAFD [50].

When planning a spring ligament operation, the surgeon should address several questions (Fig. 17.5).

The ligament is approached surgically through the classical medial incision used to expose the tibialis posterior tendon, medial navicular and FDL tendon. Placing the ankle in full inversion and retracting the TPT inferiorly improves visualisation [14].

Spring Ligament Repair

Direct repair is possible if the injury is relatively recent with no chronic degeneration and/or attenuation.

Various techniques have been described in case reports and small series:

- Direct repair +/− resection of lesion ends [20, 29, 37, 51, 52].
- 'Vest over pants' repair [26].
- Ligament advancement and plication +/− trans-osseous navicular drill holes [32, 53].
- Endoscopic repair using the TPT endoscopy portal [54].

However, most techniques described above had additional reinforcement or protective procedures, including FDL transfer [20, 26, 29], medialising calcaneal osteotomy [29], and reinforcement with either the tendon graft used to reconstruct the incompetent PTT [53], a Cobb

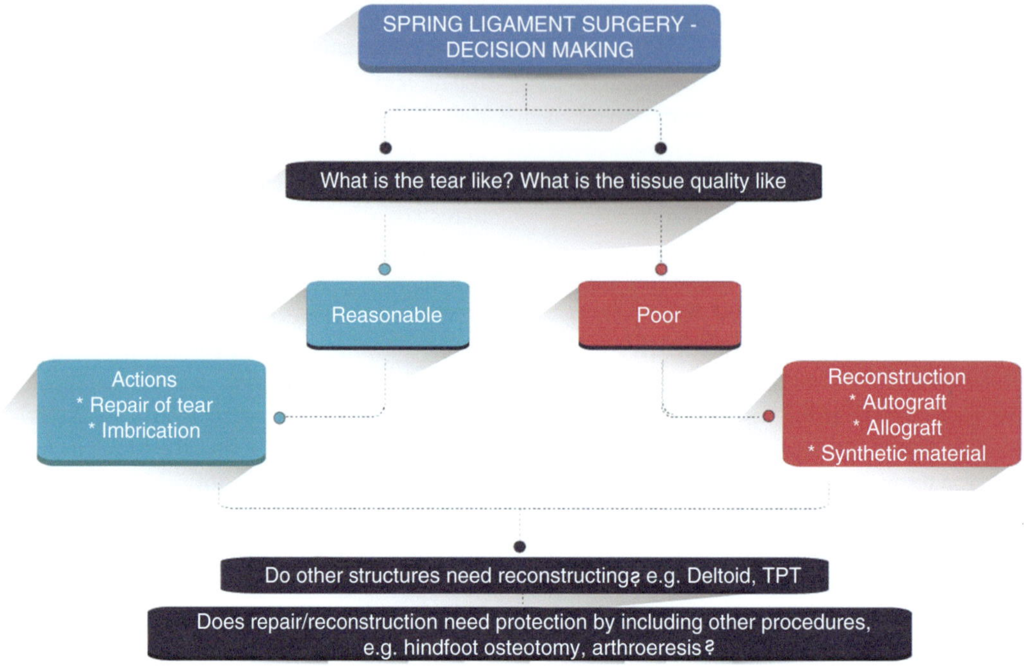

Fig. 17.5 Considerations for surgical repair of spring ligament

repair modification (split tibialis anterior tendon) [20], or use of the distal stump of the TPT [20].

Gazdag [20] reported 78% had excellent results with a follow-up between 24 and 40 months using a combination of spring ligament repair and FDL transfer.

Spring Ligament Reconstruction

Many times, direct repair will not be possible because of the poor quality of the damaged ligament. Therefore, various techniques for reconstruction using autografts, allografts or synthetic materials have been described.

Cadaver Studies

Different tissue types have been tested experimentally using cadavers but have either failed initial biomechanical testing or not translated into viable options for patients. These include the use of the anterior fibres of the deltoid ligament [55] Achilles tendon transfer [56] and tibialis anterior tendon transfer [56].

Various techniques using the peroneus longus tendon (PLT) have been described. These involve different harvesting, routing and fixation techniques in both cadavers and patients [18, 49, 56–58]. Baxter compared different methods of medial ligament reconstruction using PLTs and found that anatomic reconstruction of the spring ligament provided the least correction. Conversely, combined reconstruction of the SMCNL and anterior superficial components of the deltoid ligament provided 2–4 times the amount of hindfoot and talonavicular deformity correction [58].

Choi [57] and Thordarson [56] described spring ligament reconstruction using PLT in cadavers. Choi divided the PLT proximal to the lateral malleolus and passed it through a medial incision retaining its attachment to the first metatarsal base. By harvesting the PLT, it loses first ray plantar flexion function but is balanced by the loss of PLT's eversion and abduction activity.

Tan used a split tibialis anterior tendon to span from the talar neck to the medial cuneiform and reported radiographic improvement in key AAFD parameters [59].

Clinical Studies

Autograft Transfers

Deland [18] described one patient who had undergone a reconstruction using PLT, and Williams [49] described a series of 14 feet (13 patients) who had a spring ligament reconstruction using a PLT autograft. The technique was utilised in patients with persistent forefoot abduction or talonavicular sag after hindfoot osteotomies, including lateral column lengthening. In Williams' series, 11 patients (79%) obtained satisfactory or excellent results [49].

Lee used the FHL tendon to replace both the diseased spring ligament and TPT. In 23 patients, they transected the FHL distally and rerouted it through the medial cuneiform and navicular before anchoring it to the sustentaculum tali. This provided a static substitute for the spring ligament and dynamic substitute for TPT. Both clinical and radiological parameters improved at follow-up [60].

The diseased TPT is usually resected and discarded during surgery to correct AAFD. However, several authors have advocated using its distal portion to reconstruct the spring ligament [3, 61].

Synthetic Materials

Use of autografts during TPT reconstructive surgery involves additional operative time and potential harvest site morbidity and weakness following tendon transfer. Interest has turned to the use of synthetic materials to reconstruct/augment the spring ligament.

One of the authors (WJR) has used a polycaprolactone-based polyurethane scaffold (*Artelon, Lavender Medical*) to allow for host tissue ingrowth to reconstruct a torn or incompetent spring ligament and overlain it with the distal part of TPT [62].

FibreTape as part of the *Internal*Brace construct (Arthrex, Naples, Florida) has been developed in conjunction with one of the authors (GM) for a range of uses in orthopaedics and has been adapted for spring ligament reconstruction.

Acevedo described combining direct ligament repair and augmentation for both SMCNL and ICNL elements. Following proximal FibreTape anchoring, one limb is passed dorsal and the other inferior to the navicular. Both limbs are passed through the same tunnel as the FDL transfer and anchored together. All 26 patients had an additional FDL transfer, and 25 had a medial displacement calcaneal osteotomy (MDCO). All but one procedure was successful, and improved deformity correction was reported with the addition of the FibreTape [63]. Palmanovich [64] used the FibreTape with different distal anchoring position to augment direct repairs of the spring ligament. In five isolated spring ligament injuries, the author reported excellent long-term improvement in function [33] (Fig. 17.6).

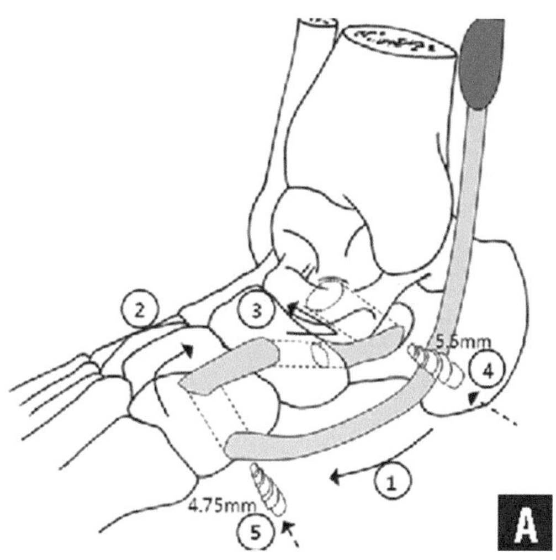

Fig. 17.6 Schematic illustration showing the FHL tendon transfer graft insertion sequence. First, the flexor hallucis longus tendon is passed from plantar to dorsal through the medial cuneiform. Next, the graft is passed from dorsal to plantar through the navicular. This is followed by going medial to lateral through the sustentaculum tali. The graft is secured to the sustentaculum tali with a 5.5 mm bioabsorbable interference screw. Additional fixation can be applied to the medial cuneiform and navicular to ensure stability of the graft. (From: Lee WC, Yi Y. Spring ligament reconstruction using the autogenous flexor hallucis longus tendon. Orthopedics 2014;37(7):467–71)

Combined Spring and Deltoid Ligament Repair

In the knowledge that the spring-deltoid ligament complex acts in unison, concomitant injuries to both structures are often observed on imaging and there is improved correction in cadaver models following combined reconstruction with PL tendon [58], recent authors have advocated extending the surgery to involve reinforcement of the deltoid ligament.

Brodell [65] used an allograft to reconstruct the tibiocalcaneonavicular ligament (TCNL) (combined anterior superficial deltoid and SMCNL) combined with osseous reconstructions. In 14 cases of peri-talar instability in the presence of AAFD, the authors reported significant improvement in clinical and radiographic parameters.

Nery [46] and Bastias [9] have described the use of FibreTape to augment the spring and deltoid ligaments. Nery reported successful outcomes in ten cases (Figs. 17.7 and 17.8).

Additional Procedures

Most cadaveric and clinical work involving spring ligament surgery has included additional procedures.

These include tendon transfers (e.g. FDL) for TPT pathology and additional bone procedures (MDCO, lateral column lengthening, medial cuneiform osteotomy) for protection of soft-tissue work and to promote deformity correction. Otis [66] produced cadaver evidence that MDCOs unload the spring ligament. Lateral column lengthening reduces talonavicular abduction and SMCNL tension [49].

Post-Operative Rehabilitation

The various combinations of procedures to stabilise failing medial column structures are major operations for patients to recover from. There is no consensus as to the length of time patients should spend in each stage of post-operative recovery.

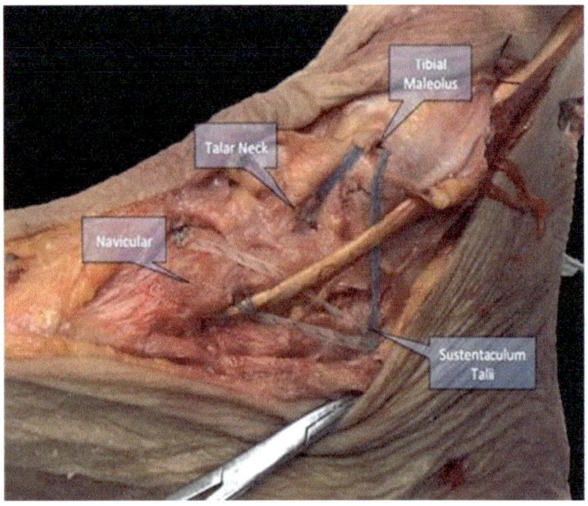

Fig. 17.8 Internal bracing of spring ligament (Figs. 17.7a) and in combination with deltoid ligament (Figs. 17.7b). (Courtesy of Dr. Caio Nery, Sao Paulo, Brazil)

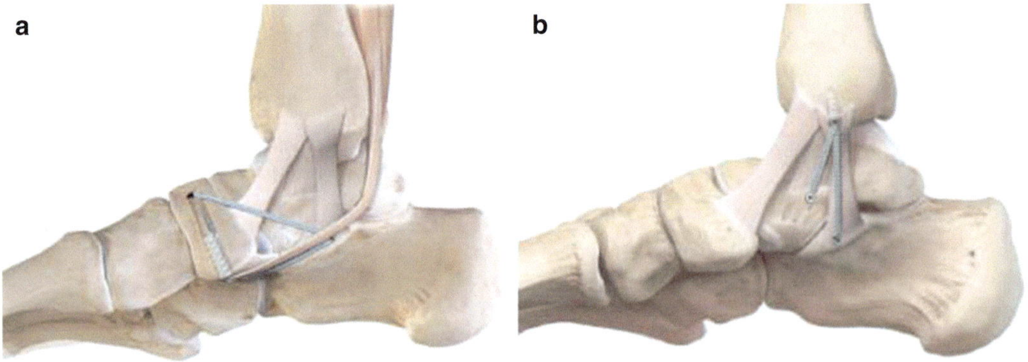

Fig. 17.7 (**a**) Spring ligament augmentation with InternalBrace. (**b**) Deltoid ligament augmentation with InternalBrace. (Courtesy Arthrex Inc., Naples, Florida)

It is imperative that additional osseous procedures are given time to heal and tendon transfers and ligament reconstructions should not be placed under undue strain before adequate integration has taken place – particularly at anchoring points.

The authors' preferred programme involves protection of the operated foot for 6 weeks. The timing of commencement of progressive weight-bearing depends upon the extent of procedures undertaken and the quality of host tissue. Some form of more prolonged protection may be required for up to a further 6 weeks. Progression should be judged on a combination of satisfactory wound healing, overall foot appearance and satisfactory radiographs. Physiotherapy should commence at a minimum of 6 weeks. It should progressively aim to maintain and then improve strength and proprioception. Some orthotic provision can help provide further protection going forward. Patients should be advised that recovery to their ultimate level of functioning may not be achieved for 1 year.

Conclusions

Our understanding and recognition of spring ligament pathology has evolved enormously since the 1990s. Its importance in the genesis of AAFD and, more rarely, as an isolated injury is acknowledged.

In acute partial injuries, conservative treatment may suffice. In acute full ruptures, surgery is advocated for the active patient. It is rarely sufficient to simply repair the ligament. Augmentation is commonly performed.

More commonly the spring ligament is involved in AAFD pathology. Stabilisation of the ligament in combination with other procedures to reconstruct the TPT and perform osseous corrections is required. However, by combining procedures, it has been difficult to isolate the contribution of each to the overall outcome.

Scientific knowledge has evolved through cadaveric studies involving both sectioning the spring ligament and its adjacent structures and examining the effects of different reconstructions using various tendons and fixation points.

However, clinical outcomes remain at the stages of Level IV (small cohort studies) and Level V (expert opinion). Initial work involved the outcomes of autograft, and to lesser extent allograft, tendon reinforcement. More latterly, the use of FibreTape has increased in popularity. There is to date no clearly accepted superior surgical procedure. The need for future well-designed large long-term studies with results combining clinical outcome scores, radiographic parameters and patient reported outcome measures is required.

References

1. Sarrafian SK. Anatomy of the foot and ankle: descriptive, topographic, functional. Philadelphia: Lippincott; 1983. p. 159–282.
2. Patil V, Ebraheim NA, Frogameni A, Liu J. Morphometric dimensions of the calcaneonavicular (spring) ligament. Foot Ankle Int. 2007;28(8):927–32.
3. Mousavian A, Orapin J, Chinanuvathana A, et al. Anatomic spring ligament and posterior tibial tendon reconstruction: new concept of double bundle PTT and a novel technique for spring ligament. Arch Bone Jt Surg. 2017;5(3):201–5.
4. Davis WH, Sobel M, DiCarlo EF, et al. Gross, histological, and microvascular anatomy and biomechanical testing of the spring ligament complex. Foot Ankle Int. 1996;17(2):95–102.
5. Steginsky B, Vora A. What to do with the spring ligament. Foot Ankle Clin. 2017;22(3):515–27.
6. Cromeens BP, Kirchhoff CA, Patterson RM, et al. An attachment-based description of the medial collateral and spring ligament complexes. Foot Ankle Int. 2015;36(6):710–21.
7. Taniguchi A, Tanaka Y, Takakura Y, Kadono K, Maeda M, Yamamoto H. Anatomy of the spring ligament. J Bone Joint Surg. 2003;85:2174–8.
8. Hintermann B, Golano P. The anatomy and function of the deltoid ligament. Tech Foot Ankle Surg. 2014;13(2):67–72.
9. Bastias GF, Dalmau-Pastor M, Astudillo C, Pellegrini MJ. Spring ligament instability. Foot Ankle Clin North Am. 2018;23:659–78.
10. Milner CE, Soames RW. The medial collateral ligaments of the human ankle joint: anatomical variations. Foot Ankle Int. 1998;19:289–92.
11. Niki H, Ching RP, Kiser P, et al. The effect of posterior tibial tendon dysfunction on hindfoot kinematics. Foot Ankle Int. 2001;22(4):292–300.

12. Jennings MM, Christensen JC. The effects of sectioning the spring ligament on rearfoot stability and posterior tibial tendon efficiency. J Foot Ankle Surg. 2008;47(3):219–24.
13. Kitaoka HB, Ahn TK, Luo ZP, An KN. Stability of the arch of the foot. Foot Ankle Int. 1997;18:644–8.
14. Iaquinto JM, Wayne JS. Computational model of the lower leg and foot/ankle complex: application to arch stability. J Biomech Eng. 2010;132(2):021009.
15. Huang CK, Kitaoka HB, An KN, et al. Biomechanical evaluation of longitudinal arch stability. Foot Ankle Int. 1993;14(6):353–7.
16. Hollinshead WH. Anatomy for surgeons, vol. 3. New York: Hoeber-Harper; 1954. p. p831–81.
17. Pasapula C, Devany A, Fischer NC, et al. The resistance to failure of spring ligament reconstruction. Foot. 2017;33:29–34.
18. Deland JT. The adult acquired flatfoot and spring ligament complex: pathology and implications. Foot and Ankle Clinics North Am. 2001;6(1):129–35.
19. Deland JT. Spring ligament complex and flatfoot deformity: curse or blessing? Foot Ankle Int. 2012;33(3):239–43.
20. Gazdag AR, Cracchiolo A. Rupture of the posterior tibial tendon. Evaluation of injury of the spring ligament and clinical assessment of tendon transfer and ligament repair. J Bone Joint Surg. 1997;79(5):675–81.
21. Balen PE, Helms CA. Association of posterior tibial tendon injury with spring ligament injury, sinus tarsi abnormality and plantar fasciitis on MR imaging. AJR Am J Roentgenol. 2001;176(5):1137–43.
22. Deland JT, de Asla RJ, Sung IH, et al. Posterior tibial tendon insufficiency: which ligaments are involved? Foot Ankle Int. 2005;26(6):427–35.
23. Williams G, Widnall J, Evans P, et al. Could failure of the spring ligament complex be the driving force behind the development of the adult flatfoot deformity? J Foot Ankle Surg. 2014;53(2):152–5.
24. Pasapula C, Cutts S. Modern theory of the development of adult acquired flat foot and an updated spring ligament classification system. Clin Res Foot Ankle. 2017;5(3):1–4.
25. Pasapula C, Shariff S, Cutts S, West J, Kobezda T. Adult acquired flat foot: a new biomechanical classification for the deformity based on two point failure of the medial column. Clin Res Foot Ankle. 2018;6(2):1–7.
26. Borton DC, Saxby TS. Tear of the plantar calcaneonavicular (spring) ligament causing flatfoot. A case report. J Bone Joint Surg. 1997;79(4):641–3.
27. Chen JP, Allen AM. MR diagnosis of traumatic tear of the spring ligament in a pole vaulter. Skelet Radiol. 1997;26(5):310–2.
28. Subhas N, Sundaram M. Diagnosis: isolated spring ligament tear demonstrated on magnetic resonance imaging. Orthopedics. 2007;30(1):70–2.
29. Tryfonidis M, Jackson W, Mansour R, Cooke PH, The J, Ostlere S, Sharp RJ. Acquired adult flat foot due to isolated plantar calcaneonavicular (spring) ligament insufficiency with a normal tibialis posterior tendon. Foot Ankle Surg. 2008;14(2):89–95.
30. Shuen V, Prem H. Acquired unilateral pes planus in a child caused by a ruptured plantar calcaneonavicular (spring) ligament. J Pediatr Orthop B. 2009;18(3):129–30.
31. Orr JD, Nunley JA 2nd. Isolated spring ligament failure as a cause of adult acquired flatfoot deformity. Foot Ankle Int. 2013;34(6):818–23.
32. Masaragian HJ, Ricchetti HO, Testa C. Acute isolated rupture of the spring ligament: a case report and review of the literature. Foot Ankle Int. 2013;34(1):150–4.
33. Palmanovich E, Shabat S, Brin YS, et al. Novel reconstruction technique for an isolated plantar calcaneonavicular (SPRING) ligament tear: a 5 case series report. Foot (Edinb). 2017;30:1–4.
34. Kavanagh EC, Koulouris G, Gopez A, Zoga A, Raikin S, Morrison WB. MRI of rupture of the spring ligament complex with talo-cuboid impaction. Skelet Radiol. 2007;36(6):555–8.
35. Yao L, Gentili A, Cracchiolo A. MR imaging findings in spring ligament insufficiency. Skelet Radiol. 1999;28(5):245–50.
36. Toye LR, Helms CA, Hoffmann BD, Easley M, Nunley JA. MRI of spring ligament tears. AJR Am J Roentgenol. 2005;184(5):1475–80.
37. Hintermann B. Medial ankle instability. Foot Ankle Clinics North Am. 2003;8(4):723–38.
38. Pasapula C, Devany A, Magan A, et al. Neutral heel lateral push test: the first clinical examination of spring ligament integrity. Foot (Edinb). 2015;25(2):69–74.
39. Saltzman CL, El-Khoury GY. The hindfoot alignment view. Foot Ankle Int. 1995;16(9):572–6.
40. Harish S, Jan E, Findlay K, Petrisor B, Popowich T, Friedman L, Wainman B, Jurriaans E. Sonography of the superomedial part of the spring ligament complex of the foot: a study of cadavers and asymptomatic volunteers. Skelet Radiol. 2007;36(3):221–8.
41. Harish S, Kumbhare D, O'Neill J, Popowich T. Comparison of sonography and magnetic resonance imaging for spring ligament abnormalities: preliminary study. J Ultrasound Med. 2008;27(8):1145–53.
42. Crim J. Medial-sided ankle pain: deltoid ligament and beyond. Magn Reson Imaging Clin N Am. 2017;25(1):63–77. 22
43. Mengiardi B, Pinto C, Zanetti M. Spring ligament complex and posterior tibial tendon: MR anatomy and findings in acquired adult flatfoot deformity. Semin Musculoskelet Radiol. 2016;20(1):104–15.
44. Williams G, Widnall J, Evans P, et al. MRI features most often associated with surgically proven tears of the spring ligament complex. Skelet Radiol. 2013;42(7):969–73.
45. Rule J, Yao L, Seeger LL. Spring ligament of the ankle: normal MR anatomy. AJR Am J Roentgenol. 1993;161(6):1241–4.
46. Nery C, Lemos AVKC, Raduan F, et al. Combined spring and deltoid ligament repair in adult-acquired flatfoot. Foot Ankle Int. 2018;39(8):903–7.

47. Mann RA. Flatfoot in adults. In: Coughlin MJ, Mann RA, editors. Surgery of the foot and ankle. St Louis: Mosby; 1999. p. 733–67.
48. Zanolli DH, Glisson RR, Nunley JA 2nd, et al. Biomechanical assessment of flexible flatfoot correction: comparison of techniques in a cadaver model. J Bone Joint Surg Am. 2014;96(6):e45.
49. Williams BR, Ellis SJ, Deyer TW, et al. Reconstruction of the spring ligament using a peroneus longus autograft tendon transfer. Foot Ankle Int. 2010;31(7):567–77.
50. Hiller L, Pinney SJ. Surgical treatment of acquired adult flatfoot deformity: what is the state of practice among academic foot and ankle surgeons in 2002? Foot Ankle Int. 2003;24(9):701–5.
51. Myerson MS, Corrigan J, Thompson F, et al. Tendon transfer combined with calcaneal osteotomy for posterior tibial tendon insufficiency: a radiological investigation. Foot Ankle Int. 1995;16:712–8.
52. Vadell AM, Peratta M. Calcaneonavicular ligament: anatomy, diagnosis, and treatment. Foot Ankle Clin. 2012;17(3):437–48.
53. Goldner JL, Keats PK, Bassett FH 3rd, Clippinger FW. Progressive talipes equinovalgus due to trauma or degeneration of the posterior tibial tendon and medial plantar ligaments. Orthop Clin North Am. 1974;5:39–51.
54. Lui TH. Endoscopic repair of the superficial deltoid ligament and spring ligament. Arthrosc Tech. 2016;5(3):e621–5.
55. Deland JT, Annoczky S, Thompson FM. Adult acquired flatfoot deformity at the talonavicular joint: reconstruction of the spring ligament in an in vitro model. Foot Ankle Int. 1992;13:327–32.
56. Thordarson DB, Schmotzer H, Chon J. Reconstruction with tenodesis in an adult flatfoot model. A biomechanical evaluation of four methods. J Bone Joint Surg Am. 2003;77:1557–64.
57. Choi K, Lee S, Otis JC, et al. Anatomical reconstruction of the spring ligament using peroneus longus tendon graft. Foot Ankle Int. 2003;24(5):430–6.
58. Baxter JR, LaMothe JM, Walls RJ, et al. Reconstruction of the medial talonavicular joint in simulated flatfoot deformity. Foot Ankle Int. 2015;36(4):424–9.
59. Tan GJ, Kadakia AR, Ruberte Thiele RA, et al. Reconstruction of the medial talonavicular joint in simulated flatfoot deformity. Foot Ankle Int. 2015;36(4):424–9.
60. Lee WC, Yi Y. Spring ligament reconstruction using the autogenous flexor hallucis longus tendon. Orthopedics. 2014;37(7):467–71.
61. Ryssman DB, Jeng CL. Reconstruction of the spring ligament with a posterior tibial tendon autograft: technique tip. Foot Ankle Int. 2017;38(4):452–6.
62. Ribbans WJ, Garde A. Tibialis posterior tendon and deltoid and spring ligament injuries in the elite athlete. Foot Ankle Clin. 2013;18:255–91.
63. Acevedo J, Vora A. Anatomical reconstruction of the spring ligament complex: "internal brace" augmentation. Foot Ankle Spec. 2013;6(6):441–5.
64. Palmanovich E, Shabat S, Brin YS, et al. Anatomic reconstruction technique for a plantar calcaneonavicular (spring) ligament tear. J Foot Ankle Surg. 2015;54(6):1124–6.
65. Brodell JD, MacDonald A, Perkins JA, Deland JT, Oh I. Deltoid-spring ligament reconstruction in adult acquired flatfoot deformity with medial Peritalar instability. Foot Ankle Int. 2019;40(7):753–61.
66. Otis JC, Deland JT, Kenneally SM, Chang V. Medial arch strain after medial displacement calcaneal osteotomy: an in vitro study. Foot Ankle Int. 1999;20(4):222–6.

18 Posterior Ankle Ligaments: The Role of Posterior Talofibular Ligament, Flexor Retinaculum, Posterior Talocalcaneal Ligament, and Fibulotalocalcaneal Ligament in Posterior Ankle Impingement

Gian Luigi Canata and Valentina Casale

Introduction

Posterior ankle impingement (PAI) is a common cause of chronic ankle pain. It is a clinical diagnosis characterized by painful limitation of motion in plantar flexion [1, 2]. It results from compression between bony and soft tissue structures during terminal plantar flexion.

Pathologic contributors to posterior impingement may be differentiated in either osseous or soft tissue disorders [3].

Osseous disorders include the *os trigonum* syndrome, prominent lateral talar tubercle (also known as Stieda's process), fractured lateral talar tubercle, posteromedial talar ossicle, and *os post peronei* [4–7]. Anatomical variations of the tibia and calcaneus may also predispose to posterior impingement [3].

Soft tissue causes of PAI include capsule and synovium disorders, tendon pathological conditions (especially the flexor hallucis longus tenosynovitis), and ligamentous conditions [3].

In particular, the capsular soft tissues involved as part of PAI include the posterior capsule and the posterior talofibular, intermalleolar, and tibiofibular ligaments. The flexor hallucis longus tendon runs between the lateral and the medial processes of the talus and may also be involved in PAI, with a consequent stenosing tenosynovitis [8].

Posterior ankle impingement syndrome clinically presents with chronic pain and swelling within the posterior ankle [9]. It is typically correlated with sports activities requiring extreme plantar flexion, such as soccer, ballet, football, javelin throwing, gymnastics, and downhill running.

The most cited mechanisms of posterior impingement are [2]:

- An acute plantar hyperflexion injury.
- A chronic repetitive microtrauma.

These two mechanisms cause the development of a secondary hypertrophy and compression between the posterior aspect of the talus and the calcaneus [9].

Such an enhanced compression may lead to lesions of the surrounding tendons and ligaments [10].

Differential diagnosis is essential, especially considering Achilles tendinosis, Achilles tendon tear, arthrosis, flexor hallucis longus tenosynovitis, Haglund's syndrome, osteochondral lesions, retrocalcaneal bursitis, and acute posterior talar process fractures [9].

G. L. Canata (✉) · V. Casale
Centre of Sports Traumatology, Koelliker Hospital, Torino, TO, Italy
e-mail: studio@ortosport.it

P. D'Hooghe et al. (eds.), *Ligamentous Injuries of the Foot and Ankle*,
https://doi.org/10.1007/978-3-031-08682-3_18

With regard to posterior soft tissue impingement, Giannini et al. differentiate between a posteromedial and posterolateral soft tissue impingement [1].

Posteromedial impingement may result from a severe inversion injury, with the ankle plantar flexed [11, 12]. It is usually caused by compression and subsequent hypertrophic changes at the posteromedial tibiotalar capsule and the posterior deltoid fibers, in particular those of the posterior tibiotalar ligament, between the talus and the medial malleolus [13]. Once the posterior tibiotalar ligament becomes hypertrophied, it may come into contact with the flexor tendons and partially encase the tibialis posterior, the flexor hallucis longus, or the flexor digitorum longus tendons [14].

Posterolateral ankle impingement is typically caused by soft tissue impingement of an accessory ligament, namely the posterior intermalleolar ligament (PIML) [15].

To date, a significant variability in the frequency of presentation of this ligament is reported, although it has been observed that the PIML is a distinct and almost constant structure with several shapes [16].

First described by Rosenberg et al. [17] and referred to as a marsupial meniscus, it originates from the superior border of the posterior tibiofibular ligament and runs transversally in a posterior recess of the ankle joint, between the posterior talofibular and the posterior tibiofibular ligaments [18]. During plantar flexion, it may protrude into the ankle joint, eventually getting entrapped and torn causing PAI [1] (Fig. 18.1).

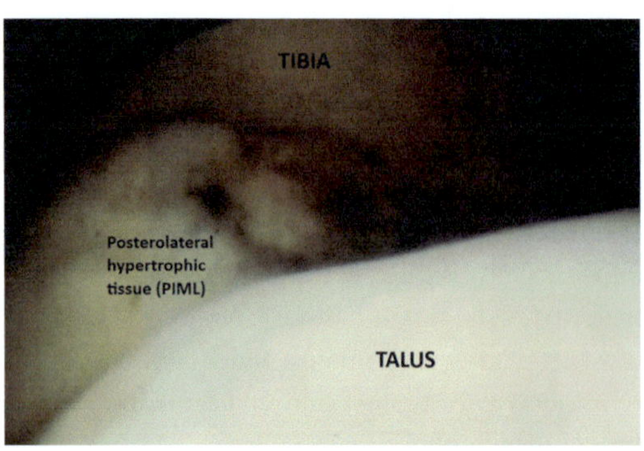

Fig. 18.1 Arthroscopic view of a posterolateral ankle impingement

Ligamentous Sources of Posterior Ankle Impingement

Several ligaments are located in the posterior ankle compartment. Given their proximity to the tibia, these ligaments are at risk of impingement when the talus and the calcaneus approximate each other during extreme plantar flexion [3].

This section deals with some of these structures, focusing on their role in the pathomechanics or management of PAI (Fig. 18.2).

Posterior Talofibular Ligament

The lateral tubercle of the posterior process of the talus is the site where part of the posterior talofibular ligament (PTFL), the posterior talocalcaneal ligament (PTCL), and the superomedial lamina of the fibulotalocalcaneal ligament (FTCL) are attached [19].

When a posterior ankle impingement develops, the PTFL is easily exposed to compression due to its horizontal position at the posterolateral aspect of the ankle; thus, it is one of the most frequently involved ligaments [8, 15].

It is an established fact that one of the main causes of posterior ankle impingement is *os trigonum*. Its presence causes a progressive bony impingement and narrows the space around the posterior soft tissues [20, 21].

In case of os trigonum surgical removal, especially with endoscopy, a partial detachment of the PTFL has been suggested, before releasing the flexor retinaculum and the PTCL, respectively [22].

Flexor Retinaculum

The flexor retinaculum of the foot is also called laciniate ligament or internal annular ligament. It is a fibrous band formed by the fusion of the superficial and deep aponeuroses of the leg. It is characterized by a triangular shape: the superficial apical fibers insert on the subcutaneous anterior and medial surfaces of the medial malleolus, while the base corresponds to the medial border of the calcaneus [23].

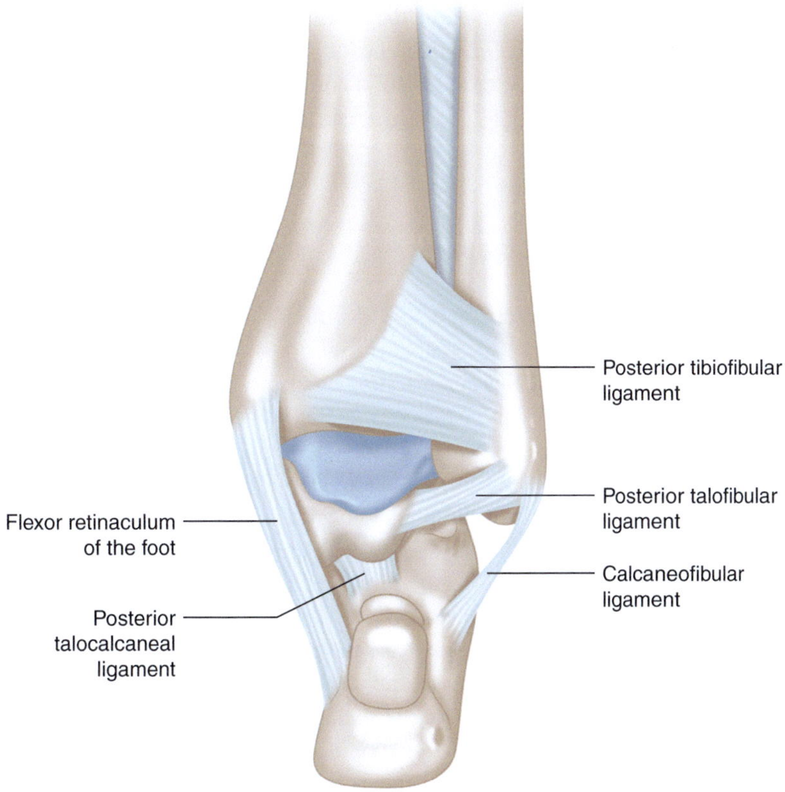

Fig. 18.2 Posterior view of the ankle

The flexor retinaculum forms the roof, the superior and the inferior margins of the tarsal tunnel, converting the bony grooves present in that area into four canals. Thus, it delimitates, from the medial side, the passage of the tibialis posterior tendon, the flexor digitorum longus tendon, the posterior artery, the vein and the posterior nerve together, and the flexor hallucis longus (FHL) tendon [23].

With regard to the posterior ankle impingement, the flexor retinaculum plays an important role, being a possible cause of FHL tenosynovitis [9].

As mentioned above, frequent consequences of the os trigonum are damages to the regional tendons and ligaments, including the FHL tendon, and then the development of the *os trigonum syndrome* [10, 20, 21].

For this reason, especially in the case of bony impingement associated with disorders of the neurovascular bundle or the flexor hallucis longus (FHL) tendon, the identification and detachment of the flexor retinaculum during surgery of the os trigonum syndrome is advisable. It has been described during both the open posteromedial and the endoscopic approaches [22, 24].

Posterior Talocalcaneal Ligament

The posterior talocalcaneal ligament (PTCL) is a short, flat, and quadrangular ligament of the ankle. It originates at the lateral tubercle on the posterior process of the talus and inserts on the superior contour of the calcaneus [25].

It may interchange fibers with the PTFL at the talar origin [23], while at its insertion, it connects with the superomedial lamina of the fibulotalocalcaneal ligament [26].

When an os trigonum is present, it has been reported that the PTCL can originate from it and then forms a trigonocalcaneal ligament [23].

For this reason, the PTCL has an important role during the surgical removal of the os trigonum. Together with the PTFL and the flexor retinaculum, in fact, it must be released for a correct procedure [22].

Rouvière Ligament or Fibulotalocalcaneal Ligament

In 1924, Dujarier first described a posterior fibulocalcaneal ligament arising from the posterior aspect of the lateral malleolus and inserting on the posterosuperior border of the calcaneus laterally [27]. He qualified it as abnormal, but in 1932, Henri Rouvière and Miguel Canela Làzaro deepened the topic and described the fibulotalocalcaneal ligament (FTCL), today also known as the Rouvière ligament [28]. It has been described as an extrinsic sheathlike ligament which occupies the posterolateral corner of the ankle and the posterior subtalar joint, independent of the capsules and ligaments of the nearby joints [23, 29] (Fig. 18.3). The FTCL originates from the medial border of the peroneal groove on the posterior aspect of the lateral malleolus, like the PTFL. Furthermore, it frequently extends up to the calcaneofibular ligament's origin [23]. It occupies the same tissue plane as the deep posterior crural fascia of the lower leg [30].

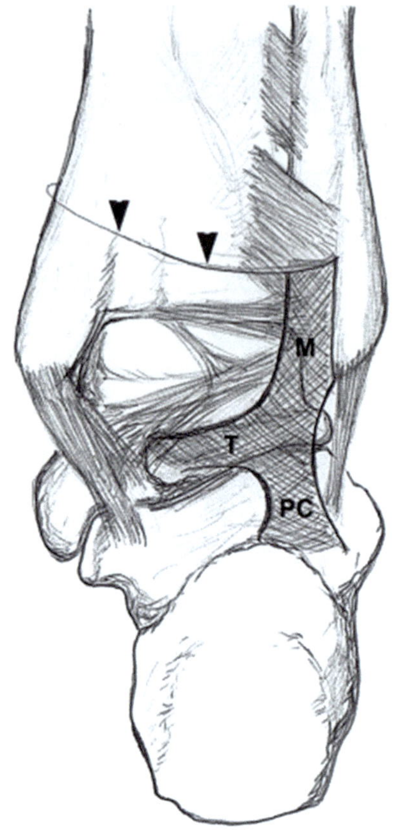

Fig. 18.3 Drawing of the posterior aspect of the ankle. The FTCL corresponds to the hatched area: the main stem (M), the talar lamina (T), and the peroneocalcaneal lamina (PC). The FTCL continues with the deep posterior crural fascia of the lower leg (arrowheads). (Reproduced with permission from Peduto AJ, Numkarunarunrote N, Trudell DJ, Resnick DL. Fibulotalocalcaneal ligament: magnetic resonance imaging findings with cadaver correlation. J Comput Assist Tomogr. 2009;33:444–8. Wolters Kluwer Health, Inc. https://journals.lww.com/jcat/Abstract/2009/05000/Fibulotalocalcaneal_Ligament__Magnetic_Resonance.21.aspx)

The main stem then divides into two fibrous laminae: the superomedial or talar lamina, which inserts on the posterolateral tubercle of the talus, and the inferolateral or peroneocalcaneal lamina, which represents the major component and inserts on almost the whole width of the superior calcaneal surface [23].

The prolongation of the superomedial lamina of the FTCL continues to the medial tubercle, limiting the osteofibrous tunnel for the FHL, and finally joins with the flexor retinaculum [26].

The superomedial lamina can be also considered as a connection between the lateral side of the ankle by means of the PTFL [25].

The FTCL is an important restraint to excessive dorsiflexion of the foot and contributes to guarantee ankle and subtalar stability in all foot positions [31].

During hindfoot endoscopy for the os trigonum syndrome management, the Rouvière ligament may be considered as a thickened part of the deep crural fascia at the lateral side of the hindfoot. The cranial part of the posterior talar process freed from this ligament provides a better identification of the FHL tendon, so as to remove the os trigonum [22].

Conclusions

Besides the most frequent causes of posterior ankle impingement, such as the presence of the *os trigonum* or Stieda's process, the posterior ligaments of the ankle may also play a role. Some of them contributes to the development of PAI, and others must be considered when operatively managing it. A thorough knowledge of their anatomical features and their role in foot dynamics is mandatory.

References

1. Giannini S, Buda R, Mosca M, Parma A, Di Caprio F. Posterior ankle impingement. Foot Ankle Int. 2013;34:459–65.
2. Hayashi D, Roemer FW, D'Hooghe P, Guermazi A. Posterior ankle impingement in athletes: pathogenesis, imaging features and differential diagnoses. Eur J Radiol. 2015;84:2231–41.
3. Russell JA, Kruse DW, Koutedakis Y, McEwan IM, Wyon MA. Pathoanatomy of posterior ankle impingement in ballet dancers. Clin Anat. 2010;23:613–21.
4. Brodsky AE, Khalil MA. Talar compression syndrome. Am J Sports Med. 1986;14:472–6.
5. Callanan I, Williams L, Stephens M. "Os post peronei" and the posterolateral nutcracker impingement syndrome. Foot Ankle Int. 1998;19:475–8.
6. Henderson I, La Valette D. Ankle impingement: combined anterior and posterior impingement syndrome of the ankle. Foot Ankle Int. 2004;25:632–8.
7. Ramsey K, Davies M, Healy J, Peckett W. Isolated ossicle causing posteromedial ankle impingement—a new diagnosis? Foot Ankle Surg. 2004;10:201–5.
8. Hamilton WG, Geppert MJ, Thompson FM. Pain in the posterior aspect of the ankle in dancers. Differential diagnosis and operative treatment. J Bone Joint Surg Am. 1996;78:1491–500.
9. Berman Z, Tafur M, Ahmed SS, Huang BK, Chang EY. Ankle impingement syndromes: an imaging review. Br J Radiol. 2020;16:90. Available from: https://www.ncbi.nlm.nih.gov/pmc/articles/PMC5685116/
10. Hedrick MR, McBryde AM. Posterior ankle impingement. Foot Ankle Int. 1994;15:2–8.
11. Liu SH, Mirzayan R. Posteromedial ankle impingement. Arthroscopy. 1993;9:709–11.
12. van Dijk CN, Bossuyt PM, Marti RK. Medial ankle pain after lateral ligament rupture. J Bone Joint Surg Br. 1996;78:562–7.
13. Donovan A, Rosenberg ZS. MRI of ankle and lateral hindfoot impingement syndromes. AJR Am J Roentgenol. 2010;195:595–604.
14. Koulouris G, Connell D, Schneider T, Edwards W. Posterior tibiotalar ligament injury resulting in posteromedial impingement. Foot Ankle Int. 2003;24:575–83.
15. Golanó P, Vega J, Pérez-Carro L, Götzens V. Ankle anatomy for the arthroscopist. Part II: role of the ankle ligaments in soft tissue impingement. Foot Ankle Clin. 2006;11:275–96, v–vi
16. Oh C-S, Won H-S, Hur M-S, Chung I-H, Kim S, Suh J-S, et al. Anatomic variations and MRI of the intermalleolar ligament. AJR Am J Roentgenol. 2006;186:943–7.
17. Rosenberg ZS, Cheung YY, Beltran J, Sheskier S, Leong M, Jahss M. Posterior intermalleolar ligament of the ankle: normal anatomy and MR imaging features. AJR Am J Roentgenol. 1995;165:387–90.
18. Chen Y. Arthroscopy of the ankle joint. Arthroscopy. 1985:104–27.
19. Bureau NJ, Cardinal E, Hobden R, Aubin B. Posterior ankle impingement syndrome: MR imaging findings in seven patients. Radiology. 2000;215:497–503.
20. Grogan DP, Walling AK, Ogden JA. Anatomy of the os trigonum. J Pediatr Orthop. 1990;10:618–22.
21. McDOUGALL A. The os trigonum. J Bone Joint Surg Br. 1955;37-B:257–65.
22. van Dijk CN, de Leeuw P, a. J, Scholten PE. Hindfoot endoscopy for posterior ankle impingement. Surgical technique. J Bone Joint Surg Am. 2009;91(Suppl 2):287–98.
23. Sarrafian SK. Anatomy of the foot and ankle: descriptive, topographic, functional. 2nd ed. Philadelphia, Pennsylvania: Lippincott; 1993.
24. Rungprai C, Tennant JN, Phisitkul P. Disorders of the flexor hallucis longus and Os trigonum. Clin Sports Med. 2015;34:741–59.
25. Pastore D, Cerri GG, Haghighi P, Trudell DJ, Resnick DL. Ligaments of the posterior and lateral talar processes: MRI and MR arthrography of the ankle and posterior subtalar joint with anatomic and histologic correlation. AJR Am J Roentgenol. 2009;192:967–73.
26. Szaro P, Polaczek M, Ciszek B. The Kager's fat pad radiological anatomy revised. Surg Radiol Anat. 2020;43(1):79–86.
27. Dujarier C. Anatomie des Membres: Dissection - Anatomie Topographique. Anat Memb. 2nd ed. Paris: Elsevier Masson; 1924. p. 403–7.
28. Rouvière H, Canela LM. Le ligament Péroneo-Astragalo-Calcanéen. Ann Anat Pathol Anat Norm Méd-Chir. 1932;9:745–50.
29. Wiegerinck JI, Somford MP, Hoornenborg D, van Dijk CN. Eponyms of the Kager triangle. J Bone Joint Surg Am. 2012;94:e67.
30. Peduto AJ, Numkarunarunrote N, Trudell DJ, Resnick DL. Fibulotalocalcaneal ligament: magnetic resonance imaging findings with cadaver correlation. J Comput Assist Tomogr. 2009;33:444–8.
31. Stephens MM, Sammarco GJ. The stabilizing role of the lateral ligament complex around the ankle and subtalar joints. Foot Ankle. 1992;13:130–6.

19 Lisfranc Injuries of the Foot and Ankle: Diagnosis and Treatment Indications

Jeremy J. McCormick and Brian M. Fisher

A Lisfranc injury refers to bony or ligamentous disruption of the tarsal-metatarsal (TMT), intercuneiform (IC), and/or naviculocuneiform (NC) joints and can range from a stable ligament sprain to a grossly displaced and unstable fracture dislocation through the midfoot. These are rare injuries which are estimated to occur in 1 of 55,000 people per year in the United States [1–4]. Lisfranc injuries are often overlooked and misdiagnosed as simply a foot sprain with 20% of injuries not identified on initial evaluation, most of these being a purely ligamentous injury [5]. Failure to properly evaluate, diagnose, and treat these injuries can be disabling and lead to midfoot arthritis and collapse of the foot into a position where the forefoot is abducted and the hindfoot shifts into a valgus position [6, 7]. Lisfranc injuries are increasingly being reported in sports [8–13]; thus, knowledge of the anatomy, proper clinical evaluation, and effective utilization of imaging modalities to assist with diagnosis are important for the clinician treating athletes.

J. J. McCormick (✉)
Department of Orthopaedic Surgery, Washington University School of Medicine, St. Louis, MO, USA
e-mail: mccormickj@wustl.edu

B. M. Fisher
Department of Orthopedic Surgery, Prisma Health-Upstate, University of South Carolina School of Medicine Greenville, Greenville, SC, USA
e-mail: brian.fisher@prismahealth.org

Anatomy

The Lisfranc joint complex refers to the articulation between the distal tarsal bones and the bases of the metatarsals. It is further divided into the medial, middle, and lateral columns consisting of the first TMT, second and third TMT, and fourth and fifth TMT joints, respectively (Fig. 19.1). The medial and middle columns are fairly rigid with minimal motion, while the lateral column maintains flexibility to assist the foot in accommodating to uneven surfaces and the normal mechanics of gait. The second and third TMT joints are most rigid with maximal sagittal motion of 0.6 mm and 1.6 mm, respectively. The first TMT joint is slightly more mobile with 3.5 mm of sagittal motion due to the ellipsoid shape of the joint compared to the flat second and third TMT joints. The fourth and fifth TMT joints maintain the most sagittal mobility with 9.6 mm and 10.2 mm, respectively [14].

The bony structure of the Lisfranc complex has inherent stability based on its Roman arch configuration. At the TMT articulations, the second metatarsal base acts as the keystone. The middle cuneiform is recessed approximately 8 mm in relation to the medial cuneiform and 4 mm to the lateral cuneiform [15]. Interosseous ligaments connect the second through fifth metatarsal bases, link the metatarsals to the cuneiforms and cuboid, and bridge the IC joints.

P. D'Hooghe et al. (eds.), *Ligamentous Injuries of the Foot and Ankle*,
https://doi.org/10.1007/978-3-031-08682-3_19

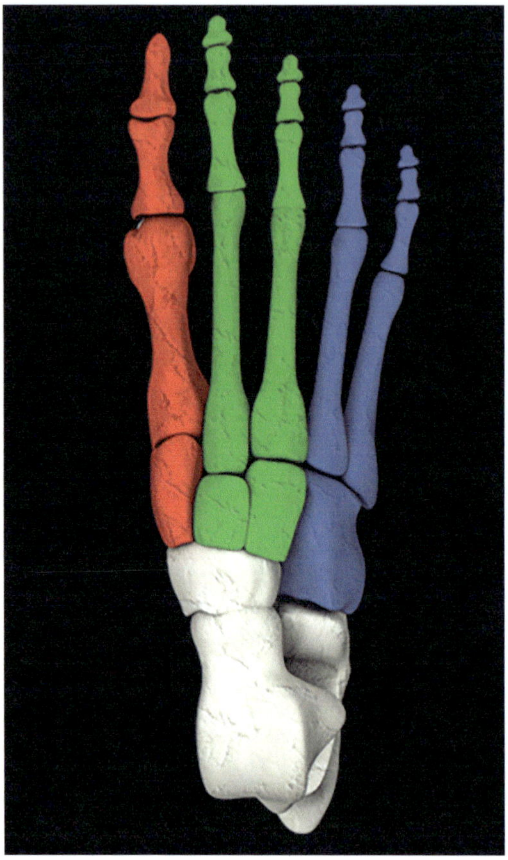

Fig. 19.1 The three columns of the midfoot are demonstrated with the medial column (red), middle column (green), and lateral column (blue) (With permission from Llopis E, Carrascoso J, Iriarte I, de Prado Serrano M, Cerezal M. Lisfranc Injury Imaging and Surgical Management. *Semin Musculoskeletal Radiol.* 2016;20(2):139–153)

The named Lisfranc ligament connects the medial column to the middle column by attaching the medial cuneiform to the base of the second metatarsal. The integrity of this ligament is critical, as there is no transverse intermetatarsal ligament attaching the first and second metatarsals. Throughout the midfoot, the plantar ligaments are more stout than the dorsal ligaments, and this is true for the Lisfranc ligament as well. The Lisfranc ligament has been described as being composed of dorsal, interosseous, and plantar elements (Fig. 19.2) [15–17], but in some anatomic studies, only a plantar and dorsal band were identified [18, 19]. In a biomechanical study investigating the mean stiffness of the dorsal and plantar elements, the dorsal element had a mean stiffness of 66.3 Newtons per millimeter, whereas the plantar ligament had a stiffness of 189.7 Newtons per millimeter. The mean load to failure of the dorsal ligament was 150.7 Newtons and 368.8 Newtons for the plantar ligament [18]. In an anatomic study, all observed feet had three components to the Lisfranc ligament. The thickest component was the interosseous at 7.68 mm, followed by the plantar portion at 3.25 mm and the dorsal at 2.62 mm. Several studies have demonstrated that the thickness of ligaments outside of the foot correlates with the strength of the ligament [20], so it may be reasonably concluded that the interosseous portion of the ligament is the strongest and contributes significant stability to the Lisfranc joint complex.

Mechanism of Injury

Lisfranc injuries involve disruption of the ligamentous stability of the TMT joints, bony injury to tarsal bones and/or metatarsal bones, and, depending on the pattern of injury, may also interrupt the intertarsal joints. Disruption of the normal TMT anatomy is typically a result of high-energy injury including motor vehicle collisions or a fall from significant height. Lisfranc injuries sustained in athletic endeavors are distinct from high-energy injuries and more commonly represent a ligamentous injury with proximal instability and fewer fractures. Thus, these athletic injuries can be more difficult to appreciate on initial evaluation.

Lisfranc injuries in athletes result from direct or indirect mechanisms. A direct mechanism includes an axial load placed on a plantarflexed foot causing plantar flexion at the TMT joints (Fig. 19.3a). This mechanism causes the weaker dorsal ligaments to fail first. The stronger plantar ligaments rupture next, and, finally, the injury culminates in dorsal displacement of the metatarsals relative to the cuneiforms. Indirect injuries occur with a twisting mechanism to the foot.

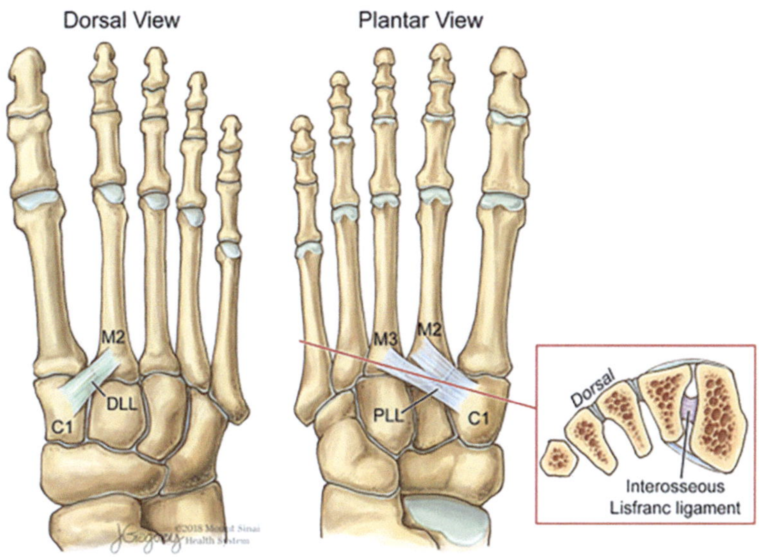

Fig. 19.2 The dorsal Lisfranc ligament (DLL) demonstrated on dorsal view extending from medial cuneiform (C1) to the second metatarsal. The plantar Lisfranc ligament (PLL) extends from C1 to the second and third metatarsals. The interosseous Lisfranc ligament is seen on cross section as a thicker band which extends between the C1 and second metatarsal (With permission from Gunio DA, Vulcano E, Benitez C. Dynamic stress MRI of Midfoot Injuries: Measurable Morphology and Laxity of the Sprained Lisfranc Ligament During Mechanical Loading: A Case Report. *JBJS Case connect.* July-Sep 2019;9(3):e0228)

Indirect injuries account for greater than 50% of injuries in collegiate football players [21]. This type of injury occurs when a planted foot sustains a twisting moment around the midfoot (Fig. 19.3b). In professional football players, 90% of Lisfranc injuries occurred while players were engaged with another player with very few being direct axial loading of the foot [21]. The degree and location of injury is dependent on the direction and magnitude of the force. The energy dispersion usually begins proximally in the NC and/or IC joints and exits distally through the TMT and intermetatarsal joints. Because of this, multiple joints may be injured and unstable, and each must be evaluated carefully to avoid the late sequela of midfoot instability such as loss of push-off strength or arthritic changes.

Some athletes may be predisposed to a Lisfranc injury not only due to their sport of choice but also because of their anatomy. It has been noted that patients who sustained Lisfranc injuries had a shallower second TMT mortise when compared to controls [22]. The medial depth of the joint was >2.5 mm shorter in the injured cohort. A shallower mortise may not convey the same degree of stability and may also indirectly decrease the amount of space for a more broad and volumetric Lisfranc ligament to form. Another risk factor predisposing an athlete to injury is a shorter second metatarsal in relation to overall foot length [23]. As the length of the metatarsal decreased, probability of Lisfranc injury was increased. It was postulated that a shortened second ray would place more stress at the midfoot that would otherwise have been absorbed by the forefoot.

Prevention of Lisfranc injuries should be a priority for all athletes but particularly professional sports organizations. In collegiate and professional football, it represents the second most common foot injury and is thus a source of lost productivity and income [12]. Demands for more flexible and lightweight cleats have diminished the ability of the shoe to support the midfoot, and longer cleats are desirable for increased grip on the playing surface. Work that continues to identify predictive

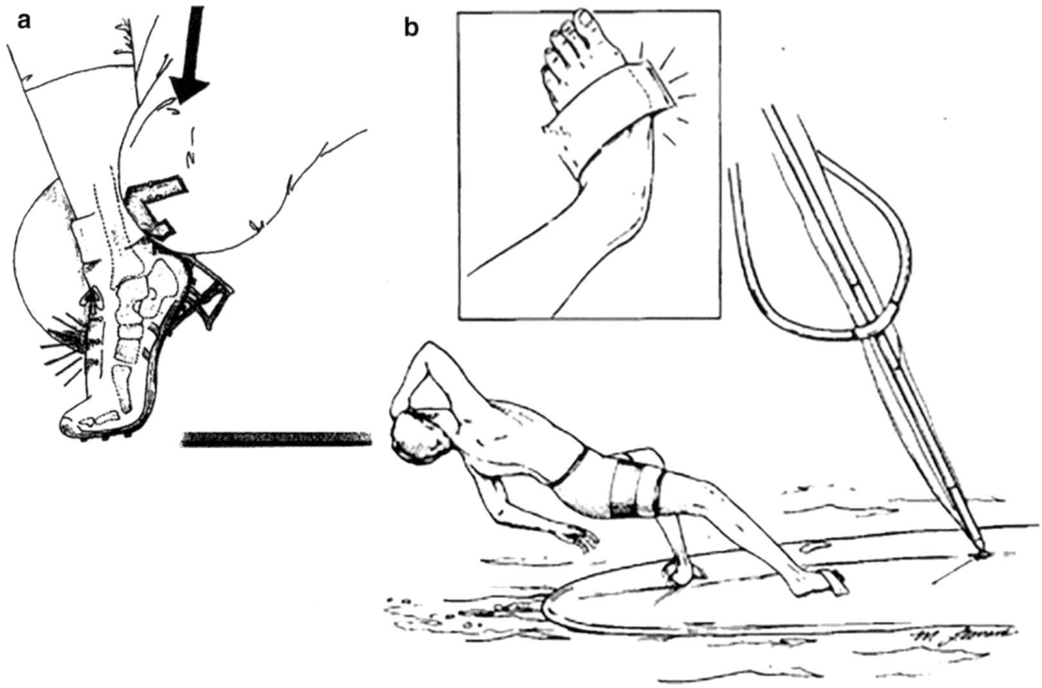

Fig. 19.3 Direct mechanism of Lisfranc injury (**a**) with axial loading of a plantarflexed foot. Indirect mechanism (**b**) with an abduction moment of a fixed, grounded foot (with permission from (**a**)Meyer SA, Callaghan JJ, Albright JP, Crowley ET, Powell JW: Midfoot sprains in collegiate football players. *Am J Sports Med* 1994;22:392–40 and (**b**) Curtis MJ, Myerson M, Szura B: Tarsometatarsal joint injuries in the athlete. *Am J Sports Med* 1993;21:497–502)

factors may assist shoe wear manufactures and orthotists to develop a better combination of both accommodating and protective footwear.

Classification

Lisfranc injuries were initially classified by Quenu and Kuss as homolateral, isolated, or divergent [24]. Myerson modified the above classification to account for proximal instability [7]. Type A describes a completely incongruent TMT joint complex with medial or lateral dislocation of the forefoot. Type B characterizes a partially incongruent injury with further sub-classifications of B1 and B2, describing medial dislocation of the first metatarsal and lateral dislocation of the second to fifth metatarsals. Divergent injuries are classified as Type C injuries with C1 for partial and C2 for total displacement (Fig. 19.4). While the aforementioned classifications are applicable to high-energy mechanisms, they do not adequately classify subtle injuries more commonly seen in athletes.

Nunley and Vertullo [25] presented a classification for ligamentous Lisfranc injuries (Fig. 19.5). Stage I is a sprain of the ligament without associated instability but increased uptake on bone scan. Stage II has 2–5 mm of diastasis between the first and second metatarsal bases but without medial column sag. Stage III presents with >5 mm widening between the first and second metatarsal bases with associated medial column sag. In their series of 15 athletes, none had a stage III injury, and there was otherwise no correlation between a higher-grade injury and worse outcome.

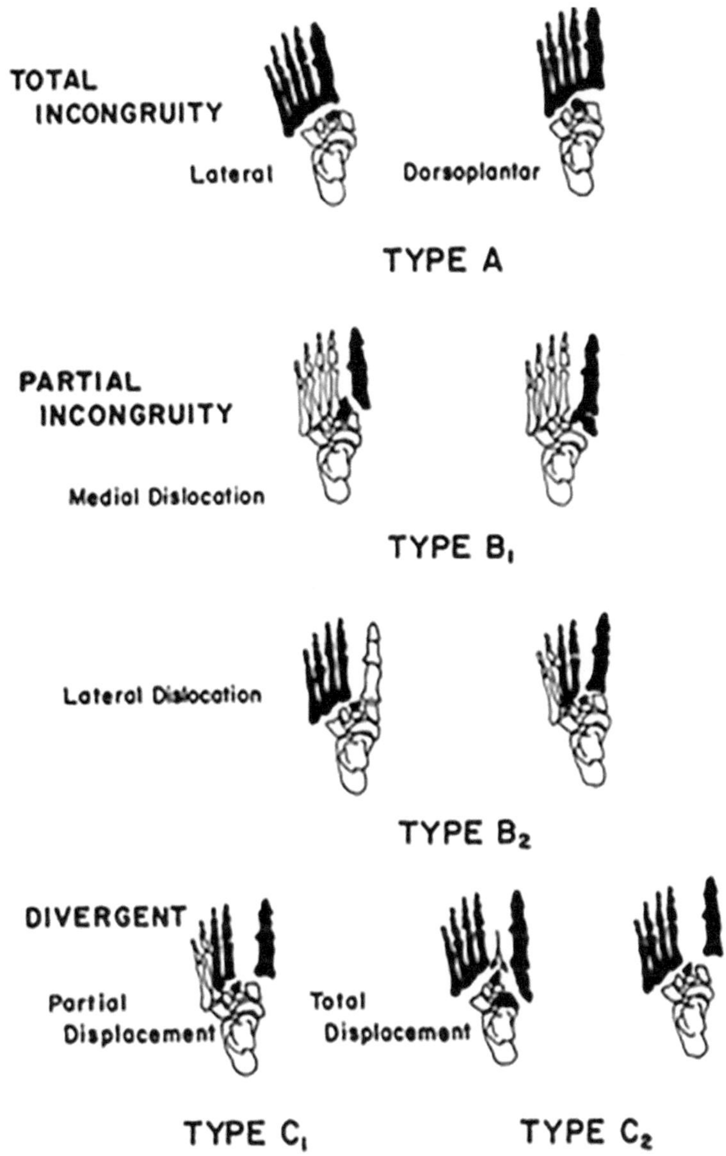

Fig. 19.4 Myerson classification of Lisfranc injury with Types A, complete incongruence; B, partially incongruent with B1 representing medial dislocation of the first metatarsal and B2 representing lateral dislocation of the second to fifth metatarsals; and C with divergent injuries with C1 for partial and C2 for total displacement. With permissions from Myerson MS, Fisher RT, Burgess AR, Kenzora JE. Fracture dislocations of the tarsometatarsal joints: end results correlated with pathology and treatment. *Foot Ankle.* 1986 Apr;6(5):225–242)

Porter [26] also described three different patterns appreciated in subtle Lisfranc injuries. Traditional (TRAD) affects the ligaments attaching the medial cuneiform and first MT, medial cuneiform and second MT, and middle cuneiform and second metatarsal. Medial column dislocation (MCD) injuries affect the ligaments attaching medial cuneiform to second MT and first IC joint. Proximal extension (PE) injuries are a combination of the TRAD and MCD. In their cohort of 82 patients, 49% were noted to have TRAD, 28% PE, and 21% MCD patterns of injury. However, there was no statistical significance in time of recovery, patient reported outcomes, or clinical management; however, the importance of recognizing and treating all unstable joints is noted.

While the current classification systems are important for describing the general pattern of injury and helping the practitioner identify injured joints of the midfoot, they lack evidence regarding their impact in the prediction of treatment or clinical and functional outcomes.

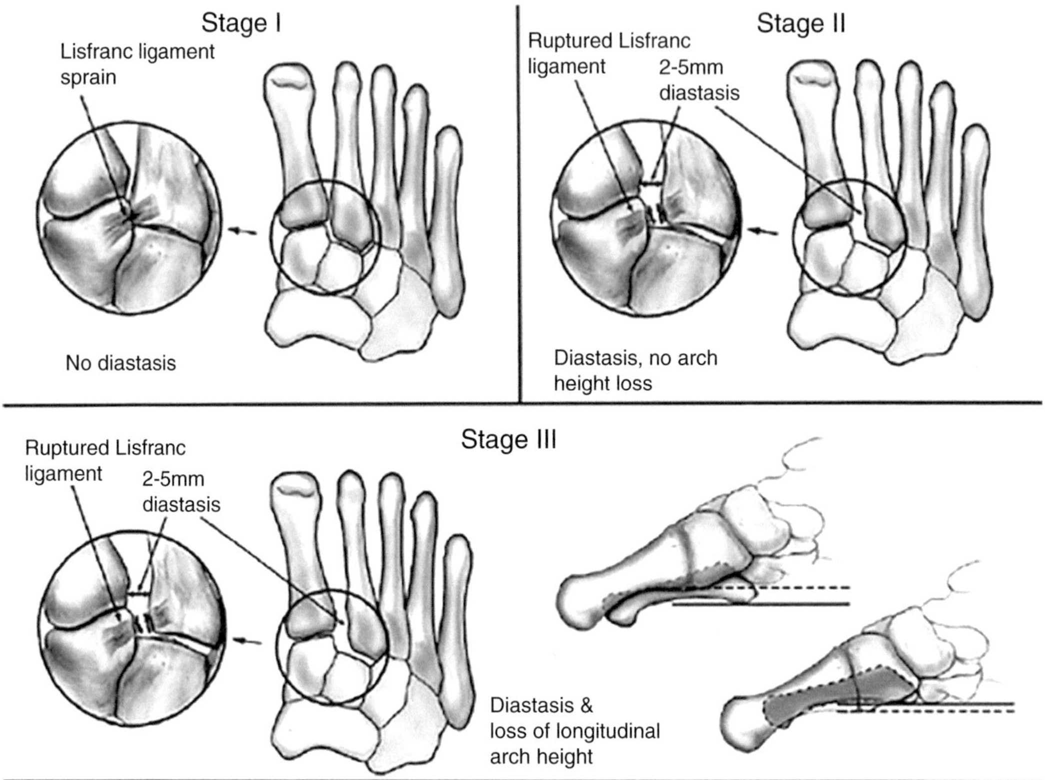

Fig. 19.5 Nunley and Vertullo classification of subtle Lisfranc injury. Stage I—sprain of the ligament without associated instability but increased uptake on bone scan. Stage II—has 2–5 mm of diastasis between the first and second metatarsal bases. Stage III—>5 mm widening between the first and second metatarsal bases with associated medial column sag. (With permissions from Nunley JA, Vertullo CJ. Classification, investigation, and management of midfoot sprains: Lisfranc injuries in the athlete. *Am J Sports Med.* 2002;30:871–878)

Clinical Evaluation

Athletes with a Lisfranc injury typically present with pain in the midfoot after an injury. The athlete is not always able to recount the mechanism of injury or position of their foot at the time of injury. They are often labelled as having had a "foot sprain." There is usually generalized foot swelling, predominantly over the midfoot. Plantar ecchymosis may be present depending on how acutely the patient presents but may not be present until several days following the injury (Fig. 19.6). The presence of plantar ecchymosis, while not specific to Lisfranc injury, should be a clue of potential midfoot injury.

A careful examination of the foot is essential to establish a diagnosis and to ensure other injuries are not missed. A motor examination of all tendons that cross the ankle and foot is important to evaluate motor nerve units but also to ensure no tendon injury. This can be accomplished by having the patient perform ankle dorsiflexion, plantarflexion, inversion, and eversion to assess the tibialis anterior, gastroc-soleus, posterior tibialis, and peroneals, respectively. Contraction of the posterior tibial tendon and anterior tibial tendon may cause pain due to attachments on the cuneiforms and motion at injured joints.

A detailed sensory evaluation should be undertaken. There are five nerves which give sensation to the foot, and each should be evaluated at the following locations: saphenous at medial heel, sural at lateral heel and lateral border of the foot, superficial peroneal nerve on the dorsal aspect of the midfoot, deep peroneal nerve in the first web space, and tibial nerve on the plantar

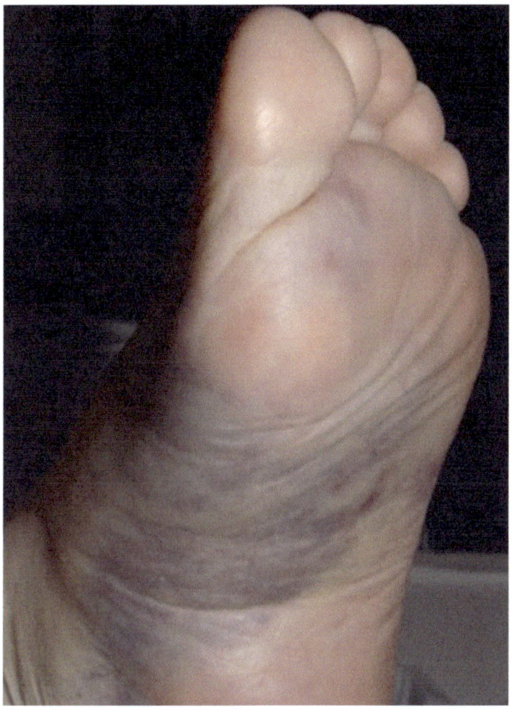

Fig. 19.6 Plantar ecchymosis indicating significant foot injury. (With permissions from Court-Brown CM, Heckman JD. *Rockwood and Green's: Fractures in Adults* eighth ed. Philadelphia: Wolters Kluwer Health;2015)

aspect of the foot. Although some abnormalities may be present due to significant swelling associated with the initial injury and not necessarily due to nerve injury, these should be documented and followed. Vascular competency of the foot should be assessed by palpating the dorsalis pedis artery on the dorsum of the foot and the posterior tibial artery posterior to the medial malleolus. With swelling of the foot, these may be difficult to palpate in which case a Doppler evaluation is appropriate. The toes may also be evaluated for perfusion with a capillary refill test, with normal reperfusion of the toes in <2 s.

Palpation at the midfoot is important in an attempt to localize the origin of foot pain. Motion of the TMT joints will often cause significant pain, and instability may be felt with piano key testing of both the first and second rays. Compression of the metatarsals may also cause pain due to ligamentous injury and possible instability.

Patients are often unwilling or unable to bear weight on the affected extremity. The patient may bear some weight but try to protect the medial midfoot and forefoot by preferentially loading the lateral aspect of the foot. If able to bear weight and stand on the injured foot, the patient may be encouraged to perform single-leg stance and if comfortable can further try single-limb heel rise. If the patient is able to perform all the above steps, suspicion for an unstable injury should be diminished. However, if a patient is unable to bear significant weight on the injured extremity and has tenderness in the midfoot, suspicion for a Lisfranc injury should be heightened.

Imaging Studies

Radiographs

Patients with the above presentation should obtain weight-bearing radiographs of the affected foot. Three views of the foot include a standard anteroposterior view, an oblique view, and a lateral view. On the AP view of the foot, a line drawn along the medial border of the second metatarsal should be congruent with the medial border of the middle cuneiform. On the oblique view of the foot, a line drawn along the medial border of the fourth metatarsal should be congruent with the medial border of the cuboid. On the lateral view, the dorsal aspect of the first and second metatarsal bases should be congruent with the dorsal aspect of the distal medial and middle cuneiforms, respectively (Fig. 19.7). Additionally there should be <2 mm widening between the bases of the first and second metatarsals on the AP view [27]. Subtle avulsion or "fleck" fractures may also be appreciated, and the cuboid may show signs of compression from an abduction moment about the midfoot [7]. Radiographs should be critically analyzed for absence of normal anatomic relationships indicating subtle signs of instability.

Non-weight-bearing (NWB) radiographs are useful for identifying any obvious fracture or unstable injury; however, they are poor tools for ruling out subtle Lisfranc injury, particularly

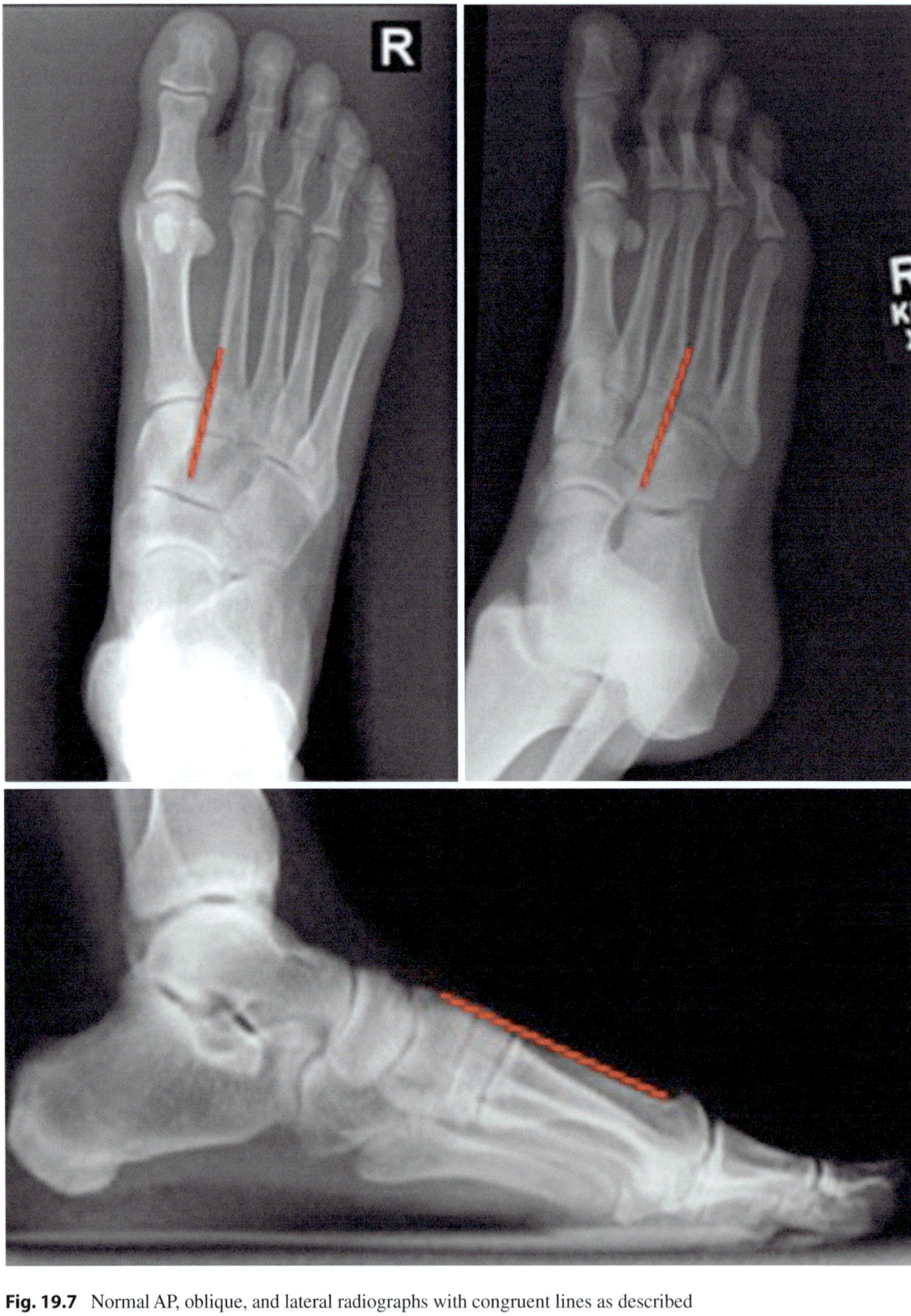

Fig. 19.7 Normal AP, oblique, and lateral radiographs with congruent lines as described

when it is a ligamentous injury. Although patients have pain and difficulty weight bearing (WB) after an acute injury, WB films are an important study for determining the presence of midfoot instability. If a patient can bear weight on their injured side, a WB radiograph must be obtained for a complete evaluation of the injury. If they are unable to bear weight, then the patient should be treated initially for comfort but return in 7–10 days for a repeat radiograph when the pain from the initial injury has subsided. Additionally, when possible, a single-leg stance, WB view of the foot should be obtained (Fig. 19.8). This view creates a weight-bearing stress through the foot and can more consistently identify the presence of a subtle ligamentous injury at Lisfranc joint. WB radiographs of the uninjured, contralateral foot are important for comparison of each patient's normal anatomy. There can be some variability in the alignment of the joints of the midfoot, and it is critical in diagnosis to assure that a perceived widening at Lisfranc interval is not, in fact, a normal anatomic variant for that patient.

If there is evidence of a subtle Lisfranc injury on plain radiographs, where the space between the first and second metatarsals is widened or the second metatarsal is laterally displaced in relation to the middle cuneiform, then the diagnosis is made. If the evidence of Lisfranc injury is inconclusive, and clinical suspicion is high, then an advanced imaging study can be ordered. Additionally, advanced imaging can also be helpful in the situation where the injury has been diagnosed, but more information about subtle fractures or extent of injury is desired. Typically, advanced imaging should be ordered when the result of that study will influence decision-making on treatment or rehabilitation after the injury.

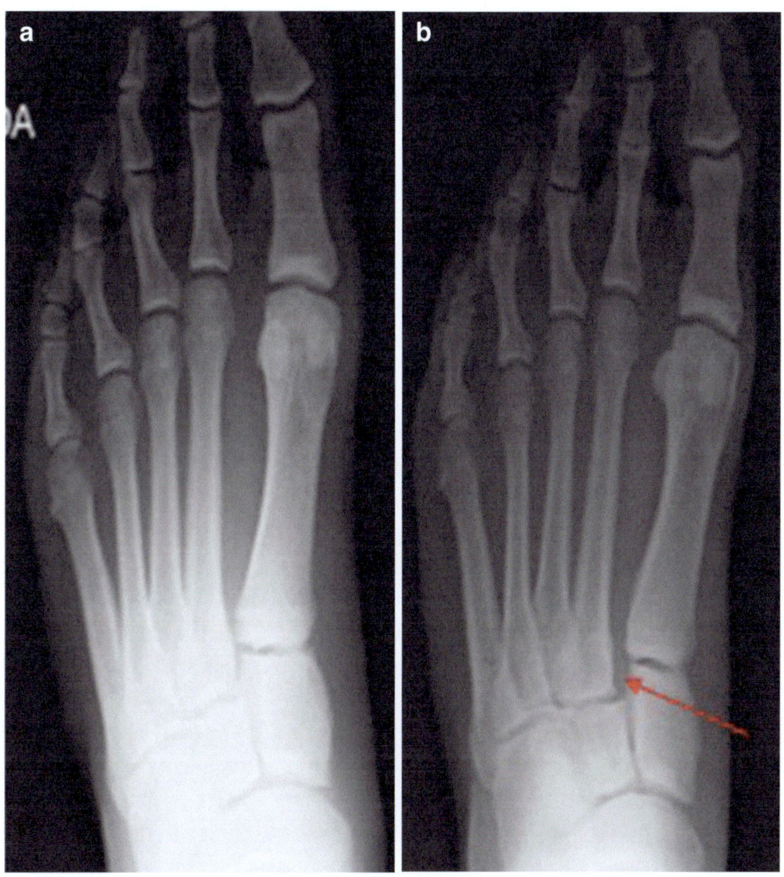

Fig. 19.8 (**a**) AP non-weight-bearing radiograph demonstrating normal-appearing radiograph without evidence of instability. (**b**) The same patient with single-leg weight-bearing AP radiograph now demonstrating widening of the interval between the medial cuneiform and second metatarsal (red arrow)

Stress Radiographs

In situations of heightened clinical suspicion with normal or equivocal weight-bearing radiographs, assessment under fluoroscopy while manipulating the foot has been advocated. This involves stabilizing the hindfoot and then placing a pronation and abduction force through the forefoot. An ankle block with local anesthetic or anesthesia sedation is typically necessary for patient tolerance. In a cadaveric study, isolated sectioning of the Lisfranc ligament resulted in disruption of the medial column line (MCL) in three of four specimens. Complete sectioning of dorsal and plantar TMT ligaments and the Lisfranc ligament demonstrated positive stress radiographs with disruption of the MCL [28]. No widening between the medial cuneiform and second metatarsal or disruption of the medial column line was appreciated on simulated weight-bearing radiographs. The utility of stress radiographs however is controversial and has largely been replaced by MRI to evaluate ligamentous injury. For the authors, manual stress exam under fluoroscopy is not a standard element in evaluation of subtle Lisfranc injury.

Computed Tomography (CT)

When compared to radiographs, CT provides clearer visualization of the midfoot, free of overlapping structures. This is a useful modality to evaluate fracture patterns, presence of additional subtle fractures, or widening of TMT and intercuneiform joints when there is evidence of fracture or concern for subtle widening on initial radiographs. The study is typically a static examination, and its utility in evaluating the stability of the Lisfranc complex when gross instability or fracture is not appreciated on initial radiographs is uncertain.

The advent of weight-bearing CT (WBCT) scan is intriguing as an additional tool to evaluate for subtle instability that is otherwise not appreciated by weight-bearing radiographs. To date, the authors are not aware of a study evaluating the utility of WBCT, and there is uncertainty whether the same radiographic measurements would indicate instability. Recently, a cadaveric study by Sripanich et al. [29] evaluated the amount of widening on the axial and coronal views of WBCT with partial weight bearing (40 kg) and full weight bearing (80 kg) after sequential sectioning of the dorsal Lisfranc ligament, interosseous Lisfranc ligament, and plantar Lisfranc ligament. The cadaver limbs were then sorted to have the first TMT, second TMT, or medial to middle intercuneiform ligament sectioned. Patients demonstrated >2 mm of widening between the first cuneiform to second metatarsal on axial images after sectioning of the three portions of the Lisfranc ligament. This study demonstrates the utilitarian nature of WBCT to be a dynamic test to assist in the assessment of subtle Lisfranc instability. It is still unclear whether WBCT would be more sensitive in assessing for Lisfranc injury.

If a CT scan, regardless of it being WB or NWB, shows evidence of abnormal alignment at Lisfranc joint, then the injury can be considered unstable. The uninjured side can also be imaged by CT scan as a means of comparison. One should be cautious in using a CT scan in isolation as the critical piece of data in determining treatment plan. While the WBCT shows promise, there is no data, as of yet, to support use in this way. CT is best utilized in combination with information gained from physical exam, weight-bearing radiographs, and potentially an MRI.

Magnetic Resonance Imaging (MRI)

MRI is not routinely performed in evaluation of Lisfranc injuries unless there is high suspicion for injury despite negative or inconclusive weight-bearing radiographs or failure to improve with conservative management. The benefit of MRI is that it is quite sensitive at determining injury to the Lisfranc ligament and can help clarify whether there is a sprain or complete disruption. Furthermore, isolated injury to the Lisfranc ligament may or may not predict some degree of instability. In a retrospective study, Raikin et al. investigated what features on MRI suggested instability of the Lisfranc joint [27]. They found the strongest predictor of instability was grade 2 sprain of the plantar ligament from the medial cuneiform to second MT with sensitivity, specificity, and positive predictive value of 94%, 75%, and 94%, respectively.

The challenge with creating an algorithm for treatment of Lisfranc injury based on MRI findings is that, like most CT scans, it is a NWB study. Despite identifying subtle injury to structures of the midfoot, the MRI cannot assess their stability. It is most useful as a tool to elevate index of suspicion for instability if WB radiographs were considered normal. Perhaps the greatest utility of an MRI in evaluation of a midfoot sprain is identifying the potential for a normal Lisfranc ligament. If the Lisfranc ligament is completely normal on MRI, then one can be much more confident that the injury can be treated non-operatively.

Authors' Diagnostic Algorithm (Fig. 19.9)

When a patient presents with pain in the midfoot after an injury, the clinician should consider the potential for significant injury. The patient's history can be important in assessing the mechanism of injury. Understanding if a patient was able to bear weight on the injured foot can also help contribute to recognizing the magnitude of the injury. Additionally, physical exam findings, including focal tests to examine the Lisfranc joint, can help narrow potential diagnoses. A high index of suspicion should always be present to avoid a missed Lisfranc injury.

Radiographs are an excellent initial diagnostic tool after physical exam, with WB radiographs being preferred when possible. Plain radiographs can be helpful in those patients who are unable to bear weight to rule out obvious fractures and obvious displacement or instability. If obvious fractures or Lisfranc instabilities are seen on NWB radiographs, the provider should obtain a CT scan at that time to better delineate fracture patterns and other sites of more subtle instability

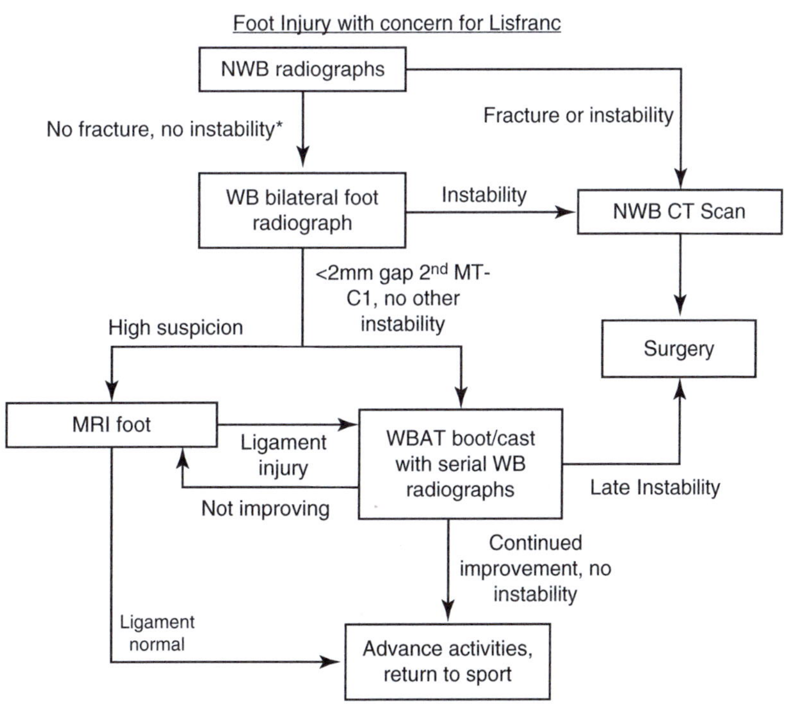

Fig. 19.9 Diagnostic algorithm for imaging of the foot for suspected Lisfranc injury. *Instability defined as >2 mm widening between the second MT base and medial cuneiform (C1), incongruence of the first TMT joint, and/or disruption of normal radiographic landmarks as noted in Fig. 19.6

to assist with operative decision-making and planning.

If no obvious bony injuries or instabilities are identified on NWB radiographs, WB radiograph of bilateral feet will allow for a stress view on the joints of the midfoot. This can show subtle widening between the second metatarsal base and the medial cuneiform on the injured side when compared to the contralateral side. If instability is then noted, the diagnosis is made, and surgical intervention would be recommended to stabilize the injury. Despite the diagnosis on plain radiographs, if there is concern for other fractures or there is value to the clinician and/or the patient in assessing the injury more completely, a CT scan may be obtained. This information can assist in surgical planning or may identify other areas of subtle displacement.

If the patient is able to bear weight and weight-bearing radiographs demonstrate no instability, patients should continue to be immobilized in a boot or cast, dependent on symptoms and degree of swelling. Weight bearing is permitted if tolerated, and the patient should be examined regularly (every 1–2 weeks) with WB radiographs to ensure improving course without radiographic signs of latent instability. If the patient is able to advance, they will typically move through a progression of full weight bearing in a boot, full weight bearing out of the boot typically with an arch support orthotic, double-limb heel rise up onto the toes, single-limb heel rise onto the toes, bicycle, elliptical, light jogging, running, and then returning to sport. The details of recovery on non-operative care of Lisfranc injuries will be covered elsewhere in this text. The key is that the patient should clinically improve, sometimes slowly, over the course of subsequent office visits with consistently stable-appearing weight-bearing radiographs. If latent Lisfranc instability is noted on plain X-ray or there is inability to progress through non-operative care, then advanced imaging should be considered and operative intervention planned.

If the athlete is unable to bear sufficient weight due to pain, one cannot reliably know if their injury is stable. The patient should be placed into a boot for a period of 1 week, weight bearing as tolerated (WBAT), and then return to the office for repeat attempt at weight-bearing radiographs and clinical evaluation. If, at follow-up appointment, the patient has not improved to a point to allow a weight-bearing radiograph and single-limb stance X-ray, then an MRI should be obtained to rule out Lisfranc injury. An MRI could be obtained in the acute phase in those patients with significant injury, inability to bear weight due to pain, or high clinical suspicion based on reported mechanism without obvious injury on non-weight-bearing radiographs. An MRI can also be obtained in the athlete who is trying to minimize time to return to play where treatment decisions are more time critical. If the MRI does not demonstrate ligamentous injury to the Lisfranc ligament, it is safe to have the patient bear weight in a boot with serial monitoring as above. If the MRI demonstrates complete injury to the Lisfranc ligament or the presence of a fleck of bone from the second metatarsal or medial cuneiform, strong consideration should be given to operative reduction and stabilization. It is still possible that a significant ligament injury on MRI can be treated non-operatively, but less likely. That patient should be monitored carefully for delayed presentation instability.

Treatment

The goal of treatment of Lisfranc injury is to correct or maintain midfoot alignment and to have a painless, plantigrade foot. In patients with a stable Lisfranc injury, this is most often obtained with non-operative management with protected weight bearing and gradual resumption of activities as symptoms allow. In patients with unstable injuries, anatomic open reduction and internal fixation are necessary to restore correct alignment. This can be undertaken utilizing a variety of techniques including screw fixation, bridge plating, or suture bridge devices. Alternatively, patients with unstable Lisfranc injuries may be treated with primary arthrodesis. Discussion of the decision-making and techniques surrounding operative fixation is beyond the scope of this chapter.

References

1. Hardcastle PH, Reschauer R, Kutscha-Lissberg E, Schoffmann W. Injuries to the tarsometatarsal joint. Incidence, classification and treatment. J Bone Joint Surg Br. 1982;64:349–56.
2. Faciszewski T, Burks RT, Manaster BJ. Subtle injuries of the Lisfranc joint. J Bone Joint Surg. 1990;72A:1519–22.
3. Lee CA, Birkedal JP, Dickerson EA, Vieta PA, Webb LX, Teasdall RD. Stabilization of Lisfranc joint injuries: a biomechanical study. Foot Ankle Int. 2004;25:365–70.
4. Anderson RB, Ardoin GT. Subtle Lisfranc injury. Tech Foot Ankle. 2010;9:100–6.
5. Perron AD, Brady WJ, Keats TE. Orthopedic pitfalls in the ED: Lisfranc fracture-dislocation. Am J Emerg Med. 2001;19:71–5.
6. Arntz CT, Veith RG, Hansen ST Jr. Fractures and fracture-dislocations of the tarsometatarsal joint. J Bone Joint Surg. 1988;70(2):173–81.
7. Myerson MS, Fisher RT, Burgess AR, Kenzora JE. Fracture dislocations of the tarsometatarsal joints: end results correlated with pathology and treatment. Foot Ankle. 1986;6(5):225–42.
8. Chilvers M, Donahue M, Nassar L, Manoli A. Foot and ankle injuries in elite female gymnasts. Foot Ankle Int. 2007;28(2):214–8.
9. Curtis MJ, Myerson M, Szura B. Tarsometatarsal joint injuries in the athlete. Am J Sports Med. 1993;21(4):497–502.
10. Clanton TO, Porter DA. Primary care of foot and ankle injuries in the athlete. Clin Sports Med. 1997;16(3):435–66.
11. DeOrio M, Erickson M, Giuseppe F, Easley M. Lisfranc injuries in sport. Foot Ankle Clin. 2009;14(2):169–86.
12. Meyer SA, Callaghan JJ, Albright JP, Crowley ET, Powell JW. Midfoot sprains in collegiate football players. Am J Sports Med. 1994;22(3):392–401.
13. Myerson MS, Cerrato RA. Current management of tarsometatarsal injuries in the athlete. J Bone Joint Surg. 2008;90(11):2522–33.
14. Hansen JST. Functional reconstruction of the foot and ankle. 1st ed. Philadelphia: Lippincott Williams & Wilkins; 2000.
15. Sarrafian SK. Anatomy of the foot and ankle: descriptive, topographic, functional. 2nd ed. Philadelphia: Lippincott Williams & Wilkins; 1993.
16. Trevino S, Kodros S. Controversies in tarsometatarsal injuries. Orthop Clin North Am. 1995;26:229–38.
17. De Palma L, Santucci A, Sabeta S, Rapali S. Anatomy of the Lisfranc joint complex. Foot Ankle Int. 1997;18:356–64.
18. Kura H, Luo Z, Kitaoka H, Smutz W, An K. Mechanical behavior of the Lisfranc and dorsal cuneometatarsal ligaments: in vitro biomechanical study. J Orthop Trauma. 2001;15(2):107–10.
19. Johnson A, Hill K, Ward J, Ficke J. Anatomy of the Lisfranc ligament. Foot Ankle Spec. 2008;1(1):19–23.
20. Sung P, Kwan M, Maldonado F, Akeson W. Adhesion strength of human ligament fibroblasts. J Biomech Eng. 1994;116:237–42.
21. Kent RW, Lievers WB, Riley PO, Frimenko RE, Crandall JR. Etiology and biomechanics of tarsometatarsal injuries in professional football players: a video analysis. Orthop J Sports Med. 2014;2(3):2325967114525347.
22. Peicha G, Lobovitz J, Seibert FJ, Grechenig W, Weiglein A, Preidler KW, et al. The anatomy of the joint as a risk factor for Lisfranc dislocation and fracture-dislocation. An anatomical and radiological case control study. J Bone Joint Surg Br. 2002;84(7):981–5.
23. Gallagher SM, Rodriguez NA, Andersen CR, Granberry WM. PAnchbhavi VK. Anatomic predisposition to ligamentous Lisfranc injury: a matched case-control study. J Bone Joint Surg Am. 2014;95(22):2043–7.
24. Quenu E, Kuss G. Etude sur les luxations du metatarse. Rev Chir Paris. 1909;39:281.
25. Nunley JA, Vertullo CJ. Classification, investigation, and management of midfoot sprains: Lisfranc injuries in the athlete. Am J Sports Med. 2002;30:871–8.
26. Porter DA, Barnes AF, Rund A, Walrod MT. Injury pattern in ligamentous Lisfranc injuries in competitive athletes. Foot Ankle Int. 2019;40(2):185–94.
27. Raikin SM, Elias I, Dheer S, Besser MP, Morrison WB, Zoga AC. Prediction of midfoot instability in the subtle Lisfranc injury: comparison of magnetic resonance imaging with intraoperative findings. J Bone Joint Surg Am. 2009;91(4):892–9.
28. Coss HS, Manos RE, Buoncristiani A, Mills WJ. Abduction stress and AP weight-bearing radiography of purely ligamentous injury in the tarsometatarsal joint. Foot Ankle Int. 1998;19(8):537–41.
29. Sripanich Y, Weinberg M, Krahenbuhl K, Rungprai C, Saltzman CL, Barg A. Change in the first cuneiform-second metatarsal distance after simulated ligamentous Lisfranc injury evaluated by weightbearing CT scans. Foot Ankle Int. 2020;41(11):1432–41.

20 Lisfranc Injuries in Athletes: Surgical Treatment Techniques

David A. Porter and Gregory J. Schmidt

Introduction

The Lisfranc joints are the primary midfoot articulations between the tarsal and metatarsal bones. These joints provide the stability of the entire midfoot. Athletic injury to the Lisfranc ligaments is career threatening and historically had been career ending. The surgical treatment of the Lisfranc injury has changed dramatically over time and has enabled the athlete to return to sports at a much higher rate. Midfoot stability is paramount for athlete performance. Surgical stabilization has become the standard to provide a rigid midfoot needed for optimal push-off. The advancement in stabilization techniques is the principal development that has allowed the competitive and recreational athlete to have a much more predictable return [1–3]. Anatomic alignment has been shown to be the principal goal of treatment in all patients [7], and the athlete is unlikely to return without an anatomic, pain-free midfoot. Anatomic reduction maintained by screw and plate fixation until complete healing of the Lisfranc ligaments has become the standard in the competitive athlete. Primary arthrodesis has gained popularity in some recreational and non-athletic populations. We will discuss this progressive approach for treatment in this chapter and familiarize the reader with historical approaches, biomechanical and physiological reasonings, and future directions for this exciting and critical area. We will also give detailed technical instructions for optimizing surgical management and state-of-the-art rehabilitation approaches.

Supplementary Information The online version contains supplementary material available at [https://doi.org/10.1007/978-3-031-08682-3_20].

D. A. Porter (✉)
Purdue University, Butler University, Wabash College, Indianapolis, IN, USA

Department of Orthopedics, Voluntary Clinical Faculty, Indiana University, Carmel, IN, USA
e-mail: dporter@methodistsports.com

G. J. Schmidt
Department of Orthopedics, Indiana University, Indianapolis, IN, USA
e-mail: gjschmid@iupui.edu

Historical Perspective on Treatment/Procedures

Historically, the Lisfranc injury was popularized by Jacques Lisfranc de St. Martin during the War of the Sixth Coalition in 1815 when a soldier fell off a horse with his foot caught in the stirrup; it was treated with an amputation procedure of the midfoot tarsometatarsal (TMT) joints due to a concurrent vascular injury [4].

As knowledge of the injury and anatomy progressed, closed reduction and non-operative treatment procedures became a mainstay. Closed treatment of the injury was then modified to a "pins and plaster" procedure approach in which the

P. D'Hooghe et al. (eds.), *Ligamentous Injuries of the Foot and Ankle*,
https://doi.org/10.1007/978-3-031-08682-3_20

closed reduction of the injury was supplemented by pins for additional fixation and placed in a plaster cast surrounding and over the pins [5–7].

Due to difficulty with achieving and maintaining a good reduction with closed treatment, open treatment of these injuries became more common. The initial approach included fixation with Kirschner wire (K-wire) or trans-articular screw fixation [3]. This technique was later modified, as the development of new, effective, rigid fixation hardware and techniques became available. Especially, screw development allowed the ability to hold fixation with the addition of a "Lisfranc" screw (later termed the "homerun" screw) which mirrors the path of the Lisfranc ligament from the medial cuneiform to the second metatarsal. Dorsal bridge plating has recently been popularized as an option for both bony and purely ligamentous Lisfranc injuries, particularly being used across the first TMT joint [1, 8–11]. Fusion has traditionally been reserved for chronic reconstructive treatment or with severe joint surface disruption. However, more recently, midfoot fusion for purely ligamentous Lisfranc injuries has been advocated in the recreational and non-athlete [26].

Epidemiology and Injury Patterns

Injuries to the Lisfranc joint are fairly uncommon with a previously reported incidence of 1 per 55,000 people per year [12]. These injuries can occur with a wide range of severity with approximately one-third of injuries classified as low-energy injuries (most sports injuries fall into this category) with the remainder attributed to high-energy mechanisms like motor vehicle accidents [13]. When deciding on a treatment strategy, it is important to note that ligamentous Lisfranc injuries can occur within a spectrum of injury type and severity. The spectrum of Lisfranc injuries includes any ligamentous or bony injury that compromises the ligament integrity between the TMT joints. This ligament compromise causes instability of the midfoot and can lead to malalignment with midfoot collapse and pain.

Due to the variety of ligamentous injuries, it is critical to precisely determine the pattern and extent of injury. We believe the classification system by Porter best describes the sports injury and best drives treatment and technique decisions. *Porter* et al. [10] evaluated 80 athletes with a ligamentous injury and created a classification system for ligamentous injuries with a focus on the extent and detail of the ligaments damaged. In that cohort, only 50% of patients presented with a "traditional" injury pattern involving the first TMT and between the medial cuneiform and second metatarsal (Fig. 20.1a). However, 50% of patients in the Porter study had proximal extension of ligament disruption into the intercuneiform (medial and middle cuneiform) joint [10]. Of the 80 athletes with proximal extension, 17 of the original cohort presented with a middle col-

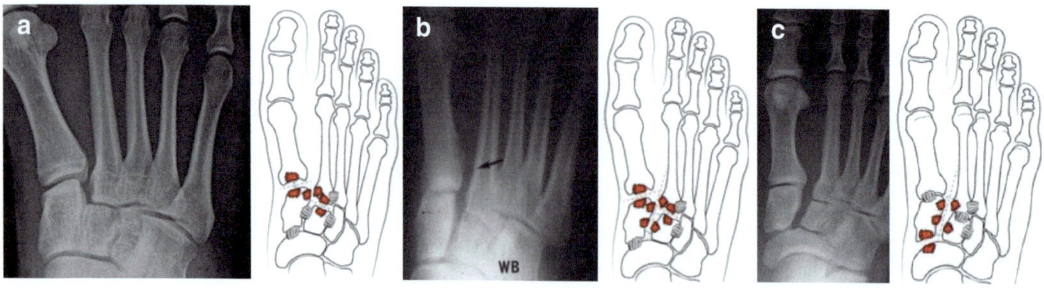

Fig. 20.1 (**a–c**) Ligamentous injury patterns in athletes as described by Porter [10]. (**a**) Traditional (TRAD) pattern of Lisfranc disruption with the first tarsometatarsal (TMT) and second TMT joints. (**b**) Proximal extension (PE) pattern of Lisfranc injury involving the first TMT and second TMT and intercuneiform disruption (medial and middle cuneiform joint disruption). (**c**) Medial column dislocation (MCD) pattern involving the navicular-medial cuneiform, medial and middle cuneiform, and medial cuneiform-second metatarsal. (Reproduced with permission from Porter DA, Barnes AF, Rund A, Walrod MT. Injury Pattern in Ligamentous Lisfranc Injuries in Competitive Athletes. *Foot Ankle Int*. 2019;40 (2):185–194. © 2019 (American Orthopaedic Foot & Ankle Society). DOI: https://doi.org/10.1177/1071100718802264)

umn dislocation (MCD) defined as intercuneiform disruption with proximal extension of the ligamentous injury leading to damage of the navicular-medial cuneiform ligamentous stability but preserved stability of the first TMT joint (Figs. 20.1c and 20.6a, b). Twenty-three of the 80 athletes had a proximal extension pattern (Fig. 20.1b). The high rate of intercuneiform instability noted by *Porter* et al. [10] increases the importance of pre- and intra-operative imaging and clinical assessment to ensure that all injured segments are properly addressed and stabilized. Lack of recognition and incomplete treatment of the intercuneiform disruption have been proposed to lead to poor outcome [1].

Evaluation

Presentation/Examination

Patients with a ligamentous Lisfranc injury typically present with midfoot pain following an acute injury. Typically, this manifests as tenderness and swelling over the tarsometatarsal joints. A classically described sign of subtle Lisfranc injury is plantar ecchymosis (Fig. 20.2a); however, this is not always present. We have also noted mild ecchymosis in the lesser toes as a subtle sign (Fig. 20.2b). Ligamentous Lisfranc injuries are commonly associated with sports, and a review of 154 ligamentous Lisfranc repairs reported 62% occurred during sports [10]. Prior chapters detail more extensively these physical findings. We have not noted any specific exam finding that delineates the pattern of disruption.

Imaging

The treatment strategy, in particular operative technique, is supported by radiographic assessment. Weight-bearing radiographs (XR) of the foot are the initial workup. Three views of the foot are recommended for full evaluation. A standard AP view allows for direct assessment of the Lisfranc joint, intercuneiform joint, and medial column of the foot. The oblique XR allows for closer evaluation of the lateral column of the foot. A diagnosis of Lisfranc injury can be made on the basis of widening between the second metatarsal and medial cuneiform on the AP view

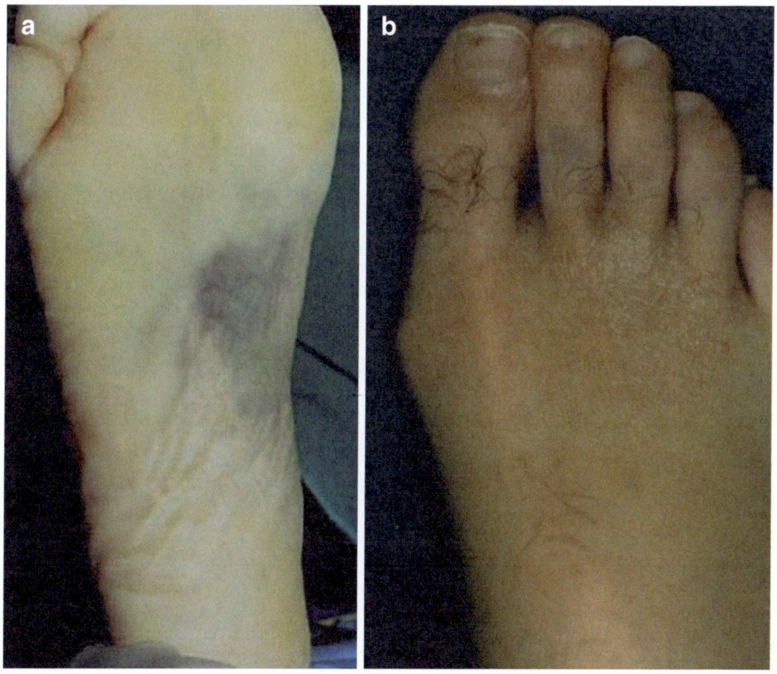

Fig. 20.2 (**a** and **b**) Clinical signs of low-energy sports Lisfranc injury. (**a**) Ecchymosis in arch of the right foot common in low-energy sports Lisfranc injury. (**b**) Clinical foot picture showing mild ecchymosis two to three toes as subtle sign of sports Lisfranc injury

(Figs. 20.1a, 20.4a and 20.25). A comparison AP image is helpful to detect subtle malalignment (Fig. 20.4a and 20.25). In the case of subtle Lisfranc injury, stress radiographs have been shown to be more sensitive in the evaluation of midfoot instability as compared to weight-bearing X-ray alone (Figs. 20.4b and 20.6a, b) [14]. A medial column dislocation as described by *Porter* et al. [10] is best seen on the AP image also (Fig. 20.3a, b). Chronic Lisfranc disruption in athletes can demonstrate dorsal subluxation of the metatarsal(s) on the cuneiforms seen best on the weight-bearing lateral. We propose standing one-legged AP and comparison AP on all athletes with suspected Lisfranc injuries. Occasionally, local anesthetic infiltration can help with full weight-bearing status.

Computed tomography (CT) is commonly performed for evaluation of Lisfranc injuries. A weight-bearing CT allows for a close evaluation of the Lisfranc joint to assess for widening or dorsal subluxation and can provide additional detail on the extent of bony injury. CT may be used for ligamentous Lisfranc injuries if the patient is unable to bear weight on the injured foot due to pain or in cases where the XR findings are equivocal for widening at the Lisfranc joint or intercuneiform joint. A non-weight-bearing (NWB) CT shows small avulsion chip fractures and more significant intra-articular fractures but does not always demonstrate subtle instability.

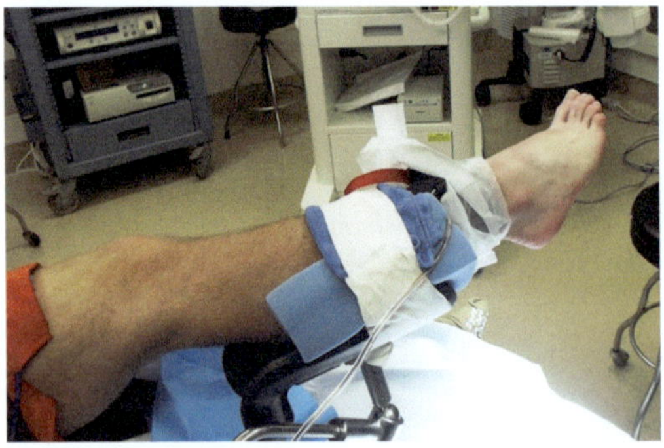

Fig. 20.3 Setup of right lower extremity with leg holder under calf and lower leg to allow circumferential access to the foot with physician-run mini C-arm. Left, unoperated leg flexed slightly to give better access to the foot

Magnetic resonance imaging (MRI) is another imaging option for evaluation of the Lisfranc injuries that can provide additional information for planning the appropriate techniques for treatment. Like CT, it may be used for a closer evaluation of tarsometatarsal joint alignment to assess for subtle subluxation when evaluating for Lisfranc injury. As it provides visualization of the ligaments of the foot, MRI may also be used to assess the extent of damage following injury and plan the extent of operative fixation, that is, which joints are unstable. Furthermore, we use the MRI scan to assess for bone edema, especially if we plan non-operative treatment for the stable injury. Evidence of disruption of the plantar ligament between the medial cuneiform and second and third metatarsals has been shown to be highly predictive of midfoot instability requiring surgical intervention [15]. Additionally, a normal-appearing ligament is suggestive of a stable midfoot and may be a safer alternative to stress radiograph evaluation under anesthesia. We do not believe it is mandatory to obtain an MRI if plain or stress imaging confirms instability. An MRI is also helpful in the chronic setting to determine if there are signs of early arthritis which would preclude reconstruction of the Lisfranc ligament and support secondary fusion.

Treatment Principle

Today, treatment of unstable ligamentous Lisfranc injuries requires surgical intervention. While stable injuries may be amenable to non-operative treatment, most athletic injuries with even mild instability typically will benefit from surgical stabilization techniques. Non-operative techniques for unstable Lisfranc often result in continued pain, midfoot collapse, and significant midfoot arthritis [3, 16, 17]. Prior clinical studies have demonstrated the importance of anatomic reduction and restoration of midfoot stability on clinical outcomes [3, 9, 18]. This finding is further supported by the increased joint contact forces noted in the setting of mild biomechanical malalignment [19]. Surgical techniques must reliably reduce and maintain anatomic alignment. Also, ideal techniques will restore the ligamentous integrity and thus stability. Anatomic reduction may be achieved through closed manipulation and percutaneous fixation, but it is important to be very careful to verify anatomic reduction and have a low threshold for open reduction and verification of alignment.

Principles for stabilization techniques of Lisfranc injuries involve balancing care for the soft tissues and articular surfaces of the foot and maximizing stability of the repair. The importance of stability is twofold. First, it increases the likelihood of maintaining anatomic reduction throughout the healing process and beyond. Second, it makes it safer to quickly allow non-weight-bearing motion in patients after surgery in an attempt to prevent forefoot stiffness.

Repair of the affected ligaments can be performed in addition to the placement of hardware for additional stability. It is not recommended to solely attempt ligament repair without the use of stabilizing implants/hardware.

Primary arthrodesis for purely ligamentous injuries has recently become more popular in the non-athlete. This is largely based on the prolonged healing time of the damaged ligaments and the limited motion in the medial tarsometatarsal joints [20]. Ligamentous Lisfranc injuries have also been reported to lead to posttraumatic arthritis rates as high as 40% following open reduction and internal fixation [21]. However, not all radiographic osteoarthritis leads to clinical symptoms [22]. Ly and Coetzee [23] performed a randomized controlled study of primary arthrodesis vs. open reduction and internal fixation and showed higher AOFAS midfoot scores and a higher rate of return to preoperative level of activity (92% vs. 65%) in the arthrodesis group. The open reduction and internal fixation group also had a higher rate of reoperation with 5 of the 20 patients in the open reduction and internal fixation group undergoing secondary arthrodesis at an average of 42.5 months of follow-up. A similar randomized trial of primary arthrodesis vs. ORIF by Henning et al. [24] showed equivalent physical functioning, Short Form 36 (SF-36) scores, and Selective Functional Movement Assessment (SMFA) scores between the two treatments. The study did show a high rate of reoperations following ORIF compared to arthrodesis. However, DeGiovanni's group [29] showed no greater reoperation rate with ORIF compared to primary arthrodeses if the planned removal of hardware after ORIF was taken into consideration.

One concern following primary arthrodesis in the athlete is first metatarsal stress fracture in patients who continue to have a high level of activity. It is hypothesized to be related to increased stress in the first ray after fusion with loss of the normal motion present in the first TMT joint. Furthermore, fusion will increase the total lever arm of the first ray by 25–30%. This has led some authors to advocate for a hybrid approach to ligamentous Lisfranc injuries involving ORIF with dorsal bridge plating of the first TMT with fusion of other affected joints. *Stødle* et al. [25] performed a randomized trial comparing temporary bridge plating vs. primary arthrodesis of the first metatarsal joint in ligamentous Lisfranc injuries and showed equivalent outcome scores at 2 years between the groups. The study did demonstrate improved alignment of the first metatarsal in the bridge plating group, but 46% of patients in the dorsal bridge plating group had evidence of radiographic arthritis.

The Argument of Fixation Versus Fusion in the Athlete

Many authors continue to recommend ORIF as opposed to primary arthrodesis for ligamentous Lisfranc injuries in athletes. A review of patients treated with partial primary arthrodesis for ligamentous injuries by MacMahon et al. [26]. showed that 25% of the patients were unable to return to the same level of activity, whereas Porter [10] and McHale [2] both reported a greater than 90% rate of return to competitive sports, even at an elite level, after ORIF. It is also important to consider the extent of the injury in athletes before proceeding with arthrodesis. For example, an abduction and midfoot flexion injury (axial load) through the Lisfranc joint when playing sports typically causes disruption of the dorsal ligamentous structures with preservation of the plantar ligaments. The intact plantar ligaments prevent multidirectional instability in the midfoot, and these injuries can be well treated with ORIF [27]. We personally have seen a few athletes that have had primary arthrodesis and developed first metatarsal stress fractures. It is rare for elite athletes to return to pre-injury level of play after primary arthrodesis.

Increased reoperation rates following ORIF have been an argument for primary arthrodesis. However, as mentioned earlier, further analysis by Buda et al. [28] indicated this is largely due to the frequency of planned operations for hardware removal in the fixation cohort. They found a reoperation rate of 75.5% for fixation and 31.5% for arthrodesis when including all planned and unplanned operations. After excluding planned reoperations, they showed no significant difference in reoperation rates for ORIF (29.5%) and primary arthrodesis (29.6%). While many will retain hardware indefinitely in patients treated with fusion, it is common in the senior author's practice, and others, to remove hardware once a stable non-fusion fixation has been achieved. Anecdotally, patients respond well to removal of the hardware after ORIF with decreased pain around the area of hardware placement. And, we believe this low-risk ROH is a small inconvenience to produce a more "normal" foot for return to play.

Treatment Options: Acute

The Principles and Techniques for Open Reduction and Internal Fixation (ORIF) with Rigid Hardware

Technique No. 1: ORIF (Video 20.1)

Open reduction and internal fixation (ORIF) with rigid hardware has become the mainstay treatment approach in ligamentous Lisfranc injuries. It allows for direct visualization of the injury and verification of anatomic reduction. Internal fixation of the injury can be completed with different forms of rigid fixation, but it is imperative to restore stability of the medial column (first and second TMT and intercuneiform joints) of the foot while limiting damage to the articular surfaces and soft tissues. Rigid fixation has involved trans-articular screws most commonly, and it has been recommended to leave the fixation for 3–4 months to allow for ligamentous healing. Bridge plating has become popular for the first TMT joint in the athlete. This technique described is the current technique we use for the majority of our athletic population [10] (Fig. 20.4).

Technique

Appropriate anesthesia is supplied. We utilize an ankle block with sedation. The patient is supine. We utilize a unilateral leg holder under the involved calf to allow circumferential access for imaging (Fig. 20.3). We utilize an ankle tourniquet to allow sufficient anesthesia with an ankle block and dorsal foot field block. Others could use a general anesthetic or regional block and use a thigh or calf tourniquet. The opposite extremity has a sequential compression device (SCD) for thromboprophylaxis. A small bump is placed under the ipsilateral hip. The foot of the bed is flexed to allow easy circumferential physician-directed mini C-arm access (Fig. 20.3).

Many different open approaches have been described. We utilize a primary dorsal curvilinear incision starting over the midshaft of the first metatarsal and extending dorsally and proximally moving laterally at the first TMT joint to track over the second TMT and then proximally and slightly medially over the intercuneiform joint (medial and middle cuneiforms). To visualize and access the lateral foot (if needed), a second dorsal incision is utilized for fixation while limiting soft tissue damage. In addition, a small percutaneous incision is utilized over the medial foot for medial to lateral intercuneiform screw (if needed) and MC-second MT screw placement. In the athlete, often open exposure is not required of the third–fifth TMT joints if these joints are aligned well after medial reduction. The interval between the extensor hallucis longus and brevis is utilized to access the first TMT joint (Fig. 20.15). Once the approach has been completed, it should be possible to visualize the dorsal midfoot and fully assess the extent

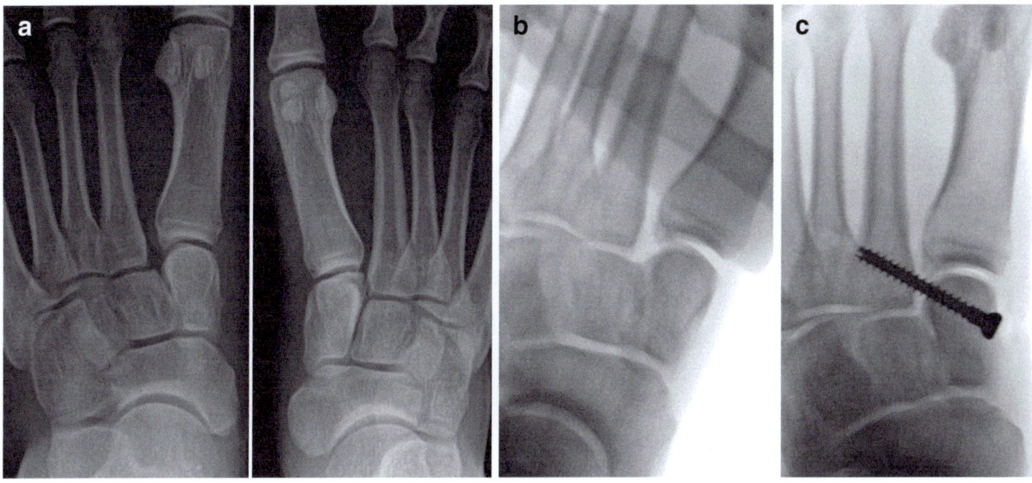

Fig. 20.4 (**a**–**c**) Technique for assessing instability and sequence of fixation in ORIF traditional Lisfranc. (**a**) Comparison anterior and posterior (AP) radiographic views of the foot. Right is normal foot and left is unstable midfoot. See the lateral shift of the second metatarsal on the middle cuneiform and mild lateral shift of the first metatarsal on medial cuneiform. (**b**) AP radiograph with intraoperative abduction stress image showing tilting and instability of the first and second TMT joints. (**c**) AP radiograph demonstrating anatomic alignment of the second TMT joint with 4.5 mm fully threaded "homerun" screw from medial cuneiform to the second metatarsal base

of ligamentous injury. We confirm if the first TMT is disrupted (traditional pattern and proximal extension pattern) or if the first TMT is stable, as in the medial column dislocation pattern. It is especially important to assess the medial cuneiform-middle cuneiform ligament since this ligament is not well assessed with preoperative plain radiographs. Intraoperative stress testing with a blunt Freer elevator under fluoroscopy should be used to evaluate and confirm the extent of the injury and document ligamentous damage (Fig. 20.5b and Porter [10], Video 20.1).

Intercuneiform ORIF

We prefer to start proximally first and then work distally and medial to lateral (intercuneiform, second TMT, and first TMT and then determine if the third–fifth TMT require fixation). If the intercuneiform joint is disrupted (proximal extension and medial column dislocation), we stabilize that joint first. We reduce and/or confirm the navicular-cuneiform joint (Nav-cun) is reduced. Stabilization of the navicular-cuneiform joint is undertaken first if needed. We do not typically find fixation is required, but use screw fixation if required (4.0 mm). A second small medial incision as mentioned above is undertaken along the dorsal border of the anterior tibial tendon (ATT). A medial to lateral partially threaded screw is placed to reduce the intercuneiform joint. You must be careful to not overtighten the screw and compress the cartilage. We use a 4.0 or 4.5 mm screw depending on the size of the athlete. If the patient is large or the pattern is a medial column dislocation, we often use two intercuneiform screws (Fig. 20.5c, d).

Second TMT ORIF

The second TMT joint is addressed next. We dissect just lateral to the base of the second metatarsal and use a tenaculum reduction forceps (a Lisfranc-specific reduction clamp can also be used but we find it a bit bulky) between the medial cuneiform and the lateral second metatarsal base to snuggly reduce the second metatarsal on the middle cuneiform's lateral edge. This maneuver takes the foot out of abduction, and the surgeon should see the foot move out of a pronated and abducted position and restore the arch and slight adduction of the midfoot. Next is placement of the guide pin from the medial cuneiform to the base of the second MT. It is paramount to carefully plan and evaluate the trajectory

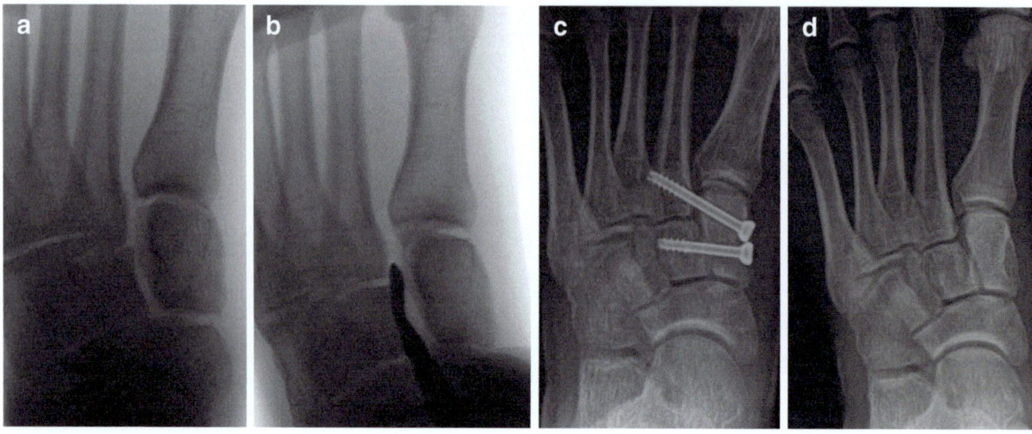

Fig. 20.5 (**a**–**d**) Technique for assessing and performing ORIF medial column dislocation (MCD). (**a**) Preoperative anterior-posterior (AP) image of the left foot showing well-aligned first and second tarsometatarsal (TMT) joints but wide at MC-second MT and intercuneiform joint as well as subluxation at Nav-med cuneiform joint. (**b**) Intraoperative AP stress imaging of medial column with Freer elevator between the medial cuneiform and second metatarsal base showing MCD instability. (**c**) AP radiograph demonstrating two-screw fixation of MCD with anatomic midfoot alignment. (**d**) 1-year postoperative AP image demonstrating maintained anatomic midfoot alignment without arthritis or complication

of the guidewire placement to ensure accurate, centered placement. Cadaveric studies have shown a significant increase in the amount of articular surface damage when two pin passes were required. Additionally, 40% of the specimens with two passes of the guidewire prior to screw fixation demonstrated fracture of the articular surfaces [8]. A cannulated drill is used to predrill for the screw, and a solid or cannulated screw is then inserted. We initially used a partially threaded screw but now prefer a fully threaded screw for better long-term stability (Fig. 20.4c). Imaging should demonstrate ideal screw placement both on the anterior-posterior (AP) (Fig. 20.4c) and lateral views. The lateral is crucial to confirm centralized placement in the base of the second metatarsal dorsal to plantar. Too dorsal or too plantar can result in poor bone purchase and inadequate stabilization.

First Tarsometatarsal ORIF

If the pattern is NOT a medial column dislocation, then the first TMT is stabilized with either a single distal to proximal trans-articular screw or a dorsal four- or five-hole bridge plate. The first TMT joint is typically well reduced after the second TMT (and proximal IC joint if necessary) is reduced and stabilized. The instability is then primarily in the sagittal plane. Traditionally, the first TMT stabilization has been with a distal to proximal 4.0 or 4.5 mm trans-articular screw. It is important to countersink the distal insertion point after drilling to make room for the head to sit flush with the cortex and decrease the risk for dorsal breakout. The surgeon must be careful to not "overcompress" the joint and lead to early osteoarthritis (OA).

Alternatively, dorsal bridge plating (especially in the first TMT) has gained popularity as a method to achieve TMT stability while preserving the articular surfaces. This obviates the need to place a screw through the chondral surface and eliminates the risk of intra-articular screw breakage. Additionally, cadaveric biomechanical testing has shown an equivalent ability of dorsal bridge plates to maintain anatomic reduction with loading in comparisons to trans-articular screws [29]. We prefer a 2.7 mm low-contour, dynamic compression (LCDC) dorsal bridge plate, contoured and stabilized with 2.7 mm screws (Fig. 20.6a, b). We find two screws are often adequate (one proximal and

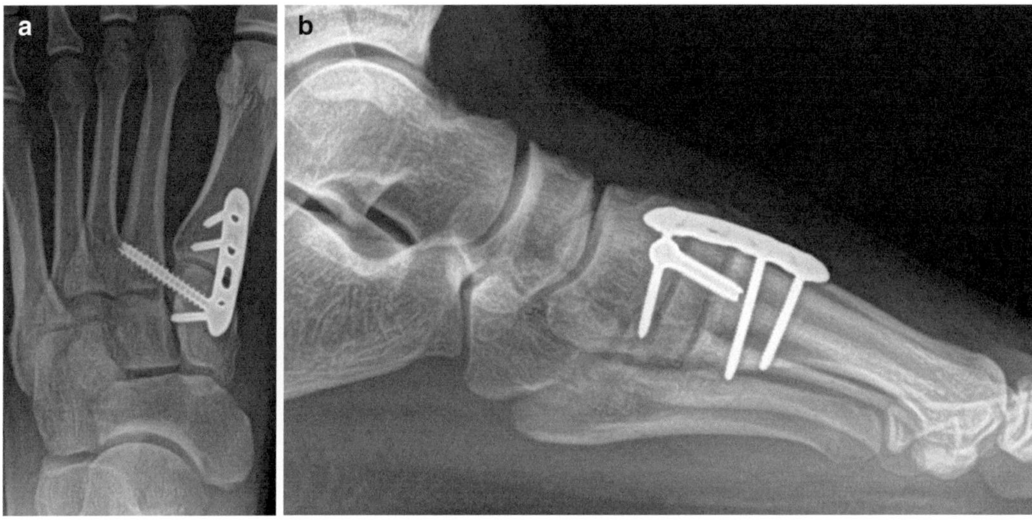

Fig. 20.6 (**a**, **b**) Postoperative images after ORIF traditional Lisfranc stabilization. (**a**) Anterior-posterior (AP) radiograph after ORIF with the first tarsometatarsal (TMT) 2.7 mm five-hole "bridge" plate with dorsal to plantar 2.7 mm screws. Also, note 4.5 mm fully threaded "homerun" screw from medial cuneiform to the base of the second metatarsal. (**b**) Lateral radiograph of the foot demonstrating the same first TMT plate and 4.5 mm "homerun" screw

one distal to the first TMT joint). If there was dorsal subluxation noted on the preoperative imaging, or if a chronic case, we may use three to four screws and occasionally a five-hole plate to increase sagittal stabilization. Hu has shown improved alignment and less arthritic changes after a minimum of 2-year follow-up, but the patients were not athletes and were actually more high-energy injuries [11]. The difference in outcome in the athlete has not been reported between a dorsal bridge plate and trans-articular screw.

The Principles of Fixation and Technique for PRIF (Percutaneous)

Technique No. 2: Percutaneous Lisfranc Fixation (Video 20.2)

Percutaneous fixation has the stated advantage of smaller incisions in an attempt to decrease skin and wound complications. Percutaneous treatment is relatively simple and can be a reasonable option for treatment of these injuries, and meta-analysis revealed the procedure was safe and effective as long as anatomic reduction was obtained and maintained [31]. The meta-analysis did not specifically look at results in athletes. There are no clear, agreed-upon indications for closed reduction and percutaneous fixation, but it is paramount to achieve and verify an anatomic reduction. It is important to have a low threshold for converting to an open approach if the surgeon is unable to achieve an anatomic reduction. Setup is in the supine position with either a general or regional anesthetic. The involved leg is prepped and draped up above the knee, so the knee can be flexed and extended to obtain appropriate mini fluoroscopy views (Fig. 20.7).

When performing percutaneous treatment, instability of the TMT joints is first confirmed fluoroscopically. Closed reduction is performed in a medial to lateral fashion. We like to start proximally and clamp the medial and middle cuneiforms to allow placement of a medial to lateral cannulated screw (Fig. 20.8a, b). The first ray is first reduced by applying an adduction and plantar flexion force. Once reduction of the first ray is confirmed, it can be provisionally fixed in

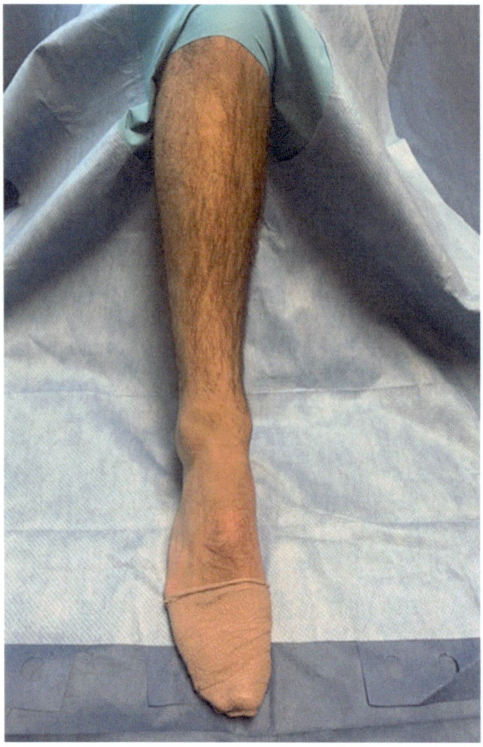

Fig. 20.7 Setup and draping technique used in percutaneous fixation Lisfranc

place with percutaneous Kirschner wires (K-wires). Following fixation of the first ray, attention is then turned to the second metatarsal. The second metatarsal can be reduced with the use of a percutaneously inserted clamp from the base of the second metatarsal to the medial cuneiform recreating the course of the Lisfranc ligament (Figs. 20.9a, b and 20.7a). Reduction is then verified fluoroscopically, and the second MT fixation can be placed with the use of screws (Fig. 20.10a–d). If instability of the lateral column persists following stabilization of the medial TMT joints, K-wire fixation would then be used to stabilize the lateral TMT joints (Fig. 20.9c, d). Once the affected joints have been stabilized with the use of clamps and provisional K-wire fixation, screw fixation can be performed (Fig. 20.10c–d). Fixation can be achieved with the use of cannulated screws inserted over the previously placed guidewires. The "homerun" screw between the medial cuneiform and second metatarsal is placed first and followed by trans-articular screws at the unstable TMT joints (Fig. 20.11, Video 20.2) [30].

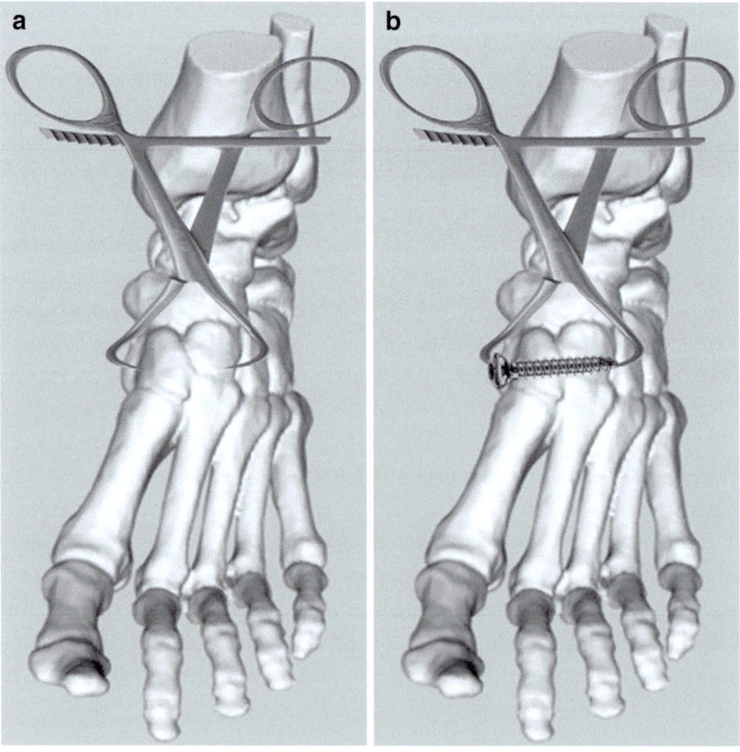

Fig. 20.8 (**a**, **b**) Percutaneous fixation of intercuneiform joint as described by Sharma [30]. (Reproduced with permission from Sharma S, Dhillon MS, Arora C, Patel S. Percutaneous fixation of Lisfranc injuries. *J Clin Orthop Trauma*. 2020;11 (3):487–491. © 2020 (Delhi Orthopedic Association). DOI: https://doi.org/10.1016/j.jcot.2020.03.018)

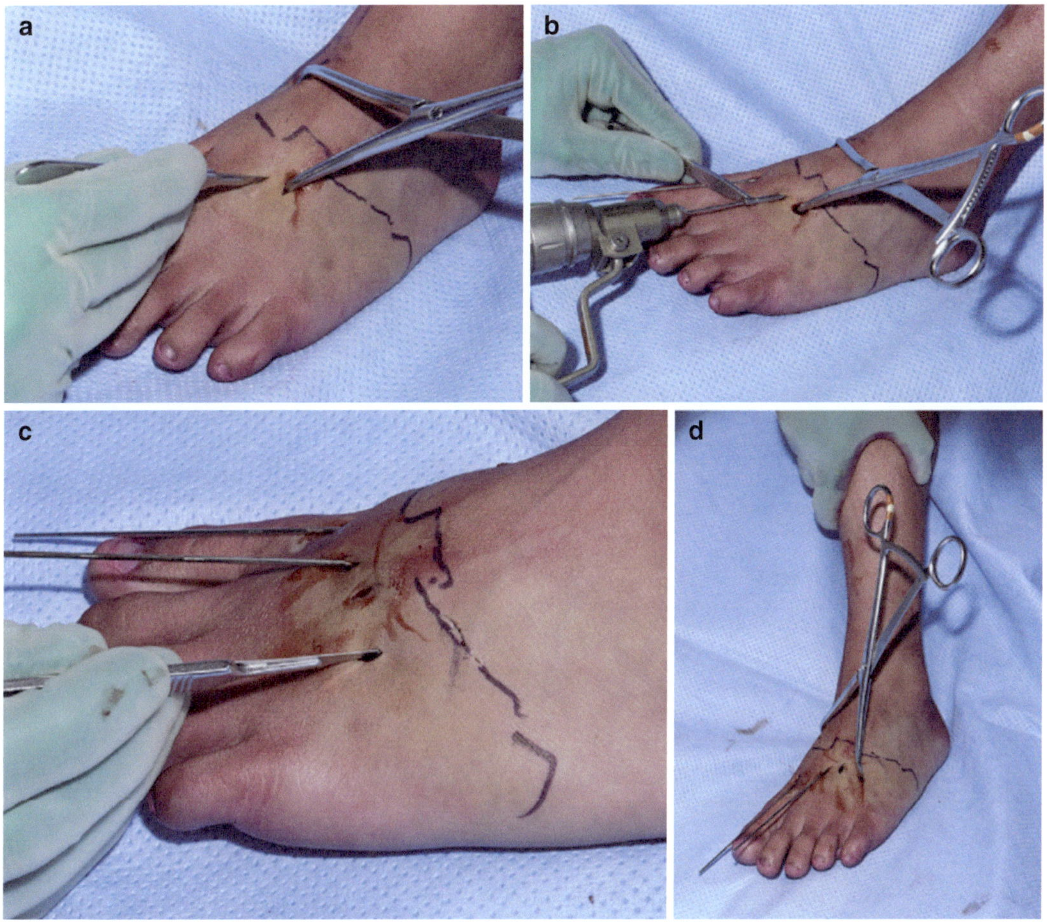

Fig. 20.9 (**a**–**d**) Sequential wires are then placed across the second (**a**, **b**) and third metatarsal bases. The clamp can be moved more laterally to reduce the third metatarsal base (**c**, **d**) as described by Sharma [30]

The Principles of Fixation and Technique for Suture Button Flexible Fixation for Isolated Lisfranc Ligament Injury

Technique No. 3: Primary Open Flexible Fixation with Suture Button(s) by Cho et al. [32]

Positioning is supine and diastasis is confirmed with image intensification. An isolated MC1-MT2 instability is confirmed in order to use this technique (Fig. 20.12a). Two short longitudinal incisions are made, one over the medial border of the medial cuneiform and the second over the dorsal lateral base of the second MT base (Fig. 20.14a–b).

Reduction can be attempted via a closed mechanism but commonly requires a large tenaculum reduction clamp between the lateral base of the second metatarsal base and medial cortex of the medial cuneiform (Fig. 20.13a, b). Anatomic reduction of the medial MT2 base on the MC1 is mandatory (Fig. 20.13b). The suture button itself cannot be relied upon to further reduce the diastasis. The suture button can only be expected to maintain reduction (unlike a partially threaded trans-articular screw which can be utilized to "dial in" the final reduction – though not recommended by this author). Further open extraction of interposed soft tissue or a small osteochondral fragment can be accessed through the dorsal incision if unsatisfactory reduction is initially not obtained.

The TightRope (Arthrex, Naples, LF) guidewire is placed from the posteromedial cortex of

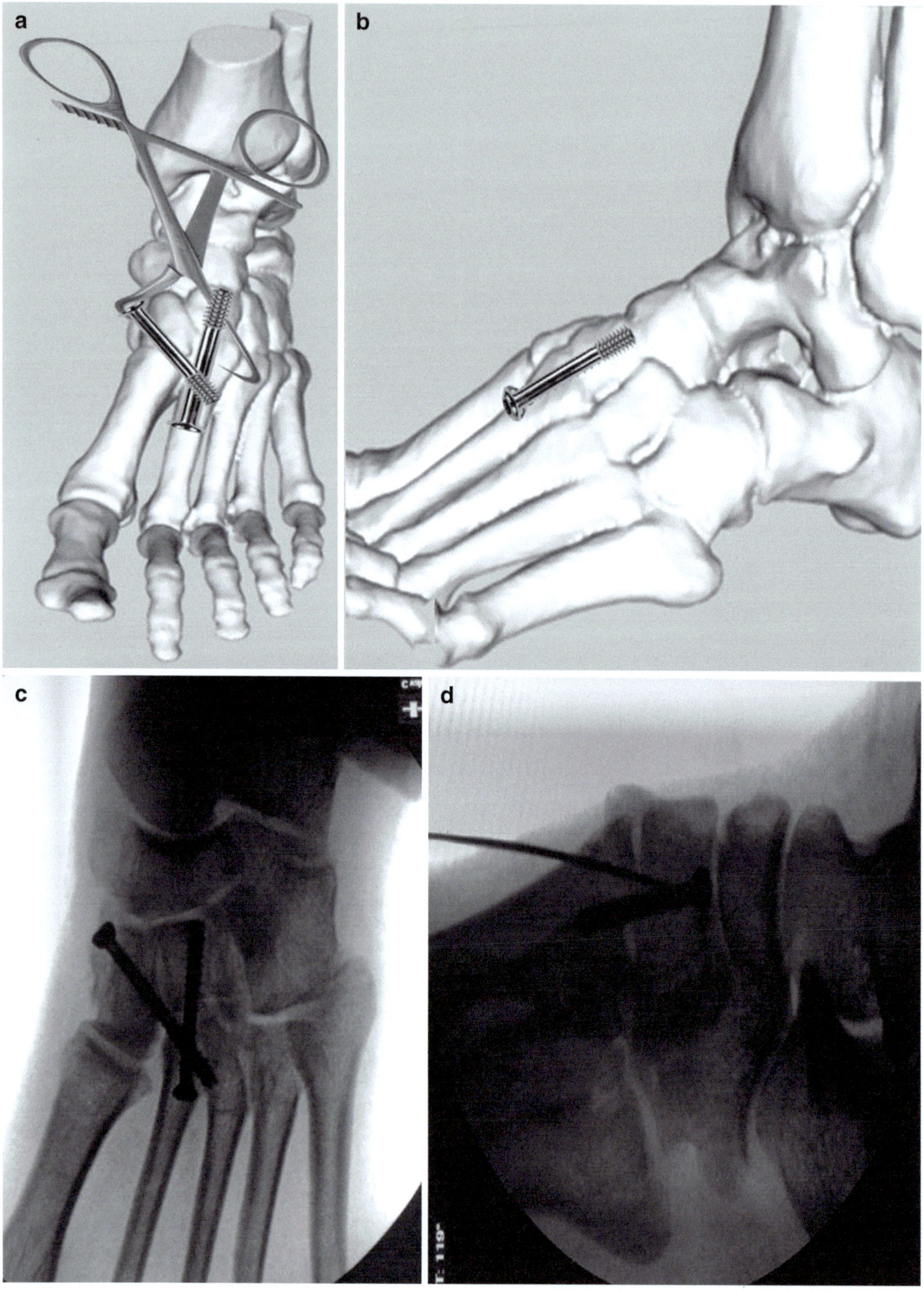

Fig. 20.10 (**a**–**d**) Percutaneous fixation of the second metatarsal to reduce the second MT to the medial cuneiform and stabilize the second TMT joint as described by Sharma [30]. (Reproduced with permission from Sharma S, Dhillon MS, Arora C, Patel S. Percutaneous fixation of Lisfranc injuries. *J Clin Orthop Trauma*. 2020;11 (3):487–491. © 2020 (Delhi Orthopedic Association). DOI: https://doi.org/10.1016/j.jcot.2020.03.018)

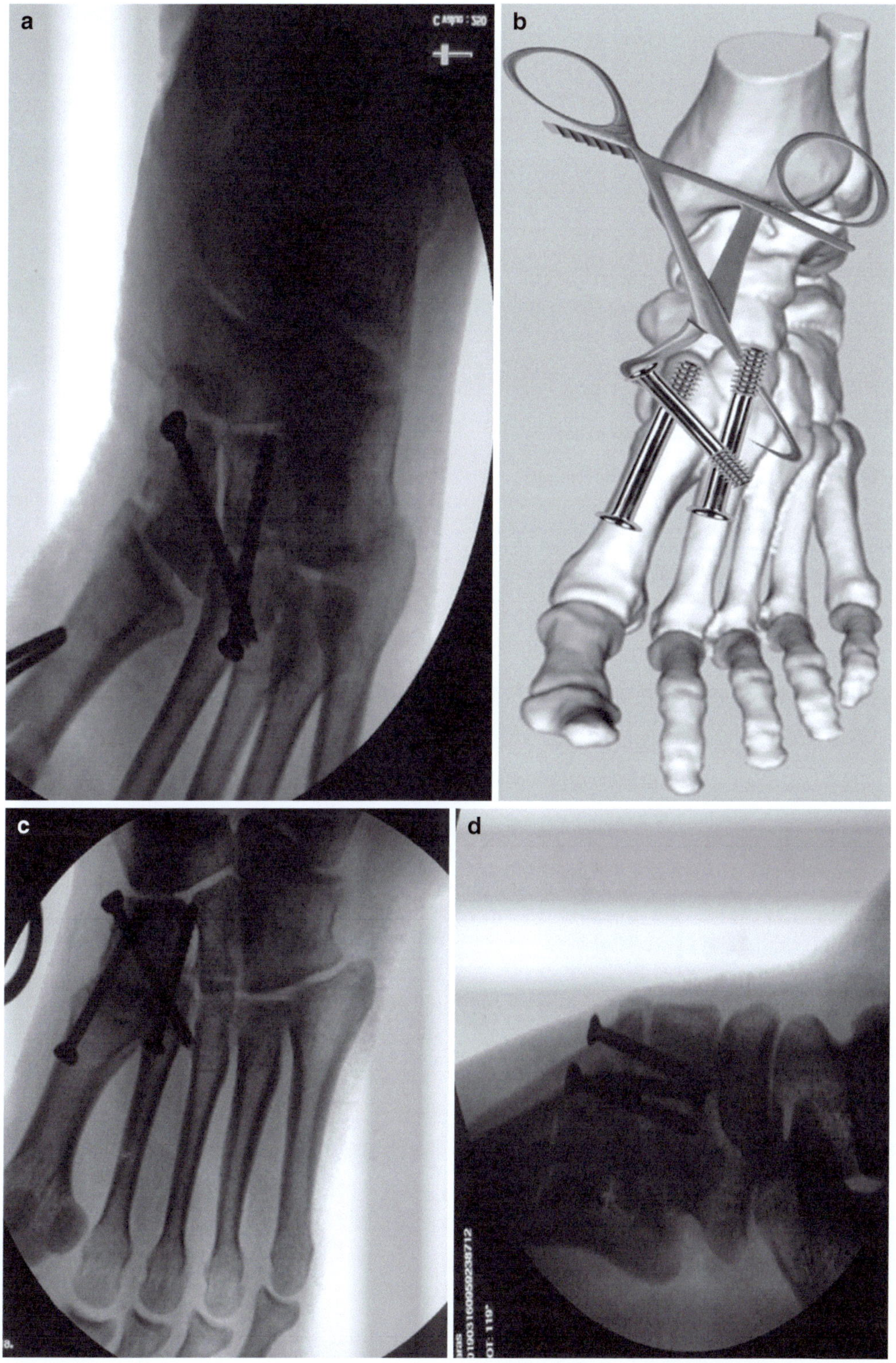

Fig. 20.11 (**a–d**) ORIF first TMT percutaneous fixation as illustrated by Sharma [30]. (Reproduced with permission from Sharma S, Dhillon MS, Arora C, Patel S. Percutaneous fixation of Lisfranc injuries. *J Clin Orthop Trauma*. 2020;11(3):487–491. © 2020 (Delhi Orthopedic Association). DOI: https://doi.org/10.1016/j.jcot.2020.03.018)

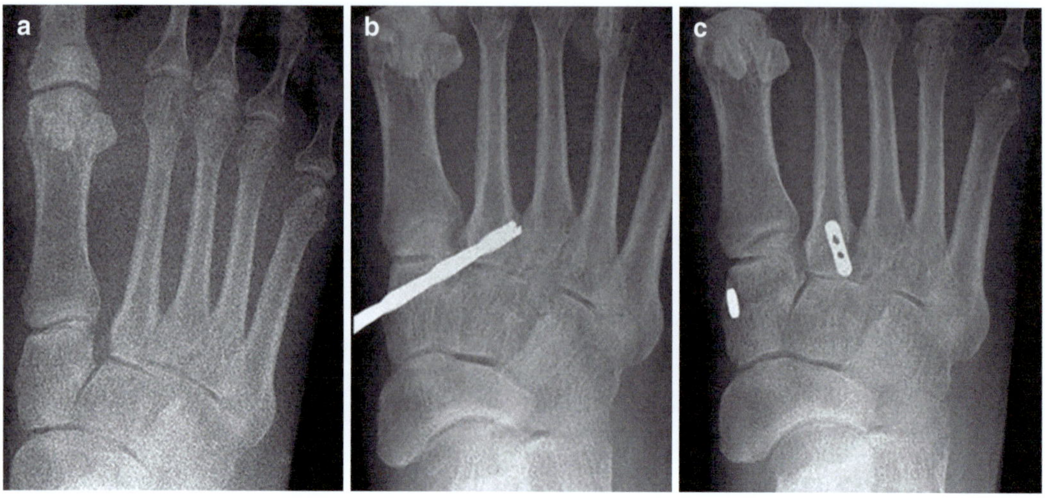

Fig. 20.12 (**a**–**c**) Intraoperative radiologic image of the Lisfranc ligament fixation using a suture button. (**a**) Preoperative evaluation of the Lisfranc joint diastasis. Note the anatomic alignment of the first tarsometatarsal joint. (**b**) Reaming along the guidewire inserted across the Lisfranc joint. (**c**) Reduced diastasis after fixation with a suture button. As shown by Cho et al. [32]. (Reproduced with permission from Cho J, Kim J, Min TH, et al. Suture Button vs Conventional Screw Fixation for Isolated Lisfranc Ligament Injuries. *Foot Ankle Int.* 2021;42(5):598–608. © 2021 (American Orthopaedic Foot & Ankle Society). DOI: https://doi.org/10.1177/1071100720976074)

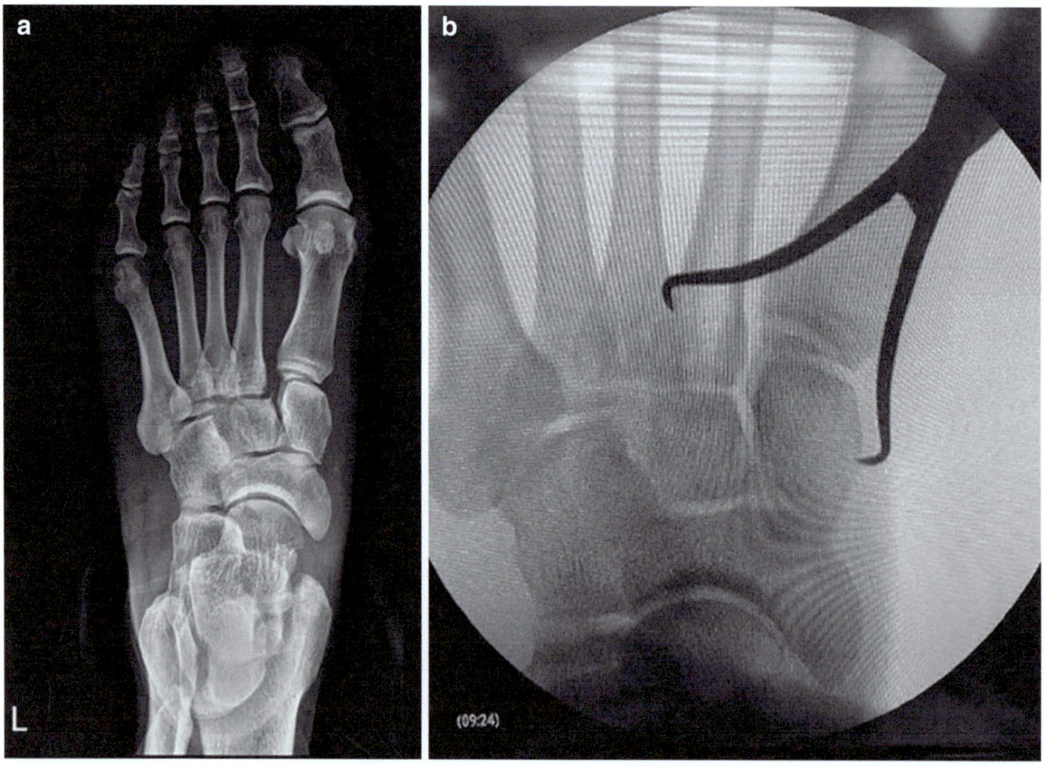

Fig. 20.13 (**a**–**b**) (**a**) Preoperative dorsoplantar foot radiograph with widened Lisfranc joint. (**b**) Following the insufficient manual reduction, additional reduction was performed with the use of a large bone-reduction clamp applied between the base of the second metatarsal and medial surface of medial cuneiform

the medial cuneiform through the base of the second metatarsal along the course of the Lisfranc ligament. AP, lateral, and oblique image intensification is utilized to confirm placement of the wire centered within the second metatarsal base 4–8 mm distal to the articular surface of MT2. A bone tunnel is then created with a 3.5 mm cannulated drill (Fig. 20.12b). A large TightRope is then threaded from medial to lateral utilizing the pass pin with two pull-through sutures through the tunnel exiting just lateral to the MT2 base through the dorsal incision (Fig. 20.14c). Of the two pull-through sutures, only the white one is pulled with tension with the other suture being slack allowing the oblong endobutton to position in line with the tunnel. When the leading edge of the oblong button clears the lateral MT2 base lateral cortex, the green and white pull-through sutures are toggled to seat the oblong button on this lateral cortex while maintaining some tension on the medial sutures. The authors recommend placing the oblong button in a longitudinal fashion along the second metatarsal to decrease stress riser and dorsal irritation. Image intensification is utilized to confirm the buttons are directly on the medial cuneiform and MT2 cortex with no soft tissue interposition (Fig. 20.12c). If required, the surgeon should clear the cortex to allow flush placement on each cortex. Soft tissue interposition can lead to soft tissue necrosis and micro-creep. The free ends of the fiber wire are tied over the washer and cut 1 cm in length and buried under the medial

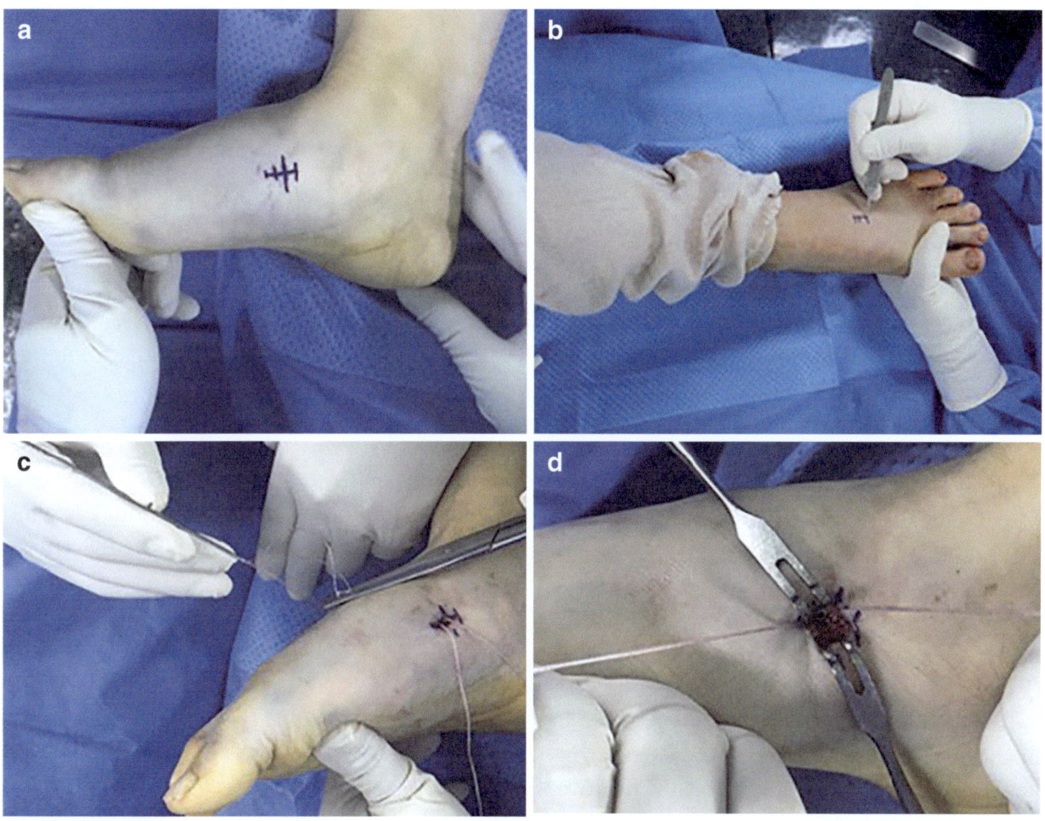

Fig. 20.14 (**a**–**d**) Intraoperative images of the Lisfranc joint fixation using a suture button. (**a**) Medial incision over the medial border of medial cuneiform. (**b**) Dorsal incision just lateral to the second metatarsal base. (**c**) Advancement of the suture button. (**d**) Knot made over the suture button. As shown in Cho et al. [32]. (Reproduced with permission from Cho J, Kim J, Min TH, et al. Suture Button vs Conventional Screw Fixation for Isolated Lisfranc Ligament Injuries. *Foot Ankle Int.* 2021;42(5):598–608. © 2021 (American Orthopaedic Foot & Ankle Society). DOI: https://doi.org/10.1177/1071100720976074)

cuneiform periosteum (Fig. 20.14d). The soft tissues are closed in layers.

Postoperative protocol involves 6 weeks of NWB with a splint (3 weeks) and then a removable cast (3 weeks). Pool therapy and range-of-motion movement are initiated after suture removal, typically 2 weeks postoperatively. Partial weight-bearing is initiated between 6 and 12 weeks with an "arch supporting removable cast" gradually advancing to full weight-bearing. The authors report "the patients return to regular sports practice in 12–16 weeks." [32]. The authors noted a more normal plantar first metatarsal head pressure when compared to conventional screw fixation of isolated Lisfranc ligament injuries.

The Principles of Fixation and Technique for Primary Arthrodeses

Technique No. 4: Primary Arthrodesis Principles of Coetzee and Ly [27] and Technique of Kuhn [33]

The patient is typically positioned supine on the operating room table, and a tourniquet is commonly used. Preoperatively, it is necessary to determine the extent of the ligamentous instability (Figs. 20.4a, 20.6a, and 20.12a). In low-energy injuries, the instability is typically limited to the medial column, which may be addressed with fusion of only the first and second tarsometatarsal (TMT) joints and the intercuneiform (IC) joint. This may be accomplished through only one dorsal-medial incision. In the setting of high-energy injuries with more extensive midfoot instability, two dorsal incisions are used (Fig. 20.15).

The medial incision is commonly between the first and second rays overlying the extensor hallucis longus. It is important to note the neurovascular bundle containing deep peroneal nerve and dorsalis pedis artery run deep to the extensor hallucis longus. Branches of the superficial peroneal nerve cross the distal aspect of the medial incision and should be carefully protected (Fig. 20.16).

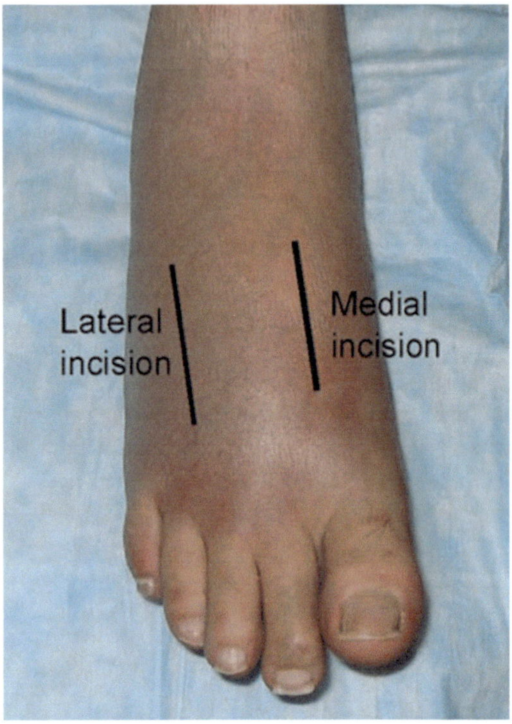

Fig. 20.15 Dorsal incision for approach to Lisfranc primary fusion for purely ligamentous injury [27]. (Reproduced with permission from Coetzee, J. Chris MD, FRCSC1; Ly, Thuan V. MD2 Treatment of Primarily Ligamentous Lisfranc Joint Injuries: Primary Arthrodesis Compared with Open Reduction and Internal Fixation, *J Bone Joint Surg Am.* 2007;89(2):122–127. © 2007 (The Journal of Bone and Joint Surgery, Incorporated). DOI: https://doi.org/10.2106/JBJS.F.01004)

Once satisfactory exposure has been obtained and the instability confirmed (Fig. 20.17), meticulous preparation of the involved joints is paramount. Cartilage should be removed from the entire joint surface with the use of curettes and small osteotomes. Using of a saw or burr for joint preparation can lead to increased bone loss, which is not desired. Due to its depth, the first TMT joint requires particular attention to the plantar aspect of the joint to ensure complete preparation and avoid a dorsiflexion deformity. A Hintermann distractor or lamina spreader can be used to aid visualization of the plantar joint surfaces (Fig. 20.18).

Once the articular surfaces have been denuded of cartilage, the subchondral surface should be penetrated to increase surface area and promote

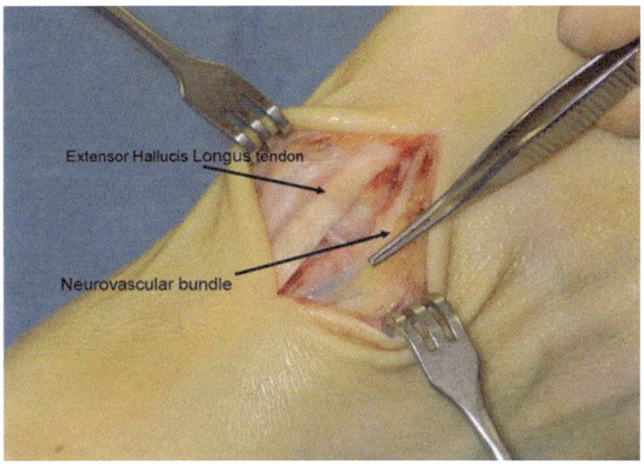

Fig. 20.16 A close-up view of a left foot demonstrating the extensor hallucis longus tendon lying medial. The dorsalis pedis artery and the deep peroneal nerve are lateral to the tendon and will be encountered during the exposure. A branch of the superficial peroneal nerve usually runs from the lateral to medial across the distal portion of the exposure. These structure should be identified and protected [27]. (Reproduced with permission from Coetzee, J. Chris MD, FRCSC1; Ly, Thuan V. MD2 Treatment of Primarily Ligamentous Lisfranc Joint Injuries: Primary Arthrodesis Compared with Open Reduction and Internal Fixation, *J Bone Joint Surg Am.* 2007;89(2):122–127. © 2007 (The Journal of Bone and Joint Surgery, Incorporated). DOI: https://doi.org/10.2106/JBJS.F.01004)

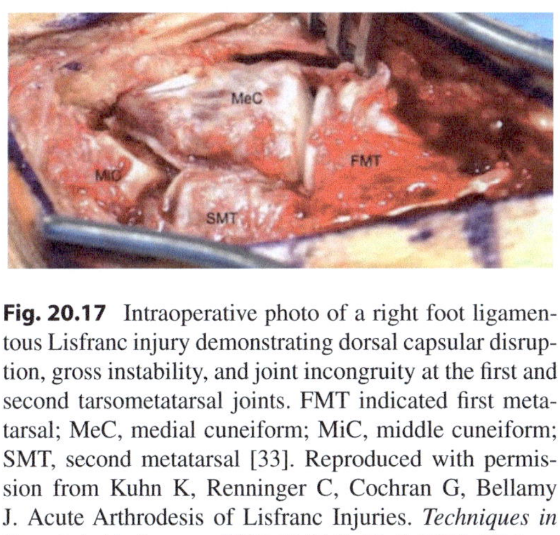

Fig. 20.17 Intraoperative photo of a right foot ligamentous Lisfranc injury demonstrating dorsal capsular disruption, gross instability, and joint incongruity at the first and second tarsometatarsal joints. FMT indicated first metatarsal; MeC, medial cuneiform; MiC, middle cuneiform; SMT, second metatarsal [33]. Reproduced with permission from Kuhn K, Renninger C, Cochran G, Bellamy J. Acute Arthrodesis of Lisfranc Injuries. *Techniques in Foot & Ankle Surgery*. 2019;18(1):8–15. © 2018 (Wolters Kluwer Health, Inc.). DOI: https://doi.org/10.1097/BTF.0000000000000200)

fusion. A 2.0 mm drill bit may be used for this step, and we like to irrigate while drilling to decrease bone temperature. We also do a "shingling" technique on the surface with a 4 mm osteotome to provide additional cancellous expo-

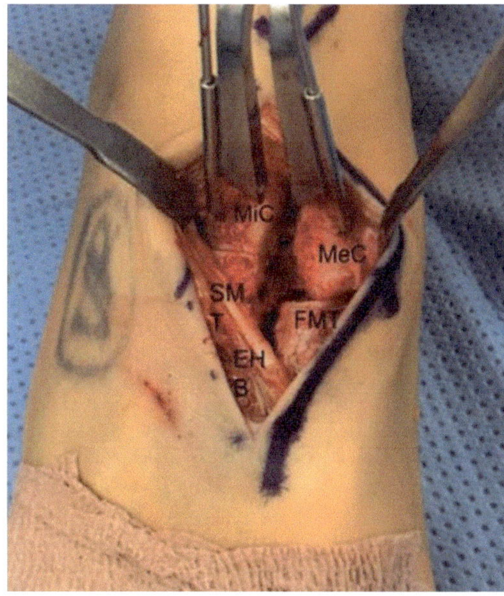

Fig. 20.18 Intraoperative photo demonstrating dorsal exposure and distraction of the intercuneiform (IC) joint with a Hintermann distractor. EHB indicated extensor hallucis brevis; FMT, first metatarsal; MeC, medial cuneiform; MiC, middle cuneiform; SMT, second metararsal [33]. (Reproduced with permission from Kuhn K, Renninger C, Cochran G, Bellamy J. Acute Arthrodesis of Lisfranc Injuries. *Techniques in Foot & Ankle Surgery*. 2019;18(1):8–15. © 2018 (Wolters Kluwer Health, Inc.). DOI: https://doi.org/10.1097/BTF.0000000000000200)

sure. A small arthroscopy "micro-fracture" pick could be used in place of the 2.0 drilling (Fig. 20.19).

If necessary, a lateral incision overlying the fourth ray can be made to provide exposure of the third TMT and lateral aspect of the second TMT. The third TMT would then be prepared in a similar fashion to the first and second.

Bone graft is placed following preparation of the joint. Autogenous bone graft is recommended, and it may be obtained from multiple places including the calcaneus, distal or proximal tibia, and iliac crest. The prepared joints are then reduced following graft placement (Fig. 20.20). Dorsiflexion of the toes can be used to activate the "windlass" mechanism, which aids in avoiding TMT dorsiflexion deformity. The use of a clamp across the Lisfranc joint aids in reducing the lateral subluxation following Lisfranc injuries. Once the reduction has

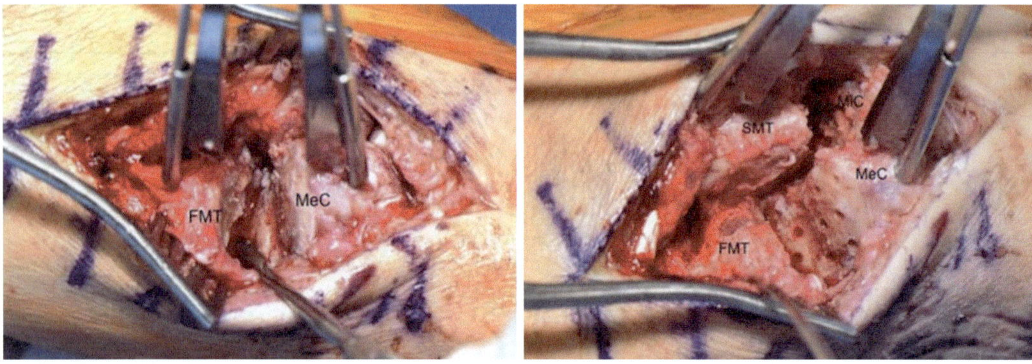

Fig. 20.19 (Left image) Intraoperative photo demonstrating distraction of the first tarsometatarsal joint. The Freer elevator is inserted to demonstrate the plantar extent of this joint. (Right image) Photograph demonstrating the prepared articular surface of the MeC after cartilage removal and trephination with a 2 mm drill. FMT indicated first metatarsal; MeC, medial cuneiform; MiC, middle cuneiform; SMT, second metatarsal [33]. (Reproduced with permission from Kuhn K, Renninger C, Cochran G, Bellamy J. Acute Arthrodesis of Lisfranc Injuries. *Techniques in Foot & Ankle Surgery*. 2019;18(1):8–15. © 2018 (Wolters Kluwer Health, Inc.). DOI: https://doi.org/10.1097/BTF.0000000000000200)

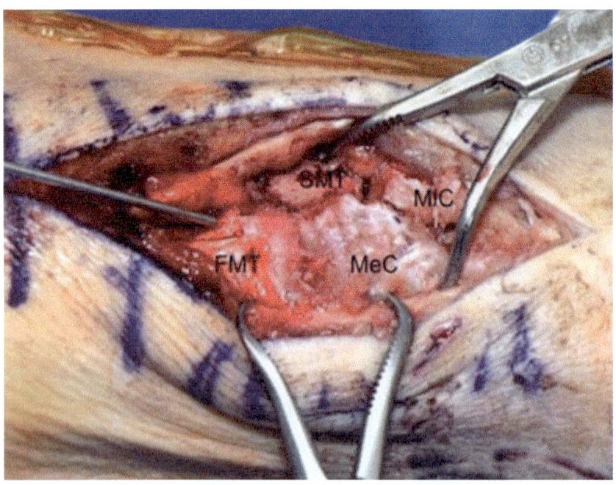

Fig. 20.20 Intraoperative photo demonstrating reduction, compression, and provisional fixation of the first tarsometatarsal joint using pointed reduction clamps and Kirschner wire. FMT indicated first metatarsal; MeC, medial cuneiform; MiC, middle cuneiform; SMT, second metatarsal [33]. (Reproduced with permission from Kuhn K, Renninger C, Cochran G, Bellamy J. Acute Arthrodesis of Lisfranc Injuries. *Techniques in Foot & Ankle Surgery*. 2019;18(1):8–15. © 2018 (Wolters Kluwer Health, Inc.). DOI: https://doi.org/10.1097/BTF.0000000000000200)

been achieved and confirmed fluoroscopically, the joints can then be provisionally fixed with K-wires (Fig. 20.20).

Multiple fixation constructs for midfoot fusion have been described, but they typically include a combination of solid or cannulated lag screws and dorsal compression plates. A "Lisfranc screw" may be placed to recreate stability of the Lisfranc joint. If instability of the IC joint is present, it should be stabilized with lag screw fixation following joint preparation and graft placement. Commonly, the first TMT joint is fixed with retrograde lag screws that may be inserted over the previously placed K-wires for provisional fixation. This provides compression while ensuring the reduction of the first TMT is maintained. Some prefer a dorsal plate fixation or hybrid lag screw and dorsal plate. Working from medial to lateral, the second TMT joint can be fixed with dorsal compression plating. Prior to placement, the plate should be pre-contoured in slight flexion to avoid a dorsiflexion deformity. Additionally, a lag screw can be placed through the second TMT joint to prevent dorsiflexion with plate placement (Fig. 20.21).

If necessary, the third TMT could then be stabilized with either screw or plate fixation in a similar manner to the second TMT. Further bone graft is placed after definitive fixation (Figs. 20.21 and 20.22).

Once fixation is in place, the reduction is confirmed fluoroscopically (Fig. 20.23). The wounds are then closed, and the patient is placed in a splint or boot.

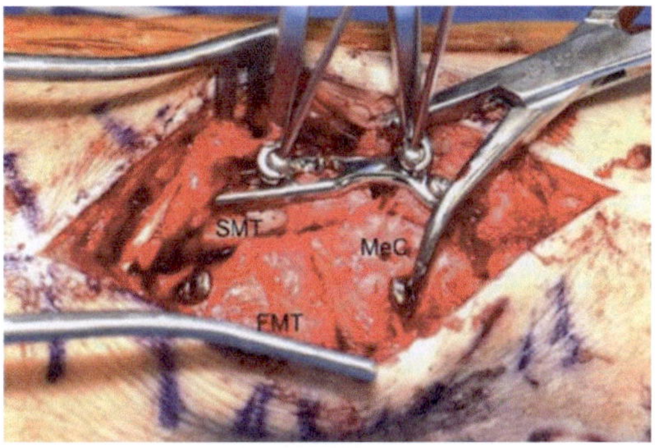

Fig. 20.21 Intraoperative photo demonstrating application of compression and fixation of the second tarsometatarsal joint. FMT indicated first metatarsal; MeC, medial cuneiform; SMT, second metatarsal [33]. (Reproduced with permission from Kuhn K, Renninger C, Cochran G, Bellamy J. Acute Arthrodesis of Lisfranc Injuries. *Techniques in Foot & Ankle Surgery*. 2019;18(1):8–15. © 2018 (Wolters Kluwer Health, Inc.). DOI: https://doi.org/10.1097/BTF.0000000000000200)

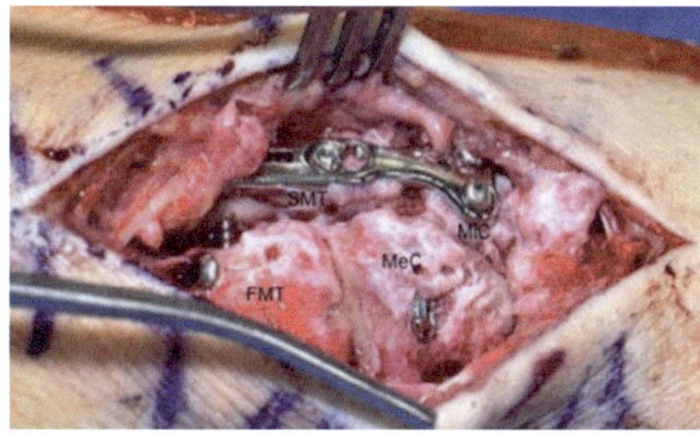

Fig. 20.22 Intraoperative photo demonstrating final fixation construct. FMT indicated first metatarsal; MeC, medial cuneiform; MiC, middle cuneiform; SMT, second metatarsal [33]. Reproduced with permission from Kuhn K, Renninger C, Cochran G, Bellamy J. Acute Arthrodesis of Lisfranc Injuries. *Techniques in Foot & Ankle Surgery*. 2019;18(1):8–15. © 2018 (Wolters Kluwer Health, Inc.). DOI: https://doi.org/10.1097/BTF.0000000000000200)

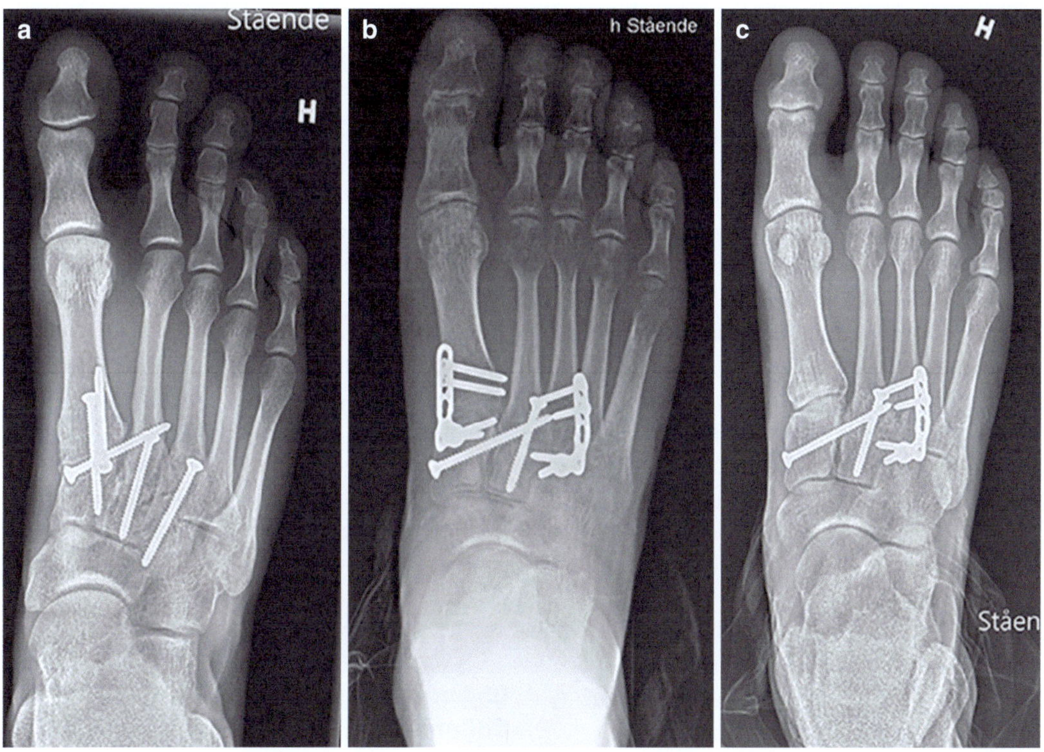

Fig. 20.23 (**a**–**c**) (**a**) Primary arthrodesis of the three medial TMT joints. (**b**) Temporary bridge plating of the first TMT joint using locking plate and primary arthrodesis of the second and third TMT joint. (**c**) The same patient as in panel **b**, but after removal of the temporary bridge plating. TMT, tarsometatarsal [25]. (Reproduced with permission from Stødle AH, Hvaal KH, Brøgger HM, Madsen JE, Husebye EE. Temporary Bridge Plating vs Primary Arthrodesis of the First Tarsometatarsal Joint in Lisfranc Injuries: Randomized Controlled Trial. *Foot Ankle Int*. 2020;41(9):901–910. © 2020 (American Orthopaedic Foot & Ankle Society). DOI: https://doi.org/10.1177/1071100720925815)

Additional Considerations for Primary-Hybrid Arthrodeses

Technique No. 4: Hybrid-Primary Arthrodesis (Stødle Technique [25])

The positioning and anesthesia approaches are similar to a primary fusion. A two-incision technique is utilized with a 4 cm distance between incisions to decrease wound complications (Fig. 20.15). The three medial tarsal-metatarsal joints are exposed and visualized. The second and third TMT joints are prepared and stabilized similar to the primary arthrodesis technique (Fig. 20.23a, b). Stødle [28] utilizes a 2.7 or 3.5 mm lag screw across the second and third TMT joints and does not use bone graft. For severely comminuted joints, a 2.7 mm locking plate is utilized. The first TMT joint however is approached similar to ORIF technique, that is, the cartilage is left intact and a dorsal bridge plate is applied after anatomic reduction (Fig. 20.23b). Stødle [28] utilizes a 2.7 mm locking plate for stabilization of the first TMT joint (LCP Compact Foot 2.4/2.7, DePuy Synthes, Oberdorf, Switzerland – Fig. 20.23b). A "homerun screw" is also used to "secure the Lisfranc mortise." Stødle [28] also recommends temporary K-wire fixation for the fourth and fifth TMT joint if unstable after first and second TMT fixation.

Postoperative care is similar to the primary arthrodeses with NWB for 6–8 weeks. Any temporary K-wire fixation of the fourth and fifth TMT joint is removed at 12 weeks. The dorsal bridge plate is removed at 4.5 months (Fig. 20.18c). Alignment of the first TMT joint is noted to be superior to the PA group, but radiographic early OA was noted at the first TMT joint.

Treatment Options: Chronic

Chronic Lisfranc Dislocation (>4 Weeks After Injury)

In the high-demand patients or elite athletes who are poor candidates for arthrodesis, reconstruction rather than arthrodesis has been advocated [34]. Reconstruction of the Lisfranc ligament provides the opportunity for permanent restoration of the stability of the Lisfranc joint due to concerns over the native ligament's healing capacity. Multiple methods and types of reconstruction have been described. Some authors advocate suture button fixation, while others have described techniques for free tendon autograft reconstruction [34–37].

Suture button fixation has been biomechanically shown to have similar resistance to displacement of the Lisfranc joint to screw fixation [38]. Unlike screws, suture button fixation does allow mobility in the joints and does not require removal. *Charlton* et al. [34] reported the results of seven high-level athletes (five professional dancers and two Division 1 soccer players) with chronic Lisfranc injuries who were treated with suture button fixation, and all patients returned to their prior level of activity within 6 months of surgery. However, these athletes were treated in the acute phase of the injury, not in the chronic time period.

Free tendon reconstruction of the Lisfranc ligament has also been advocated for chronic Lisfranc injuries with a variety of different techniques reported. *De los Santos-Real* et al. [35] described a reconstruction technique using a gracilis graft. They reported good results in three patients at 2 years of follow-up. Similarly, *Miyamoto* et al. [36] described a reconstruction technique using gracilis graft in five athletes and showed significant improvement in AOFAS scores and return to prior activities in all patients. *Zwipp and Rammelt* [37] described the use of an extensor hallucis brevis tendon to reconstruct the Lisfranc ligament in four patients including an elite gymnast resulting in a stable joint and a return to competition (Figs. 20.24 and 20.25).

Chronic Lisfranc Injury Without Collapse (4–12 Weeks Post Injury)

Technique No. 1: Fixation (ORIF with Suture Button Augmentation)

The preparation and approach are identical in the chronic setting as in the acute setting noted above (**Technique No. 1:** ORIF). However, after utiliz-

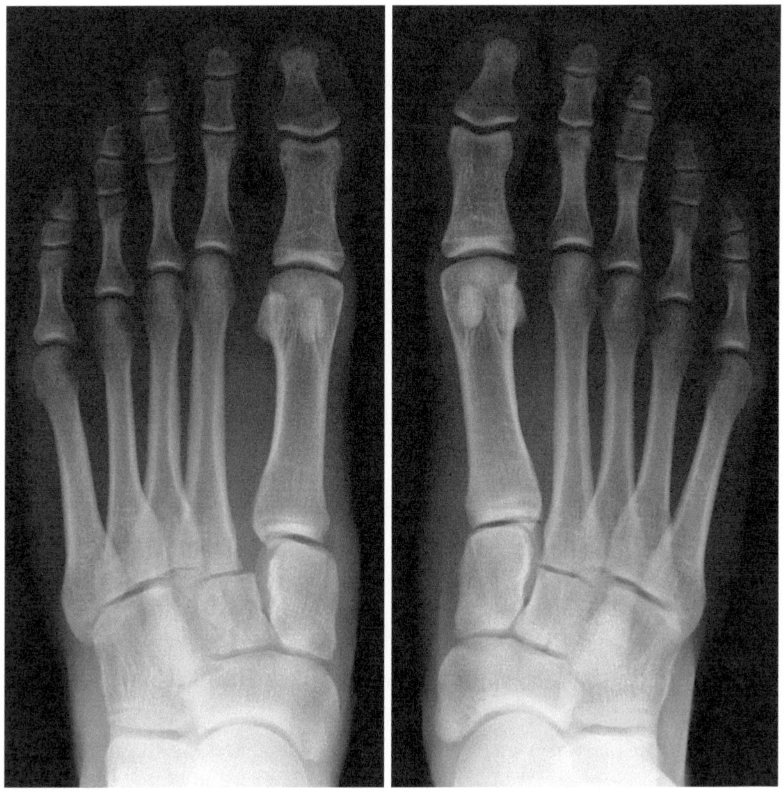

Fig. 20.24 Bilateral AP foot imaging demonstrating left severe chronic lateral shift and instability in chronic Lisfranc injury in elite high school running back. Right side demonstrates normal midfoot Lisfranc alignment

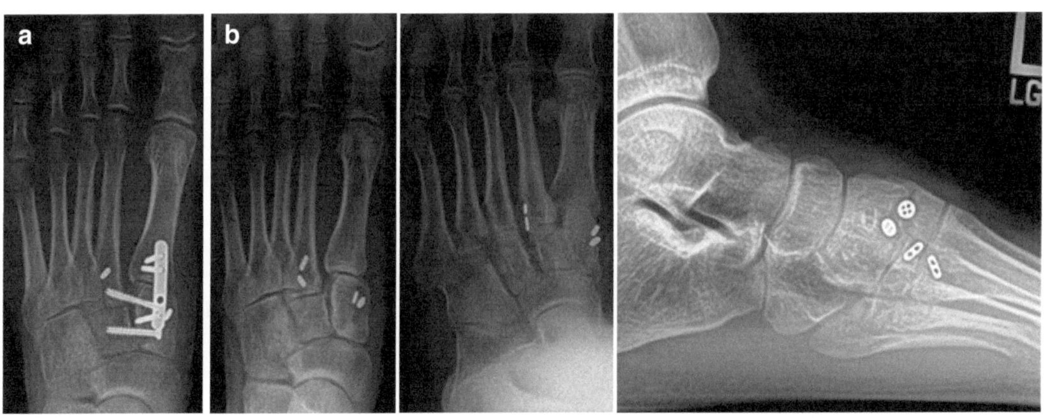

Fig. 20.25 (**a**–**b**) Reconstruction of chronic left Lisfranc in high school (HS) running back. (**a**) AP image 3.5 months postoperative after suture button augmentation of the second tarsometatarsal (TMT) joint with rigid trans-articular screw for intercuneiform and second TMT. Trans-articular bridge plating for the first TMT joint. (**b**) AP, oblique, and lateral image of the same HS athlete 6 months after initial reconstruction and 3 months after removal of rigid fixation and addition of second suture button from medial cuneiform to the second TMT base. Note on the oblique image the appropriate position of lateral endobutton on the base of the second MT despite it appearing to have subsidence on AP image. Lateral image demonstrates the two suture buttons "stacked" dorsal to plantar

ing the EHL and EHB interval, the scarred ligaments are then evaluated. The true "Lisfranc" ligament is typically enveloped into the interval between the medial cuneiform and the base of the second metatarsal causing a rigid, stiff malalignment. Comparison AP imaging clearly shows malalignment, and severe lateral shift is often seen in the chronic setting (Fig. 20.24). Time must be spent to remove the scarred ligament from in between the medial cuneiform and the second metatarsal base to allow reduction of the second metatarsal on the medial cuneiform. Failure to remove this scarred ligament will compromise the complete reduction of the second MT base on the cuneiform. The accurate reduction typically will bring the second TMT joint into alignment, and the first TMT joint is then more easily reduced. Also, we believe the ligament placed back in its original location improves the healing potential of the ligament.

At this time, the decision has to be made if the scarred ligament is still a viable reconstructive tissue or if new tissue must be brought into this location to recreate this dorsal ligament [25–27]. We typically find the ligament is adequate for reconstruction as long as it can be removed from its interval between the second metatarsal and medial cuneiform. Usually, the ligament is well attached to the second metatarsal base and requires lifting the scarred and torn ligament from the interval between the two bones and off of the medial cuneiform. We then roughen the medial cuneiform at this location with a 4.0 egg burr to create a reattachment site for the ligament.

Depending on the ease of reduction and the degree of preoperative malalignment, we determine if we augment the medial cuneiform-second metatarsal fixation with a more plantar positioned suture button. If the reduction has been more difficult and/or if the preoperative lateral displacement of the second metatarsal was greater than 4 mm, we first place a suture button from the medial cuneiform to the base of the second metatarsal with the endobutton secured at the lateral second metatarsal base. This requires an additional incision dorsally at the lateral base of the second metatarsal. We use a regular-sized suture button rather than the mini suture button. We place a tenaculum reduction forceps from the medial cuneiform into the base of the second metatarsal as described under the acute ORIF (Figs. 20.9a, 20.10a, b, 20.13b) to hold position and full reduction while tightening the knotless tight rope medially (Fig. 20.25a). A more dorsal position is then utilized for insertion of a 4.5 mm partially threaded screw. The partially threaded screw can allow additional "dialing in" of the reduction to the medial cuneiform. However, just as in an acute fixation, it is imperative to not overtighten this screw and create pressure necrosis of the cartilage.

If mild collapse has occurred through the midfoot as noted on the lateral image, we use a dorsal 2.7 mm four-hole LCDC plate with four 2.7 mm screws at the second TMT joint in addition to the tight rope from the medial cuneiform into the base of the second metatarsal. We also utilize a five-hole, 2.7 mm LCDC plate on the first TMT joint with four screws to help restore the midfoot arch and the natural inclination of the first TMT joint. If the third TMT joint is involved, we commonly use a similar dorsal plate in that location also.

We confirm the reduction with intraoperative mini C-arm imaging in all three views and confirm anatomic position of each TMT joint and restoration of the arch (Fig. 20.25a).

Postoperative management is similar to the acute approach with some minor alterations. We have a low threshold for utilizing a well-molded short-leg cast at weeks 2–6 to help support the arch, especially if there was any loss of arch preoperatively. In the immediate post-op period, we still utilize cold compression therapy inside a long, knee-high boot to help with management of pain, edema, and nerve sensitivity. Non-weight-bearing is still 6 weeks, but we wean off the crutches over 4 weeks rather than 2 weeks and always use a custom orthotic with a well-molded arch to help support the midfoot. We also use the boot until at least 3 months postoperatively before weaning out of the boot over a 4-week period of time rather than a 2-week period of time. We follow closely with X-ray imaging at 1 week, 6 weeks,

3 months, and 4.5 to 5 months postoperatively, to make sure there is no loss of alignment. Once the screws show lucency on X-ray and the patient is greater than 4 months postoperatively, we offer hardware removal of all the plate and screws. However, we leave the tight rope in place, and the medial cuneiform-second metatarsal base screw is replaced with a regular-sized TightRope suture button to support the alignment and MC-second MT ligament in the long term (Fig. 20.25b). We have not found leaving the suture button in place leads to any higher risk of fracture or pain.

Technique No. 2: Fixation (ORIF Chronic Lisfranc with Suture Button – Charlton [34])

Charlton [33] describes their suture button fixation used in elite dancers [5] and soccer players [2]. Their technique was used in athletes that had failed 6 months of conservative treatment and had disabling pain with point tenderness at the Lisfranc ligament and no signal change in the second metatarsal base which would have suggested arthritis. The athletes were positioned supine and an ankle tourniquet is utilized. A 2 cm dorsal incision was undertaken (Fig. 20.26) to allow exposure of the dorsal cutaneous nerve. The interval between the EDL and EHB was utilized and the neurovascular bundle retracted laterally. The Lisfranc ligament can then be evaluated with a Freer elevator. Easy penetration between the MC1 and MT2 base confirms instability.

Under fluoroscopic guidance, a 1.6 mm Kirschner wire (K-wire) is placed from the medial cuneiform, across the "Lisfranc" joint and into the base of the second metatarsal (Fig. 20.27). AP and lateral imaging is used to confirm appropriate position. The authors note that medial to lateral trajectory allows easier positioning without blockage by the third metatarsal. Careful attention to the starting point is stressed to avoid damage to the anterior tibial tendon (ATT) and to not be too close to the first TMT joint which could lead to bone breakout. A 2.7 mm cannulated drill is used over the K-wire from medial to lateral.

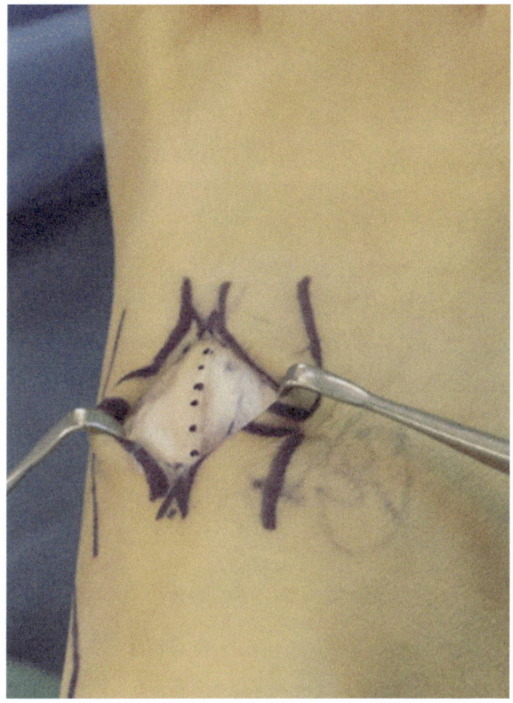

Fig. 20.26 The dorsal cutaneous nerve is predictably in the field and should be avoided. The EHL and EHB tendons are retracted to show the deep peroneal nerve [34]. (Reproduced with permission from Charlton T, Boe C, Thordarson DB. Suture Button Fixation Treatment of Chronic Lisfranc Injury in Professional Dancers and High-Level Athletes. *J Dance Med Sci.* 2015;19 (4):135–139. Copyright © 2015 J. Michael Ryan Publishing, Inc.)

A suture lasso is positioned through the drill hole medial to lateral and is exposed between the second and third MT base (Fig. 20.28). The suture button is then advanced from lateral to medial, from the second metatarsal to medial cuneiform. A small incision is made to facilitate and confirm the endobutton sits flush on the medial cuneiform and no entrapment of the ATT. The suture button is then tied over the washer at the lateral edge of the second MT base (Fig. 20.29). The authors used this direction (lateral to medial) to eliminate the knot on the medial cuneiform which could rub on the shoe of the dancer (knotless suture anchors may obviate this concern, and non-dancer athletes may tolerate the suture button device in either direction). AP (Fig. 20.30) and lateral imaging (Fig. 20.31) is undertaken to confirm reduction and position of

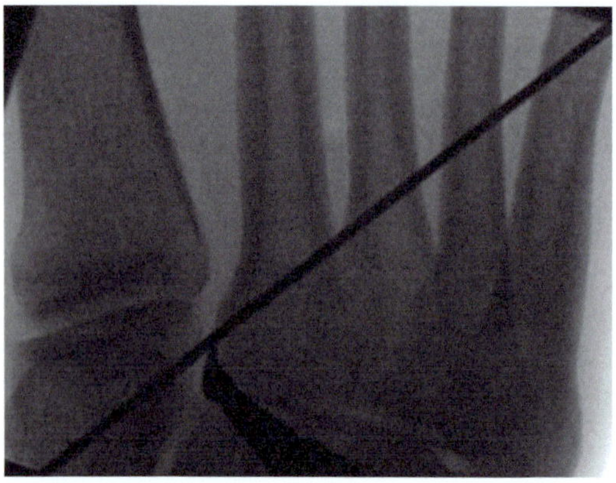

Fig. 20.27 Intraoperative imaging demonstrating guide placement from the medial cuneiform to the base of the second metatarsal. Three elements in this pin placement are (1) avoiding the tibialis anterior tendon, (2) bisecting the articular surface of the medial cuneiform and the first intermetatarsal joint, and (3) avoiding the articulation between the second and third metatarsals while terminating in the space between these two bones [34]. (Reproduced with permission from Charlton T, Boe C, Thordarson DB. Suture Button Fixation Treatment of Chronic Lisfranc Injury in Professional Dancers and High-Level Athletes. *J Dance Med Sci.* 2015;19(4):135–139. Copyright © 2015 J. Michael Ryan Publishing, Inc.)

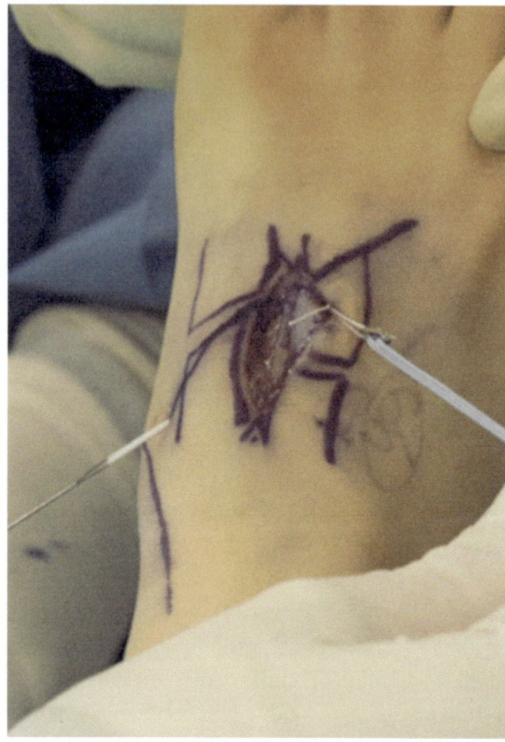

Fig. 20.28 A passing loop is placed after drill holes are created [34]. Reproduced with permission from Charlton T, Boe C, Thordarson DB. Suture Button Fixation Treatment of Chronic Lisfranc Injury in Professional Dancers and High-Level Athletes. *J Dance Med Sci.* 2015;19(4):135–139. Copyright © 2015 J. Michael Ryan Publishing, Inc.)

suture button device. The authors mention nonabsorbable suture can be used to augment the dorsal ligament but was not used in their series.

Technique No. 3: Use of Free Tendon Graft for Chronic Lisfranc Ligament Reconstruction

Miyamoto Technique [36]

A general anesthetic is utilized to allow harvesting of a gracilis autograft from a 3 cm medial knee incision. The gracilis graft is prepared. A thigh tourniquet is required because of the graft harvest (Fig. 20.32). A longitudinal (or a curvilinear) skin incision is utilized between the first and second metatarsal bases and a medial incision just dorsal to the ATT. A large tenaculum clamp is used to obtain and maintain reduction with the graft is placed (Fig. 20.33). A guide pin is placed medial to lateral along the course of the Lisfranc ligament between the medial cuneiform and the second MT base similar to techniques described above (Acute **Technique No. 3** and Chronic **Technique No. 2**). "Over-drilling was performed along this guide wire to create a bone tunnel using a cancellous bone-harvesting drill with a bit diameter of 4.2 mm (Meira Co., Ltd., Nagoya, Japan)" (Fig. 20.33). A 2–0 nylon suture passer is introduced lateral to medial through completed drill hole, and the prepared gracilis tendon graft is then inserted medial to lateral, secured medially at the medial cuneiform with a 4–0 solid interference screw (Meira Co., Ltd) (Fig. 20.33). The graft end laterally is pulled out the incision between the first and second MT bases (Fig. 20.33). The authors use a cannulated screw across the intercuneiform joint as needed, similar to that discussed under Acute **Technique No. 1**: ORIF. The end of the graft lateral to the

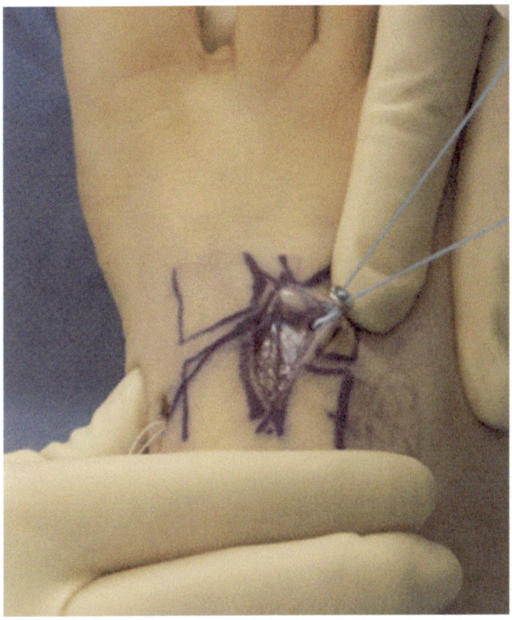

Fig. 20.29 The suture button fixation is passed with attention to making the knot on the second metatarsal side to avoid irritation with the dance pointe shoe, for example. A small incision is made medially to confirm the button fixation is not entrapping the tibialis anterior tendon [34]. (Reproduced with permission from Charlton T, Boe C, Thordarson DB. Suture Button Fixation Treatment of Chronic Lisfranc Injury in Professional Dancers and High-Level Athletes. *J Dance Med Sci.* 2015;19(4):135–139. Copyright © 2015 J. Michael Ryan Publishing, Inc.)

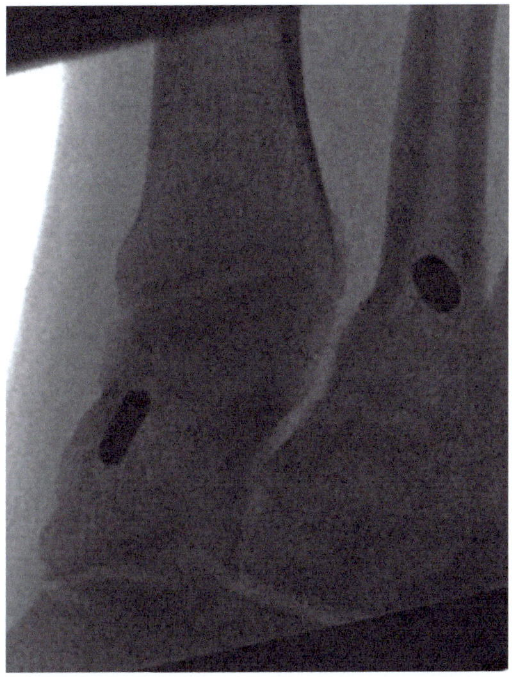

Fig. 20.30 Radiographic confirmation of appropriate placement [34]. Reproduced with permission from Charlton T, Boe C, Thordarson DB. Suture Button Fixation Treatment of Chronic Lisfranc Injury in Professional Dancers and High-Level Athletes. *J Dance Med Sci.* 2015;19 (4):135–139. Copyright © 2015 J. Michael Ryan Publishing, Inc.)

base of the second MT is tensioned and secured with a suture anchor in the second MT base (Fig. 20.34). The medial and lateral free loose ends of the gracilis are tensioned and tied onto one another with 3-0 absorbable suture (permanent suture could be used also) (Figs. 20.32 and 20.34). The authors reported their technique used in five athletes (three rugby, one American football, one judo). All athletes failed 5–24 months of non-operative treatment, and all returned to pre-injury activity at an average of 4.1 months.

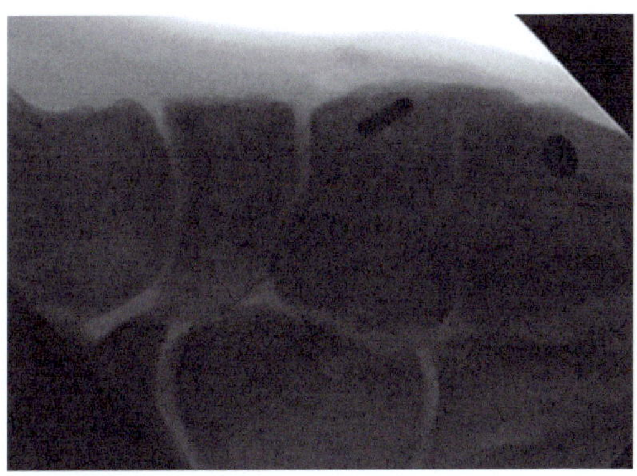

Fig. 20.31 Care is taken to avoid dorsal cortex disruption, as the tendency is for "high" placement of the device [34]. (Reproduced with permission from Charlton T, Boe C, Thordarson DB. Suture Button Fixation Treatment of Chronic Lisfranc Injury in Professional Dancers and High-Level Athletes. *J Dance Med Sci.* 2015;19(4):135–139. Copyright © 2015 J. Michael Ryan Publishing, Inc.)

De los Santos-Real Technique [35]

De los Santos-Real [35] describes a free gracilis tendon autograft reconstruction of the Lisfranc ligament and first-second MT base sling to augment the reconstruction. Also, these authors supplement their technique with temporary screw

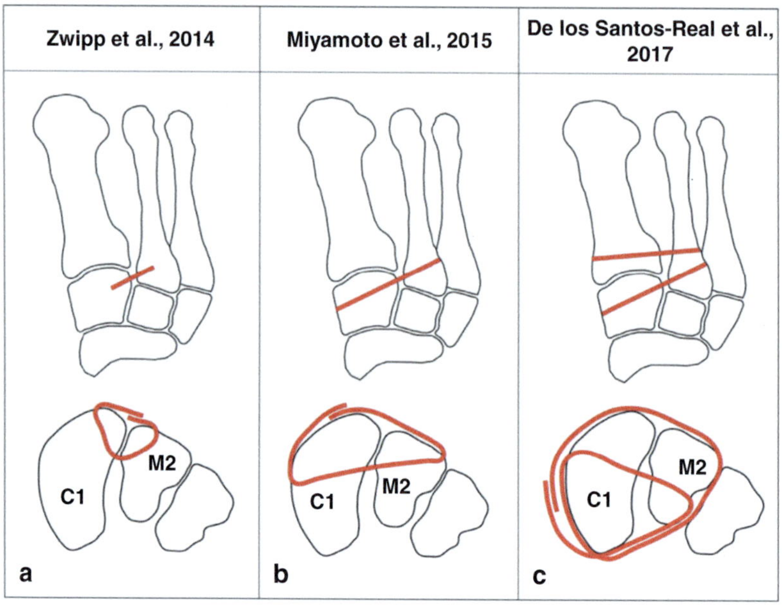

Fig. 20.32 Techniques for Lisfranc ligament reconstruction in chronic Lisfranc injury without secondary degenerative arthritis by using different types of autograft and configuration [39]. (**a**) Zwipp technique [37]. (**b**) Miyamoto technique [36]. (**c**) De los Santos-Real technique [35]. (Reproduced with permission from Sripanich, Y., Weinberg, M. W., Krähenbühl, N., Rungprai, C., Haller, J., Saltzman, C. L., Barg, A. Surgical Outcome of Chronic Lisfranc Injury without Secondary Degenerative Arthritis: A Systematic Literature Review. *Injury.* 2020;51(7):1258–1265. © 2020 (Elsevier Ltd). DOI: https://doi.org/10.1016/j.injury.2020.04.005)

fixation. The technique involves circumferential routing of the tendon graft around the first and second MT base and bone tunnels through the MC and second MT base to route the graft between these bones. The graft is actually used as one continuous free graft, and the two ends are tied through the medial incision. The authors described their technique but only reported on three cases, and it was not noted if the patients were athletes.

Zwipp Technique [37]

The Zwipp technique [37] (Fig. 20.32) is similar to the Miyamoto technique (Fig. 20.32), but the drill holes are through the dorsal first and second MT base, rather than completely through the MT as described by Miyamoto [36]. I would have some concern with dorsal bone break through with the small dorsal bone bridge.

Technique No. 4: Secondary Arthrodeses for Chronic Lisfranc

Chronic Lisfranc injuries may occur due to a delay in care or missed injuries with subtle findings on initial radiographs. After a significant delay in treatment following injury to the tarsometatarsal ligaments or a failure of non-operative treatment, it is important to closely examine the patient's radiographs for arthritic changes. In patients with significant arthritic changes, the most reliable treatment is secondary arthrodesis. Also, we use MR imaging to assess for physiologic arthroses noted with severe peri-articular edema and cartilage disruption or thinning. A CT can be used to assess subtle spurring and joint space narrowing, but does not address bone edema/stress from early OA. In this reconstructive situation, the arthrodesis is similar to the PA, but the reduction and joint preparation are more tedious and involved. It is critical to get full reduction out of abduction and to attempt to restore the anatomic arch (longitudinal and transverse). Fixation is the same as outlined above for PA. If there is more involved abduction deformity, some will be more inclined to use a first TMT plate and move the plate more medial to help draw the foot out of abduction and secure

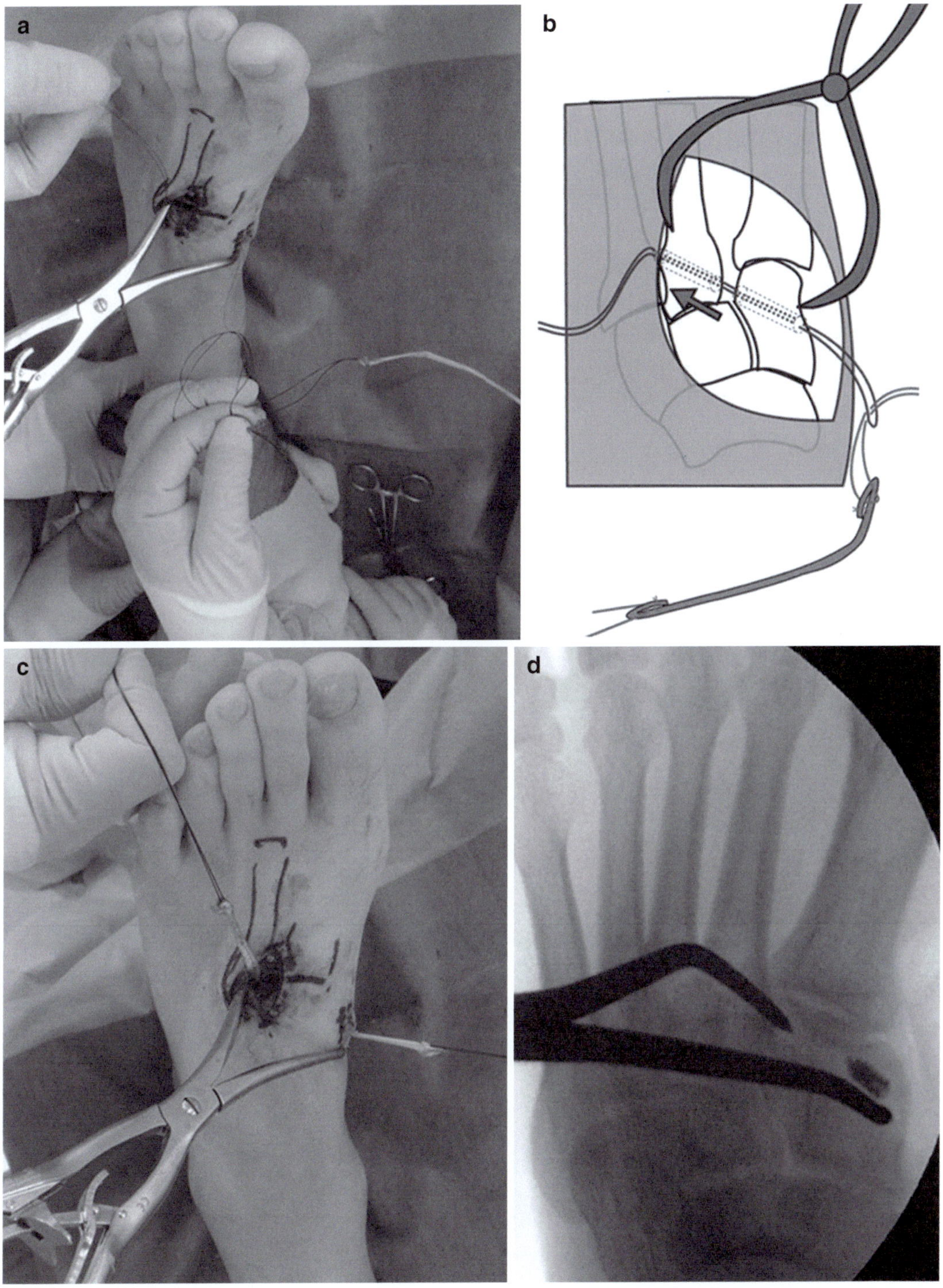

Fig. 20.33 (**a**–**d**) (**a**) Intraoperative photograph showing introduction of the autograft into the bone tunnel through the 2-0 nylon loop. (**b**) Schematic diagram of the intraoperative photograph of **a**. (**c**) Intraoperative photograph showing the introduced autograft. (**d**) Image intensifier view showing fixation of the autograft at the proximal part of the bone tunnel by a solid interference screw with a diameter of 4.0 mm [36]. (Reproduced with permission from Miyamoto, W., Takao, M., Innami, K. et al. Ligament Reconstruction with Single Bone Tunnel Technique for Chronic Symptomatic Subtle Injury of the Lisfranc Joint in Athletes. *Arch Orthop Trauma Surg*. 2015;135(9):1063–1070. DIO: 10.1007/s00402-015-2250-6)

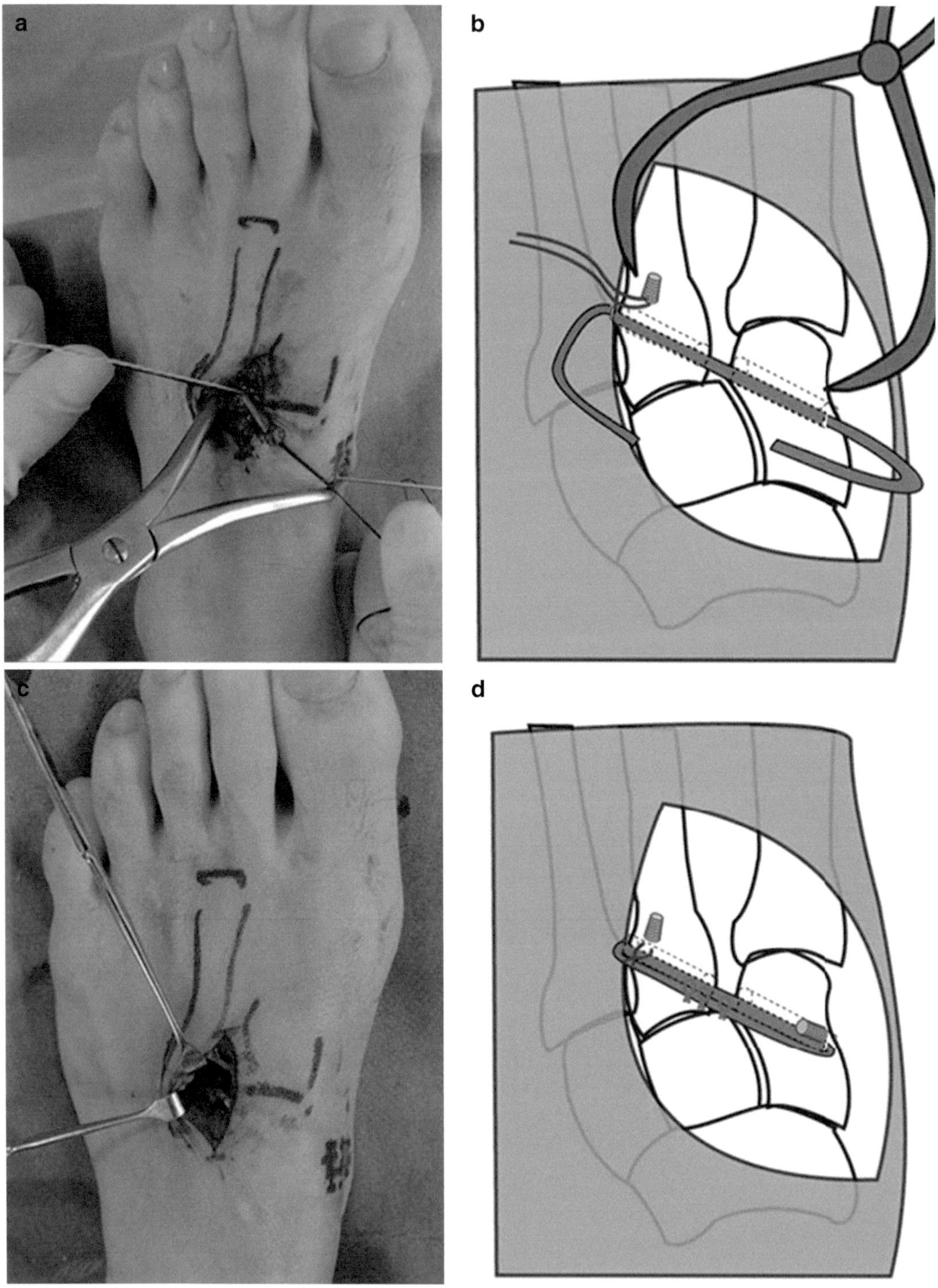

Fig. 20.34 (**a**–**d**) (**a**) Intraoperative photograph and (**b**) schematic diagram (of **a**) showing insertion of a suture anchor into the base of the second metatarsal bone perpendicular to its long axis. (**c**) Intraoperative photograph and (**d**) schematic diagram (of **c**) showing fixation of the tensioned distal end of the autograft by the suture anchor and suturing of the tensioned ends using 3-0 absorbable sutures [36]. (Reproduced with permission from Miyamoto, W., Takao, M., Innami, K. et al. Ligament Reconstruction with Single Bone Tunnel Technique for Chronic Symptomatic Subtle Injury of the Lisfranc Joint in Athletes. *Arch Orthop Trauma Surg.* 2015;135 (9):1063–1070. DIO: 10.1007/s00402-015-2250-6)

the reduction better. The athlete should be counseled that return to high-level competitive sports at the pre-injury state is doubtful.

Hardware Removal

Hardware removal is commonly performed following surgical treatment of Lisfranc injuries, particularly in the setting of acute (and often with chronic also) ORIF. As the hardware spans the TMT joints, it is recommended to remove after the ligaments have healed and the athlete desires to return to activity. Typically, any K-wires used to stabilize the lateral column of the foot would be removed 6 weeks postoperatively. Plates and screws would be removed 3–4 months postoperatively and/or after clear lucency around the screws. Some surgeons will leave the screw across the intercuneiform joint even when removing the remaining hardware. There are no reports to support or refute this approach to the intercuneiform screw(s). If there is a broken solid screw in the dorsal bridge plate, we have seen no ill effects of leaving the distal portion within the medial cuneiform (most common location of breakage). If a 4.0 or 4.5 mm screw is broken, and it is cannulated, a reverse threaded "easy out" can be used to get a deep broken portion of screw. Solid broken deep portion of screws are left in place if they do not impinge or interfere with the involved joint. While arthrodesis is associated with lower rates of hardware removal due to most surgeons leaving the hardware indefinitely, the senior author commonly removes the hardware after arthrodesis in hopes of preventing soft tissue irritation [23].

Rehabilitation

Because of the advancement of surgical stabilization, the athlete can begin early NWB ROM exercises. Rigid screw and plate fixation allows ankle and toe movement, pool therapy, and muscle stimulation to counteract disuse atrophy. In the immediate postoperative period, patients are recommended to remain non-weight-bearing for 6 weeks. As patients progress, they are typically moved through a graduated postoperative protocol (Table 20.1).

Expected Outcomes

Expected outcomes following operative treatment of Lisfranc injuries have been shown to be most dependent on the accuracy of the reduction [3, 9]. In the setting of anatomic reduction, *Nunley and Vertullo* [40] reported excellent results in 93% of patients following operative treatment in athletes. The authors noted an average return to sport in 14.4 weeks. *Deol* et al. [41] showed an average return to competition of 22.5 weeks following ligamentous Lisfranc in elite soccer and rugby players. Alternatively, other authors have noted an expectation of return to sport taking at least 6 months [42]. McHale noted an average of 11.1 months to return to professional American football but reported a 90% return rate [2]. An analysis of low-energy Lisfranc injuries in active-duty military members showed a return to full duty in 4.5 months following arthrodesis and 6.7 months following ORIF. Both groups had an increase in their average mile time at 1 year (arthrodesis, 9 s; ORIF, 39 s). [43] Injury pattern also can affect outcomes and return to sport with medial column dislocation being associated with a prolonged return to sport [3] (see Table 20.2).

Complications

A variety of complications have been reported following surgical fixation of Lisfranc injuries. The most common complication following ORIF is posttraumatic radiographic arthritis which has been reported in up to 72.1% of patients [44]. Rates of symptomatic arthritis following ORIF are typically much lower. *Kuo* et al. [21] reported radiographic arthritis in 25% of patients but noted that only half of those patients had significant symptoms from arthritis leading them to request secondary arthrodesis. Loss of sensation in the deep peroneal nerve distribution has also been reported in as many as 17.6% of patients [41]. Also, deep peroneal nerve sensation deficits have also been reported in 15% of patients following

Table 20.1 Rehabilitation protocol after Lisfranc fixation in athlete as presented by Porter [10]. (Reproduced with permission from Porter DA, Barnes AF, Rund A, Walrod MT. Injury Pattern in Ligamentous Lisfranc Injuries in Competitive Athletes. *Foot Ankle Int.* 2019;40(2):185–194. © 2019 (American Orthopaedic Foot & Ankle Society). DOI: https://doi.org/10.1177/1071100718802264)

Phase	Phase 1(1–6 weeks)	Phase II (6–12 weeks)	Phase III (12–16 weeks)	Phase IV (3.5–9 months)
Clinical goals	• Full ROM ankle (DF, PF, IV, EV)	• Strength comparable to opposite side	• Full ROM, strength and flexibility	• ROH typical at 3.5–5 month PO if needed
	• Full ROM MTPjt toes control swelling	• Bilateral double to single toe raise	• Restore normal PRT at rest/ standing	• RTS is 4-6 month for H S
	• Desensitize foot	• Wean out-of-boot into CFP and the orthotic/athletic shoe	• Begin running, and sports-specific training	• 5–8 month for college
		• PRT activity in shoe		• 6–10 month for professional
Exercise	• NWB for full 6 weeks	• Wean off crutches over 10–14 days	• Advanced PRT	• Sports-specific performance exercises and conditioning for full play
	• Toes curls (active and passive)	• Stationary bike in boot until 8–10 week PO	• Increase from biking to SM/ elliptical/AlterG to running	
	• ATS with towel strengthening with theraband at 2 weeks all directions of ankle	• PRT (boot 6–10 weeks PO and in shoe 8–12 week PO)	• Can begin leg press when can do SM/elliptical	
	• All UE lifting—sitting)	• Bilateral standing TR work to STR	• Can do squats/ clings/lunges after can run	
	• Leg extension and curls, seated calf raises (no weight bearing)			

ATS, Achilles tendon stretching CFP, carbon fiber plate; DF, dorsiflexion; EV, eversion; HS, high school; IV, inversion; MTPjt, metatarsophalangeal joint; NWB, nonweightbearing; PF, plantarflexion; PO, postoperative; PRT, proprioception retraining; ROH, removal of hardware; ROM, range-of-motion; SM, stair stepper machine; STR, single toe raise; TR, toe raises; UE, upper extremity

hardware removal [45]. Infection rate requiring ROH and/or IV antibiotics should be less than 1%.

Authors' Preferred Approach

1. Acute, purely ligamentous dislocation: TRAD or PE pattern.
   (a) ORIF—Intercuneiform (as indicated) 1–2, 4.0 or 4.5 mm screw (depending on the size of the athlete).
   (b) ORIF—MC1-MT2: 4.0 or 4.5 mm "home run" screw.
   (c) ORIF—first TMT: 4-hole 2.7 mm dorsal bridge plate.
   (d) ROH—3–4 months: RTS 6–12 months.
2. Acute, purely ligamentous dislocation: MCD pattern.
   (a) ORIF—Intercuneiform 1 or 2, 4.0 or 4.5 mm screw (depending on the size of the athlete).
   (b) ORIF—MC1-MT2: 4.0 or 4.5 mm "home run" screw.
   (c) ROH—4 months: RTS 7–12 months.
3. Chronic dislocation (> 4 weeks): no arthritis and negative MRI.
   (a) ORIF—Intercuneiform 2, 4.5 mm screw.
   (b) ORIF—MC1-MT2: 4.5 mm "home run" screw.
   (c) ORIF—first TMT: 5-hole, 2.7 mm dorsal bridge plate.

Table 20.2 Demographics, outcomes, and return to sport in competitive athletes with ORIF after differing patterns of low-energy, purely ligamentous Lisfranc injuries [3]. ORIF, open reduction internal fixation; AAOS, American Academy of Orthopaedic Surgeons; mo, months; y, years [10]. (Reproduced with permission from Porter DA, Barnes AF, Rund A, Walrod MT. Injury Pattern in Ligamentous Lisfranc Injuries in Competitive Athletes. *Foot Ankle Int*. 2019;40(2):185–194. © 2019 (American Orthopaedic Foot & Ankle Society). DOI: https://doi.org/10.1177/1071100718802264)

A. Traditional 1–2 Dislocation[a]
Return to sports: 7.6 mo
Age: 20.6 year (14–37)
Male: 27, Female: 13
Sport: football 20, basketball 7, 13 others
AAOS Score ($n = 5$), >1 year postoperation
• AAOS lower limb: 100
• AAOS foot pain: 99.3
• AAOS foot/ankle function: 96.0
B. Medial Column Dislocation[b]
Return to sports: 8.4 month
Age: 22.7 year (16–40)
Male: 15, Female: 2
Sport: football 9, wakeboarding 3, basketball 2, cheer/soccer/motorcross 1 each
AAOS Score ($n = 8$), >1 year postoperation
• AAOS lower limb: 99.4
• AAOS foot pain: 92.1
• AAOS foot/ankle function: 95.0
C. Proximal Extension Dislocation[c]
Return to sports: 7.2 month
Age: 21.1 year (15–31)
Male: 21, Female: 2
Sport: football 18, basketball 3, wrestling/track 1 each
AAOS score ($n = 8$), 6 month–1 year postoperation
• AAOS lower limb: 100
• AAOS foot pain: 98.3
• AAOS foot/ankle function: 95.8

[a]Fig 20.1a Lisfranc disruption pattern
[b]Fig 20.1b Lisfranc disruption pattern
[c]Fig 20.1c Lisfranc disruption pattern

(d) Flexible hardware: Use TightRope MC1–MT2 to augment at index procedure;

TightRope at ROH through hole of MC1–MT2 screw (Fig. 20.27b).

(e) ROH—4–6 months: RTS 8–12 months.

4. <u>Chronic dislocation (>4 weeks or posttraumatic): +arthritis and/or ± MRI.</u>
   (a) Fusion—first, second TMT: 2, 3.5 cortical screws first, bridge plate second to third TMT.
   (b) Fusion—intercuneiform as indicated with 3.5 mm trans-articular screw.
   (c) Fusion—first TMT: NOTE: use dorsal medial plate if abduction deformity.
   (d) Bone graft: Calcaneal, distal tibia or proximal tibia (surgeon choice).
   (e) NO ROH: RTS after fusion—recreational only!
5. <u>Future directions and other considerations.</u>
   (a) Flexible fixation: NOT used in high-level or competitive athlete for acute.

   Used for augmentation and post ROH now.

   Further research needed to confirm adequacy and efficacy.

   Advantage of no second surgery for ROH.

   (b) Absorbable fixation: Not currently adequate and risk of reaction

   If right material, more rigid and no ROH

   (c) Ligament recon.: Free tendon reconstruction has promise

   Needs rigid fixation also to maintain anatomic reduction.

   Use in chronic dislocation without arthritis as augment.

   (d) Rehabilitation: Currently every procedure: <u>at least 6 weeks NWB.</u>

   Critical to get ROM in forefoot, full strength.

   Techniques cannot compromise anatomic alignment.

   CAN we get to point we don't need NWB after fixation?

   CAN we avoid posttraumatic arthritis?

Conclusions

Lisfranc injury and dislocations continue to be a potentially disabling injury for athletes. Increased recognition and advancement in diagnosis and management of Lisfranc injuries have made tremendous strides. Just in the last 50 years, this injury has gone from a career-ending injury to one with proper surgical techniques as described, and careful rehabilitation can allow the athlete to return to high-level activities. This continues to be an exciting area of research and treatment.

This chapter has addressed the historical perspective and development of treatment techniques. Rigid fixation after anatomic alignment has become the mainstay for treatment in the competitive athlete. Midfoot fusion has gained interest in the non-athlete but is today reserved for posttraumatic arthritis in the post-athletic career. The potential for this injury to be career threatening still exists, but the techniques described in this chapter are encouraging and give hope for even further advancement, reliable return to activity, and lessened risk for posttraumatic changes and degenerative arthritis. Our goal remains developing techniques for treatment that provide and maintain anatomic alignment with full range of motion and no risk for long-term compromise in the athlete. It is exciting to spend our time and effort pursuing this ultimate goal. We have not yet reached that goal, but the trajectory of recent advancements gives hope for the future.

References

1. Lewis JS Jr, Anderson RB. Lisfranc injuries in the athlete. Foot Ankle Int. 2016;37(12):1374–80.
2. McHale KJ, Rozell JC, Milby AH, Carey JL, Sennett BJ. Outcomes of Lisfranc injuries in the National Football League. Am J Sports Med. 2016;44(7):1810–7.
3. Curtis MJ, Myerson M, Szura B. Tarsometatarsal joint injuries in the athlete. Am J Sports Med. 1993;21(4):497–502.
4. de St L, Martin J. Nouvelle méthode opératoire pour l'amputation partielle du pied dans son articulation tarso-métatarsienne: méthode précédée des nombreuses modifications qu'a subies celle de Chopart (in French). Paris: L'imprimerie de Feuguery; 1815.
5. Aitken A, Poulson D. Dislocations of the tarsometatarsal joint. J Bone Joint Surg Am. 1963;45:246–60.
6. English TA. Dislocations of the metatarsal bone and adjacent toe. J Bone Joint Surg. 1964;46-B(4):700–4.
7. Resch S, Stenström A. The treatment of tarsometatarsal injuries. Foot Ankle. 2016;11(3):117–23.
8. Gaines RJ, Wright G, Stewart J. Injury to the tarsometatarsal joint complex during fixation of Lisfranc fracture dislocations: an anatomic study. J Trauma. 2009;66(4):1125–8.
9. Lau S, Guest C, Hall M, Tacey M, Joseph S, Oppy A. Functional outcomes post Lisfranc injury-Transarticular screws, dorsal bridge plating or combination treatment? J Orthop Trauma. 2017;31(8):447–52.
10. Porter DA, Barnes AF, Rund A, Walrod MT. Injury pattern in ligamentous Lisfranc injuries in competitive athletes. Foot Ankle Int. 2019;40(2):185–94.
11. Hu SJ, Chang SM, Li XH, Yu GR. Outcome comparison of Lisfranc injuries treated through dorsal plate fixation versus screw fixation. Acta Ortop Bras. 2014;22(6):315–20.
12. Ponkilainen VT, Laine HJ, Maenpaa HM, Mattila VM, Haapasalo HH. Incidence and characteristics of midfoot injuries. Foot Ankle Int. 2019;40(1):105–12.
13. Vuori JP, Aro HT. Lisfranc joint injuries: trauma mechanisms and associated injuries. J Trauma. 1993;35(1):40–5.
14. Kaar S, Femino J, Morag Y. Lisfranc joint displacement following sequential ligament sectioning. J Bone Joint Surg Am. 2007;89(10):2225–32.
15. Raikin SM, Elias I, Dheer S, Besser MP, Morrison WB, Zoga AC. Prediction of midfoot instability in the subtle Lisfranc injury. Comparison of magnetic resonance imaging with intraoperative findings. J Bone Joint Surg Am. 2009;91(4):892–9.
16. Lattermann C, Goldstein JL, Wukich DK, Lee S, Bach BR. Practical Management of Lisfranc Injuries in athletes. Clin J Sport Med. 2007;17(4):311–5.
17. Hesp WLEM, Van Der Werken C, Goris RJA. Lisfranc dislocations: fractures and/or dislocations through the Tarso-metatarsal joints. Injury. 1984;15(4):261–6.
18. Ghate SD, Sistla VM, Nemade V, Vibhute D, Shahane SM, Samant AD. Screw and wire fixation for Lisfranc fracture dislocations. J Orthop Surg. 2012;20(2):170–5.
19. Ebraheim NA, Yang H, Lu J, Biyani A. Computer evaluation of second tarsometatarsal joint dislocation. Foot Ankle Int. 1996;17(11):685–9.
20. Clare MP. Lisfranc injuries. Curr Rev Musculoskelet Med. 2017;10(1):81–5.
21. Kuo RS, Tejwani NC, Digiovanni CW, et al. Outcome after open reduction and internal fixation of Lisfranc joint injuries. J Bone Joint Surg Am. 2000;82(11):1609–18.
22. Marin-Pena OR, Viloria Recio F, Sanz Gomez T, Larrainzar GR. Fourteen years follow up after Lisfranc fracture-dislocation: functional and radiological results. Injury. 2012;43(Suppl 2):S79–82.
23. Ly TV, Coetzee JC. Treatment of primarily ligamentous Lisfranc joint injuries: primary arthrodesis compared with open reduction and internal fixation. A prospective, randomized study. J Bone Joint Surg Am. 2006;88(3):514–20.
24. Henning JA, Jones CB, Sietsema DL, Bohay DR, Anderson JG. Open reduction internal fixation versus primary arthrodesis for lisfranc injuries: a prospective randomized study. Foot Ankle Int. 2009;30(10):913–22.
25. Stødle AH, Hvaal KH, Brogger HM, Madsen JE, Husebye EE. Temporary bridge plating vs primary

arthrodesis of the first tarsometatarsal joint in Lisfranc injuries: randomized controlled trial. Foot Ankle Int. 2020;41(8):901–10.
26. MacMahon A, Kim P, Levine DS, et al. Return to sports and physical activities after primary partial arthrodesis for Lisfranc injuries in young patients. Foot Ankle Int. 2016;37(4):355–62.
27. Coetzee JC, Ly TV. Treatment of primarily ligamentous Lisfranc joint injuries: primary arthrodesis compared with open reduction and internal fixation. Surgical technique. J Bone Joint Surg Am. 2007;89(Suppl 2 Pt.1):122–7.
28. Buda M, Kink S, Stavenuiter R, et al. Reoperation rate differences between open reduction internal fixation and primary arthrodesis of Lisfranc injuries. Foot Ankle Int. 2018;39(9):1089–96.
29. Alberta FG, Aronow MS, Barrero M, Diaz-Doran V, Sullivan RJ, Adams DJ. Ligamentous Lisfranc joint injuries: a biomechanical comparison of dorsal plate and transarticular screw fixation. Foot Ankle Int. 2005;26(6):462–73.
30. Sharma S, Dhillon MS, Arora C, Patel S. Percutaneous fixation of Lisfranc injuries. J Clin Orthop Trauma. 2020;11(3):487–91.
31. Stavrakakis IM, Magarakis GE, Christoforakis Z. Percutaneous fixation of Lisfranc joint injuries: a systematic review of the literature. Acta Orthop Traumatol Turc. 2019;53(6):457–62.
32. Cho J, Kim J, Min TH, et al. Suture button vs conventional screw fixation for isolated Lisfranc ligament injuries[formula: see text]. Foot Ankle Int. 2020:1071100720976074.
33. Kuhn K, Renninger C, Cochran G, Bellamy J. Acute arthrodesis of Lisfranc injuries. Techn Foot Ankle Surgery. 2019;18(1):8–15.
34. Charlton T, Boe C, Thordarson DB. Suture button fixation treatment of chronic Lisfranc injury in professional dancers and high-level athletes. J Dance Med Sci. 2015;19(4):135–9.
35. De Los S-RR, Canillas F, Varas-Navas J, Morales-Munoz P, Barrio-Sanz P, Medina-Santos M. Lisfranc joint ligament complex reconstruction: a promising solution for missed, delayed, or chronic Lisfranc injury without arthritis. J Foot Ankle Surg. 2017;56(6):1350–6.
36. Miyamoto W, Takao M, Innami K, Miki S, Matsushita T. Ligament reconstruction with single bone tunnel technique for chronic symptomatic subtle injury of the Lisfranc joint in athletes. Arch Orthop Trauma Surg. 2015;135(8):1063–70.
37. Zwipp H, Rammelt S. Anatomical reconstruction of chronically instable Lisfranc's ligaments. Unfallchirurg. 2014;117(9):791–7.
38. Panchbhavi VK, Vallurupalli S, Yang J, Andersen CR. Screw fixation compared with suture-button fixation of isolated Lisfranc ligament injuries. J Bone Joint Surg Am. 2009;91(5):1143–8.
39. Sripanich Y, Weinberg MW, Krähenbühl N, et al. Surgical outcome of chronic Lisfranc injury without secondary degenerative arthritis: a systematic literature review. Injury. 2020;51(6):1258–65.
40. Nunley JA, Vertullo CJ. Classification, investigation, and management of midfoot sprains: Lisfranc injuries in the athlete. Am J Sports Med. 2002;30(6):871–8.
41. Deol RS, Roche A, Calder JD. Return to training and playing after acute Lisfranc injuries in elite professional soccer and Rugby players. Am J Sports Med. 2016;44(1):166–70.
42. Myerson MS, Cerrato RA. Current management of tarsometatarsal injuries in the athlete. J Bone Joint Surg Am. 2008;90(11):2522–33.
43. Cochran G, Renninger C, Tompane T, Bellamy J, Kuhn K. Primary arthrodesis versus open reduction and internal fixation for low-energy Lisfranc injuries in a young athletic population. Foot Ankle Int. 2017;38(9):957–63.
44. Dubois-Ferriere V, Lubbeke A, Chowdhary A, Stern R, Dominguez D, Assal M. Clinical outcomes and development of symptomatic osteoarthritis 2 to 24 years after surgical treatment of tarsometatarsal joint complex injuries. J Bone Joint Surg Am. 2016;98(9):713–20.
45. Meyerkort DJ, Gurel R, Maor D, Calder JDF. Deep peroneal nerve injury following hardware removal for Lisfranc joint injury. Foot Ankle Int. 2020;41(3):320–3.

21 Lisfranc Injury in Athletes: Return to Play and Rehabilitation

Ahmed K. Attia and Pieter D'Hooghe

Return to Play Following Lisfranc Injury

Introduction

Traditionally, the Lisfranc injury was thought to be an isolated rupture of the stout ligament connecting the medial cuneiform and the second metatarsal base with or without associated fractures (metatarsal and cuneiform fractures). However, as our understanding of the complexity of the midfoot has evolved, we now know that the midfoot acts as a functional unit rather than an isolated anatomical structure as a Lisfranc injury is primarily the loss of midfoot stability. In the uninjured midfoot, the lateral column is flexible and accommodates for uneven surfaces, and the middle column (the most stable) transmits forces to forefoot to allow for foot toe-off while the medial column bears the majority of the forces during stance [1–3]. A stable and pain-free midfoot is necessary for athletic activities and is the ultimate treatment goal after injury.

Fortunately, reported return to play (RTP) after Lisfranc injury in athletes has remained excellent with many authors reporting a 100% RTP rate in athletes [4–9], while others report a RTP rate above 80% which is still considered high [10–16]. However, the performance of the player after return, time necessary to attain per-injury level, competitions missed, and effect of the injury on the player's career need to be part of the discussion and treatment decision-making between the player and the medical team. This chapter aims to provide an overview on Lisfranc injuries in athletes with specific focus on rehabilitation and RTP. Table 21.1 highlights some of the common questions regarding Lisfranc injuries that the medical team should be prepared to answer.

It is not Uncommon!
Lisfranc injury is increasingly diagnosed in athletes, and it affects up to 4% of collegiate American football players in comparison to 0.2% of all fractures in the general population. Offensive players specifically quarterbacks are at an increased risk of sustaining such an injury [14, 16].

A. K. Attia
Department of Orthopaedic Surgery, Hamad General Hospital, Hamad Medical Corporation, Doha, Qatar

P. D'Hooghe (✉)
Department of Orthopaedic Surgery, Aspetar Orthopaedic and Sports Medicine Hospital, Doha, Qatar
e-mail: pieter.dhooghe@aspetar.com

P. D'Hooghe et al. (eds.), *Ligamentous Injuries of the Foot and Ankle*,
https://doi.org/10.1007/978-3-031-08682-3_21

Table 21.1 Common concerns of injured players

What is a Lisfranc injury exactly?
When will I be able to play again?
Will I be able to perform at the same level? How long will it take?
Does my position on the field play a role?
Will the injury affect my career on the long term?
When can I return to practice?
Will I have problems in the future?

Anatomical Characteristics of the Injury and Return to Play Parameters

The commonly used categorization of Lisfranc injuries is a ligamentous versus a bony type (see Fig. 21.1). However, this represents an oversimplification of a variable and complex injury to a

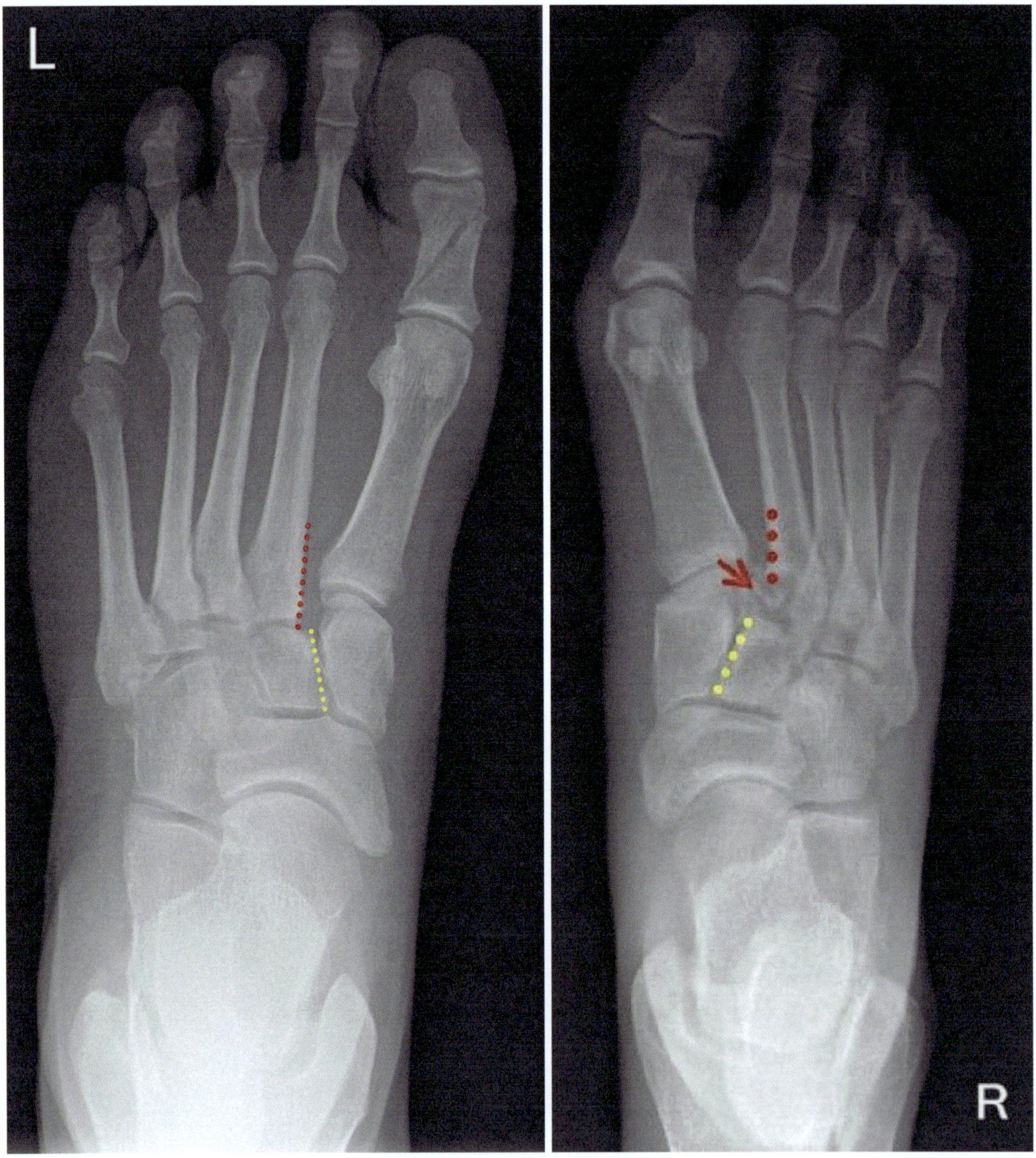

Fig. 21.1 Radiographs of the left **ligamentous** (left panel) and right **bony** Lisfranc injuries (right panel). Note the displacement of the medial border of the base of the MT-2 (red dotted line) from the medial border of the medial cuneiform (yellow dotted line). The arrow marks the comminution of the proximal second metatarsal which poses a management challenge

unique anatomical foot structure. While a consensus on classification for Lisfranc injuries in the foot would be optimal, such a consensus does not exist currently. However, two current classification systems used together have proven useful in approaching these injuries. Nunley and Vertullo described a classification system for low-energy Lisfranc injuries in 2002 [5]. In their series of 15 athletes, they classified the injury based on the presence or absence of diastasis between the base of MT-1 and MT-2 on anteroposterior weight-bearing radiographs and preservation of the midfoot arch on lateral weight-bearing radiographs. An earlier classification system was described by Myerson et al. in 1986, using the description of the segmental pattern of injury (with excellent interobserver reliability) [17].

While evidence comparing bony to ligamentous Lisfranc injuries in athletes concluded that bony injuries take 4–8 weeks longer to return to play [10, 15], the overall RTP rate was shown not to be affected by the type of the injury. However, there is a significant variability reported in recovery time within either ligamentous or bony injuries, based on injury severity and other factors. Some athletes with ligamentous injuries were able to return as early as 13 days [11] while others required up to 9 months. Those athletes with bony injuries returned no sooner than 8 weeks and up to 11 months from surgery.

A longer recovery time is reported for bony Lisfranc foot injuries, but this could also be explained by the fact that ligamentous injuries are more often treated non-operatively compared to bony injuries.

Does Management Strategy Impact RTP Parameters?

The management of each Lisfranc injury should be determined on a case-by-case basis taking into consideration the anatomic nature of the injury, the severity of the injury, as well as the players' expectations. Unfortunately, there are no evidence-based treatment guidelines that indicate one uniform type of management for these injuries. As Coetzee commented, not all Lisfranc injuries are created equal and there will never be a single treatment option for these types of injuries. Many athlete Lisfranc injuries are managed non-operatively with excellent outcomes and expedited recovery. Interestingly, rugby players are more likely to be treated non-operatively in comparison to American football players. This points out the different body demands and mechanics for each individual sport and the geographical different management styles used. Moreover, the conservative management might be simply a surrogate of the severity of the injury rather than the outcome of the treatment itself. In other words, grade I and II injuries treated non-operatively result in a significantly shorter recovery compared to grade III injuries that are treated surgically [11]. Many techniques have been described, and a myriad of implants are used; hence, any comparison between operative and non-operative management should be interpreted with caution.

Operative vs. Non-operative

Both operative and non-operative treatments are shown to have an excellent and comparable RTP rate, similar midfoot degenerative joint disease (DJD), and reoperation rate [5, 8–11, 16]. The main difference reported is the time needed to return to sports practice and play. Collegiate football players who underwent surgery missed at average almost 8 times the amount of games missed by those who were managed non-operatively. Surgical management was also correlated with a higher chance of being undrafted, and when they did, they had a worse overall National Football League (NFL) draft position [16]. Similar studies in the NFL show that players need an average of 10 months to RTP postoperatively, while conservative management allowed for a return after an average of 6 months. This can partially be explained by the severity of the initial injury. Interestingly, both groups had comparable drop in performance after return to full play [10].

It is worth mentioning that time till full recovery and return to practice are not uniformly reported in literature. Some athletes return as soon as 13 days after non-operative management, and others need up to several months. In summary, there is a clear trend in literature toward a longer time to recovery with operative management.

ORIF vs. PA Is Still Controversial

The two broad categories are either temporary fixation with open reduction and internal fixation (ORIF) or permanent fixation with primary arthrodesis (PA). The landmark study on PA in high-energy Lisfranc is the randomized clinical trial published by Ly and Coetzee in 2006 [18]. They concluded that PA is superior to ORIF in purely ligamentous Lisfranc injuries in the short and medium term. It is noteworthy that their technique in the ORIF group involved transarticular screw fixation violating a considerable portion of the articular cartilage. However, their result was not reproducible in another randomized clinical trial [19] and a systematic review by Sheibani-Rad [20] which showed no difference between both techniques. It is also important that none of those studies included any athletes.

To date, there are a limited number of comparative studies in the athletic population with very small sample size to detect any differences. The power analysis of one study demonstrated the need of 400 patients to allow for detection of any statistically significant difference in return to duty and 31,000 patients to detect any effect of early vs. delayed surgery [21].

However, some lessons can be learned from the studies on military personnel. While not necessarily a sports injury, Lisfranc injuries in young military personnel share many comparisons with those in athletes. They both are low-energy injuries resulting from axial loading of a plantarflexed foot. Moreover, they also have high functional demands such as running, jumping, and general fitness. Similar to professional athletes, they are motivated and incentivized to return to active-duty participation.

Three studies compared ORIF to PA of low-energy Lisfranc injuries in an active-duty military population [3, 14, 21]. These studies showed satisfactory return to duty rates (RTD) that was comparable to athletes. Both procedures resulted in similar pain scores at final follow-up and comparable scores of all components of the Foot and Ankle Ability Measure (FAAM). PA was superior in terms of time to RTD and running speed at fitness testing. PA returned 2 months sooner and was 29 s faster per mile compared to ORIF. Salvage arthrodesis, on the other hand, had a significantly worse return to duty rates (only 29%).

It is important (when comparing PA to ORIF in reoperation rates and time needed for recovery) to consider that removal of hardware is a planned part of ORIF and not a complication. Recovery after a hardware removal procedure might lead to a longer overall recovery time from the injury. When planned hardware removal is excluded, PA and ORIF have comparable reoperation rates. This needs to be discussed with the players and coaches as a part of the decision-making process.

To sum up, PA is a viable option in a high-demand population, but there is insufficient evidence to argue for superiority of either ORIF or PA. However, Myerson has recommended against PA in athletes believing that it may prevent restoration of normal foot function [22]. Moreover, there are no studies on the long-term consequences in midfoot fusion neither in general population nor athletes. The current suggested indications for primary arthrodesis are major ligamentous disruption with multidirectional instability, inability to obtain anatomical reduction with ORIF, comminuted intraarticular fractures of the first and second metatarsals, and significant delay in management although a clear cutoff is controversial [18, 22–24]. The optimal management remains debatable, and anatomical reduction remains the goal, regardless of the chosen procedure type.

Primary Arthrodesis in Athletes

In high-energy (purely ligamentous) Lisfranc injuries, level I evidence published by Ly and Coetzee shows that PA results in better functional outcomes than ORIF [18]. *However, the current literature does NOT provide sufficient evidence of compelling superiority of either options in elite and professional athletes. This topic is further explored in Chap. 20.*

Anatomical Reduction and Residual Displacement Matter the Most

A general rule in orthopedic fracture treatments is anatomical reduction of intraarticular injuries, and Lisfranc injuries are no exception. Myerson et al. and Kuo et al. highlighted the paramount importance of anatomical reduction for satisfactory outcomes [17, 25]. Patients who had non-anatomical reduction had higher odds of developing post-traumatic arthritis of the midfoot. Interestingly, the severity of the initial injury was not a predictor of DJD if anatomical reduction was achieved. However, over 40% of football players who suffer from a Lisfranc injury have residual displacement. A displacement of just over 2 mm strongly correlates with an inferior performance including games started, games missed, and draft position [16].

> ***Quality of Reduction Is Crucial!***
> *Residual displacement of more than 2 mm leads to a significant decline in the performance of the NFL Scouting Combine players in the following 2 years of their career. They started fewer games, missed more games, and had a worse overall draft position* [16].

The Players' Position Does Matter

While the athlete's position on the field may not affect the overall RTP progress, it might be related to the odds of sustaining a Lisfranc injury as well as performance after RTP. In American football, certain offense positions have a statistically significant higher correlation with Lisfranc injuries in comparison to defense positions. Quarterbacks are found to have the greatest risk of sustaining a Lisfranc injury (estimated at 6.8%), over three times the mean risk for all football players in the NFL Scouting Combine [16].

Postoperatively, offensive players in the NFL suffer a significantly greater decline in their performance in comparison to their defensive counterparts one season after the injury. Offensive players also need a longer time to regain their pre-injury level. Interestingly, there is no difference in RTP rates, recovery time, and career length between both groups [10]. Offensive players played a mean of 48 regular season games in comparison to 50 games for the defensive players, a difference that is neither clinically nor statistically significant [26] (Table 21.2).

So What Matters?

Conclusion

Athletic Lisfranc injuries possess features that separate them from those in the general population. While return to play to pre-injury level is excellent, the initial time to return to play is variable from weeks to months depending on the severity of the initial injury. The strongest predictor of performance remains anatomical reduction, regardless of the surgical procedure chosen, and a residual gap of 2 mm and more is poorly tolerated in high-demand athletes. The published literature remains relatively underpowered and of low level of evidence. Studies with superior methodology are required with specific focus on the athletic population.

Rehabilitation of Lisfranc Injuries

Introduction

While criteria for safe return to play have been described in detail for many sports injuries such as ACL, Lisfranc injury rehabilitation has received little attention. Most rehabilitation protocols focus on allowing gradual progression of weight bearing to allow adequate healing, ankle range of motion, and plantar flexion strengthening. However, there is no clear agreement on the specifics. It is crucial to seek input from the physical therapy and rehabilitation team to allow the players back on the field.

Table 21.2 Literature summary of the effect of selected variables on the outcome of Lisfranc injuries in athletes

	Return to play %	Recovery time	Games missed	Drop in performance	Games played	Games started	Overall pick	Draft position	DJD	Reoperation	Career length
Operative/ non-operative	N	**Y**	**Y**	N	N	N	**Y**	**Y**	N	N	N
ORIF/PA	N	Y	N	Y	–	–	–	–	N	N	N
Offense/defense	N	N	N	Y	N	N	N	N	–	–	N
Residual displacement	**Y**	N	**Y**	**Y**	N	**Y**	**Y**	–	**Y**	**Y**	–
Bony/ligamentous	N	**Y**	**Y**	–	–	–	–	–	–	–	–

Y yes, *N* no, – not reported

Protocol Depends on the Management

Non-operative Rehabilitation

Immobilization in CAM walker and protected weight bearing to progress to full weight bearing by 3 weeks as tolerated. Once asymptomatic, a supervised gradual rehab protocol can begin.

Postoperative Rehabilitation

Non-weight bearing for 4–6 weeks followed by partial weight bearing for another 4–6 weeks. At 8–12 weeks postoperatively depending on healing, hardware should be removed if needed, and progression to full weight bearing can be allowed. Once asymptomatic, rehabilitation can commence in the form of range of motion, strengthening, proprioception, and gradual return to play along with a supervised home exercise program. These home programs include elastic band exercises for plantar flexion strengthening and ankle stretching, standing bilateral heel raises, and generalized lower extremity stretching and strengthening. Players need to achieve full range of motion and strength to be allowed to return to full participation (see Fig. 21.2).

While a detailed rehabilitation protocols specifically for Lisfranc injuries are rarely reported, a few programs have been described in detail.

LERC Milestones Program [7]

Structured rehab programs such as Lower Extremity Return to Competition (LERC) – Iowa Football consists of five stages of milestone activities that are completed sequentially. A player graduates to the next phase based on supervised, confident, and pain-free completion of activities.

Phase 1: Begin weight bearing, toe raises, cycling, StairMaster, step-ups, and treadmill.

Phase 2: Bounding activities, jump rope, plyometrics, jogging, and buildups.

Phase 3: Full-speed straight-ahead sprints, backpedaling, and buildups.

Phase 4: Functional activities, Figure 8s, running and cutting, and carioca and sport-specific drills.

Phase 5: Return to full team activities.

Lorenz and Beauchamp [27]

In their articles, they described a detailed rehabilitation approach for a football player who sus-

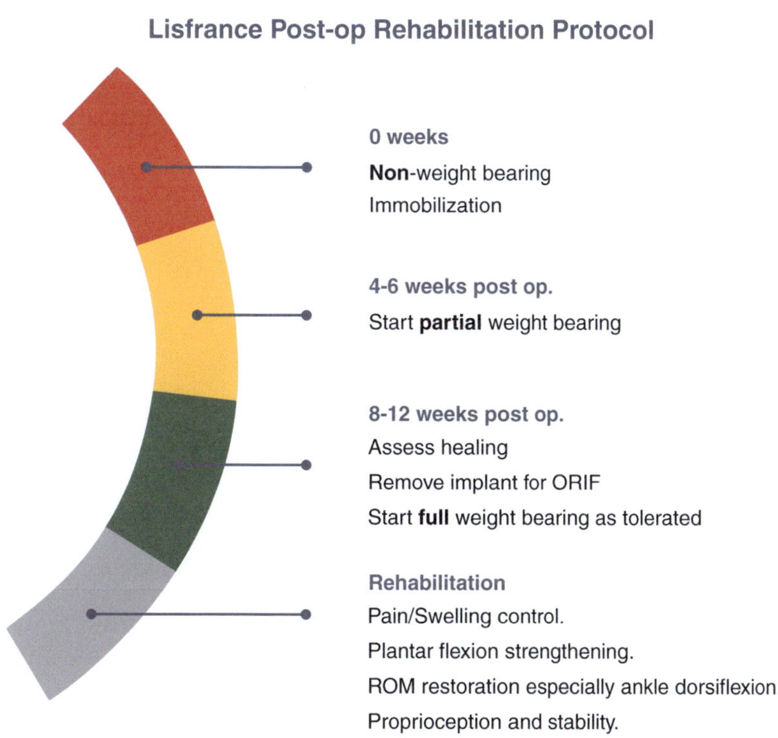

Fig. 21.2 Timeline of authors' preferred postoperative rehabilitation protocol of Lisfranc injuries in athletes

tained a Lisfranc injury who underwent ORIF. Their protocol focused on restoring the ankle range of motion and progressive closed-chain strengthening of the plantar flexion. They utilized standing heel rises (bilateral then single) that progressed to leaning heel rises and eventually hopping in a twice weekly program over 8 weeks. Activities otherwise are similar to LERC.

Return to Play Criteria and Testing

While criteria for diagnosis and operative intervention are well described, criteria for when to release the player back to sports and objective testing to guide that decision are not as clear. However, the Lower Extremity Functional Scale (LEFS) [28] can be used in athletes with Lisfranc injuries to provide an objective assessment of progression throughout rehabilitation. Moreover, tests to assess strength on plantar flexion such as single-leg hop, triple hop, and 6-meter timed hop can be used along with assessing the gait and ability to hop in multiple planes without pain or instability [27]. Figure 21.3 shows various tests to assess the strength of plantar flexion and the stability of the forefoot.

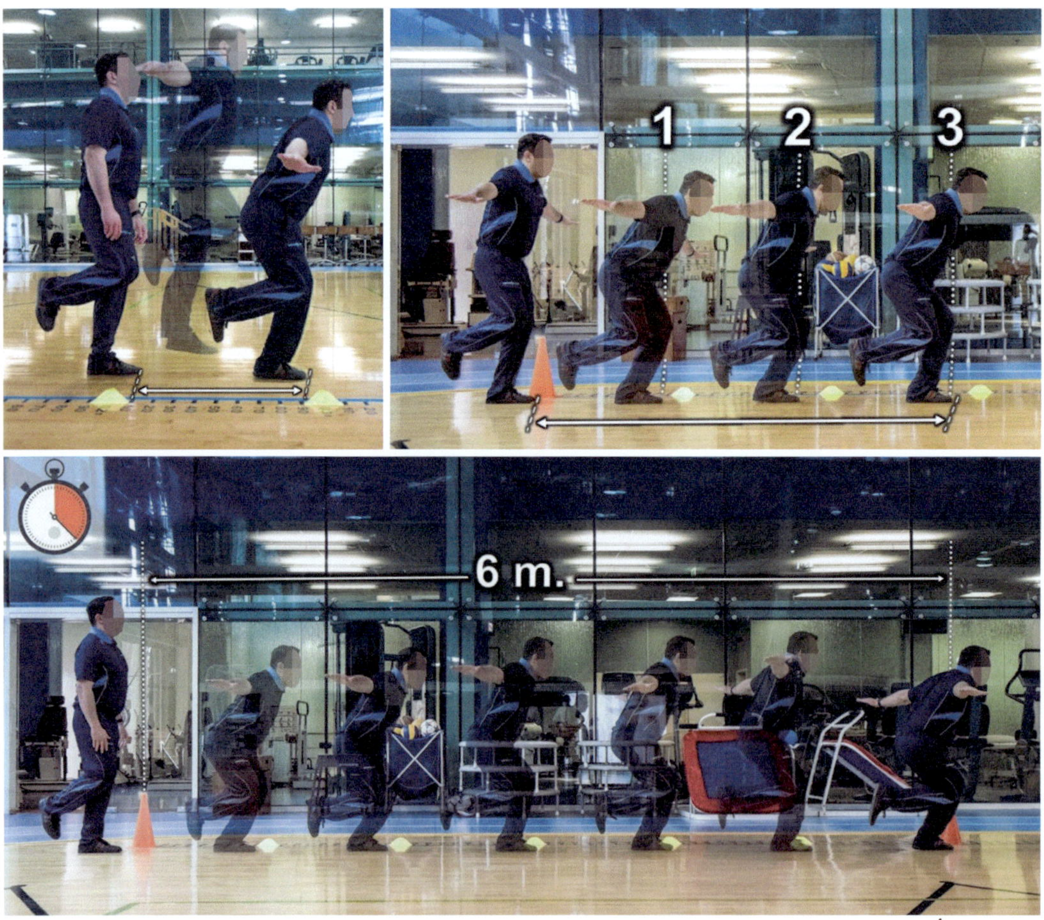

Fig. 21.3 **Single-leg hop** (upper right panel) and **triple hop tests** (upper left panel): the athlete is asked to hop forward on one leg as far as possible, and the distance is compared to that of the unaffected side. The **timed 6 m single-leg hop test** (lower panel): the patient is asked to hop on one leg for 6 m, and the time needed to complete the test is compared to that of the unaffected side

Conclusion

Criteria for return to play after Lisfranc injuries in athletes represent a gap in orthopedic knowledge. Superior-quality studies are needed to provide an evidence-based approach to allow safe return of athletes with such injuries. At the moment, rehabilitation should focus on pain and swelling control, strengthening of plantar flexion, and restoring range of motion and proprioception in a supervised and gradual approach.

References

1. Myerson MS. The diagnosis and treatment of injury to the tarsometatarsal joint complex. J Bone Joint Surg Br. 1999;81:756–63.
2. Eleftheriou KI, Rosenfeld PF, Calder JD. Lisfranc injuries: an update. Knee Surg Sports Traumatol Arthrosc. 2013;21:1434–46.
3. Balazs GC, Hanley MG, Pavey GJ, Rue JPH. Military personnel sustaining lisfranc injuries have high rates of disability separation. J R Army Med Corps. 2017;163:215–9. https://doi.org/10.1136/jramc-2016-000681.
4. Wagner E, Ortiz C, Villalón IE, Keller A, Wagner P. Early weight-bearing after percutaneous reduction and screw fixation for low-energy lisfranc injury. Foot Ankle Int. 2013;34:978–83. https://doi.org/10.1177/1071100713477403.
5. Nunley JA, Vertullo CJ. Classification, investigation, and management of midfoot sprains: Lisfranc injuries in the athlete. Am J Sports Med. 2002;30:871–8. https://doi.org/10.1177/03635465020300061901.
6. Cottom JM, Hyer CF, Berlet GC. Treatment of Lisfranc fracture dislocations with an interosseous suture button technique: a review of 3 cases. J Foot Ankle Surg. 2008;47:250–8. https://doi.org/10.1053/j.jfas.2008.01.004.
7. Meyer SA, Callaghan JJ, Albright JP, Crowley ET, Powell JW. Midfoot sprains in collegiate football players. Am J Sports Med. 1994;22:392–401. https://doi.org/10.1177/036354659402200316.
8. Curtis MJ, Myerson M, Szura B. Tarsometatarsal joint injuries in the athlete. Am J Sports Med. 1993;21:497–502. https://doi.org/10.1177/036354659302100403.
9. Shapiro MS, Wascher DC, Finerman GAM. Rupture of Lisfranc's ligament in athletes. Am J Sports Med. 1994;22:687–91. https://doi.org/10.1177/036354659402200518.
10. Singh SK, George A, Kadakia AR, Hsu WK. Performance-based outcomes following lisfranc injury among professional American football and rugby athletes. Orthopedics. 2018;41:e479–82. https://doi.org/10.3928/01477447-20180424-03.
11. Osbahr DC, O'Loughlin PF, Drakos MC, Barnes RP, Kennedy JG, Warren RF. Midfoot sprains in the National Football League. Am J Orthop (Belle Mead NJ). 2014;43:557–61.
12. Bleazey ST, Brigido SA, Protzman NM. Technique tip: percutaneous fixation of partial incongruous Lisfranc injuries in athletes. Foot Ankle Spec. 2013;6:217–21. https://doi.org/10.1177/1938640013486515.
13. Chilvers M, Donahue M, Nassar L, Manoli A. Foot and ankle injuries in elite female gymnasts. Foot Ankle Int. 2007;28:214–8. https://doi.org/10.3113/FAI.2007.0214.
14. Cochran G, Renninger C, Tompane T, Bellamy J, Kuhn K. Primary arthrodesis versus open reduction and internal fixation for low-energy Lisfranc injuries in a young athletic population. Foot Ankle Int. 2017;38:957–63. https://doi.org/10.1177/10711.
15. Deol RS, Roche A, Calder JDF. Return to training and playing after acute Lisfranc injuries in elite professional soccer and Rugby players. Am J Sports Med. 2016;44:166–70. https://doi.org/10.1177/0363546515616814.
16. McHale KJ, Vopat BG, Beaulieu-Jones BR, Sanchez G, Whalen JM, McDonald LS, et al. Epidemiology and outcomes of Lisfranc injuries identified at the National Football League Scouting Combine. Am J Sports Med. 2017;45(8):1901–8. https://doi.org/10.1177/0363546517697297.
17. Myerson MS, Fisher RT, Burgess AR, et al. Fracture dislocations of the tarsometatarsal joints: end results correlated with pathology and treatment. Foot Ankle. 1986;6:225–42.
18. Ly TV, Coetzee JC. Treatment of primarily ligamentous Lisfranc joint injuries: primary arthrodesis compared with open reduction and internal fixation. A prospective, randomized study. J Bone Joint Surg Am. 2006;88:514–20.
19. Henning JA, Jones CB, Sietsema DL, Bohay DR, Anderson JG. Open reduction internal fixation versus primary arthrodesis for Lisfranc injuries: a prospective randomized study. Foot Ankle Int. 2009;30(10):913–22.
20. Sheibani-Rad S, Coetzee JC, Giveans MR, et al. Arthrodesis versus ORIF for Lisfranc fractures. Orthopedics. 2012;35:e868–73.
21. Hawkinson MP, Tennent DJ, Belisle J, Osborn P. Outcomes of Lisfranc injuries in an active duty military population. Foot Ankle Int. 2017;38:1115–9. https://doi.org/10.1177/1071100717719532.
22. Myerson MS, Cerrato RA. Current management of tarsometatarsal injuries in the athlete. J Bone Joint Surg Am. 2008;90(11):2522–33.
23. Seybold JD, Coetzee JC. Lisfranc injuries: when to observe, fix, or fuse. Clin Sports Med. 2015;34(4):705–23. https://doi.org/10.1016/j.csm.2015.06.006.
24. Trevino SG, Kodros S. Controversies in tarsometatarsal injuries. Orthop Clin North Am. 1995;26(2):229–38.
25. Kuo RS, Tejwani NC, Digiovanni CW, et al. Outcome after open reduction and internal fixation

of Lisfranc joint injuries. J Bone Joint Surg Am. 2000;82A(11):1609–18.
26. McHale KJ, Rozell JC, Milby AH, Carey JL, Sennett BJ. Outcomes of Lisfranc injuries in the National Football League. Am J Sports Med. 2016;44(7):1810–7. https://doi.org/10.1177/0363546516645082.
27. Lorenz DS, Beauchamp C. Functional progression and return to sport criteria for a high school football player following surgery for a lisfranc injury. Int J Sports Phys Ther. 2013;8(2):162–71.
28. Binkley JM, Stratford PW, Lott SA, Riddle DL. The lower extremity functional scale (LEFS): scale development, measurement properties, and clinical application. North American Orthopaedic rehabilitation research network. Phys Ther. 1999;79:371–83.

Management of Turf Toe and Sesamoid Injuries

22

Benjamin J. Ebben and Robert B. Anderson

Introduction

The connective tissue integrity of the plantar hallux metatarsophalangeal (MTP) joint is critical to normal foot function and is relied upon heavily, particularly in athletic populations, for sports-related activities demanding explosive push-off and high-speed directional changes. Injuries to this region can lead to significant pain and impairment and potentially chronic instability, deformity, and secondary joint degeneration, given the loss of normal ligament and tendon balance. The plantar anatomy supporting the hallux MTP joint is complex, and trauma to these structures manifests as a heterogeneous group of injury patterns. Collectively, these injuries are often denoted as "turf toe."

The term "turf toe" was first coined by Bowers and Martin in 1976 and originally referred to a sprain of the plantar hallux MTP joint capsuloligamentous complex resulting from forced hyperextension of the joint with a fixed forefoot and elevated heel [1]. They described this injury as a comparatively novel entity among West Virginia University football players and observed an increased incidence (5.4 turf toe injuries per season) in association with the installation of an AstroTurf artificial playing surface over a 5-year period. The authors also postulated that a simultaneous shift toward the utilization of increasingly flexible footwear compounded the increase in plantar hallux MTP joint sprains observed over that time span. These hypotheses were not entirely new, however, as plantar hallux MTP joint sprains had first garnered recognition a year earlier as a focal topic in a round-table discussion on football injuries and artificial turf between prominent members of the collegiate- and professional-level sports medicine physician community [2].

Since the first reports of turf toe injury, our understanding of hallux MTP joint injuries and pathophysiology has advanced. Although not exclusively a sports-related condition, much of our comprehension of plantar hallux MTP joint injuries has been afforded through the study of these injuries and treatment strategies in an elite-level athlete population, most commonly in football players. Over time, the diagnosis of turf toe has evolved to encompass a wide variety of traumatic lesions all involving the hallux MTP joint plantar structures, but with varying degrees and locations. This chapter will focus on the diagnosis, management, and rehabilitation of these inju-

B. J. Ebben
Department of Orthopedics and Rehabilitative Medicine, University of Wisconsin School of Medicine and Public Health, Madison, WI, USA

Department of Orthopedics, University of Colorado School of Medicine, Aurora, CO, USA

R. B. Anderson (✉)
Titletown Sports Medicine & Orthopedics, Green Bay, WI, USA

P. D'Hooghe et al. (eds.), *Ligamentous Injuries of the Foot and Ankle*,
https://doi.org/10.1007/978-3-031-08682-3_22

ries with a precursory review of the epidemiology of turf toe as well as anatomy and biomechanics of the hallux MTP joint.

Epidemiology

The incidence of turf toe injuries varies throughout the literature and over time. To the best of our knowledge, there have been no general population-based assessments. The available estimates have been the product of smaller-scale investigations isolated to sports teams and leagues. Like Bowers and Martin, Coker et al. reported on their own experience with injuries to the hallux MTP joint in college football players at the University of Arkansas in 1978 [3]. They treated six hallux MTP joint injuries per season over their study period of three seasons and noted that, although ankle sprains occurred more frequently (almost 25 per year), turf toe injuries were more disabling and accounted for disproportionately more missed practices and games. Again, these observations were attributed, in part, to conversion to an artificial playing surface and changes in footwear flexibility.

Another collegiate athlete study at Rice University in 1986 observed 56 isolated hallux MTP joint injuries severe enough to warrant treatment over a 15-year study period [4]. Ninety-six percent of these injuries occurred in football players, all on synthetic turf. Two injuries occurred in track and field athletes. Hallux MTP joint injuries accounted for over 80% of all the forefoot injuries which ranked third behind ankle and knee injuries as the most common time-loss injuries at Rice University over that time span. In 1990, Rodeo et al. surveyed 80 active professional football players from two different teams and found that 45% ($N = 36$) had incurred a turf toe injury over their professional careers averaging 5.2 years in length [5]. In instances where it could be determined, 83% of affected players identified the initial injury as having occurred while playing on an artificial surface. The authors also analyzed the effect of a previous turf toe injury on subsequent hallux MTP joint motion relative to the uninjured contralateral hallux and found significant decreases in both dorsiflexion and plantar flexion revealing the possibility of long-term sequelae such as hallux rigidus following this type of injury.

A few larger-scale and more contemporary investigations suggest that the incidence of turf toe injuries may be decreasing, potentially secondary to advances in footwear and artificial playing surface technology in the decades succeeding the initial reports. At the 2006 National Football League (NFL) Combine, Kaplan et al. evaluated all 320 participating prospective professional football players and reported on the incidence and variance of foot and ankle injuries in this group [6]. Seventy-two percent of players ($N = 231$) reported a history of a foot and ankle injury with lateral ankle sprain and syndesmotic sprain being the most common injuries at 31% and 15% of players, respectively. Turf toe injuries ranked third most common and were reported by 35 of 320 (11%) Combine participants, occurring most frequently in the running back position. In perhaps the largest epidemiologic study to date on the topic of turf toe, George and colleagues examined five seasons (2004–2009) worth of injury-related data across all of college football using the National Collegiate Athletic Association (NCAA) Injury Surveillance System (ISS) [7]. Team athletic trainers report injuries to the ISS when they occur during an organized NCAA practice or competition, require medical attention, and result in restriction from practice or competition beyond the initial injury date. Collegiate football players sustained 147 turf toe injuries during roughly 2.2 million athlete-exposures over the study period yielding an estimated incidence rate of 0.46–0.53 turf toe injuries per team per season or 0.062 injuries per 1000 athlete-exposures. Hallux MTP joint injuries accounted for 0.83% of all football-related injuries. The authors also investigated the role of playing surface and calculated an 85% higher risk of turf toe injury on artificial surfaces. Again, the running back position was afflicted most and was responsible for 23.3% of the injuries sustained during competition. Similar to previously mentioned literature, this study also demonstrated the disabling nature of this injury concluding that players averaged missing more than 10 days of athletic participation.

Anatomy

Metatarsophalangeal and Metatarsal-Sesamoidal Articulations

The hallux MTP joint is anatomically complex with multiple surrounding connective tissue structures imparting varying degrees of stability. It is injuries to the plantar supporting structures, specifically, which can result in joint instability patterns and secondary symptomology consistent with a turf toe designation. The hallux metatarsal and proximal phalanx bones form a condyloid articulation with little inherent osseous stability due to the shallow concavity at the base of the proximal phalanx and the wide and relatively flat metatarsal head.

Plantar to this MTP articulation are two sesamoid bones. These osseous structures are considered intracapsular as they have a superior articular surface composed of hyaline cartilage that directly apposes the undersurface of the hallux metatarsal head and exist within the same synovial membrane encapsulating the MTP articulation [8]. The medial sesamoid, also known as the tibial sesamoid, is typically larger and situated slightly more distal than its lateral counterpart called the lateral or fibular sesamoid. A strong intersesamoid ligament runs transversely between and links the tibial and fibular sesamoids. The sesamoids are accommodated by two corresponding grooves within the plantar aspect of the metatarsal head that are divided by a sagittally oriented crest of the bone called the crista [9]. During flexion and extension of the hallux MTP joint, the sesamoid bones glide within their respective grooves forming medial and lateral metatarsal-sesamoidal joints. One function of these joints is to dissipate force at the MTP joint during weight bearing. The sesamoids are encased within paired flexor hallucis brevis (FHB) tendons.

The FHB muscle originates from the plantar aspects of the cuboid and lateral cuneiform and separates into medial and lateral tendinous heads as it courses distally beneath the hallux MTP joint. Continuations of these tendons ultimately insert at the medial and lateral plantar tubercles at the base of the proximal phalanx. The FHB functions primarily in MTP joint plantar flexion and also serves as a dynamic stabilizer of the joint. The configuration of the sesamoid apparatus produces a mechanical advantage for hallux plantar flexion and push-off strength by increasing the plantar flexion load imparted by FHB muscle pull through hallux metatarsal head elevation and creation of a longer moment arm.

Plantar Plate and Other Capsuloligamentous Structures

The plantar plate is a confluence of multiple structures that, together, provide the critical stabilization function to the hallux MTP joint. It is difficult to differentiate distinct contributions to the plantar plate even with advanced imaging or surgical dissection. The term is generally used to describe the capsular and ligamentous tissue connecting the distal margin of the sesamoid bones and intersesamoid ligament to the plantar base of the proximal phalanx. The terminal portions of the medial and lateral FHB tendon heads distal to the sesamoids contribute to the plantar plate via the medial and lateral phalangeosesamoid ligaments. Thickened fibrous capsular tissue spans the interval between the phalangeosesamoid ligaments from the intersesamoid ligament to the plantar base of the proximal phalanx (Fig. 22.1). Together these robust plantar plate structures firmly anchor to the proximal phalanx, while the more proximal capsular tissue is thinner with a weaker metatarsal neck attachment [10]. The plantar plate proper affords stability mainly in the sagittal plane and resists MTP joint hyperextension. Disruptions of the plantar plate, often in combination with deformations in closely associated structures like the collateral ligaments, are typically implicated in turf toe injuries.

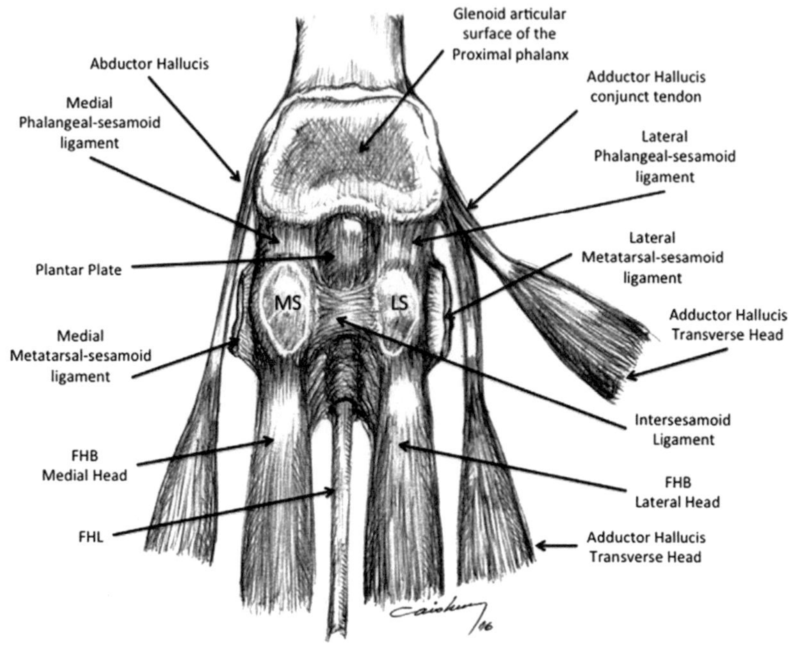

Fig. 22.1 Anatomy of the hallux metatarsophalangeal joint supporting plantar structures viewed from dorsal with the metatarsal removed. (*Reprinted from*: Nery C, Baumfeld D, Umans H, Yamada AF. MR imaging of the plantar plate: normal anatomy, turf toe, and other injuries. *Magnetic Resonance Imaging Clinics of North America*. 2017;25:127–144. Copyright (2017), with permission from Elsevier)

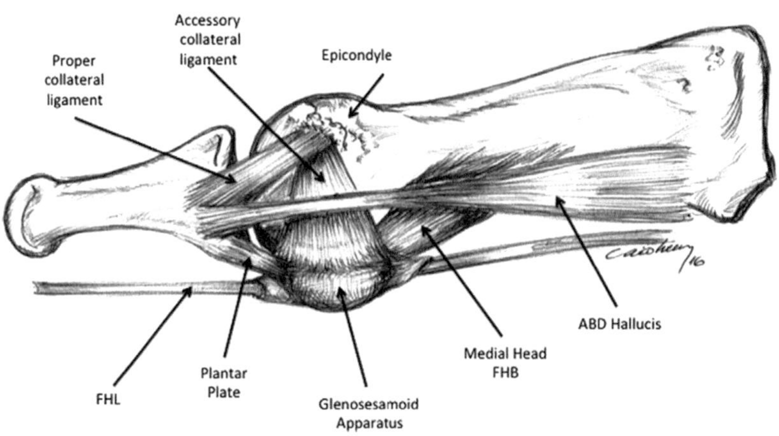

Fig. 22.2 Anatomy of the hallux metatarsophalangeal joint supporting structures viewed from medially. (*Reprinted from*: Nery C, Baumfeld D, Umans H, Yamada AF. MR imaging of the plantar plate: normal anatomy, turf toe, and other injuries. *Magnetic Resonance Imaging Clinics of North America*. 2017;25:127–144. Copyright (2017), with permission from Elsevier)

The collateral ligaments converge with the plantar plate and sesamoid apparatus on the medial and lateral sides of the MTP joint and provide stability in a more transverse plane. The collaterals include two unique components: the proper and accessory ligaments. The proper collaterals or metatarsophalangeal ligaments originate from the dorsal aspect of the metatarsal head and fan out in an oblique manner to insert on the plantar base of the proximal phalanx and predominantly resist varus and valgus stress at the MTP joint. The accessory collaterals are also commonly referred to as the metatarsosesamoid ligaments or sesamoid suspensory slips (Fig. 22.2). These bands also originate dorsally from the metatarsal head tubercle but course more plantarly than their counterparts to insert on the sesamoids and plantar plate (the phalangeosesamoid ligaments). Relative to the proper collaterals, the accessory ligaments confer additional sagittal plane stability.

Dynamic Stabilizers

Lastly, both intrinsic and extrinsic hallucal musculotendinous units provide dynamic support to the plantar MTP joint, outside of the FHB, which has previously been discussed. The flexor hallucis longus (FHL) is an extrinsic muscle that originates from the posterior fibula and distal interosseus membrane. It courses through the medial hindfoot beneath the sustentaculum tali, and its tendon inserts to the plantar base of the hallux distal phalanx. At the level of the MTP joint, the FHL tendon rests just plantar to the intersesamoid ligament. It serves primarily as a flexor of both the hallux MTP and interphalangeal joints. The abductor hallucis is an intrinsic muscle that arises from the medial process of the calcaneal tuberosity. It functions to abduct the MTP joint and resist valgus. The terminal portion of the abductor hallucis merges with a number of structures on the plantar medial aspect of the MTP joint including the medial head of the FHB, the tibial sesamoid medial margin, the medial phalangeosesamoid ligament and plantar plate, as well as the plantar medial base of the proximal phalanx. A similar confluence arrangement occurs with the insertion of the adductor hallucis tendon on the lateral side of the hallux MTP joint. This muscle has two origins: a transverse head that arises from each lesser MTP joint and an oblique head that originates from the bases of the second through fourth metatarsals. The adductor hallucis exerts an adduction force on the MTP joint and resists varus. An appreciation of this delicate tendon balance is mandatory given the recent increase in medial sided turf toe injuries: those rupturing the abductor hallucis tendon and then having an unopposed force from the adductor tendon that may create a progressive hallux valgus deformity.

Biomechanics

Motion through the hallux MTP joint predominantly occurs in the sagittal plane. Numerous investigators have reported on or attempted to quantify this motion in normal subjects, and a review of the literature suggests a total passive allowance of approximately 110 degrees in this plane (75 degrees of dorsiflexion and 35 degrees of plantar flexion) [1, 4, 5, 11, 12]. Active sagittal motion is generally considered to be much less with healthy subjects able to generate about 50–60 degrees of active dorsiflexion and about 20–30 degrees of active plantar flexion. Motion in the transverse plane is quite minimal. Shereff and colleagues found that the hallux MTP joint maximally translates approximately 15% of the diameter of the metatarsal head in the transverse plane during the entire arc of motion in the sagittal plane using fresh-frozen cadaveric specimens [11]. In the same study, the authors determined that motion between the hallux proximal phalanx and metatarsal occurs through tangential sliding from maximal plantar flexion to moderate dorsiflexion. Through construction of surface velocity vectors, they were able to demonstrate compressive motion at the dorsal aspect of the MTP joint in extreme dorsiflexion. This late hyper-dorsiflexion-range compressive force is likely the source of concomitant dorsal articular and periarticular damage sometimes incurred with a turf toe injury.

The position of the hallux MTP joint within the medial forefoot subjects it to substantial stress with normal gait and especially with athletic activity. The first ray disproportionately bears the majority load relative to the remainder of the forefoot during the later stages of forefoot contact and push-off in normal feet. Multiple authors have attempted to quantify load distributions under the foot during normal barefoot walking using strain gauges in force platforms. These works have generated consistent results suggesting that the mean peak resultant force experienced by the hallux MTP joint is roughly equal to that of subject body weight [13–15]. Stokes et al. conducted a similar investigation but reported on the joint reaction force at the hallux MTP joint and estimated it to be about 80% of body weight during normal gait [16].

The implication of sesamoid complex positioning as it relates to hallux push-off strength has also been established in the literature. Aper and colleagues conducted mechanical testing on 12 cadaveric specimens and measured the effects of selective sesamoid resections on the hallux MTP joint moment arm of the FHL tendon [17]. The authors discovered a significant 10% decrease in the FHL tendon effective moment arm when the tibial sesamoid, alone, was excised. When the fibular sesamoid, alone, was excised, there was a 16% decrease, and excisions of both the tibial and fibular sesamoids resulted in a 30% reduction in FHL tendon effective moment arm. Interestingly, no significant change was observed with hemiresection of either sesamoid. This study did not emphasize the resultant "cock-up" deformity of the hallux when both sesamoids are resected, one that leads to further impairment.

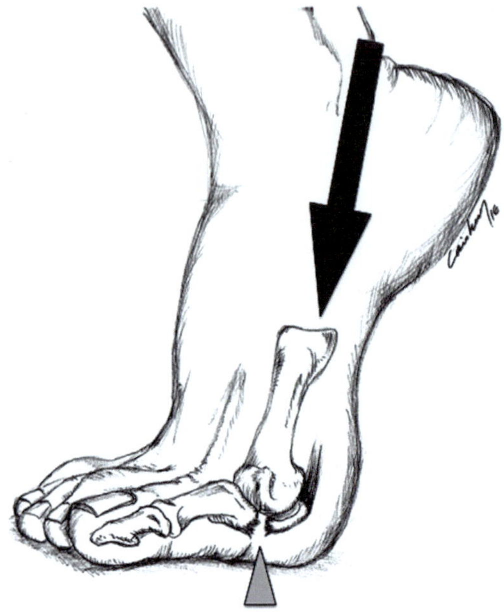

Fig. 22.3 Depiction of the classic turf toe injury mechanism involving an axially directed force onto a hyper dorsiflexed hallux metatarsophalangeal joint with an elevated heel. (*Reprinted from*: Nery C, Baumfeld D, Umans H, Yamada AF. MR imaging of the plantar plate: normal anatomy, turf toe, and other injuries. *Magnetic Resonance Imaging Clinics of North America*. 2017;25:127–144. Copyright (2017), with permission from Elsevier)

Mechanism of Injury and Pathoanatomy

The hallux MTP joint is susceptible to hyper-dorsiflexion injuries especially during athletic participation involving explosive movement patterns and physical contact. This risk can be further compounded by less forgiving, often artificial, playing surfaces and footwear with increased forefoot flexibility. The classic turf toe injury mechanism involves the delivery of an axial load onto a foot that is positioned in equinus with the heel elevated (Fig. 22.3). The axial load drives the hallux MTP joint beyond physiologic range dorsiflexion, and this can lead to a spectrum of tension-related failures to the plantar supporting structures as well as potential compression-type injuries to the dorsal joint surfaces. Prieskorn and colleagues developed a mechanical model to recreate the classic turf toe injury mechanism by applying uniplanar hyper-dorsiflexion loads to the MTP joint of fresh-frozen cadaveric specimens [18]. The specimens were then dissected and injury patterns elucidated. The authors discovered ruptures distal to the sesamoids involving the plantar plate in two specimens, ruptures primarily involving the medial joint capsule and collateral ligaments in another two specimens, and failure of the capsule proximal to the sesamoids in a final specimen. Hyper-dorsiflexion can also lead to tension-related failures of the bone and can be manifested as hallux proximal phalanx or metatarsal neck avulsion fractures, acute sesamoid fractures, or diastasis at the synchondrosis of a bipartite sesamoid [19].

Not all turf toe injuries are uniplanar and the result of pure hyper-dorsiflexion. Other variants have been described and attributed to the relative position of the hallux and the external force vector. The addition of a valgus load component to the dorsiflexed MTP joint, such as during lateral cutting, can lead to disruption of the medial collateral ligaments in combination with varying degrees of plantar medial capsuloligamentous complex deformation. Covell and colleagues referred to this pattern as traumatic hallux valgus and recognized the susceptibility for acute or progressive bunion deformity [20]. This may well be the most common injury pattern in football as an increased incidence has been noted in the past 10 years.

It is important to distinguish injuries sustained predominantly to the dorsal aspect of the hallux MTP joint from lesions with origins involving the plantar structures. These dorsal patterns are not categorized as turf toe injuries as the mechanism of injury involves forced MTP joint plantar flexion and the treatment strategy completely differs. Frey and his colleagues described this distinct dorsal capsuloligamentous sprain pattern in 1996 and coined the term "sand toe" due to the propensity for these injuries to occur in sand volleyball players [21].

Diagnosis and Classification

Athletes presenting with medial forefoot pain must be approached with a high index of suspicion for a turf toe injury, as findings can be subtle and the exam often challenging in the acute setting due to pain intolerance. The athlete may provide a history consistent with the typical mechanism of injury. Begin with an assessment for gait disturbances and ability to bear weight through the injured forefoot. Clinical exam continues with inspection of the hallux for obvious gross deformity, MTP joint swelling, and plantar ecchymosis. Point tenderness can aid in delineating involved areas, and palpation should be performed along the length of the plantar sesamoid complex and medial and lateral collateral ligaments and over the dorsal aspect of the MTP joint. Passive joint motion should be assessed with acknowledgment of abnormalities such as crepitus, mechanical blocks to motion, and hypermobility in dorsiflexion. The MTP drawer test gauges dorsoplantar stability and laxity in this plane suggesting disruption of the plantar capsuloligamentous complex. It is important to evaluate joint stability in the transverse plane as well with varus and valgus stress tests. Instability could indicate a concomitant collateral ligament disruption. Valgus instability or a finding of asymmetric hallux valgus in an athlete with progression of deformity shortly following an injury should prompt consideration of a medial turf toe variant or traumatic hallux valgus. Hallux flexor and extensor tendon integrity should be confirmed with active MTP joint motion against resistance. Importantly, the physical examination is not complete without a systematic comparison to the contralateral uninvolved hallux. A clinical grading classification was first introduced by Clanton et al. in 1986 and later modified to include pathoanatomy and treatment guidelines (Table 22.1) [22]. A **grade 1** injury is considered a plantar plate strain, **grade 2** injuries involve partial tearing, and **grade 3** represents a complete rupture.

A complete radiographic evaluation of the hallux MTP joint is mandatory starting with weight-bearing anteroposterior (AP), lateral, and sesamoid axial views. Direct osseous indicators of a turf toe injury may be detectable including plantar plate avulsion fractures from the plantar base of the proximal phalanx or distal pole of the sesamoids, proximal capsular avulsion fractures from the metatarsal neck, and acute midportion sesamoid fractures. Intra-articular bony flecks could represent osteochondral fragments. Attention should be paid to MTP joint space maintenance and congruity. Malalignment can be observed on both AP and lateral projections. In cases of recurrent injury and chronic instability, a dorsal metatarsal head osteophyte may suggest early hallux rigidus. A dedicated assessment of the sesamoids is paramount. Slight discrepancies in the relative positioning of these osseous structures can indirectly signify an underlying soft tissue lesion. It is preferable to scrutinize sesamoid position with weight-bearing AP views of bilateral feet taken simultaneously on the same cassette [23]. Proximal migration of one or both sesamoids suggests plantar plate rupture (Fig. 22.4). Prieskorn and colleagues established the normal relationship between the hallux MTP joint line and sesamoids in their morphometric

Table 22.1 Turf toe clinical grading classification. *Adapted from:* McCormick JJ, Anderson RB. (Rehabilitation following turf toe injury and plantar plate repair. *Clinics in Sports Medicine.* 2010;29 (2):313–323. Copyright (2010), with permission from Elsevier)

Summary system for turf toe injury grading				
Grade	Clinical findings	Activity level	Pathology	Treatment
1	Localized plantar or medial tenderness Minimal swelling No ecchymosis	Continued athletic participation	Stretching of capsuloligamentous complex	Symptomatic
2	More diffuse and intense tenderness Mild to moderate swelling Mild to moderate ecchymosis Painful and restricted range of motion	Loss of playing time up to 2 weeks	Partial tear of capsuloligamentous complex No articular injury	Walking boot and crutches as needed
3	Severe and diffuse tenderness Marked swelling Moderate to severe ecchymosis Range of motion very painful and limited Hallux flexion weakness Instability of hallux MTP joint	Loss of playing time 6–10 weeks depending on sport and position	Complete disruption of plantar structures	Long-term immobilization in boot or cast *OR* Surgical reconstruction

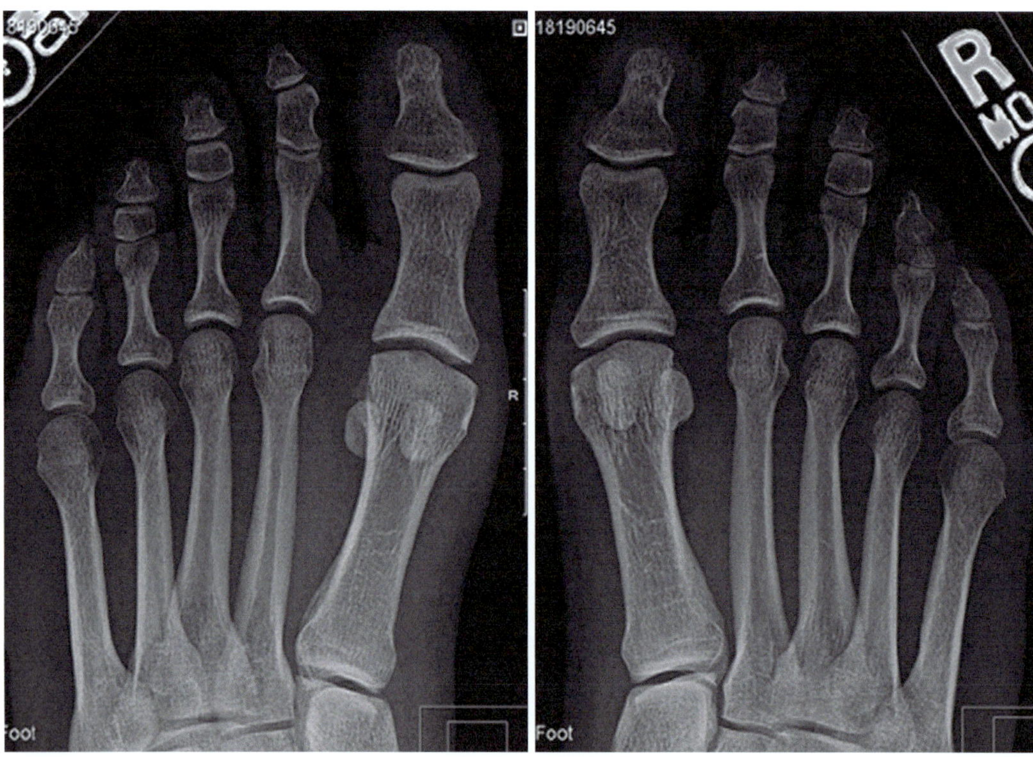

Fig. 22.4 Bilateral weight-bearing AP foot radiographs demonstrating proximal migration of both tibial and fibular sesamoids (left). (*Reprinted from:* McCormick JJ, Anderson RB. Rehabilitation following turf toe injury and plantar plate repair. *Clinics in Sports Medicine.* 2010;29 (2):313–323. Copyright (2010), with permission from Elsevier)

analysis of 100 asymptomatic adult patients and found a 99.7% likelihood of plantar plate disruption when the absolute distance from the distal aspect of the sesamoid to the MTP joint line exceeded 10.4 millimeters (mm) and 13.3 mm for the tibial and fibular sesamoids, respectively [24].

A forced dorsiflexion lateral stress radiograph of the hallux MTP joint can be obtained with detection of decreased distal sesamoid excursion in plantar plate ruptures when compared to the contralateral uninjured side [5, 19]. Joint subluxation can also be identified with this technique. When available, fluoroscopic dynamic dorsiflexion stress assessments have become standard practice in many diagnostic algorithms. Waldrop et al. showed that a 3 mm decrease in distal sesamoid movement on lateral dorsiflexion stress fluoroscopy, relative to the intact state, is highly predictive of severe turf toe injury and disruption to at least three plantar ligaments [25]. Radiographs may also reveal diastasis through bipartite sesamoids representing injury to the fibrocartilagenous synchondrosis (Fig. 22.5).

Magnetic resonance imaging (MRI) is a powerful adjunct and is considered by many to be the gold standard for diagnosing the extent of soft tissue disruption in turf toe injuries. It is highly reproducible with superior specificity compared to ultrasonography and superior soft tissue resolution relative to computed tomography (CT) [9]. MRI is typically recommended with grade 2 or 3 findings on clinical exam (Table 22.1) and in any patient with radiographic or fluoroscopic abnormalities. Normally, the plantar plate appears as a dense low-signal band connecting the sesamoids to the plantar base of the proximal phalanx. Fluid-sensitive sequences detect edema patterns and can signify strains or partial tears in this tissue. Discontinuity of the plantar plate low-signal band with a fluid gap likely indicates a complete rupture (Fig. 22.6). The integrity of the MTP joint and metatarsal-sesamoid joint chondral surfaces can also be assessed with unequaled detail on MRI.

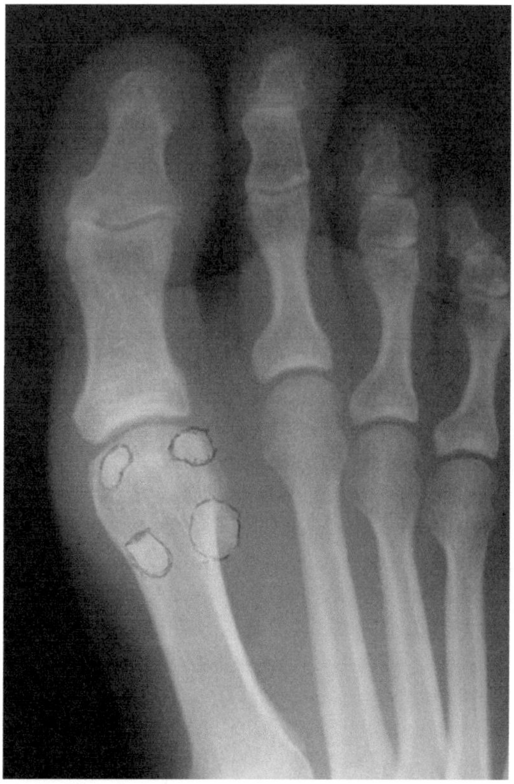

Fig. 22.5 Standing AP radiograph demonstrating diastasis of both the tibial and fibular sesamoids indicating failure of the plantar sesamoid apparatus through bipartite synchondroses

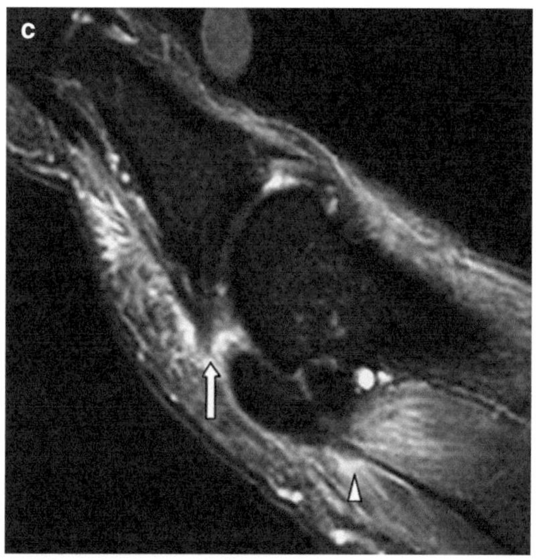

Fig. 22.6 Sagittal short tau inversion recovery (STIR) MRI illustrating a complete rupture of the plantar plate (tibial phalangeosesamoid ligament) with proximal migration of the tibial sesamoid. Edema within the medial head of the FHB tendon is also depicted. (*Adapted from:* Crain JM, Phancao JP, Stidham K. MR imaging of turf toe. *Magnetic Resonance Imaging Clinics of North America.* 2008;16:93–103. Copyright (2008), with permission from Elsevier)

Management/Rehabilitation

After the diagnosis of a turf toe injury is made, the initial management is generally conservative, regardless of clinical severity. Many patterns of hallux plantar capsuloligamentous trauma are amenable to entirely nonsurgical care. In a large epidemiological study using the NCAA ISS, George et al. found that only 1.74% of collegiate-level football players who sustained a turf toe injury ultimately required operative intervention [7]. Indications for surgical repair (Table 22.2) have been established by McCormick and Anderson based upon considerable personal experience with the treatment of these injuries [26]. These include findings of gross MTP joint instability, sesamoid displacement, intra-articular loose bodies, and failure of conservative management. These indications have been generally accepted but have not been the subject of rigorous scientific inquiry. Much of our knowledge regarding the treatment of these injuries is based on small case series and case reports.

Nonoperative

The conservative treatment of an athlete with a turf toe injury progresses through three basic phases much like the management of most other musculoskeletal conditions. Variations in the rate of progression through each phase are typically predicted by the initial clinical grade of the injury with more guarded expectations established in the highest severity athletes. The early phase is one of protection with implementation of rest, ice, compression, and elevation principles. The goal is to prevent a repetitive insult to the MTP joint and supporting structures and to combat inflammation. Protection can be accomplished with a stiff-soled shoe, walking boot, or even a short leg cast with a toe spica extension promoting hallux MTP joint plantar flexion. For example, a diastasis of both the tibial and fibular sesamoids poses a unique treatment challenge. In this instance, the application of a toe spica apparatus maintaining plantar flexion has anecdotally achieved apposition of the fragments and scar stabilization over a period of 6–8 weeks.

With immobilization, a period of non-weight bearing or partial weight bearing may be necessary based on symptoms. Physiologic forefoot push-off and dorsiflexion through the joint should be avoided. Nonsteroidal anti-inflammatory medications are recommended. Local anesthetics and corticosteroid injections are contraindicated in the acute setting and are especially discouraged in an effort to keep an athlete on the playing field, as masking the symptoms can lead to cumulative irreparable joint damage.

The second phase of care involves reintroducing hallux MTP joint range of motion. This phase is critical to minimizing arthrofibrosis. Athletes with **grade 1** plantar attenuations may be appropriate to advance to this phase within the first several days following injury, whereas **grade 2** and **3** tears may be delayed multiple days to multiple weeks, respectively. Passive motion should be initiated first in plantar flexion followed by gentle dorsiflexion as symptoms permit. It is not advised to test dorsiflexion limits prematurely as stressing the traumatized plantar capsuloligamentous structures can impede healing. For global conditioning purposes, low-impact activities such as bicycling, elliptical training, and pool therapy should be initiated during this phase with the hallux protected from dorsiflexion using footwear modifications. These include plated turf toe shoes and custom Morton extension orthotic devices. Even when not actively rehabilitating

Table 22.2 Surgical indications for turf toe injury. (*Adapted from:* McCormick JJ, Anderson RB. The great toe: failed turf toe, chronic turf toe, and complicated sesamoid injuries. *Foot and Ankle Clinics of North America*. 2009;14:135–150. Copyright (2009), with permission from Elsevier)

Indications for surgical reconstruction of turf toe injury
1. Large capsular avulsion with unstable MTP joint
2. Diastasis of bipartite sesamoid
3. Diastasis of sesamoid fracture
4. Proximal retraction of one or both sesamoids
5. Traumatic hallux valgus deformity
6. Vertical MTP joint instability
7. Loose intra-articular body
8. Chondral injury
9. Failure of conservative management

under the discretion of a therapist, the athlete should continue to protect with these same devices for day-to-day activities. The athlete should not participate in any higher-level activities until low-impact exercise is tolerated without pain or limitation.

The final phase of treatment features functional training and position-specific rehabilitation activities and, ultimately, return to sport. Running, cutting, and more explosive drills can be incorporated only if tolerated without discomfort. It has been suggested that 50–60 degrees of painless passive hallux MTP joint dorsiflexion be achieved prior to advancing to this phase [27]. The hallux MTP joint should continue to be protected, and, as a general rule, the athlete can be counseled that protective footwear will likely be necessary for 6 months from the time of injury, even after unrestricted release to play. Compliance with these recommendations can be challenging in the athlete who perceives these modifications as potentially restrictive to athletic performance. The ability to reach pre-injury level of functioning dictates return to play, and this will be heavily influenced by player position. In football, for example, a skill position athlete such as a defensive back can be expected to advance slower through this functional progression due to the forefoot demands associated with specialized movements such as backpedaling. The overall recovery process or loss of playing time for grade 2 partial tears ranges from a few days to 2 weeks, while complete grade 3 ruptures can require up to 3 or 4 months of rehabilitation. Time lost to injury tends to be minimal with **grade 1** sprains.

Operative

Acute turf toe reconstruction is generally reserved for the most severe turf toe injuries presenting with obvious gross hallux MTP joint instability and proximal sesamoid migration, which are findings inherent to many of the accepted surgical indications previously referenced. Occasionally, delayed reconstruction is pursued for cases that prove recalcitrant to conservative management efforts. The primary surgical objective is to reconstruct the failed portion of the plantar apparatus and reestablish MTP joint stability. The surgical management of intra-articular pathology will sometimes be necessary and may involve retrieval of loose bodies or stabilization of concomitant chondral defects. The highest-grade injury patterns command the full complement of diagnostic imaging, and this serves to guide surgical planning.

The plantar hallux is classically approached plantarmedially with a longitudinal incision or a "J-shaped" incision with a transverse plantar limb projecting from medial to lateral across the MTP joint flexion crease. The longitudinal portion of this incision is typically performed in line with the abductor hallucis tendon. If needed, a capsulotomy can be made dorsal to this tendon insertion to gain intra-articular visualization of the plantar structures and MTP joint. When approached medially, care must be taken to identify and protect the plantarmedial cutaneous nerve to the hallux that courses adjacent to the tibial sesamoid. An accessory plantar lateral approach can be made for improved access to the lateral MTP joint and fibular sesamoid, if needed. The common plantar digital nerve and its proper digital branch to the lateral hallux should be visualized and protected with this approach. With the more common medial-based injury pattern, a single medial approach is sufficient.

In an acute setting, the plantar defect is usually readily identifiable, and the tissue ends will mobilize. In operative scenarios, it is most common for the capsuloligamentous complex to rupture distal to the sesamoids through the plantar plate. When adequate proximal and distal stumps of tissue are available, a direct end-to-end primary repair with non-absorbable suture can be completed [28]. If the injury to the plantar plate is very distal and the remnant attached to the proximal phalanx base is inadequate for primary repair, then suture anchors can be utilized to ensure fixation (Fig. 22.7) [26]. Alternatively, horizontal mattress sutures can be passed from plantar to dorsal through the proximal stump of plantar plate tissue and guided through drill tunnels out the dorsum of the proximal phalanx and tensioned over bone bridges [29]. When there is a

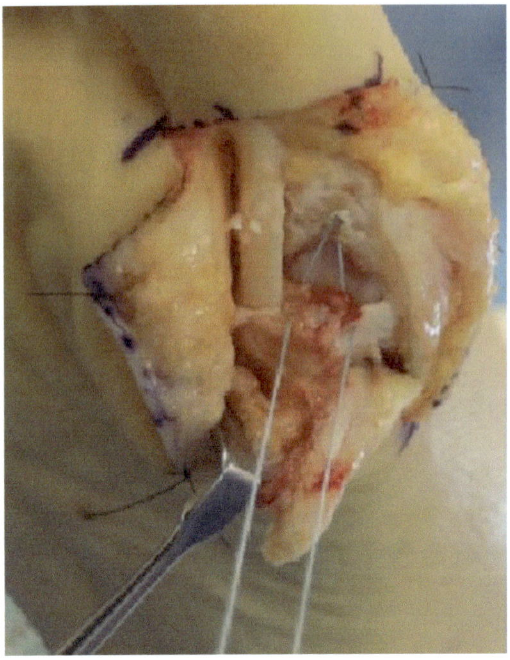

Fig. 22.7 Intraoperative photograph demonstrating the "J-shaped" plantarmedial surgical approach to the hallux MTP joint. Suture anchor fixation of ruptured medial plantar plate directly to base of proximal phalanx. (*Adapted from:* Nery C, Fonseca LF, Goncalves JP, Mansur N, Lemos A, Maringolo L, Fonseca LF. First MTP joint instability - Expanding the concept of "Turf-toe" injuries. *Foot & Ankle Surgery*. 2020;26 (1):47–53. Copyright (2020), with permission from Elsevier)

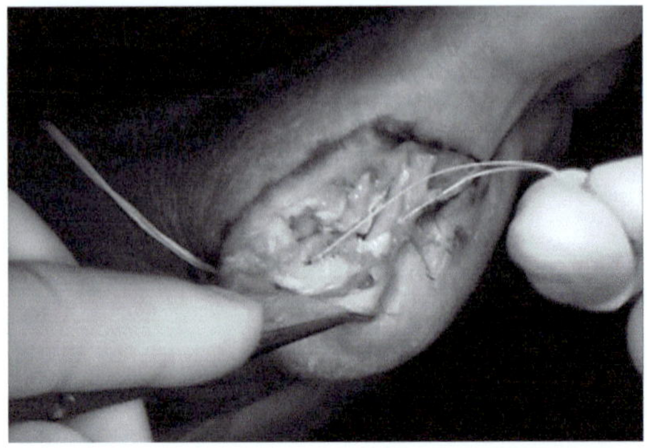

Fig. 22.8 Intraoperative photograph demonstrating a transverse drill hole with suture passed through the tibial sesamoid. This technique can be utilized to advance the sesamoid distally toward the plantar plate in the setting of complete soft tissue avulsion from the distal pole of the sesamoid

soft tissue avulsion off the tibial sesamoid, a drill hole can be placed into the sesamoid to help it advance distally to the base of the phalanx (Fig. 22.8).

In cases of complete rupture, it is recommended to repair the plantar plate from lateral to medial. Both sesamoids will typically be retracted in this situation. In chronic settings, this retraction can be difficult to overcome due to fibrosis. Reapproximation of the plantar plate may not be possible without additional excursion provided through fasciotomies or fractional lengthenings of the FHB and abductor hallucis proximal to the sesamoids [27]. Plantar flexion of the hallux MTP joint will aid in tissue reapproximation and should always be performed with final tensioning of the repair, generally 10–15 degrees.

Failure of the hallux MTP joint plantar complex through the sesamoids, by way of fracture or bipartite diastasis, presents a unique set of surgical challenges. Open and percutaneous sesamoid fixation methods have been described, but these techniques require simple fracture patterns with good proximal and distal bone stock. If the sesamoid disruption leaves small pole fragments or there is significant comminution or degenerative changes, excision of part or all of the sesamoid is the recommended surgical strategy. Ideally, the smaller pole can be excised with preservation of its capsuloligamentous envelope. Soft tissue repair of this tissue to the preserved larger pole can then be facilitated through drill tunnels. Occasionally, a complete tibial sesamoidectomy will be required, and an abductor hallucis tendon transfer can be employed to close the plantar soft tissue defect and reconstitute the plantarmedial restraint [27].

Medial turf toe variants with hallux valgus deformity warrant additional transverse plane soft tissue stabilization. These injuries are associated with disruption of medial joint capsule, ligaments, and even tendon attachments. Covell and Anderson published on their preferred surgical technique for this specific injury pattern in a case series of elite-level football players [20]. In addition to reconstruction of the plantar structures as previously described, the authors advise adding a modified McBride bunionectomy. This consists of a medial metatarsal head eminence resection, a medial capsular reefing, and a separate first dorsal webspace approach for an adductor hallucis tenotomy. Together, these additional procedures balance the deforming forces in the transverse plane and resist progressive hallux valgus.

Postoperative Rehabilitation

Multiple, comprehensive postoperative rehabilitation protocols for turf toe reconstruction have been developed and presented in the literature [30, 31]. These protocols generally parallel the phases of nonoperative management with longer intervals and a greater emphasis on early protection of the surgical repair. Rigid immobilization of the hallux MTP joint in slight plantar flexion (5–10 degrees) is typically employed for the first 7–10 days following surgery utilizing a toe spica cast or splint. At the first postoperative visit, this can be exchanged for a controlled ankle motion (CAM) boot, but the athlete should expect to be non-weight bearing with crutches for a period of 4 weeks. After that, a gradual return to full weight bearing is allowed within the confines of the walking boot. In medial turf toe variant injury patterns, a toe spacer or bunion splint can be utilized between the hallux and second toe to combat valgus drift and to take tension off the medial capsular repair. Gentle passive motion in plantar flexion should be initiated early in the postoperative course always under the supervision of an athletic trainer or physical therapist. Passive dorsiflexion past neutral and active plantar flexion should be avoided for at least the first 4–6 weeks postoperatively. At around 8 weeks, athletes can be transitioned out of the walking boot and into accommodative stiff-soled footwear with protective taping techniques. Passive range of motion exercises continue during this phase with limitations dictated only by symptoms. Active and active-assisted exercises are advanced, and, if tolerated, the athlete is gradually re-introduced to low-impact activities. The 8–12-week period should feature a straight-line running program with incorporation of some agility and plyometric training as symptoms allow. Many athletes are appropriate to begin more explosive sport-specific exercises including contact drills around 4 months out from surgery. The establishment of realistic recovery expectations is paramount, and athletes must anticipate at least 6 months and sometimes an entire year before achieving full recovery.

References

1. Bowers KD, Martin BR. Turf-toe: a shoe-surface related football injury. Med Sci Sports. 1976;8(2):81–3.
2. Ryan AJ, McColl W, Behling F, Garrick JG. Artificial turf: pros and cons. Phys Sportsmed. 1975;2:41–50. https://doi.org/10.1080/00913847.1975.11948143.
3. Coker TP, Arnold JA, Weber DL. Traumatic lesions of the metatarsophalangeal joint of the great toe in athletes. Am J Sports Med. 1978;6(6):326–34. https://doi.org/10.1177/036354657800600604.
4. Clanton TO, Butler JE, Eggert A. Injuries to the metatarsophalangeal joints in athletes. Foot Ankle. 1986;7(3):162–76. https://doi.org/10.1177/107110078600700306.
5. Rodeo SA, O'Brien S, Warren RF, Barnes R, Wickiewicz TL, Dillingham MF. Turf-toe: an analysis of metatarsophalangeal joint sprains in professional football players. Am J Sports Med. 1990;18(3):280–5. https://doi.org/10.1177/036354659001800311.
6. Kaplan LD, Jost PW, Honkamp N, Norwig J, West R, Bradley JP. Incidence and variance of foot and ankle injuries in elite college football players. Am J Orthop. 2011;40(1):40–4.
7. George E, Harris AHS, Dragoo JL, Hunt KJ. Incidence and risk factors for turf toe injuries in intercollegiate football. Foot Ankle Int. 2014;35(2):108–15. https://doi.org/10.1177/1071100713514038.
8. Schein AJ, Skalski MR, Patel DB, White EA, Lundquist R, Gottsegen CJ, Forrester DM, Matcuk GR. Turf toe and sesamoiditis: what the radiologist needs to know. Clin Imaging. 2015;39:380–9. https://doi.org/10.1016/j.clinimag.2014.11.011.
9. Nery C, Baumfeld D, Umans H, Yamada AF. MR imaging of the plantar plate: normal anatomy, turf toe, and other injuries. Magn Reson Imaging Clin N Am. 2017;25:127–44. https://doi.org/10.1016/j.mric.2016.08.007.
10. Clanton TO, Ford JJ. Turf toe injury. Clin Sports Med. 1994;13(4):731–41.
11. Shereff MJ, Bejjani FJ, Kummer FJ. Kinematics of the first metatarsophalangeal joint. J Bone Joint Surg. 1986;68(3):392.
12. Frimenko RE, Lievers B, Coughlin MJ, Anderson RB, Crandall JR, Kent RW. Etiology and biomechanics of first metatarsophalangeal joint sprains (turf toe) in athletes. Crit Rev Biomed Eng. 2012;40(1):43–61.

https://doi.org/10.1615/CritRevBiomedEng.v40.i1.30.
13. McBride ID, Wyss UP, Cooke T, Chir B, Murphy L, Phillips J, Olney S. First metatarsophalangeal joint reaction forces during high-heel gait. Foot Ankle. 1991;11(5):282–8. https://doi.org/10.1177/107110079101100505.
14. Hutton WC, Dhanendran M. The mechanics of Normal and hallux valgus feet—a quantitative study. Clin Orthop Relat Res. 1981;157:7–13.
15. Hetherington VJ, Chessman GW, Steuben C. Forces on the first metatarsophalangeal joint: a pilot study. J Foot Surg. 1992;31(5):450–3.
16. Stokes IA, Hutton WC, Stott JR. Forces acting on the metatarsals during normal walking. J Anat. 1979;129(3):579–90.
17. Aper RL, Saltzman CL, Brown TD. The effect of hallux sesamoid excision on the flexor hallucis longus moment arm. Clin Orthop Relat Res. 1996;325:209–17.
18. Prieskorn D, Graves S, Yen M, Ray J, Schultz R. Integrity of the first metatarsophalangeal joint: a biomechanical analysis. Foot Ankle Int. 1995;16(6):357–62. https://doi.org/10.1177/107110079501600608.
19. Rodeo SA, Warren RF, O'Brien SJ, Foot HP. 1993. Diastasis of bipartite sesamoids of the first metatarsophalangeal joint. Foot Ankle Int. 1993;14(8):425–34. https://doi.org/10.1177/107110079301400801.
20. Covell DJ, Lareau CR, Anderson RB. Operative treatment of traumatic hallux valgus in elite athletes. Foot Ankle Int. 2017;38(6):590–5. https://doi.org/10.1177/1071100717697961.
21. Frey C, Andersen GD, Feder KS. Plantarflexion injury to the metatarsophalangeal joint ("sand toe"). Foot Ankle Int. 1996;17(9):576–81. https://doi.org/10.1177/107110079601700914.
22. McCormick JJ, Anderson RB. Rehabilitation following turf toe injury and plantar plate repair. Clin Sports Med. 2010;29(2):313–23. https://doi.org/10.1016/j.csm.2009.12.010.
23. Graves SC, Prieskorn D, Mann RA. Posttraumatic proximal migration of the first metatarsophalangeal joint sesamoids: a report of four cases. Foot Ankle. 1991;12(2):117–22. https://doi.org/10.1177/107110079101200210.
24. Prieskorn D, Graves SC, Smith RA. Morphometric analysis of the plantar plate apparatus of the first metatarsophalangeal joint. Foot Ankle. 1993;14(4):204–7. https://doi.org/10.1177/107110079301400405.
25. Waldrop NE III, Zirker CA, Wijdicks CA, LaPrade RF, Clanton TO. Radiographic evaluation of plantar plate injury: an in vitro biomechanical study. Foot Ankle Int. 2013;34(3):403–8. https://doi.org/10.1177/1071100712464953.
26. McCormick JJ, Anderson RB. The great toe: failed turf toe, chronic turf toe, and complicated sesamoid injuries. Foot Ankle Clin. 2009;14:135–50. https://doi.org/10.1016/j.fcl.2009.01.001.
27. Anderson RB. Turf toe injuries of the hallux metatarsophalangeal joint. Techn Foot Ankle Surg. 2002;1(2):102–11.
28. McCormick JJ, Anderson RB. Turf toe: anatomy, diagnosis, and treatment. Sports Health. 2010;2(6):487–94. https://doi.org/10.1177/1941738110386681.
29. Doty JF, Coughlin MJ. Turf toe repair: a technical note. Foot Ankle Spec. 2013;6(6):452–6. https://doi.org/10.1177/1938640013507107.
30. Faltus J, Mullenix K, Moorman CT III, Beatty K, Easley ME. Case series of first metatarsophalangeal joint injuries in division 1 college athletes. Sports Health. 2014;6(6):519–26. https://doi.org/10.1177/1941738114527546.
31. Drakos MC, Fiore R, Murphy C. DiGiovanni CW. Plantar-Plate Disruptions: "The Severe Turf-Toe Injury." Three Cases in Contact Athletes. J Athl Train. 2015;50(5):553–60. https://doi.org/10.4085/1062-6050-49.6.05.

23 Lesser Toe Plantar Plate Injuries and Angular Deformities: Indications, Techniques, and Outcomes

James R. Jastifer, Christopher Traynor, and Homer Stryker

Lesser Toe Plantar Plate Tears

Introduction

Lesser toe MTP joint instability is a common clinical problem encountered by the practicing foot and ankle surgeon. Coughlin in 1987 first described the term "second crossover toe" to characterize the clinical deformity of the second toe with dorsiflexion at the MTP joint and medially directed crossing over the great toe [1]. However, early in the disease process, the second toe does not always cross over. Swelling at the MTP joint with associated pain or subtle deviations through the joint may be indicative of MTP instability. Although the second toe is most commonly involved, it is known that the pathology may exist in any of the other lesser toes. Multifactorial causes have linked to both acute and chronic cases of MTP joint instability. Clinical and surgical staging systems have recently been developed to help guide treatment.

J. R. Jastifer (✉)
Ascension Borgess Orthopaedics, Kalamazoo, MI, USA

School of Medicine, Department of Orthopaedic Surgery, Western Michigan University, Kalamazoo, MI, USA
e-mail: jrjast@gmail.com

C. Traynor · H. Stryker
School of Medicine, Department of Orthopaedic Surgery, Western Michigan University, Kalamazoo, MI, USA
e-mail: Christopher.traynor@med.wmich.edu

Pathophysiology and Anatomy

The plantar plate plays a pivotal role in the stabilization of the lesser toe MTP joint. The stout plantar plate originates on the metatarsal head, just proximal to the articular surface, and inserts plantarly at the base of proximal phalanx [2–4]. It functions to dampen forces the MTP joint experiences during weight bearing and provide tensile strength in the sagittal plane. The key to its function as a stabilizer is likely to its central and plantar location and multiple attachments. There has been a clear link between attenuation of the plantar plate and subsequent instability of the MTP joint [5–9]. Pathology of the plantar plate is typically noted near its insertion at the proximal phalanx.

The plantar plate, along with the intrinsic musculature including the lumbricals and interossei, provides a stabilizing resistance against the dorsiflexion experienced at the MTP joint during the terminal stance phase of gait. Without plantar plate stabilization, the proximal phalanx will begin to sublux dorsally. Furthermore, it is felt that this deformity places the interossei dorsal to the axis of rotation, prohibiting their ability to plantarflex at the MTP joint. The lumbricals act to medially deviate the toe as it is tethered by the deep metatarsal ligament creating an adduction force.

MTP joint instability has been linked to several causes including acute trauma, chronic inflammation, hallux valgus, hallux varus, pes planus, hal-

P. D'Hooghe et al. (eds.), *Ligamentous Injuries of the Foot and Ankle*,
https://doi.org/10.1007/978-3-031-08682-3_23

lux rigidus, interdigital neuromas, and hammertoe deformities. In athletes, Coughlin reported 100% of the patients to have an elongated second metatarsal in relation to adjoining metatarsals [9]. Instability at the MTP joint can be seen following an acute injury but more commonly is noted insidiously, most likely from chronic attenuation of the plantar plate. Plantar plate pathology most commonly affects the second MTP joint but can affect other lesser toes as well [10].

History and Exam

On history and exam, MTP instability can be hard to differentiate from other forefoot pathologies. Typically, patients will complain of pain at the base of the involved proximal phalanx. Commonly, patients may also complain of neuroma pain or pain within the metatarsal interspaces. Sagittal and coronal plane deformity usually presents over time following capsuloligamentous attenuation and altered biomechanical forces. Initially, there is medial deviation of the affected toe, and oftentimes in the later stage of the disease process, a hyperextension deformity occurs [9–12].

The drawer test is the classic physical exam finding that is pathognomonic for MTP joint instability (Fig. 23.1). The examiner performs this test by grasping the proximal phalanx of the involved digit and applying a vertical stress in a dorsal direction. A positive test will reproduce the patient's discomfort. Additionally, the exam-

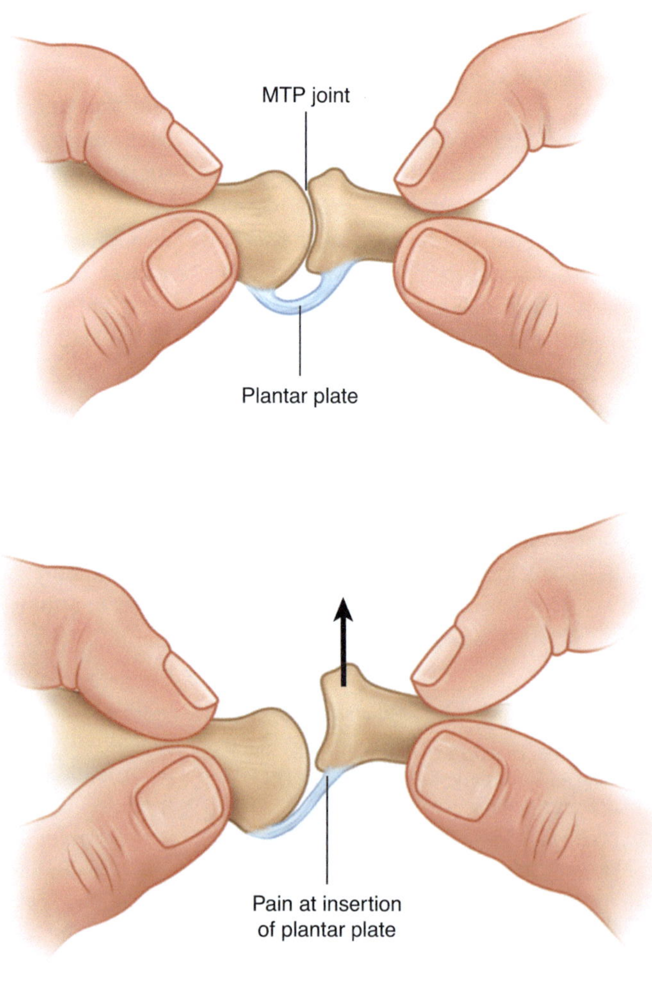

Fig. 23.1 Anatomic drawing of dorsal drawer test for MTP joint instability

iner may feel MTP joint subluxation or dislocation. Other exam findings include weakness with toe grip or a lack of toe purchase on the ground from decreased plantar flexion strength of the affected digit [10–12].

Imaging

Radiographic evaluation involves routine anterior-posterior (AP) and lateral radiographs. Common radiographic signs in MTP joint instability include widening of the joint space or malalignment in relationship to the adjoining MTP joints including medial deviation of the affected toe and splaying of the digits [11, 12]. MRI has also been shown to be reliable in the diagnosis plantar plate tears [10].

Classification

Two staging systems are available to help guide the treatment of plantar plate tears. First, a clinical staging system can be useful based on physical exam and which incorporates many of the principles of previously developed rating systems [4, 10, 13–16] (Table 23.1). Second, an anatomic grading system has been developed based on dissection of cadaveric specimens noted to have plantar plate tears and crossover second toes (Table 23.2). These systems address plantar plate dysfunction and can be helpful in quantifying the magnitude of the deformity and the preoperative planning for surgical repair of the specific type of tear.

Table 23.1 Clinical staging for plantar plate tears [4, 10, 13–16]

Grade	Alignment	Physical examination
0	No MTP joint malalignment; prodromal phase with pain but no deformity	MTP joint pain, thickening or swelling of the MTP joint, diminished toe purchase, negative drawer
1	Mild malalignment of MTP joint; widening of the webspace; medial deviation	MTP joint pain, swelling of MTP joint, reduced toe purchase, mildly positive drawer (<50% subluxable)
2	Moderate malalignment; medial, lateral, dorsal, or dorsomedial deformity; hyperextension of the MTP joint	MTP joint pain, reduced swelling, no toe purchase, moderately positive drawer (>50% subluxable)
3	Severe malalignment; dorsal or dorsomedial deformity; the second toe can overlap the hallux; may have flexible hammertoe	Joint and toe pain, little swelling, no toe purchase (dislocatable MTP joint), flexible hammertoe

Table 23.2 Surgical grading of plantar plate tears [4, 10, 13–16]

Grade	Patterns of tears
0	Plantar plate or capsular attenuation and/or discoloration
1	Transverse distal tear adjacent to insertion into proximal phalanx (<50%)
2	Transverse distal tear adjacent to insertion into proximal phalanx (>50%)
3	Transverse and/or longitudinal extensive tear. Frequently a distal transverse tear present also
4	Extensive tear with dislocation; inadequate residual tissue to repair

Treatment

Nonsurgical treatment is often the first line of treatment for management of lesser toe MTP joint instability. Conservative treatment may help symptomatically painful toes but often fail to alter progression or the associated deformities. There are a number of nonsurgical treatment options available. Shoe-wear modifications with a wide toe box may decrease pressures on the affected digit. A rigid graphite insert will limit hyperextension at the MTP joint during terminal stance phase and may lessen stress. Soft inserts have been described as well, helping to pad the plantar aspect of the metatarsal head and redistribute pressures [17, 18]. To improve sagittal plane stability, taping has been described. However, as noted by Coughlin, this may only work to decrease symptoms and prevent progression but will not correct an underlying deformity [1]. Lastly, NSAIDs and intraarticular corticosteroid injections have been utilized to systemically and locally reduce inflammation and diminish symptoms but, again, fail to correct malalignment or alter disease progression [18, 19].

Several surgical options are available for those that fail non-operative measures. For those with synovitis and a mild deformity, surgical treatment can consist of capsular reefing and synovectomy alone. If the deformity is more severe, a flexor tendon transfer can be added as well. A metatarsal shortening (e.g., Weil) osteotomy may be included for patients with severe painful instability and a long metatarsal. Additionally, a direct plantar plate repair is a surgical option [1, 7, 10, 16].

Plantar Plate Repair [2, 10] (Fig. 23.2)

- The patient is placed supine on the operating room table. An Esmarch bandage can be used to exsanguinate the limb and may be used as a tourniquet as well.
- A skin incision is made approximately 3 cm in length. This can either be straight dorsally over the MTP joint or in the adjacent webspace depending on the need for concomitant procedures.
- The extensor tendons are retracted medially or elongated via z-plasty. An MTP joint arthrotomy is made, and the collateral ligaments are released off the proximal phalanx.
- A metatarsal shortening osteotomy is utilized if a shortening procedure is indicated. The metatarsal head is translated approximately 8 mm and pinned in place utilizing a k-wire.
- Utilizing a second k-wire midline in the proximal phalanx, a distractor is used to better expose the plantar aspect of the MTP joint.
- The plantar plate is inspected and lesion type defined.

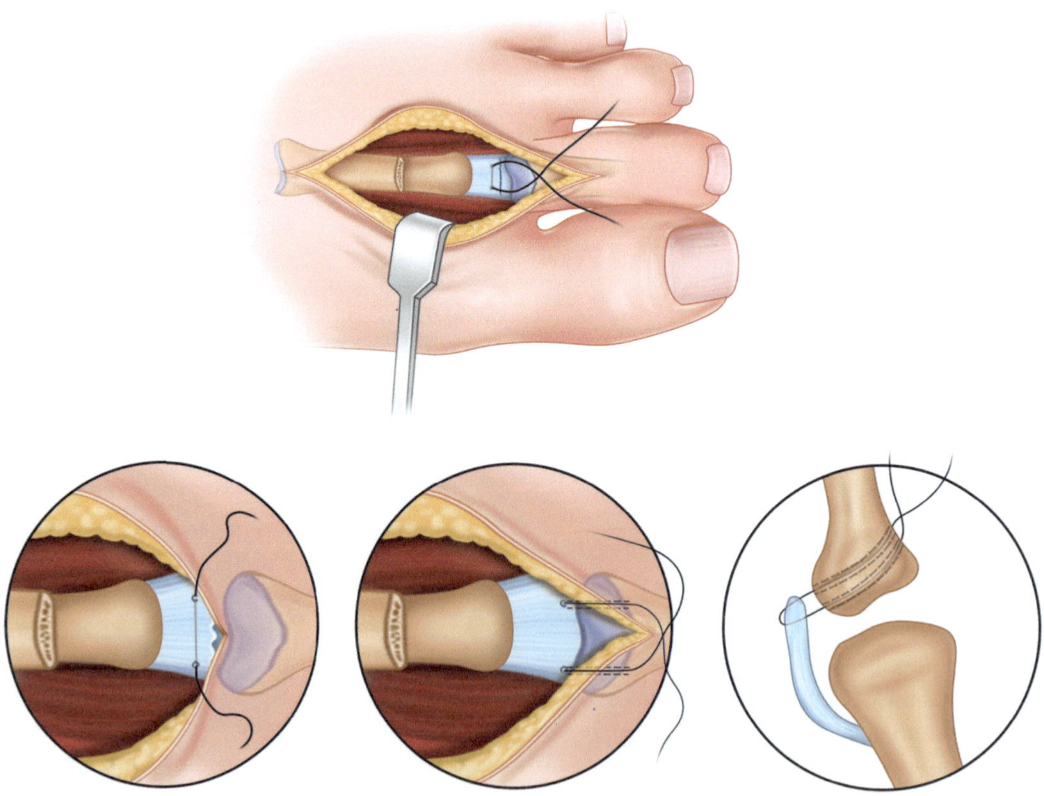

Fig. 23.2 Anatomic drawing of plantar plate repair. Suture is passed through the plantar plate and the proximal phalanx from plantar to dorsal

- The plantar plate tear is captured utilizing a small, non-absorbable suture. Longitudinal split tears were secured utilizing horizontal sutures. A mechanical suture passer can be useful for purely transverse tears.
- Once the plantar plate is captured, two small vertical drill holes are created in the proximal phalanx, medially and laterally. A small k-wire (i.e., 1.5 mm) works well for this.
- A suture passer is used to pass the sutures from plantar to dorsal.
- The sutures are then tied over the dorsal phalangeal cortex, making sure to hold the digit in approximately 20–30 degrees of plantar flexion.
- The metatarsal shortening osteotomy is secured in place utilizing a vertical screw.
- If a sagittal plane deformity still persists, capsular reefing is undertaken on the convex side of the deformity.
- A standard closure is then performed.
- Limited heel weight bearing is initiated immediately post-surgically with full weight bearing beginning 6 weeks after surgery.

Outcomes

The most frequently reported surgical techniques included MTP joint synovectomy, capsular soft tissue release with reefing, extensor and flexor tendon transfers, and phalangeal and metatarsal osteotomies [9, 11, 16, 19, 20]. These techniques, although frequently performed, demonstrate mixed results [1, 16, 19, 20]. Twenty-four out of 30 patients were completely satisfied with flexor-to-extensor and extensor brevis tendon transfers utilized in the series by Haddad et al. [16]. Trnka et al. described 15 toes treated with a metatarsal shortening (e.g., Weil) osteotomy and noted all subluxated or dislocated MTP joints were successfully reduced and demonstrated satisfactory AOFAS scores [20]. Coughlin was able to demonstrate good to excellent results in 93% of cases utilizing the previously mentioned techniques [1]. However, more recent results may indicate that outcomes from classical operative treatments appear little better when compared to non-operative treatments [19].

Techniques that involve direct repair of plantar plate tears have recently emerged as viable surgical options for treatment of MTP joint instability. Cadaveric studies have obtained MTP joint stability with direct plantar plate repair in a comparable fashion to flexor tendon transfers. Both dorsal and plantar incisions have been described as ways to approach the plantar plate. Plantar incisions intuitively make sense; however, advocates for dorsally based incisions argue that it may be difficult to expose multiple MTP joints and place patients at risk for uncomfortable plantar scars. Cooper and Coughlin were able to demonstrate sufficient MTP joint exposure while combining a dorsal approach with a metatarsal shortening osteotomy [2]. Clinically, this technique has been shown to provide satisfactory pain relief and overall good relief [10]. At least one study with 1-year follow-up demonstrated 80% good to excellent results utilizing a dorsal approach to the repair [21].

Continued pain and discomfort, recurrent deformity, limited range of motion, and transfer metatarsalgia have all been described as complications following treatment of MTP joint instability [17].

Toe Deformities

Introduction

Lesser toe deformities are a common foot problem. There is a wide array of pathologies associated with, and classified as, lesser toe deformities. They can be static or dynamic. The most common nomenclature utilized are hammertoes, claw toes, and mallet toes. Hammertoes are defined as a flexion contracture at the PIP joint. Oftentimes they are associated with dorsiflexion at the MTP joint and DIP joint dorsiflexion. Claw toe deformities are characterized as PIP and DIP flexion contractures with MTP hyperextension. Flexion deformity at the DIP joint describes a mallet toe deformity [17, 22, 23]. Causes of lesser toe deformities are multifactorial but can include ill-fitting shoe wear, trauma, genetics, inflammatory arthropathies, and neuromuscular diseases [22–24].

Anatomy

To understand the deformities of the lesser toes, it is important to appreciate the underlying anatomy and normal interplay of forces acting on the toes. With each lesser ray, there are a metatarsal bone and three phalanges creating the metatarsal phalangeal joints, proximal interphalangeal joints, and distal interphalangeal joints. These joints have minimal inherent bony stability and are stabilized primarily by the collateral ligaments, the plantar plate, the joint capsule, and the interplay between the extensor and flexor tendons of the toe [22]. The extensor and flexor musculature are comprised of the extensor digitorum longus (EDL), extensor digitorum brevis (EDB), flexor digitorum longus (FDL), and flexor digitorum brevis (FDB) which act to extend the MTP joint and flex the PIP and DIP joints. The interossei muscles will flex and stabilize the MTP joint as well. Lastly the lumbricals will act to plantarflex at the MTP join and while extending the PIP and DIP joints [25]. Complex neuromuscular control of these muscles creates "normal" toe alignment, and an imbalance in these forces contributes to deformity.

Hammertoes

Hammertoe deformities can be fixed or flexible. Commonly a callus or skin irritation may be noted overlying the dorsal aspect of the PIP joint causing the patient discomfort [17, 22]. On exam, it is important to assess the rigidity of the deformity as well the presence of deformities on other toes.

Nonsurgical treatment of hammertoes consists of symptomatic management. Shoe modifications with wide and/or high shoe boxes will decrease pressure on the dorsum of the PIP joint. Padding of the painful areas may help redistribute pressure. Occasionally, shaving of the painful callosity may remove keratotic buildup. Lastly, toe splints can be used to help reduce the PIP joint and stabilize the MTP joint [17, 22].

Surgical treatment of hammertoes depends on the flexibility of the deformity. Flexible deformities can be corrected with FDL tendon transfers. Fixed deformities typically require bony treatment in the form of PIP resection arthroplasty or fusion. Additionally, it is important to consider concurrent forefoot deformities. In the setting of hallux valgus, the deformity of the first ray must be accounted for in order to prevent recurrence. Amputations have been described in this setting for patients unwilling to undergo reconstruction [22, 24, 26].

Outcomes for hammertoe correction have generally been positive. Boyer et al. reported with flexor-to-extensor tendon transfer 89% of patients were satisfied and would elect to undergo the procedure again. Complications noted in their study included recurrence of deformity, persistent corn, open traumatic dislocation of PIP fibrous union, and subungual hematoma [26]. Classic techniques for resection arthroplasty involved k-wire fixation. Using this technique, Coughlin reported subjective satisfaction in 84% of patients with 92% pain relief. Patients rated subjective alignment as acceptable in 86% of cases, and radiographic alignment was rated as good in 79% in this series [24]. Citing concerns for complication rates related to k-wire fixation, techniques have been developed utilizing intramedullary fixation. A recent retrospective review evaluated outcomes comparing k-wire fixation and intramedullary fixation, utilizing two different products. In their study of 182 feet, no difference in functional outcomes or complications was noted. However, they did notice a difference in radiographic unions and patient satisfaction favoring intramedullary devices [27].

FDL Tendon Transfer [26]

- The patient is placed supine on the operating room table. An Esmarch bandage can be used to exsanguinate the limb and may be used as a tourniquet as well.
- A longitudinal incision along the plantar aspect of the proximal phalanx is utilized to identify the FDL tendon. Care is taken with limited lateral dissection to avoid neurovascular injury.

- The tendon sheath is longitudinally opened and the FDL tendon isolated with a small hemostat or Ragnell retractor.
- Using a small incision at the plantar aspect of the DIP joint, the FDL tendon is released while under tension with the toe in extension.
- The end of the tendon is brought through the proximal incision, and the tendon is longitudinally split creating two limbs.
- A dorsally based incision is created longitudinally over the proximal phalanx and the extensor tendon identified. If an extensor tendon lengthening is indicated, a z-cut is performed.
- Utilizing a small curved hemostat, the two limbs of the flexor tendon are passed around either side of the proximal phalanx to the dorsal wound.
- The limbs of the FDL tendon are sutured into the extensor tendon dorsally with the toe held in approximately 20 degrees of plantar flexion.
- A 0.045 mm k-wire is often utilized to stabilize the repair. It can be inserted through the MTP joint, advanced in an antegrade fashion out the distal phalanx, and then driven back through the metatarsal head with the joint reduced.
- Incisions are closed in standard suture fashion.
- Postoperatively, patients were allowed to heel weight bearing in stiff-soled postoperative shoe. Pins can be removed at 4 weeks and patients weaned into supportive shoes as tolerated.

PIP Joint Arthrodesis [24, 27] (Fig. 23.3)

- The patient is placed supine on the operating room table. An Esmarch bandage can be used to exsanguinate the limb and may be used as a tourniquet as well.
- A dorsally based incision is created longitudinally (or in an elliptical fashion) over the PIP joint and proximal phalanx. Dissection is taken plantarly through the extensor tendon and capsule to expose the joint.
- The collateral ligaments and plantar plate are released.
- The proximal phalangeal head is exposed and delivered through the wound with plantar flexion of the toe.
- Utilizing a bone cutting forceps or small bone saw, the phalangeal head is resected at the head/neck junction.
- A rongeur is used to resect the articular surface of the middle phalanx.
- The joint is then reduced and stabilized utilizing a 0.045 k-wire or intramedullary implant.
- An FDL to extensor tendon transfer can be added for cases of severe deformity.
- The wound is closed in a standard suture fashion.
- Postoperatively, the patient was allowed full weight bearing in a postoperative shoe for 2–6 weeks. If a k-wire was utilized, it should be removed 3–6 weeks following surgery.

Claw Toes

Claw toe deformities tend to be less frequent but more severe than hammertoe deformities. They are characterized by MTP hyperextension in addition to PIP flexion and possibly DIP joint flexion. These too are classified as rigid or flexible. Callosities can develop overlying the dorsum of the PIP joint, and IPKs are often noted at the plantar aspect of the metatarsal head. Occasionally, a callus will develop at the tip of the distal phalanx. Patients may describe pain overlying the callosities. Claw toes can be associated with underlying neurologic diseases such as Charcot-Marie-Tooth disease or prior trauma such as compartment syndrome which may cause an imbalance between the intrinsic and extrinsic musculature [17, 22, 28].

Nonsurgical treatment of claw toes mimics that of hammertoes. Shoe modifications with large shoe boxes can decrease pressure over painful prominences. Padding these areas may help redistribute pressure. Additionally, toe splints can be used to help reduce the PIP joint and stabilize the MTP joint. Taping around the proximal pha-

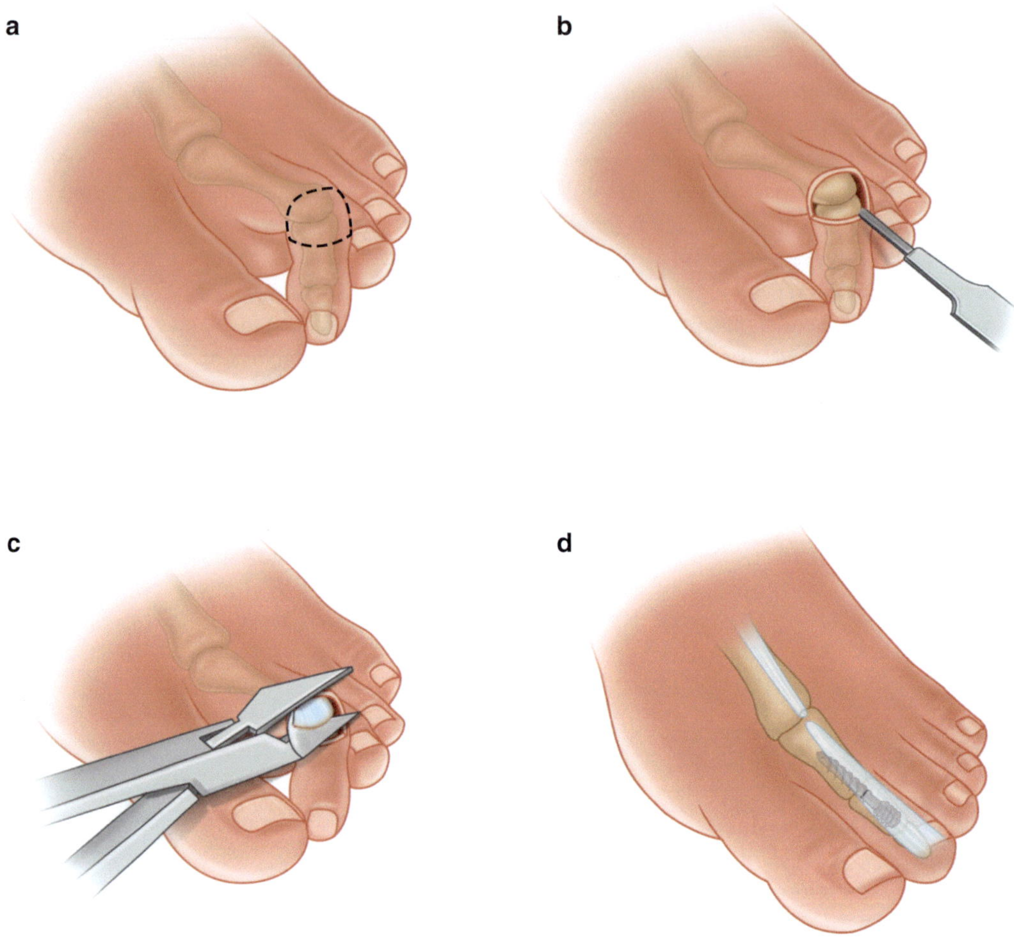

Fig. 23.3 Anatomic drawing of PIP joint resection arthrodesis. Fixation includes a k-wire or alternatively an intramedullary implant. (**a**) an elliptical incison is made over the PIP joint and (**b**) the dorsal capsular and tendon are excised. (**c**) the distal aspect of the proximal phalanx and the proximal aspect of the middle phalanx are resected before (**d**) and intramedullary device is placed or alternatively a K-wire

lanx base has been described to help pull the toe down out of MTP extension [17, 22, 28].

Surgical treatment of claw toes again follows a similar algorithm as hammertoes. Flexible deformities can be managed with soft tissue procedures including flexor-to-extensor tendon transfers. To correct the MTP extension deformity, often a release at that joint is indicated as well [28]. For rigid contractures, PIP joint resection arthroplasty vs. arthrodesis with MTP joint contracture release and possible metatarsal osteotomy is the preferred procedure (Fig. 23.4) [22, 24].

There are few outcome studies looking at treatment of claw toes in isolation. In their study of 39 feet with claw toes, Barbari and Brevig utilized flexor-to-extensor transfer with MTP joint capsulotomies or extensor tenotomies as indicated. Thirty-five patients expressed satisfaction with their procedure and general improvement of their symptoms [28]. In a study by Coughlin, nine out of ten patients who underwent procedures to address MTP hyperextension in addition to a PIP joint arthroplasty were satisfied with their surgeries [24].

MTP Joint Contracture Release

- A longitudinal incision is made over the dorsum of the MTP joint.

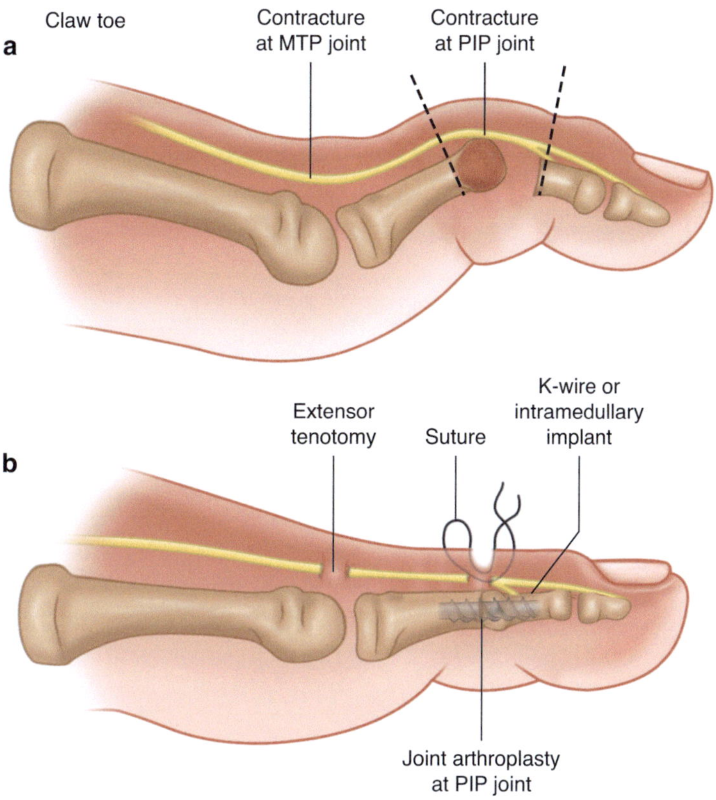

Fig. 23.4 (**a**) Anatomic drawing of (**b**) surgical correction of a claw toe deformity often including a dorsal release of contracted tissues at the MTP joint in addition to the PIP joint arthrodesis

- The extensor tendon is released. If lengthening is desired, a z-cut is made.
- The dorsal joint capsule is opened and the joint exposed.
- Sequentially the medial and lateral capsular and collateral attachments are released.
- The plantar plate may be released using an elevator if needed.
- The joint is reduced, and a 0.045 k-wire is used to maintain reduction.
- The wound is closed in standard suture fashion.
- The patient is allowed to weight bear as tolerated in a postoperative shoe for 4 weeks.
- K-wire removal at 3–4 weeks postoperatively.

Mallet Toe

Mallet toes are characterized by flexion contracture of the DIP joint and can either be flexible or rigid in nature. These are noted to be less common than other lesser toe deformities such as hammertoes [29]. Frequently patients develop calluses over the dorsum of the DIP joint or plantar tip of the distal phalanx. These may or may not be painful. Additionally, nail deformities are common. It is important to assess for ulceration at the tip of the toe, notably in diabetics. This may place them at risk for an amputation [30, 31].

Nonsurgical management addresses symptoms via pressure relief from painful areas. Shoes with increased toe box height can help. Padding will assist to redistribute pressures as well offloading painful areas. Callus shaving or trimming has been described as well [22, 30].

Flexible mallet toes can be treated surgically with a flexor tenotomy. Open and percutaneous approaches have been described [22, 30, 31]. For rigid deformities, resection arthroplasty of the DIP joint is typically indicated [22, 29, 30]. Lastly, amputation is an option for those at risk for complications to the other procedures [31].

In general, good results have been reported for surgical treatment of mallet toes. Kearney et al. were able to demonstrate an ulcer healing rate of

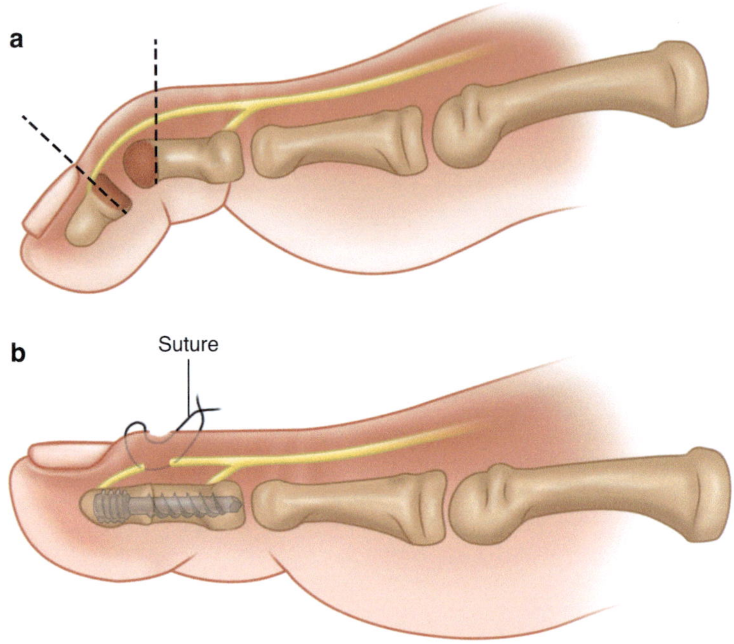

Fig. 23.5 Anatomic drawing of mallet toe correction. (**a**) A resection arthrodesi of the DIP joint is performed with either (**b**) an intramedullary screw or a temporary K-wire

98.3% among diabetic patients undergoing a percutaneous flexor tenotomy [31]. In his study evaluating outcomes for patients treated with DIP resection arthroplasty, Coughlin was able to demonstrate bony arthrodesis in 72% with fibrous union in the remaining patients. Overall, there was an 86% satisfaction rate [29].

DIP Joint Resection Arthroplasty [29] (Fig. 23.5)

- The patient is placed supine on the operating room table. An Esmarch bandage can be used to exsanguinate the limb and may be used as a tourniquet as well.
- An elliptical incision is made dorsally over the DIP joint.
- Extensor tendon and capsule are excised.
- The collateral ligaments and plantar plate are released.
- The middle phalangeal head is delivered through the incision.
- Utilizing a bone-cutting forceps, the phalangeal head is resected at the head/neck junction.
- A small rongeur is used to resect the articular surface of the distal phalanx.
- If needed for more severe deformity, FDL tendon can be released within the depths of the wound.
- The prepared surfaces are compressed and held in satisfactory alignment with a 0.045 Kirschner wire.
- Close wound in standard suture fashion.
- Heel weight bearing in postoperative shoe for 4 weeks.
- K-wire removed 3–4 weeks after surgery.

References

1. Coughlin MJ. Crossover second toe deformity. Foot Ankle. 1987;8(1):29–39. Available from: https://pubmed.ncbi.nlm.nih.gov/3623359/
2. Cooper MT, Coughlin MJ. Sequential dissection for exposure of the second metatarsophalangeal joint.

Foot Ankle Int. 2011;32(3):294–9. Available from: https://pubmed.ncbi.nlm.nih.gov/21477549/
3. Gregg J, Marks P, Silberstein M, Schneider T, Kerr J. Histologic anatomy of the lesser metatarsophalangeal joint plantar plate. Surg Radiol Anat. 2007;29(2):141–7.
4. Mendicino RW, Statler TK, Saltrick KR, Catanzariti AR. Predislocation syndrome: a review and retrospective analysis of eight patients. J Foot Ankle Surg. 2001;40(4):214–24.
5. Deland JT, Lee KT, Sobel M, Dicarlo EF. Anatomy of the plantar plate and its attachments in the lesser metatarsal phalangeal joint. Foot Ankle Int. 1995;16(8):480–6.
6. Brunet JA, Tubin S. Traumatic dislocations of the lesser toes. Foot Ankle Int. 1997;18(7):406–11.
7. Bouché RT, Heit EJ. Combined plantar plate and hammertoe repair with flexor digitorum longus tendon transfer for chronic, severe sagittal plane instability of the lesser metatarsophalangeal joints: preliminary observations. J Foot Ankle Surg. 2008;47(2):125–37.
8. Coughlin MJ, Baumfeld DS, Nery C. Second MTP joint instability: grading of the deformity and description of surgical repair of capsular insufficiency. Phys Sportsmed. 2011;39:132–41.
9. Coughlin MJ. Second metatarsophalangeal joint instability in the athlete. Foot Ankle Int. 1993;14(6):309–19.
10. Nery C, Coughlin MJ, Baumfeld D, Mann TS. Lesser metatarsophalangeal joint instability: Prospective evaluation and repair of plantar plate and capsular insufficiency. Foot Ankle Int. 2012;33(4):301–11. Available from: https://pubmcd.ncbi.nlm.nih.gov/22735202/
11. Kaz AJ, Coughlin MJ. Crossover second toe: Demographics, etiology, and radiographic assessment. Foot Ankle Int. 2007;28(12):1223–37. Available from: https://pubmed.ncbi.nlm.nih.gov/18173985/
12. Klein EE, Weil L, Weil LS, Coughlin MJ, Knight J. Clinical examination of plantar plate abnormality: A diagnostic perspective. Foot Ankle Int. 2013;34:800–4. Available from: https://pubmed.ncbi.nlm.nih.gov/23696184/
13. Yu GV, Judge MS, Hudson JR, Seidelmann FE. Predislocation syndrome: Progressive subluxation/dislocation of the lesser metatarsophalangeal joint. J Am Podiatr Med Assoc. 2002;92:182–99. Available from: https://pubmed.ncbi.nlm.nih.gov/11961086/
14. Powless SH, Elze ME. Metatarsophalangeal joint capsule tears: An analysis by arthrography, a new classification system and surgical management. J Foot Ankle Surg. 2001;40(6):374–89. Available from: https://pubmed.ncbi.nlm.nih.gov/11777233/
15. Couglin MJ. In: Couglin MJ, Mann RA, Saltzman CL, editors. Surgery of the Foot and Ankle. 8th ed. Philidelphia, PA: Mosby Elsevier Inc; 2007. p. 363–464.
16. Haddad SL, Sabbagh RC, Resch S, Myerson B, Myerson MS. Results of flexor-to-extensor and extensor brevis tendon transfer for correction of the crossover second toe deformity. Foot Ankle Int. 1999;20(12):781–8. Available from: https://pubmed.ncbi.nlm.nih.gov/10609706/
17. Coughlin MJ. Common causes of pain in the forefoot in adults. J Bone Joint Surg Br. 2000;82:781–90. Available from: https://pubmed.ncbi.nlm.nih.gov/10990297/
18. Trepman E, Yeo SJ. Nonoperative treatment of metatarsophalangeal joint synovitis. Foot Ankle Int. 1995;16(12):771–7. Available from: https://pubmed.ncbi.nlm.nih.gov/8749348/
19. Peck CN, Macleod A, Barrie J. Lesser metatarsophalangeal instability: Presentation, management, and outcomes. Foot Ankle Int. 2012;33(7):565–70. Available from: https://pubmed.ncbi.nlm.nih.gov/22835394/
20. Trnka HJ, Mühlbauer M, Zettl R, Myerson MS, Ritschl P. Comparison of the results of the Weil and Helal osteotomies for the treatment of metatarsalgia secondary to dislocation of the lesser metatarsophalangeal joints. Foot Ankle Int. 1999;20(2):72–9. Available from: https://pubmed.ncbi.nlm.nih.gov/10063974/
21. Flint WW, Macias DM, Jastifer JR, Doty JF, Hirose CB, Coughlin MJ. Plantar Plate Repair for Lesser Metatarsophalangeal Joint Instability. Foot and Ankle International. 2017;38(3):234–42. Available from: https://pubmed.ncbi.nlm.nih.gov/27852647/
22. Shirzad K, Kiesau CD, DeOrio JK, Parekh SG. Lesser toe deformities. J Am Acad Orthop Surg. 2011:505–14. Available from: https://pubmed.ncbi.nlm.nih.gov/21807918/
23. Angirasa AK, Augoyard M, Coughlin MJ, Fridman R, Ruch J, Weil L. Hammer toe, mallet toe, and claw toe. Foot Ankle Spec. 2011;4(3):182–7. Available from: https://pubmed.ncbi.nlm.nih.gov/21697399/
24. Coughlin MJ, Dorris J, Polk E. Operative repair of the fixed hammertoe deformity. Foot Ankle Int. 2000;21(2):94–104. Available from: https://pubmed.ncbi.nlm.nih.gov/10694020/
25. Dalmau-Pastor M, Fargues B, Alcolea E, Martínez-Franco N, Ruiz-Escobar P, Vega J, et al. Extensor apparatus of the lesser toes: Anatomy with clinical implications - Topical review. Foot Ankle Int. 2014;35:957–69. Available from: https://pubmed.ncbi.nlm.nih.gov/25228309/
26. Boyer M, De Orio J. Transfer of the flexor digitorum longus for the correction of lesser-toe deformities. Foot Ankle Int. 2007;28(4):422–30. Available from: https://pubmed.ncbi.nlm.nih.gov/17475135/
27. Obrador C, Losa-Iglesias M, Becerro-de-Bengoa-Vallejo R, Kabbash CA. Comparative study of intramedullary hammertoe fixation. Foot Ankle Int. 2018;39(4):415–25. Available from: https://pubmed.ncbi.nlm.nih.gov/29337598/
28. Barbari SG, Brevig K. Correction of Clawtoes by the Girdlestone-Taylor Flexor-Extensor Transfer Procedure. Foot Ankle Int. 1984;5(2):67–73. Available from: https://pubmed.ncbi.nlm.nih.gov/6500412/

29. Coughlin MJ. Operative repair of the mallet toe deformity. Foot Ankle Int. 1995;16(3):109–16. Available from: https://pubmed.ncbi.nlm.nih.gov/7599726/
30. Molloy A, Shariff R. Mallet toe deformity. Foot Ankle Clin. 2011;16:537–46. Available from: https://pubmed.ncbi.nlm.nih.gov/22118227/
31. Kearney TP, Hunt NA, Lavery LA. Safety and effectiveness of flexor tenotomies to heal toe ulcers in persons with diabetes. Diabetes Res Clin Pract. 2010;89(3):224–6. Available from: https://pubmed.ncbi.nlm.nih.gov/20580458/

Returning to Sport: Tips and Techniques for Safe Transition to Sports Participation

24

Norman E. Waldrop III, Charles C. Pitts Jr, and Yvonne C. Conway

Returning to Sport: Introduction

Foot and ankle injuries are common, often significantly affecting athletes and their ability to return to play. These injuries can lead to substantial disability and frequently lead to missed playing time. While there have been many advancements in the rehabilitation protocols and techniques of treating these injuries, there still is substantial missed playing time as a result of foot and ankle injuries.

It has been implied that the lateral ankle sprain is the most common injury in sports [14]. In fact, injuries to the foot and ankle comprise nearly 25% of all athletic injuries. Garrick and Requa reported that more than 25% of the 1600 athletic injuries in their series involved the foot and ankle [21]. These injuries can be acute or chronic in nature; however, either can lead to disability that affects the athlete.

The foot and ankle play a pivotal role in connecting the athlete with the ground. Because of this, the intricate collection of bones, ligaments, muscles, and tendons allows for highly specialized and efficient activities that provide athletes with their platform for performance. Even in the case of minor injuries, disability of the foot and ankle can significantly hamper performance in high-level athletes. Thus, rehabilitation of the injured athlete has taken on a new role in the recent past. Advancements in technology and procedures have allowed for the improvement of the care of the athlete. The same holds true for the rehabilitation of those athletes. These advances have led to improved outcomes, quicker return to sport without functional limitations, and less long-term disability. The principles of rehabilitation, while remaining consistent with the goals of the safe return of the athlete to the field, must continue to advance through improving technologies. Incorporating proven techniques and technologies into rehabilitation will provide the athlete with a complete functional recovery without long-term consequences.

Phases of Rehabilitation

Athletic injuries to the foot and ankle are among the most common and most variable in sports at all levels of play. Hunt et al. reported on 3861 injuries to collegiate athletes at a single division one institution over a 2-year period. The study found that 1035 (27%) of the injuries were located in the foot and ankle. 218 (21%) of the injuries kept the athlete from play for at least

N. E. Waldrop III (✉)
Andrews Sports Medicine, American Sports Medicine Institute, Birmingham, AL, USA
e-mail: norman.waldrop@andrewssm.com

C. C. Pitts Jr · Y. C. Conway
Department of Orthopaedic Surgery, University of Alabama—Birmingham, Birmingham, AL, USA
e-mail: charles.pitts@andrewssm.com; ychodaba@uabmc.edu

P. D'Hooghe et al. (eds.), *Ligamentous Injuries of the Foot and Ankle*,
https://doi.org/10.1007/978-3-031-08682-3_24

1 day, with an average time of 12.3 days lost from sports participation for all foot and ankle injuries [28]. Furthermore, observed injuries in the population spanned 30 discrete anatomical locations within the foot and ankle [28]. This study highlighted not only the high incidence but also the variability of foot and ankle injuries in sport that a physician may encounter. Although the athlete, the injury, or the clinician's specific protocols may vary, the general principles of rehabilitation following foot and ankle injury remain the same.

In general, a rehabilitation program allows a graduated and stepwise return to pre-injury levels of function and activity while also avoiding and preventing re-injury. This is typically approached initially by decreasing swelling, pain, and inflammation while protecting the injured anatomic structure [4, 39, 57]. Next, the athlete undergoes range of motion (ROM), strength, power, and endurance training that may be specific to sport in order to regain or even exceed pre-injury functional levels [4, 39, 57]. We list three specific phases of rehabilitation in this chapter. Each phase presents specific goals for the patient and physician, and advancement from one phase to the next should not be held to a specific time interval. Rather, advancement should be dependent on the injury, the patient, and the physician's interpretation of the patient's progress through each phase. This makes an accurate diagnosis of the specific injury paramount to the success of the protocol.

Phase I

The primary goals of phase I of rehabilitation are to decrease inflammation and restore pre-injury range of motion. Initially, whether in a post-injury or postoperative period, this phase involves protection, rest, ice, compression, and elevation (PRICE). A number of protective devices may be used such as a splint, cast, or removable walking boot to prevent re-injury or secondary inflammation to the affected extremity. The other components of PRICE, along with analgesic medication if necessary, will assist in controlling pain and inflammation and allow the athlete to better participate in exercises aimed at restoring range of motion. Restoration of normal foot and ankle ROM is emphasized following the initial period, and it will allow optimal performance once isolated and functional exercises have begun. Progression to phase II necessitates normal to near-normal foot and ankle range of motion with minimal pain and inflammation.

Phase II

Flexibility and functional strengthening are the hallmarks of phase II. Cardiovascular conditioning and proprioceptive training should also be initiated during this phase. The main goals of phase II are improving flexibility, restoring strength, and beginning light, sport-specific functional training exercises. The patient may wean away from protective devices at this stage. Progression to phase III can be considered when the patient is ready for a gradual return to light activity and sports participation.

Phase III

In general, phase III promotes a functional return to activities of daily living and previous levels of sports participation through advanced activity-specific exercise. An emphasis on proper sports-specific techniques and mechanics, in addition to building on the strength and flexibility acquired in phase II, will accelerate return to pre-injury capability and prevent re-injury. A functional progression should be performed. Additionally, external support devices such as braces, ankle straps, taping, or orthotics can be used at this time as indicated to confer stability and alleviate pain while the patient participates in his or her sport or activity.

Range of Motion/Mobilization

The need for early range of motion (ROM) versus immobilization of the ankle after surgery to protect against pathologic motion and promote tissue healing is a long disputed topic. Studies across various orthopedic subspecialties have shown improved results with early ROM protocols following injury or surgery [29, 33].

Early studies investigated the value of early motion after flexor tendon repairs of the hand with the goal of reducing stiffness and postoperative adhesions without impairing tendon healing ability. Gelberman et al. demonstrated early protected mobilization of the healing tendon to have superior strength, improved healing response, and a more natural pattern of vascularity in the healing tendon [22, 23]. Additional studies have shown that early ROM has a positive effect on tendon healing and decreased adhesions surrounding the repaired tendon [9–11, 24, 53]. It is now a standard of care to incorporate early ROM in rehabilitation of the hand after flexor tendon repair. Likewise, several studies have demonstrated that exercise and motion encourage healing and strengthening of ligaments after injury [9–11, 24, 53].

Early mobilization after various ankle injuries has been studied and found to be a valuable aspect of rehabilitation. In a prospective randomized study, Eiff et al. found that early mobilization in first-time lateral ankle sprains allows for earlier return to work and can be more comfortable for patients than prolonged immobilization [18]. Compared with immobilization with casting in the treatment of ankle sprains, early mobilization has been shown to result in quicker patient return to work and daily activities, better mobility, and less muscle atrophy [24]. Another study found that early ROM after anterior talofibular ligament reconstruction for chronic ankle instability led to a 5-week earlier return to full athletic activity when compared to a 4-week period of immobilization, with no cases of re-injury or differences in postoperative outcomes [42].

In a multicenter randomized controlled trial, Dehghan et al. found that early ankle ROM after surgical fixation of unstable ankle fractures resulted in increased patient convenience, early improved functional outcomes, and no increased complication rate [17]. With respect to ROM exercises, both active and passive ROM are utilized in a progressive manner to ultimately regain full motion. Passive ROM allows the muscles to be stretched while relaxed, while active ROM incorporates muscle re-education and requires independent muscle action. In order to protect soft tissue healing, ROM should initially be worked in the opposite direction of the mechanism of injury (i.e., focus on dorsiflexion and eversion and initially after a lateral ankle sprain). Once the injury has healed, ROM should include all directions.

The superior clinical results that have been demonstrated with early mobilization have led us to incorporate accelerated ROM exercises into the rehabilitation protocol for almost all foot and ankle injuries in our practice.

Strengthening

Once the patient has recovered 95–100% of joint ROM, muscle strengthening should be incorporated into their rehabilitation program. If strengthening is initiated too early, muscle strength can compromise joint ROM leading to joint stiffness and overall decreased function.

The most commonly performed method of strengthening focuses on isotonic muscle strengthening. Isotonic movements involve a muscular contraction against a constant force while the length of the muscle changes. The two different types of isotonic muscular contractions, concentric and eccentric, refer to the direction in which the muscle contracts. A concentric contraction causes the muscle to shorten (i.e., tibialis anterior shortens with dorsiflexion against a force). An eccentric contraction causes the muscle to lengthen (i.e., slowly releasing a dorsiflexed ankle back to neutral against a force causes the tibialis anterior to slowly lengthen while maintaining muscle contraction). It is extremely important to incorporate concentric and eccentric movements into a comprehensive rehabilitation program.

Foot and ankle strengthening can utilize several different methods including resistance bands, weights, and water resistance. Resistance bands provide dynamic resistance strengthening and are made in different levels of resistance to aid progression in strength. Once the athlete can complete 3 sets of 15 repetitions through a full range of movement, the next level of resistance should be started. This same concept can be used with ankle weights. In addition to strengthening of the primary extrinsic muscles responsible for inversion/eversion, supination/pronation, and dorsiflexion/plantar flexion, it is important to include strengthening of the foot intrinsic muscles to improve overall function.

Functional Progression

Successful completion of a clinic-based rehabilitation protocol should achieve pre-injury levels of range of motion, strength, proprioception, and endurance; however, it may not appropriately address sport-specific exercises, which are crucial for preparing an athlete for return to competition. Functional progression in the rehabilitation of athletes is composed of a series of sport-specific exercises that gradually increase in difficulty in order to prepare an athlete for safe return to sport. Yamamoto et al. described a functional progression used in the rehabilitation of injured West Point cadets that focused on using dynamic exercise for restoring agility after knee injury [56]. Tippett and Voight described functional progression in the athletic setting as a series of sport-specific, basic exercises advanced according to the difficulty of the skill and the athlete's tolerance [52]. Kegerreis et al. described effective rehabilitation, including sport-specific functional progression, as obeying the SAID principle, an acronym for specific adaptations to imposed demands, which states that when stress and overload are placed on the body, the body will adapt to the demands over time [32]. Functional progression subjects the injured area and body to the demands which will be required upon returning to competitive activity, including addressing the psychological needs of the injured athlete.

Each sport has varying skills required of the foot and ankle – functional progression provides an athlete with the opportunity to advance one step at a time as they prepare to return to their specific game. As the athlete progressively improves, he or she becomes more mentally prepared and confident to play without apprehension or fear, which plays an important role in restoring readiness to play at a competitive level. An athlete may return to full athletic activity once they have completed movements pertinent to their specific sport without pain or apprehension.

Return to Play

The treatment of any injury in an athlete necessitates recommendations on when it is safe to return to participation in his or her sport. Return to play (RTP) decisions are among the most crucial in sports medicine practice and, at times, some of the most difficult for the physician to make. In a study by Fong et al., the ankle was the most commonly injured site in 24 of 70 sports [19]. A previous injury is associated with as high as a fourfold increased risk of re-injury [20]. With this in mind, the RTP decision involves the patient's ability to not only safely participate in sports but also avoid re-injury at his or her level of play.

In 2002, the American College of Sports Medicine (ACSM) issued criteria to provide physicians a resource and guideline for returning athletes to sport following injury. Per the ACSM, the criteria in Table 24.1 must be confirmed by the team physician prior to RTP [2].

Clearly, the decision for RTP is multifactorial and will vary according to patient, injury, sport, and level of play. Typically, athletes would like to return to play as quickly as possible, and it is the role of the physician to recommend when it is safest to do so with regard to the above criteria.

RTP decisions can often result in disagreements between athletes, coaches, physicians,

Table 24.2 Return to Play criteria utilized by the American College of Sports Medicine

ACSM criteria for return to play
Anatomical and functional healing
Recovery from acute illness and associated sequelae
Status of chronic injury or illness
Risk to the safety of other participants
Restoration of sports-specific skills
Psychosocial readiness
Ability to perform safely with equipment modification, bracing, and orthoses
Compliance with applicable federal, state, local, and governing body regulations

families, teammates, and administration. Currently, there is little standardization in the RTP decision-making process, as there is little scientific evidence available to physicians to guide treatment [8, 15, 41]. This lack of standardization and evidence-based practice can lead to controversy and confusion, and it can allow decisions to be influenced by parties not trained in sports medicine or rehabilitation [40, 54]. Furthermore, the decision can be affected by external pressures from teammates, coaches, fans, families, or the media [8, 41, 54]. In order to assist the physician in the process, Creighton et al. developed a three-stage model for RTP decision-making [16]. This model is able to be modified for variations in sport, athlete, injury/illness, and external factors affecting the decision [16]. Somewhat unique to RTP considerations is the fact that the decision affects not only the patient but also other individuals that may be associated with a team, sport, school, or franchise [16].

The first step in the "decision-based RTP model" is the evaluation of the athlete's health status. This evaluation is complex and involves interpreting patient demographics, medical history, symptoms, physical exam, laboratory tests, imaging studies, functional tests, psychological state, and gravity of the injury (e.g., open fracture versus sprain). In this step of evaluation, and throughout rehabilitation, functional testing provides crucial information to the physician with regard to the healing process. A battery of functional tests provides the physician with information to assess the athlete's ability to perform activities that simulate sport-specific actions [16]. An effective schedule of tests will relay information regarding the patient's strength, range of motion, proprioception, and endurance [7, 43]. Functional testing will also challenge the athlete's confidence in his or her abilities and recovery [16]. Although biologic healing of injured tissue may have occurred, secondary functional deficits may remain. Tests within the battery should mimic the forces and stresses to which the athlete will be exposed in his or her sport at the competitive level, as this will help the physician and patient identify and address secondary deficits [7, 10, 34, 47]. Overall, Creighton et al. recommended that RTP begin when there is "no pain, no instability, normal kinematics, and near symmetrical performance compared with the contralateral limb" [12, 16, 35, 41].

Clanton et al. described a battery of functional tests specific to the rehabilitation of foot and ankle injuries. This battery is a validated method for evaluating a functional return of pre-injury performance. The four exercises in the series gauge ROM, balance and proprioception, agility, and strength [13]. They are as follows:

Dorsiflexion Lunge Test: Range of Motion (Fig. 24.1) [13]

With the foot flat and the subtalar joint locked, the foot is placed perpendicular to the wall, and

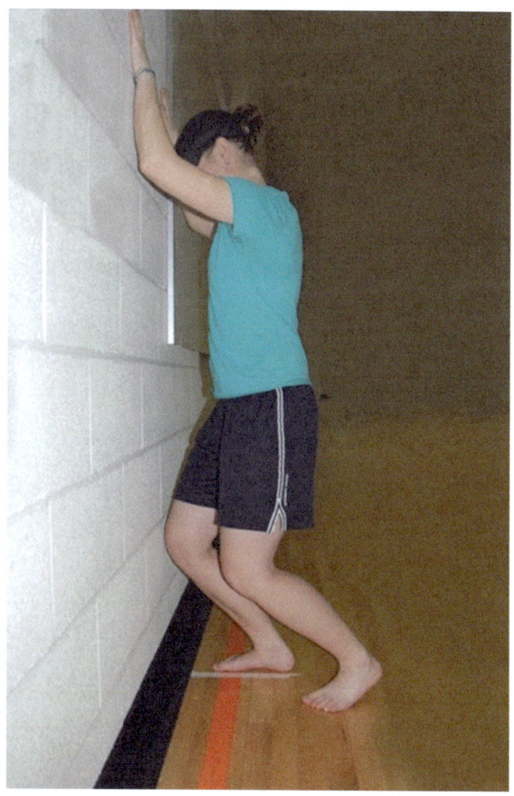

Fig. 24.1 Patient performing the Dorsiflexion Lunge Test. (Reproduced with permission from: Clanton T, Matheny L, Jarvis H, Jeronimus A. Return to play in athletes following ankle injuries. Sports Health. Nov 2012; 4(6):471–474)

the knee is bent until contact is made with the wall. The foot is moved sequentially away from the wall until maximum dorsiflexion with foot flat is achieved. Dorsiflexion is considered restricted with a distance from foot to wall of <9–10 cm or a measured angle of tibia shaft to wall of <35°–38° [13].

Star Excursion Balance Test (SEBT): Balance and Proprioception
(Fig. 24.2) [13].

This test demonstrates "unilateral balance and dynamic neuromuscular control" [13]. It involves balancing on the affected leg while reaching for and touching eight maximally defined points (eight-point star) with the contralateral leg. This test is sensitive for ankle instability if the athlete is unable to complete the test and reach all eight points [13, 45].

Agility T-Test: Agility (Fig. 24.3) [13]

In this test, the athlete navigates a T-shaped course with horizontal and longitudinal arms of 10 yards each. To begin, he or she sprints forward from the base of the longitudinal arm to the midpoint of the horizontal arm. The athlete then sidesteps, without crossing feet, to one end of the horizontal arm, then to the other end, and then back to the midpoint. The athlete subsequently backpedals to the start point of the longitudinal arm. Usual times can be between 8.9 and 13.5 s [13, 50].

Vertical Jump Test: Strength
(Fig. 24.4) [13]

This test evaluates the explosive power of the extremity and muscle strength balance. The athlete squats and jumps upward into full extension with both legs, touching the highest cardboard disk he or she can reach [13]. The patient's strength/efficiency is calculated [49]:

$$\text{Efficiency index} = \left[\text{weight}\left(\text{lbs}\right) \times \text{jump}\left(\text{in}\right)\right] / \text{patient height}\left(\text{in}\right)$$

This test can also be performed with a single leg, and a normal test is pain-free and at least 90% of the unaffected limb.

In addition to the functional progression battery, the physician should assess the athlete's mental health status. Following injury, 5–19% of athletes experience psychological distress similar

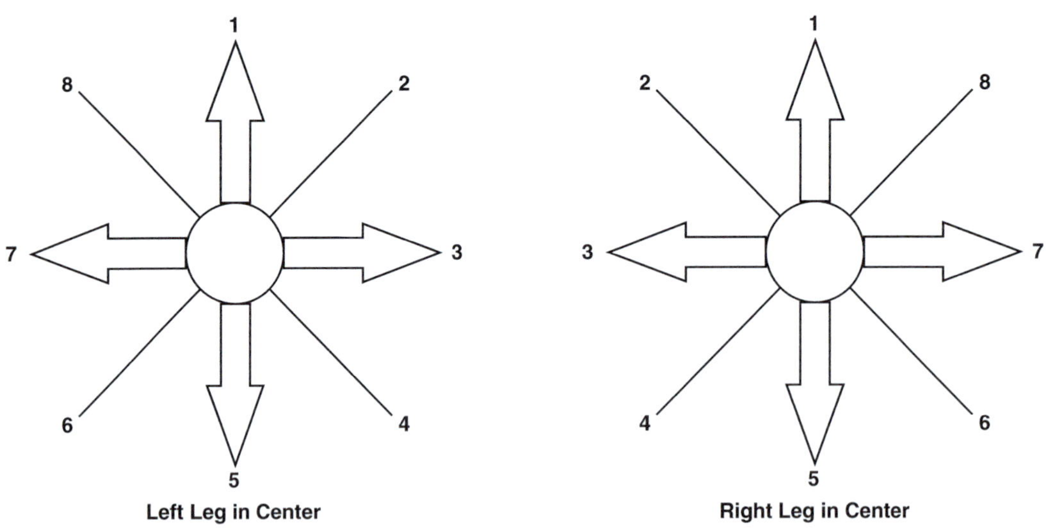

Fig. 24.2 Schematic diagram of the Star Excursion Balance Test

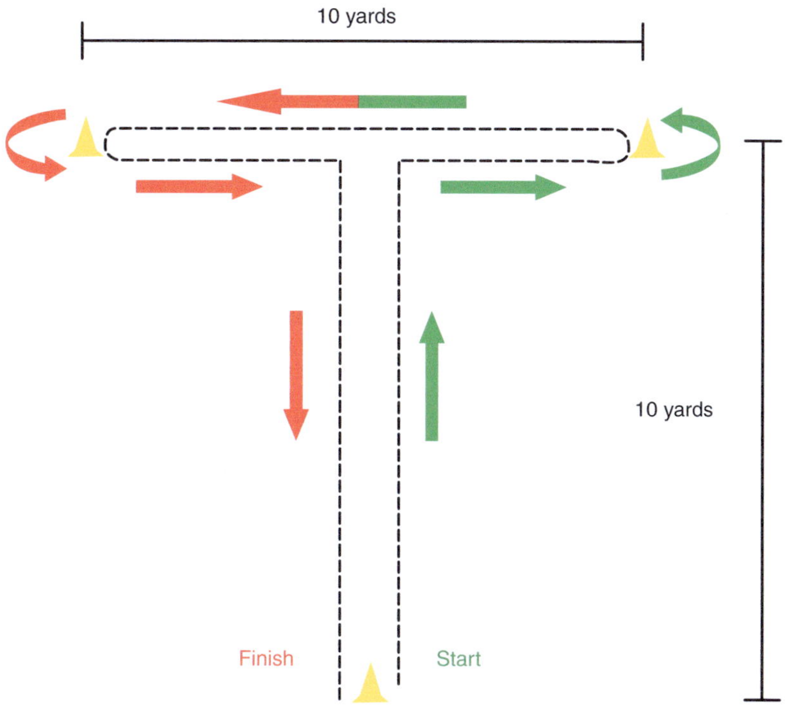

Fig. 24.3 Schematic diagram of the Agility T-Test. (Reproduced with permission from: Clanton T, Matheny L, Jarvis H, Jeronimus A. Return to play in athletes following ankle injuries. Sports Health. Nov 2012; 4(6):471–474)

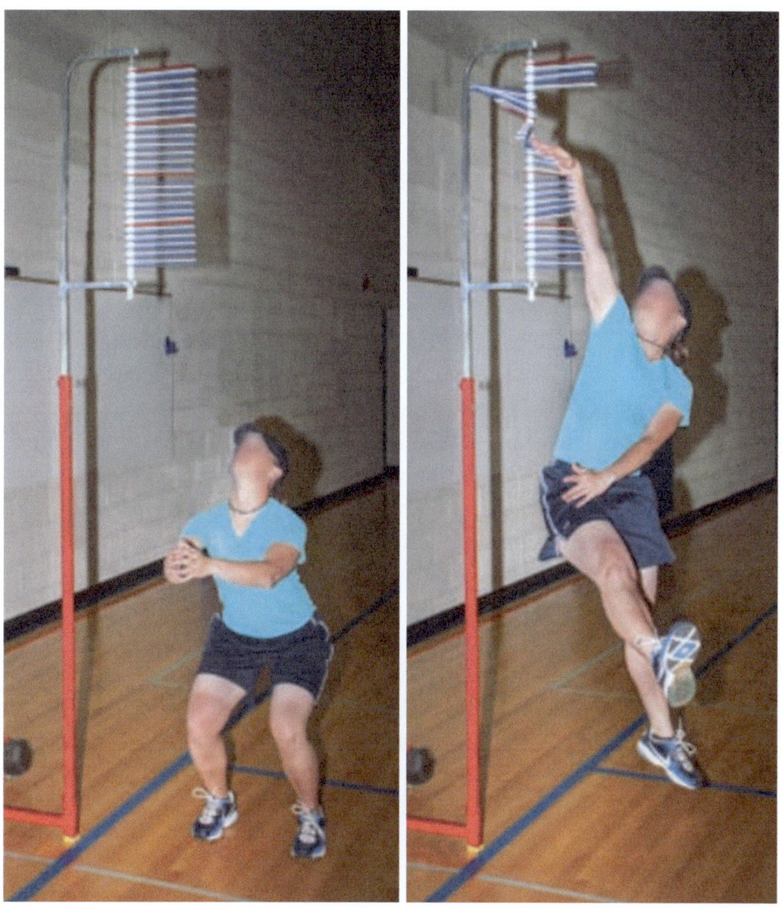

Fig. 24.4 Patient performing the Vertical Jump Test. (Reproduced with permission from: Clanton T, Matheny L, Jarvis H, Jeronimus A. Return to play in athletes following ankle injuries. Sports Health. Nov 2012; 4(6):471–474)

to patients receiving treatment for mental health illnesses [25]. In addition to physical readiness, the athlete must show psychosocial readiness for RTP. Athletes with fear, apprehension, or anxiety about their injury or recovery are at substantial risk of both re-injury and poor athletic performance [1, 13, 19]. Scoring systems such as the Trait Sport Confidence Inventory, the State Sport Confidence Inventory, and the Injury Psychological Readiness to Return to Sport Scale can be implemented to evaluate a patient's psychological state [1, 13].

Step 2 of the RTP model evaluates the athlete's participation risk in his or her particular sport. First, the physician must consider the type of sport played. Contact sports may present higher risks of acute injury or re-injury, while other sports may put a patient more at risk of repetitive overuse injuries. The physician must also consider position played and limb dominance (e.g., dominant foot of a kicker), as well as the patient's competitive level (amateur versus professional) and ability to protect the injury with padding, bracing, taping, etc. [16]. Athletes at higher levels of competition may push themselves beyond the normal levels of force and stress across the foot and ankle [16]. Rules concerning padding and protection typically are governed by the particular sport, but it is known that higher levels of competition are associated with increased health risks to the athlete [5, 16, 44]. All of these considerations may cause a physician to either delay or accelerate a particular athlete's RTP.

The final step of the RTP model involves "decision modifiers" that may affect RTP. Examples of decision modifiers may be the timing of injury (e.g., playoffs versus offseason) or external pressure from the patient's coaches, family, or teammates who may benefit from a player's participation. There may also be other conflicts of interest that play into decision-making such as a player's potential financial incentives, scholarship opportunities, or recruitment efforts. Finally, there is the potential for re-injury, which may incur further damages to the patient's health, function, or future participation in sport at the same or higher levels of competition [16].

Overall, RTP decision-making is complex, but the foremost concerns are the health and safety of the athlete and restoration of his or her ability to function at or above pre-injury levels of performance.

Achilles Tendon Injuries

Historically, treatment principles of Achilles tendon ruptures were immobilization with long- and then short-leg casting along with a slow return to weight-bearing and range of motion. Recently, treatment standards and evidence have shown benefits with early weight-bearing, early motion, and accelerated functional rehabilitation [6, 27, 31, 37]. Early functional rehabilitation allows the athlete a more rapid return to sports, without reported increased risk of re-rupture or complications [36]. Unfortunately, even with optimal surgical care and rehabilitation, many athletes experience long-term detrimental effects to their strength and athletic performance following this injury [3, 36, 46].

Mandelbaum et al. showed excellent results when an early motion protocol was initiated for patients who underwent surgical repair of the Achilles tendon. Ninety-three percent of the 29 patients had returned to full activity at 6 months with minimal functional deficit [38]. In their protocol, patients began range of motion on postoperative day 3, and weight-bearing was initiated at 2 weeks following surgery. Suchak et al. advocated for early protected motion using a walking boot with a dorsiflexion block at −20° [51]. Multiple recent protocols with a similar emphasis on early ROM and weight-bearing have similar favorable results [26, 27, 31, 36, 37]. There are a variety of protocols for return to sport and activity following surgical repair of Achilles rupture, and this chapter will describe the current preferred method of this author.

Postoperatively, phase I of rehabilitation is initiated, and the patient is splinted in slight equinus to relieve tension on the repair and protect the soft tissues. The patient returns to clinic after 10–12 days, and sutures are removed. With a healed incision, the patient is placed into a walking boot with two 0.25-in. heel lifts, and a progressive weight-bearing protocol is begun (Table 24.2). Compression and elevation are stressed during this initial phase, as the control of swelling is critical to rehab progression. Formal physical therapy (PT) is also begun with an exercise bike program in the boot and active ROM exercises. To protect the repair, it is very important that passive ROM or stretching exercises are avoided past neutral dorsiflexion. In addition to formal PT, a home therapy program utilizes toe curls and active plantar flexion with resistance bands and seated calf raises. Exercises are carried out with high frequency and low load, emphasizing early motion and stimulating a more robust and consistent healing response.

Typically, phase II begins at about 6 weeks postoperatively. With phase II, an increase in weight-bearing and the initiation of proprioceptive training seek to return the patient to normal gait and activity. Athletes come out of the boot and into a regular athletic shoe with one 9/16-in. heel lift. This transition can give patients a false sense of comfort and security, and it is important to inform the patient of the dangers of overtraining or pushing therapy faster than intended. Athletes comprise a very motivated patient population, and stressing protocol compliance can prevent re-injury or complication. Once in a regular shoe, calf raises are initiated, balance and strengthening exercises progress, and elliptical/anti-gravity treadmill/underwater treadmill programs begin. Once a normal gait is reached, proprioceptive strengthening exercises are emphasized. Dorsiflexion exercise past neutral is allowed at 8 weeks, with a slow progression toward full ROM over the course of 4 weeks. Jumping and explosive activity is prohibited in this phase. It is also important to continue to avoid forced dorsiflexion, as the final few degrees of ROM will be gained in the final phase of rehab.

Table 24.2 Postoperative weight-bearing progression protocol for Achilles tendon repair and lateral ankle ligament reconstruction

Days 1–2	25 lbs. of pressure in boot, 2 crutches
Days 3–5	50 lbs. of pressure in boot, 2 crutches
Days 6–8	75–100 lbs. of pressure in boot, 1 crutch
Days 9–11	100–125 lbs. of pressure in boot, 1 crutch
Days 12–14	150 lbs. to full weight-bearing, wean from crutch, ankle brace with boot only in times of excessive walking

Phase III begins at 3 months postoperatively. Balance, ankle strengthening, and unilateral calf raises continue to be emphasized, and full lower-extremity strengthening is initiated. Exercises such as step-downs, leg press, knee extensions, and hamstring curls are added to the regimen as the patient tolerates. Explosive exercises are not begun until at least 4 months postoperatively, as these exercises put the tendon most at risk for re-rupture. Once the athlete is able to perform a double-leg heel rise, walk without an altered gait, and use the elliptical for 30 min daily, he or she may begin light jogging outside of the anti-gravity treadmill. He or she should begin sport-specific activities at 4 months following surgery. Once the patient is nearing the end of rehabilitation, the functional progression battery discussed prior should be implemented in order to use objective, validated tests and data to make a return to play decision. RTP usually occurs at 5–8 months following surgery.

Lateral Ankle Instability

Similar to the care of Achilles tendon ruptures, lateral ankle ligament reconstruction was characterized by prolonged periods of immobilization and non-weight-bearing in the past. More recent trends favor early mobilization for accelerated recovery. It has been well established in animal models that stress deprivation of ligaments leads to a detrimental effect on their mechanical properties [26, 55]. For this reason, early motion and graduated stress on the ligaments are pursued following repair. The goals of rehabilitation of ankle sprains, or lateral ligament reconstruction, are to place the ankle in a healing position that avoids tension on the lateral ligament complex. In both cases, reducing stress on the injured ligaments initially with subsequent graduated stress and strengthening allows for optimal healing. Splints, casts, or removable walking boots, which orient the ankle in a stable, neutral position, can help avoid compromising positions that may damage the injured ligaments. These devices allow the athlete to ambulate with the mortise immobilized in its most stable orientation.

In contemporary studies, early mobilization and weight-bearing protocols have shown favorable results when compared to periods of immobilization in patients undergoing lateral ankle ligament reconstruction [30, 42, 48]. Some of these studies have resulted in an accelerated return to sports and enhanced mechanical stability in the early mobilization cohorts [30, 42]. Our protocol encourages early ROM and weight-bearing with these results in mind.

After surgery and in the beginning of phase I, the patient is placed in a splint in a position of eversion and neutral dorsiflexion. Elevation is emphasized to reduce swelling. He or she returns to clinic after 10–12 days, the splint is removed, and sutures are removed. At this visit, the patient is also transitioned to a CAM walking boot. Supervised PT is begun with a focus on swelling control, dorsiflexion and eversion ROM, and restoration of normal gait. Subsequently, light strengthening can commence, with care to avoid positions of plantar flexion and inversion. Swelling control continues to be encouraged with elevation and cold compression. Along with supervised PT, a home exercise program is implemented with the use of resistance bands for early ROM and strengthening. ROM limits are set prior. Additionally, cardiovascular exercise is begun with an exercise bike while wearing the boot.

In addition to the above, a progressive weight-bearing regimen is initiated starting 2 weeks from surgery (Table 24.2). The progression allows the patient to gradually reintroduce stress across the foot and ankle. Once full weight-bearing is achieved, the patient can wean from the boot and into athletic shoes with a lace-up ankle brace. During the transition phase from boot to shoes (Table 24.3), strengthening and ROM exercises in all planes are begun, with a goal of restoring full, pain-free ROM. Once completely out of the boot, more aggressive therapy is begun.

Table 24.3 Boot wean protocol for lateral ankle ligament reconstruction

Days 1–2	1 h out in morning/1 h out in afternoon
Days 3–5	2 h out in morning/2 h out in afternoon
Days 6–8	3 h out in morning/3 h out in afternoon
Days 9–11	4 h out in morning/4 h out in afternoon
Days 12–14	Progress to full-time weight-bearing out of boot

The final component of phase I is light, desensitization massage. Patients often experience surface hypersensitivity following lateral ligament reconstruction, and these symptoms can be abated with light massage and tactile stimulation to desensitize the tissue to normal touch and pressure. This tissue re-education regimen is best carried out with light massage for 3–5 min several times daily.

Phase II begins at 4–6 weeks postoperatively. Exercises during this phase include ROM/strengthening in all four directions (plantar flexion, dorsiflexion, inversion, eversion), aggressive Achilles stretching, calf raises, and proprioceptive training. Dorsiflexion and eversion strengthening are still performed with resistance bands. Peroneal strengthening is achieved by having the athlete lie in the lateral position with the affected side up. Weights are then hung over the end of the foot with toes pointed to isolate the peroneal muscles, and the foot is brought into an everted position against resistance. Calf raises are progressed from double- to single-leg raises. To do this, the patient initially does a double-leg raise followed by slowly lowering to foot flat with weight on the affected side only, strengthening in the eccentric phase. Once the patient can perform the eccentric phase without difficulty, he or she can progress to an isolated single-leg heel raise. Proprioception training is initiated with one-foot balance and then progressed to one-foot balance with simultaneous contralateral hip/leg exercise. Cardiovascular exercise is advanced from the bike to the elliptical machine at 4–6 weeks postoperatively and subsequently to light jogging at 6–10 weeks.

Phase III occurs during weeks 10–14 and focuses on sport-specific exercise. The hallmarks of this phase are ankle/leg strengthening, restoration of flexibility, and proprioception. No restrictions are placed on the athlete, and explosive activity can begin if swelling and pain are controlled. The patient begins on-field activity with a stirrup brace, and the functional progression battery program should be used to ensure a safe return to play. Full RTP is typical at 12–14 weeks.

Syndesmosis Injuries

The diagnosis and treatment of high ankle sprains has been a topic that has gained a significant amount of attention in recent years. For years, the standard treatment of ligamentous syndesmosis injuries, or high ankle sprains, has been conservative treatment. Recently, surgical stabilization of syndesmosis injuries has become more common. Operative stabilizations with endobutton constructs have changed how we treat this injury in athletes. These types of constructs have enabled physicians to return athletes to sport in less time because of evolving rehabilitation techniques that promote earlier mobilization.

Chronic syndesmosis injuries can be difficult to treat, and with a rising incidence in this problem, a growing number of physicians are treating severe Grade II and all Grade III syndesmosis injuries with operative stabilization. As with any injury, the goal is to restore stability and normal mechanics of the joint so the athlete can be rehabilitated at a quicker pace, without compromising the health and safety of the athlete. In doing so, the safe return of the athlete to competition is our primary goal, and with advancement of both surgical and rehabilitation techniques, we are able to do so in a much more timely and efficient manner.

In a patient with a syndesmosis injury that is deemed stable and not in need of surgical stabilization, the rehabilitation protocol closely resembles the postoperative protocol detailed below, but at an accelerated pace. The patient is initially placed in a CAM boot and made non-weight-bearing for 4–7 days, though this amount of time is largely patient-dependent. In addition to immobilization, swelling control modalities are utilized. After this initial period, the patient can progress into phase II and subsequently phase III at his or her own pace, depending on symptoms. Though there is no anatomic instability, the patient can return to sport once symptomatically and psychologically ready.

In our practice, unstable Grade II and all Grade III syndesmosis injuries warrant surgical stabilization. In doing so, ankle arthroscopy is performed to debride the joint, evaluate the cartilage, and assess the stability of the ankle. Once this is completed, stabilization of the syndesmosis is performed with a divergent endobutton construct over a small lateral plate. This plate is used to provide stress dissipation across the fibula, which is critical in the patients that are returning to play in an expedited manner. After surgical stabilization, the athlete is placed directly into a compressive dressing and into a cold compression device in the post-anesthesia care unit. They are placed in a CAM walker boot for comfort. Swelling control modalities are critical in the initial period to mitigate the amount of surgical swelling that can occur. The quicker the swelling decreases, the shorter the amount of time it takes the athlete to regain full motion, which plays a critical role in reducing the amount of time the athlete is sidelined. Most of the initial treatment utilizes swelling control modalities. Cold compression devices, high-volt stimulation, massage, and elevation are all components of the early treatment phase. Nonsteroidal anti-inflammatories are begun on postoperative day number 1. Initially, the athlete is kept non-weight-bearing, transitioning to weight-bearing as tolerated on postoperative day 4, though it often takes the athlete many days to become comfortable weight-bearing in the boot. This usually occurs after 7–10 days. During this period, it is important to care for the incision. Avoid direct pressure on the incision and any shearing forces that could compromise the skin and cause breakdown. Blood flow restriction is also initiated during this period to help maintain strength in the affected extremity while helping keep the swelling reduced.

One week from surgery, the anti-gravity treadmill and the exercise bike are initiated. The initial focus is on maintaining strength in the extremity and normalizing the gait. Once these occur, full weight-bearing on the affected limb is possible. Apprehension from the athlete is normal and typically occurs as the therapy becomes more aggressive. Thera-band exercises are used extensively to maintain strength. Proprioceptive exercises, which are critical to any ankle rehabilitation, are used extensively to help maintain the normal mechanics of the foot and ankle. The goal is to limit the loss of strength while restoring the normal motion of the ankle. Closed chain exercise and single-leg stance exercises are begun as soon as the athlete can tolerate them. These are often performed in conjunction with exercises that focus on the push-off phase of the gait. Once the gait is normalized, which varies of each athlete, a transition to full weight-bearing exercises occurs. This included straight-ahead running, followed by cutting and, finally, jumping exercises. This usually occurs between postoperative days 14 and 21. The athlete is protected with taping, utilizing a subtalar sling technique to stabilize the hindfoot. A brace is often used as well. Once the athletes reach this stage, their symptoms, strength, swelling, and range of motion dictate their progress (Fig. 24.5). Once the athlete can perform a single-leg hop test, which includes 15 consecutive single-leg hops, and has passed the validated return to play test as described by Clanton, they are cleared to return to play. Typically, full return to play is between 3 and 6 weeks. The athlete determines their own progress through this protocol. If the athlete is progressing at a faster pace, they are allowed to continue progressing. It is important to remember that, even if the athlete is able to return to sport at a quick pace, it remains critical to continue their treatment in order to get the best outcomes for the athlete.

Special Considerations

The ultimate goal of any athlete after injury is to return to the field with full strength, great confidence, and no limitations of function. There are many people involved in the team effort required to get an athlete back to 100%. The team of athletic trainers, therapists, physicians, coaches, and parents all play a unique role in this process. One of the difficulties of defining safe return to play is the varying definition used in the literature. Most, however, consider return to play as the safe return of the athlete to competition, either practice or games, without restrictions placed.

One of the unique issues encountered with an athlete's return to play is the multitude of con-

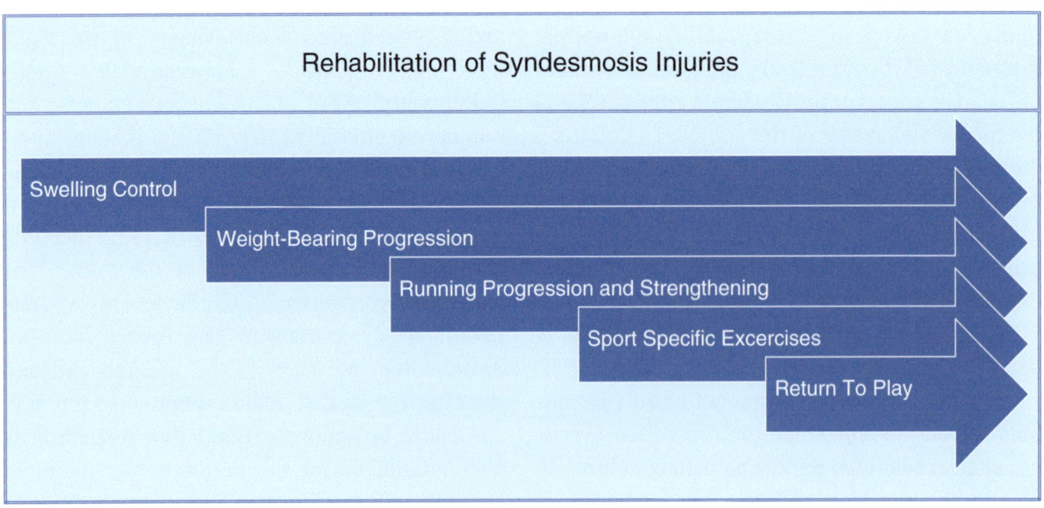

Fig. 24.5 Rehabilitation progression following syndesmosis repair

flicts of interest that are often present when making these decisions. Each member of the team faces their own unique conflicts when making these decisions. The physicians themselves often feel the pressures from their colleagues, who are sometimes providing second opinions to these athletes. They can even feel the weight of expectations from their own partners when trying to make decisions on whether or not an athlete is safe to return to play or not. Parents also provide conflict with these decisions. They can come from both sides of the spectrum. A parent may be hesitant to allow their child to return to play for fear of re-injury. That fear may be rooted in the thought that that child may be their "golden ticket." On the other hand, some parents can often pressure their child to return to play quickly, in fear that they may be lagging behind or may not be able to make up the lost ground caused from the missed time from the injury.

Coaches are also critical in these decisions. The mindset of toughness created in sports can be in direct conflict with an athlete missing time from injury. It is important to understand this distinction when making the best decision for the athlete. Lastly, the player themselves can be conflicted. They can make hasty decisions when dealing with injuries because of fear. End of career decisions as well as those athletes that have the potential to move to the next level are especially conflicted. There is the possibility that the athlete can rush their own return to sports, putting themselves at greater risk for further problems.

There are three reasons that return to play decisions can be so difficult. Firstly, there are no absolute contraindications to participation that exist. Secondly, there is often significant pressure on those making the decisions to use approaches that are non-conventional or "outside the box." Finally, these decisions are often made on a case-by-case basis, because many times, standard protocols don't exist.

A frank discussion needs to be had between all parties involved. This discussion between the player, parents, coaches, and medical staff must be honest. The risk of re-injury relative to the risk of lost time must be weighed. Can the athletes safely protect themselves? There is a real risk of re-injury, and that risk decreases with each week of return to play. Taking all of these factors into consideration is key to making the right decisions for the athlete.

The four Cs are critical to understanding the nuances of return to play after injury. Communication, consent, compassion, and competency, the four Cs, are the tenets that must provide the foundation for these decisions. Safety is required and paramount. It is vital for the physician to lead the team of decision-makers with a strong foundation that can lead to the best results for the athlete.

Conclusion

Return to competition is the goal of any athlete after injury. This requires the athlete to regain strength, motion, and full function without limitations. In doing so, it requires a full team to focus their efforts in the same direction. With each injury, the team of physicians, therapists, athletic trainers, the athlete, and their family require a coordinated response to work in conjunction with each other to allow for full return in the shortest time possible. Rehabilitation for athletes with foot and ankle injuries is evolving. Surgical techniques and therapeutic modalities have significantly changed over the past several years. The goals of rehabilitation remain the same despite efforts to continually push the envelope in terms of returning the injured athlete to competition. The goals of restoring motion of the joint, restoring strength to the affected limb, and returning the functional ability of the athlete have not changed. The progress made through both surgical techniques and advancements in the rehabilitation have allowed us to push the limits while maintaining these same principles. The process is ever-changing. Even with shortened times to return to play, the evolving process of rehabilitation of the athlete continues to be a part of the advancing technologies in medicine that guide us in returning the athlete to sport.

References

1. American College of Sports Medicine, American Academy of family physicians, American Academy of Orthopaedic surgeons, American medical Society for Sports Medicine, American Orthopaedic Society for Sports Medicine, American osteopathic academy of sports medicine. Psychological issues related to injury in athletes and the team physician: a consensus statement. Med Sci Sports Exerc. 2006;38:2030–4.
2. American College of Sports Medicine. The team physician and return-to-play issues: a consensus statement. 2002. http://www.acsm.org.
3. Amin N, Old A, Tabb L, et al. Performance outcomes after repair of complete Achilles tendon ruptures in National Basketball Association players. Am J Sports Med. 2013;41(8):1864–8.
4. Andrews J, Harrelson G, Wilk K. Physical rehabilitation of the injured athlete. 2nd ed. Philadelphia, PA: WB Saunders; 1998.
5. Bauman J. Returning to play – the mind does matter. Clin J Sports Med. 2005;15:432–5.
6. Bevoni R, Angelini A, D'Apote G, et al. Long term results of acute Achilles repair with triple-bundle technique and early rehabilitation protocol. Injury. 2014;45(8):1268–74.
7. Bowen T, Feldman D, Miller M. Return to play following surgical treatment of meniscal and chondral injuries to the knee. Clin Sports Med. 2004;23:381–93.
8. Brukner P. Return to play – a personal perspective. Clin J Sports Med. 2005;15:459–60.
9. Buckwalter JA. Activity vs rest in the treatment of bone, soft tissue and joint injuries. Iowa Orthop J. 1995;15:29.
10. Buckwalter JA. Effects of early motion on healing of musculoskeletal tissues. Hand Clin. 1996;12:13.
11. Burroughs P, Dahners LE. The effect of enforced exercise of the healing of ligament injuries. Am J Sports Med. 1990;18:376.
12. Cascio B, Culp L, Cosgarea A. Return to plate after anterior cruciate ligament reconstruction. Clin Sports Med. 2004;23:395–408.
13. Clanton T, Matheny L, Jarvis H, et al. Return to play in athletes following ankle injuries. Sports Health. 2012;4(6):471–4.
14. Clanton TO, Wood RM. Etiology of injury to the foot and ankle. In: DeLee JC, DrezJr D, Miller MD, editors. Orthopaedic sports medicine principles and practice. Philadelphia: Saunders; 2003.
15. Clover J, Wall J. Return to play criteria following sports injury. Clin Sports Med. 2010;29:169–75.
16. Creighton D, Shrier I, Shultz R, et al. Return-to-play in sport: a decision-based model. Clin J Sports Med. 2010;20:379–85.
17. Dehghan N, McKee MD, Jenkinson RJ, Schemitsch EH, Stas V, Nauth A, Hall JA, Stephen DJ, Kreder HJ. Early Weightbearing and Range of Motion Versus Non-Weightbearing and Immobilization After Open Reduction and Internal Fixation of Unstable Ankle Fractures: A Randomized Controlled Trial. J Orthop Trauma. 2016;30(7):345–52.
18. Eiff MP, Smith AT, Smith GE. Early mobilization versus immobilization in the treatment of lateral ankle sprains. Am Orthop Soc Sport Med. 1994;22:83.
19. Fong D, Hong Y, Chan L, et al. A systematic review on ankle injury and ankle sprain in sports. Sports Med. 2007;27:73–94.
20. Fuller C, Bahr R, Dick R, et al. A framework for recording recurrences, reinjuries, and exacerbations in injury surveillance. Clin J Sport Med. 2007;17:197–200.
21. Garrick JG, Requa RK. The epidemiology of foot and ankle injuries. Clin Sports Med. 1988;7:29.
22. Gelberman RH, Menon J, Gonsalves M, Akeson WH. The effects of mobilization on the vascularization of healing flexor tendons in dogs. Clin Orthop. 1980;153:283.
23. Gelberman RH, Nunley JA Jr, Osterman AL, Breen TF, Dimick MP, Woo SL. Influences of the protected passive mobilization interval on flexor tendon healing. A prospective randomized clinical study. Clin Orthop. 1991;264:189.
24. Glasoe WM, Allen MK, Awtry BF, Yack HJ. Weight-bearing immobilization and early exercise treatment following a grade II lateral ankle sprain. J Orthop Sport Phys Ther. 1999;29:394.
25. Glazer D. Development and preliminary validation of the injury psychological readiness to return to sport (I-PRRS) scale. J Athl Train. 2009;44:185–9.
26. Gomez MA, Woo SL, Amiel D, Harwood F, Kitabayashi L, Matyas JR. The effects of increased tension on healing medial collateral ligaments. Am J Sports Med. 1991;19(4):347–54.
27. Groetelaers R, Janssen L, van der Velden J, et al. Functional treatment or cast immobilization after minimally invasive repair of an acute Achilles tendon rupture: prospective, randomized trial. Foot Ankle Int. 2014;35(8):771–8.
28. Hunt K, Hurwot D, Robell K, Gatewood C, Botser I, Matheson G. Incidence and epidemiology of foot and ankle injuries in elite college athletes. Am J Sports Med. 2017;45(2):426–33.
29. Iordens G, Van Lieshout E, Schep N, De Haan J, Tuinebreijer W, Eygendaal D. Early mobilisation versus plaster immobilization of simple elbow dislocations: results of the FuncSiE multicentre randomised clinical trial. Br J Sports Med. 2017;51(6):531–8.
30. Karlsson J, Rudholm O, Bergsten T, Faxen E, Styf J. Early range of motion training after ligament reconstruction of the ankle joint. Knee Surg Sports Traumatol Arthrosc. 1995;3(3):173–7.
31. Kearney R, McGuinness K, Atchen J, et al. A systematic review of early rehabilitation methods following a rupture of the Achilles tendon. Physiotherapy. 2012;98(1):24–32.
32. Kegerreis S, Malone T, McCarroll J. Functional progressions: an aid to athletic rehabilitation. Phys Sport Med. 1984;12:67.
33. Kim S, Ha K, Jung M, Lim M, Kim Y, Park J. Accelerated rehabilitation after arthroscopic Bankart

repair for selected cases: a prospective randomized clinical study. Arthroscopy. 2003;19(7):722–31.
34. Kovacic J, Gerbfeld. Return to play issues in upper extremity injuries. Clinical. J Sports Med. 2005;15:448–52.
35. Krabak B, Kennedy D. Functional rehabilitation of lumbar spine injuries in the athlete. Sports Med Arthroscopy. 2008;16:47–54.
36. Lanitto I, Heikkinen J, Flinkkila T, et al. Early functional treatment versus cast immobilization in tension after Achilles rupture repair: results of a prospective randomized trial with 10 or more years follow up. Am J Sports Med. 2015;43(9):2302–9.
37. Lim C, Lees D, Gwynne-Jones D. 2017 functional outcome of acute Achilles tendon rupture with and without operative treatment using an identical functional bracing protocol. Foot Ankle Int. 2017;38(12):1331–6.
38. Mandelbaum B, Myerson M, Forster R. Achilles tendon ruptures: a new method of repair, early range of motion, and functional rehabilitation. Am J Sports Med. 1995;23(4):392–5.
39. Mattacola C, Dwyer M. Rehabilitation of the ankle after acute ankle sprain or chronic instability. J Athl Train. 2002;37(4):413–29.
40. McFarland E. Return to play. Clinical. Sports Med. 2004;23:15–23.
41. Miller M, Arciero R, Cooper D, et al. Doc, when can he go back in the game? Instr Course Lect. 2009;58:437–43.
42. Miyamoto W, Takao M, Yamada K, et al. Accelerated versus traditional rehabilitation after anterior talofibular ligament reconstruction for chronic lateral instability of the ankle in athletes. Am J Sports Med. 2014;42(6):1441–7.
43. Myklebust G, Bahr R. Return to play guidelines after anterior cruciate ligament surgery. Br J Sports Med. 2005;39:127–31.
44. Orchard J, Best T, Verrall G. Return to play following muscle strains. Clin J Sports Med. 2005;15:436–41.
45. Olmsted L, Carcia C, Hertel J, et al. Efficacy of the star excursion balance tests in detecting reach deficits in subjects with chronic ankle instability. J Athl Train. 1997;32:221–5.
46. Parekh S, Wray W, Brimmo O, et al. Epidemiology and outcomes of Achilles tendon ruptures in the National Football League. Foot Ankle Spec. 2006;2(6):283–6.
47. Park H, Lin S, Yokota A, et al. Return to play for rotator cuff injuries and superior labrum anterior posterior (SLAP) lesions. Clin Sports Med. 2004;23:321–34.
48. Petrera M, Dwyer T, Theodoropoulos JS, et al. Short- to medium-term outcomes after a modified Broström repair for lateral ankle instability with immediate postoperative weightbearing. Am J Sports Med. 2014;42(7):1542–8.
49. Semenick D. Testing protocols and procedures. In: Baechle TR, Earle RW, editors. Essentials of Strength Training and Conditioning. 3rd ed. Champaign, IL: Human Kinetics; 2008. p. 264.
50. Sheppard J, Young W. Agility literature review: classifications, training, and testing. J Sports Sci. 2006;24:919–32.
51. Suchak A, Bostick G, Beaupre L, et al. The influence of early weight-bearing compared with non-weight-bearing after surgical repair of the Achilles tendon. J Bone Joint Surg. 2008;90(9):1876–83.
52. Tippett SR, Voight ML. Functional progression for sport rehabilitation. Champaign, IL: Human Kinetics; 1995.
53. Vailas A, Tipton C, Matthes R, et al. Physical activity and its influence on the repair process of medial collateral ligaments. Connect Tissue Res. 1981;9:25.
54. Verrall G, Brukner P, Seward H. Doctors on the sidelines. Med J Aust. 2006;184:244–8.
55. Woo S, Gomez M, Sites T, et al. The biomechanical and morphological changes in the medial collateral ligament of the rabbit after immobilization and remobilization. J Bone Joint Surg. 1987;69(6):1200–11.
56. Yamamoto S, et al. Functional rehabilitation of the knee: a preliminary study. J Sport Med. 1975;3:288.
57. Zoch C, Fialka-Moser V, Quitten M. Rehabilitation of ligamentous ankle injuries: a review of recent studies. Br J Sports Med. 2003;37:291–5.

Index

A

Achilles stretching exercises, 67
Achilles Tendon injuries, 292, 293
Acute subtalar dislocation, 76, 77
Adult acquired flatfoot deformity (AAFD), 183–185
Aerobic training, 53
Agility T-test, 290, 291
Alterative calcaneal osteotomy techniques, 37
American Orthopaedic Foot and Ankle Society (AOFAS) scores, 102, 120
Angular measurements, 35
Ankle arthroscopy, 143
Ankle injuries, 91
Ankle lateral ligament, 9, 20, 23
Ankle, medial ankle ligaments, 21, 23
Ankle sprains, 31, 97
  athletic populations, 61
  chronic ankle instability (CAI), 61
  epidemiology of, 64
  incidence and epidemiology of, 62
  incidence of, 62
  injury prevention, 65
  nonoperative management of, 65, 68
  in USA, 63
Ankle, syndesmotic ligaments, 20–22
Anterior ankle arthroscopy, 85
Anterior drawer test (ADT), 128
Anterior inferior tibiofibular ligament (AITFL), 7, 8, 138
Anterior talar translation (ATT), 120
Anterior talocalcaneal ligament, 12
Anterior talofibular ligament (ATFL), 91, 92, 97, 175
Anterior talofibular ligament lower fascicle (ATFLlf), 9
Anterior talofibular ligament upper fascicle (ATFLsf), 9
Arthroscopic lateral ligament repair technique
  anchor placement, 99
  anesthesia, 99
  diagnostic arthroscopy, 99
  manual examination, 99
  passing sutures, 100
  portal placement, 99
  positioning, 99
  rehabilitation, 101
  repair, 100
Arthroscopy
  in lateral ligament repair, 98
  surgical techniques, 97
Athletic exposure (AE), 62, 91

B

Balance exercises, 68
Basic exercise principles, 49
Bassett's ligament, 7, 8
Biomechanical cadaveric study, 113
Biomechanical evidence, 119, 120
Biomechanical studies, 107
Blood flow-restricted exercise (BFR), 50
Broström-Evan procedure, 112
Broström-Gould anatomic repair, 132
Broström-Gould lateral ligament repair, 37
Broström-Gould procedure, 40, 42, 86
Broström ligament reconstruction, 43
Broström procedure, 97
  additional suture anchor repair augmentation, 118
  Gould modification, 117
  neoligament augmentation, 118
Broström repair, 105, 118

C

Cadaveric model, 183
Calcaneal osteotomy, 36
Calcaneal pitch, 35
Calcaneofibular ligament (CFL), 9, 84, 91, 92, 97, 115
Capsuloligamentous structures, 261, 263
Cavovarus deformity, 32, 35
Cervical ligament (CL), 12
Charcot-Marie-Tooth (CMT) population, 31
Chopart joint, 13, 14
Chronic ankle instability (CAI), 97, 171
Chronic degenerative changes, 1
Chronic instability, 1

P. D'Hooghe et al. (eds.), *Ligamentous Injuries of the Foot and Ankle*,
https://doi.org/10.1007/978-3-031-08682-3

Chronic lateral ankle instability (CLAI), 31, 45, 115
  assessment, 115
  diagnostic evaluation of, 116
  historical surgical options, 117
  nonsurgical treatment, 117
Claw toe deformities, 279–281
Clinical evidence, 120
Coleman block testing, 32, 33, 38
Common manual therapy techniques, 48
Compression garments, 49
Computed tomography (CT), 17, 77
Conventional radiographs, 77, 83
Cortical screw fixation, 41
Cryotherapy, 49

D
Daily Adjustable Progressive Resistive Exercises (DAPRE), 68
Deep anterior tibiotalar ligament (DATTL), 11
Deep posterior tibiotalar ligament (DPTTL), 11
De los Santos-Real Technique, 239
Deltoid ligament (DL) injury, 139, 190
  ankle arthroscopy, 172, 173
  arthroscopic treatment, 174–178
  CAI, 171
  clinical presentation, 172
  conservative treatment, 173, 174
  MAI, 171
  open treatment, 174, 175
  repair, 190
Denmark, 61
Distal fibula, 100
Distal tibiofibular syndesmosis, 6–8
Double limb, 51
Dwyer calcaneal osteotomy, 36
Dwyer osteotomy, 36, 40
Dynamic fluoroscopic examination, 34

E
Eccentric training, 50
Emergency center data, 61
Exercise programs, 66
Exercise rehabilitation protocols, 67

F
FibreTape, 189
Fibrous laminae, 198
Fibulotalocalcaneal ligament (FTCL), 198
First suture anchor, 100
Fixation techniques
  anatomic reconstruction, 153
  flexibility, 151
  screw, 151–153
  syndesmosis fusion, 153, 154
Flexor hallucis longus (FHL), 197
Flexor retinaculum, 196, 197
Foot and ankle
  acute subtalar dislocation, 76
  biology of, 1
  biomechanical evaluation, 32
  Chopart joint, 13, 14
  distal tibiofibular syndesmosis, 6, 7
  imaging studies, 34, 35
  lateral collateral ligaments, 9, 10
  ligamentous injuries in, 2
  lisfranc joint complex, 25, 27
  lisfranc ligamentous complex, 14, 15
  medial collateral ligaments, 10, 11
  nonoperative management, 35
  operative technique, 36, 37, 41, 42
  physical examination, 32, 34
  plantar plate, 26, 29
  subtalar instability, clinical assessment of, 76
  subtalar joint instability, 75
  subtalar joint ligaments, 12
  surgical management, 35, 36
Foot intrinsic drills and, 50
Forefoot equinus, 38
Functional instability, 125–126
Functional intraoperative tests, 142
Functional supports, 66

G
Gait, 32
Gazdag classification, 185

H
Hammertoe deformities
  clinical outcomes, 278
  FDL tendon transfer, 278, 279
  nonsurgical treatment, 278
  PIP joint arthrodesis, 279, 280
  surgical treatment, 278
Hibbs angle, 35
Hindfoot alignment, 78
Hindfoot-driven varus, 38
Hindfoot malalignment, 31
Hindfoot stability, 79
Hohmann retractors, 38
Hybrid technique, 110

I
Imaging modalities
  computed tomography (CT), 17
  conventional radiography, 17
  magnetic resonance imaging (MRI), 19
  MR arthrogram (MRA), 19
  ultrasound (US), 18
Immobilization, 66
Inferior transverse ligament (ITL), 8
Inferoplantar longitudinal calcaneonavicular ligament (ICNL), 183, 184, 186, 189
Interosseous ligament (IOL), 8
Interosseous talocalcaneal ligament (ITCL), 12, 79, 85
Intraoperative fluoroscopy, 40

K
Kirschner wire (K-wire), 41, 216

L
Larsen procedure, 107
Lateral ankle instability, 293–295
  anatomic reconstruction, 107, 108
  anatomy and biomechanics, 126
  ankle supportive devices and taping, 130, 131
  background, 125
  concomitant pathology, 128, 129
  diagnosis, 91, 92, 106
  exercise interventions, 129
  history and physical exam, 127, 128
  imaging, 128
  management, 92, 106
  manual therapy, 129
  modified Brostrom surgical technique, 93
  nonanatomic tenodesis procedures, 107
  operative treatment, 107
  rehabilitation process, 94, 110
  surgical technique, 108, 109
Lateral ankle ligaments, 108, 126
Lateral ligamentous complex, 98
Leeds-Keio artificial ligament, 119
Lesser toe plantar plate
  anatomy, 278
  classification, 275
  claw toe, 279–281
  clinical outcomes, 278
  examintion, 274, 275
  FDL tendon transfer, 278, 279
  hammertoes, 278
  history, 273–275
  imaging, 275
  mallet toes, 281, 282
  outcomes, 277
  pathophysiology and anatomy, 273, 274
  PIP joint arthrodesis, 279, 280
  treatment, 275–277
Ligament Augmentation Reconstruction System (LARS), 118
Ligamentous injury, 1, 2, 47
Lisfranc injury
  anatomy, 201–203, 215
  approaches, 244, 245
  authors' diagnostic algorithm, 212
  chronic Lisfranc dislocation, 234
  chronic Lisfranc injury without collapse
    De los Santos-Real Technique, 239
    Miyamoto technique, 238–240
    ORIF, 234–239
    secondary arthrodeses, 240, 243
    Zwipp technique, 240–242
  classification, 204–206
  clinical evaluation, 206, 207
  clinical outcomes, 243, 245
  complications, 243
  diagnostic algorithm, 211, 212
  epidemiology and clinical patterns, 216, 217
  hardware removal, 243
  history, 215, 216
  imaging
    computed tomography, 210, 218
    magnetic resonance imaging, 210, 211, 218
    radiographs, 207–210, 217, 218
  incidence, 201
  mechanism of, 202–204
  midfoot stability, 215
  ORIF
    first tarsometatarsal, 222
    intercuneiform, 221
    lower extremity, 218
    rigid fixation, 220
    second TMT, 221, 222
    technique, 220, 221, 223
  presentation/examination, 217
  PRIF, 223–227
  primary arthrodesis
    bone graft, 231
    dorsal incisions, 230
    Hintermann distractor, 230, 231
    Lisfranc screw, 232
    low-energy injuries, 230
    medial incision, 230, 231
    micro-fracture, 231, 232
    satisfactory exposure, 230, 231
    TMT joint, 232, 233
  primary-hybrid arthrodeses, 234
  rehabilitation, 243, 244, 253, 255, 256
  return to play
    characteristics, 250, 251
    medical team, 249
    midfoot, 249
    operative and non-operative treatments, 251, 252
    ORIF vs. primary arthrodesis, 252
    players' position, 253, 254
    reduction and residual displacement, 253
    treatment option, 251
  suture button flexible fixation, 225, 228–230
  treatment principle, 212, 213
    fixation vs. fusion, 219, 220
    non-operative techniques, 218
    primary arthrodesis, 219
    stabilization techniques, 219
Lisfranc ligament, 15
Loads and repetition schemes, 51
Long-term management, 49
Lower Extremity Return to Competition (LERC), 255

M
Magnetic resonance imaging (MRI), 35, 39, 92, 116, 128, 142
Mallet toes, 281, 282
Manual mobilization, 66
Manual therapy interventions, 48
Medial ankle instability (MAI), 171, 172, 177, 178
Medial ankle ligaments, 21

Medial column dislocation (MCD), 205
Medial displacement calcaneal osteotomy (MDCO), 189
Mersilene® Suture-Tape, 119
Metatarsal bones, 6
Metatarsal-sesamoidal articulations, 261
Metatarsophalangeal (MTP) joint
biomechanics, 263, 264
diagnosis and classification, 265, 267
dynamic stabilizers, 263
epidemiology, 260, 261
history, 259
management/rehabilitation
indications, 268
nonoperative, 268, 269
operative, 269–271
postoperative, 271
mechanism of injury and pathoanatomy, 264, 265
metatarsal-sesamoidal articulations, 261
plantar plate and capsuloligamentous structures, 261, 263
Minimally invasive and percutaneous techniques
arthroscopic reconstruction, 101
percutaneous anti-ROLL, 102
Miyamoto technique, 238–240
MLB Health and Injury Tracking system (HIT), 63
Modified Broström-Gould lateral ligament reconstruction, 41
Modified Brostrom-Gould Repair, 121
Modified Broström procedure, 107
Muscular foot intrinsic impairments, 50
Musculoskeletal injuries, 61
Musculoskeletal ultrasound, 93

N
National Football League (NFL), 251
Navicular-cuneiform joint (Nav-cun), 221
Navicular height, 35
Neuromuscular excitation, 49
Nonabsorbable braided suture tape, 41
Nonanatomic technique, 93
Nonoperative management, 35
Nonsteroidal anti-inflammatory drugs, 66
Non-weight-bearing (NWB) radiographs, 209

O
Objective testing, 52
Olympic Games, 63
Open reduction and internal fixation (ORIF), 219, 220
chronic Lisfranc injury without collapse, 234–239
first tarsometatarsal, 222
intercuneiform, 221
lower extremity, 218
rigid fixation, 220
second TMT, 221, 222
technique, 220, 221, 223
Orthopedic surgeon, role of, 2
os trigonum syndrome, 195, 197, 198
Ottawa ankle rules, 92

P
Painful subtalar joint instability, 85
Palpation, 92
Periodized rehabilitation, 47
Peroneus longus tendon (PLT), 188
Phalanxes, 6
Phased rehabilitation protocol, 47
Plantar plate, 261, 263
Posterior ankle impingement (PAI)
clinical diagnosis, 195
differential diagnosis, 195
flexor retinaculum, 196, 197
FTCL, 198
mechanisms, 195
osseous disorders, 195
posterolateral impingement, 196
posteromedial impingement, 196
PTCL, 197, 198
PTFL, 196
soft tissue, 195
Posterior inferior tibiofibular ligament (PITFL), 7, 138
Posterior talocalcaneal ligament (PTCL), 197, 198
Posterior talofibular ligament (PTFL), 91, 92, 115, 196
Postoperative rehabilitation protocol, 102
Progressive sporting agility, 54
Proprioceptive effect, 50
Protection, rest, ice, compression, and elevation (PRICE), 286
Provocative testing, 116
Proximal extension (PE), 205

R
Radiographic technique, 82
Rammelt's test, 80
Range of motion/mobilization (ROM), 286, 287
Rehabilitation, 65
Reparative phase, 1
Residual dorsiflexion, 32
Return to play (RTP), 160, 167, 168
ACSM, 288
agility T-test, 290, 291
decision-based model, 289
Dorsiflexion Lunge Test, 289
Lisfranc injury
characteristics, 250, 251
medical team, 249
midfoot, 249
operative and non-operative treatments, 251, 252
ORIF vs. primary arthrodesis, 252
players' position, 253, 254
reduction and residual displacement, 253
treatment option, 251
SEBT, 290
standardization, 289
vertical jump test, 290–292
Return to sport, 155, 156
Achilles Tendon injuries, 292, 293

communication, consent, compassion, and competency, 297
functional progression, 288
lateral ankle instability, 293–295
lateral ankle sprain, 285
phases of rehabilitation, 285, 286
play decisions, 297
range of motion/mobilization, 286, 287
RTP
ACSM, 288
agility T-test, 290, 291
decision-based RTP model, 289
Dorsiflexion Lunge Test, 289
SEBT, 290
standardization, 289
vertical jump test, 290–292
strengthening, 287, 288
syndesmosis injuries, 295, 296
RICE management, 65
Rotational ankle instability (RAI), 171, 172, 177, 178
Rouvière Ligament, 198

S
Silfverskiöld test, 34
Simple plyometric training, 54
Single leg exercise, 51
Small Hohmann retractors, 36
Spring ligament
anatomy, 181, 182
classification, 185
clinical features, 184, 185
clinical signs, 181
conservative treatment, 187
functions, 183, 184
ICNL, 183
imaging
MRI, 186, 187
plain X-ray, 186
ultrasound, 186
injury to, 184
SMCNL, 182
surgical treatment
autograft transfers, 189
cadaver studies, 188
deltoid ligament, 190
outcomes, 187
pathology, 187
planning, 187
post-operative rehabilitation, 190, 191
reconstruction, 188
repair, 187, 188
synthetic materials, 189, 190
tendon transfers, 190
talocalcaneonavicular joint complex, 181, 182
TCNL, 183
tibiospring ligament, 183
Star Excursion Balance Test (SEBT), 53, 290
Strength impairments, 50
Stress radiography, 78, 92, 128
Subtalar arthrography, 82
Subtalar joint, 12
Subtalar joint instability (SJI), 75
conservative treatment, 83
operative treatment, 85, 86
radiographic assessment, 76
Subtalar joint ligaments, 12
Superomedial calcaneonavicular ligament (SMCNL), 182–184, 186, 188, 189
Sural nerve, 100
Surgical management, 144
Suture knots, 101
Syndesmosis fusion, 153, 154
Syndesmosis injuries, 295, 296
Syndesmosis ligamentous tears, 139
Syndesmotic injuries, 21, 22
biomechanics, 138
classification system, 143
clinical evaluation, 140, 141
conservative treatment, 144
global perspective, 160, 161
imaging, 141–143
impact and collision sports, 147
incidence, 159
mechanism of, 138
prevalence, 147
rehabilitation
first phase, 161
guidelines, 161
last phase, 165
second phase, 162
third phase, 163, 164
return to play
protocols, 160
testing, 167, 168
stable vs. unstable syndesmotic injuries, 139, 140
surgical indications, 147–149
surgical outcomes
complications, 155
fixation, 151–155
postoperative rehabilitation, 155, 156
reduction techniques, 149, 150, 154
surgical treatment, 144
Synthetic augmentation
Arthrex® Suture-Tape (InternalBrace™), 119
LARS, 118
Leeds-Keio artificial ligament, 119
Mersilene® Suture-Tape, 119

T
Talar tilt angle (TTA), 120
Talocalcaneonavicular joint, 181, 182
Tarsal-metatarsal (TMT), 201–204, 207, 210
Tarsometatarsal joint interosseous system, 15
Tendon grafts, 105
Third (medioplantar oblique) calcaneonavicular ligament (TCNL), 183

Tibiocalcaneonavicular ligament (TCNL), 190
Tibionavicular ligament (TNL), 11
Tibiospring ligament, 183
Tibiotalar instability, 99
TightRope guidewire, 225, 229
Transosseous sutures, 86
Trans-osseous tensioning, 105
Treatment modalities, 66
Tripod Index, 35
Tryfonidis, 187

U
Ultrasound (US), 128, 141
United Kingdom, 62

V
Vertical jump test, 290–292
Volkmann's tubercle, 137

W
Water exercises, 69
Weber C fractures, 139
Weight bearing, 178
Weight bearing as tolerated (WBAT), 212
Weight-bearing computed tomography (WBCT), 80, 142
West Point Ankle Grading System, 143

X
X-rays, 141

Y
Y Balance test, 53

Z
Zwipp technique, 240–242

MIX
Papier aus verantwortungsvollen Quellen
Paper from responsible sources
FSC® C105338

If you have any concerns about our products,
you can contact us on
ProductSafety@springernature.com

In case Publisher is established outside the EU,
the EU authorized representative is:
Springer Nature Customer Service Center GmbH
Europaplatz 3, 69115 Heidelberg, Germany

Printed by Libri Plureos GmbH
in Hamburg, Germany